**Psychological Aspects and
Physiological Correlates of
Work and Fatigue**

Psychological Aspects and Physiological Correlates of Work and Fatigue

Compiled and Edited by

ERNST SIMONSON, M.D., Dr. rer. nat. h.c.

Late Director, Medical Electronic Research
Mount Sinai Hospital, Minneapolis, Minnesota
Professor Emeritus of Physiological Hygiene
University of Minnesota, Minneapolis
Professor Emeritus of Physiology
Johann-Wolfgang-Goethe Universität
Frankfurt/Main, Germany

and

PHILIP C. WEISER, Ph.D.

Postdoctoral Research Fellow
Cardiovascular Pulmonary Research Laboratory
University of Colorado Medical Center
Denver, Colorado

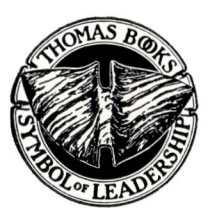

CHARLES C THOMAS · PUBLISHER
Springfield · Illinois · U.S.A.

Published and Distributed Throughout the World by
CHARLES C THOMAS • PUBLISHER
Bannerstone House
301-327 East Lawrence Avenue, Springfield, Illinois, U.S.A.

This book is protected by copyright. No part of it may be reproduced in any manner without written permission from the publisher.

© 1976, by CHARLES C THOMAS • PUBLISHER
ISBN 0-398-03430-3
Library of Congress Catalog Card Number: 75-12592

Library of Congress Cataloging in Publication Data
Main entry under title:
Psychological aspects and physiological correlates
 of work and fatigue.
 Continues Physiology of work capacity and
fatigue.
 Bibliography: p.
 Includes index.
 1. Work—Psychological aspects. 2. Work—
Physiological aspects. 3. Fatigue. I. Simonson,
Ernst, 1898-   II. Weiser, Philip C. [DNLM:
1. Fatigue. 2. Work. WE103 P975]
BF481.P8   612'.042   75-12592
ISBN 0-398-03430-3

With THOMAS BOOKS *careful attention is given to all details of manufacturing and design. It is the Publisher's desire to present books that are satisfactory as to their physical qualities and artistic possibilities and appropriate for their particular use.* THOMAS BOOKS *will be true to those laws of quality that assure a good name and good will.*

Printed in the United States of America
C-1

Contributors

S. HOWARD BARTLEY, Ph.D.
Professor Emeritus
Department of Psychology
Michigan State University
East Lansing, Michigan
Visiting Professor of Psychology
Memphis State University
Memphis, Tennessee

THOMAS A. EASTON, Ph.D.
Associate Editor
Biology, Chemistry and Geography Program
College Division, Scott, Foresman and Company
Glenview, Illinois

KEITH C. HAYES, Ph.D.
Assistant Professor
University of Waterloo
Department of Kinesiology
Waterloo, Ontario, Canada

ROBERT A. KINSMAN, Ph.D.
Chief, Psychophysiology Research Laboratories
Department of Behavioral Sciences
National Jewish Hospital and Research Center
Denver, Colorado

URSULA LEHR, Ph.D.
ord. Professor für Pädagogik und Pädagogische Psychologie
Direktor des Pädagogischen Seminars der Universität Köln
Cologne, West Germany

PATRICIA R. PALMERTON, B.A.
Abbott-Northwestern Mental Health Project
Abbott-Northwestern Hospital
Minneapolis, Minnesota

WALTER ROHMERT, Ph.D.
Professor, Director Institut für Arbeitswissenschaft
University of Technology
Darmstadt, West Germany

HANS SCHAEFER, Ph.D.
Professor, Director Physiologisches Institut der Universität
Heidelberg, West Germany

HEINZ SCHMIDTKE, Ph.D.
Professor, Director Institut für Ergonomie
Der Technischen Universität München
Munich, West Germany

OTTO H. SCHMITT, Ph.D.
Professor of Biophysics
University of Minnesota
Minneapolis, Minnesota

ERNST SIMONSON, M.D., Dr. rer. nat. h.c.
Director, Medical Electronic Research
Mount Sinai Hospital, Minneapolis, Minnesota
Professor Emeritus of Physiological Hygiene
University of Minnesota, Minneapolis
Professor Emeritus of Physiology
Johann-Wolfgang-Goethe Universität
Frankfurt/Main, Germany

HANS THOMAE, Ph.D., Dr. h.c.
Professor, Director Psychologisches Institut
Universität Bonn
Bonn, West Germany

HANS W. WENDT, Ph.D.
Professor, Department of Psychology
Macalaster College, St. Paul, Minnesota
Philipps Universität Marburg, Germany

PHILIP C. WEISER, Ph.D.
Postdoctoral Research Fellow
Cardiovascular Pulmonary Research Laboratory
University of Colorado Medical Center
Denver, Colorado

In Memoriam

ERNST SIMONSON

(1898, Tiegenhof, Germany—1975, Minneapolis, USA)

Der Vorhang fällt, das Stück is aus
(The curtain falls, the play is done)
HEINRICH HEINE, *Lamentations*

IN THE COURSE of a friendship that stretched over more than a third of a century, we wrote together numerous papers and debated weighty matters but we also had good laughs together over a cup of tea or an occasional glass of black beer. Among my most cherished memories are the occasions, altogether too rare, on which we combined not scientific disciplines or linguistic skills but musical instruments—Ernst's piano and my fiddle. Music was an expression of Ernst's innermost self, known only to his intimate friends. He loved his Bach dearly.

Ernst's first professional love was industrial physiology, and his first major piece of writing, still worth rereading, was a large chapter (pp. 519-586) on "Arbeitsphysiologie," contributed to the prestigious *Handbuch der normalen und pathologischen Physiologie* and published in 1930. In 1927, only 3 years after he had earned his M.D. at the University of Greifswald, Ernst began his academic career as a lecturer *(Privatdozent)* in industrial physiology at the University of Frankfurt. He retained his association with the University of Frankfurt until 1934 when he was removed from this position by the authorities of the Third Reich. He was reinstated, formally, to the position in 1956, with a title of full professor.

In 1931 Ernst was invited by the Soviet government to serve as scientific director of the Institute of Human Work, in Kharkov. In addition, in 1934 he became professor of normal physiology at the University of Kharkov Medical School. These were difficult years in the Soviet Union, and in 1937 Ernst left Kharkov to join the Institute of Human Work in Prague. Hitler's occupation in 1938 of the border areas of Czechoslovakia and the anticipation of worse things to come forced Ernst and his family to move again, this time to the United States. He spent the first 5 years as Research Associate at Mount Sinai Hospital, Milwaukee, Wisconsin and, in 1944 joined the Laboratory of Physiological Hygiene, a unit in the School of Public Health, University of Minnesota. And so we met again, having first crossed paths in 1937 in Zlín, Moravia, while Ernst was exploring the possibilities of establishing a Laboratory of Industrial Physiology in the Medical division of the Bat'a Shoe Company.

For a time, at Minnesota we combined our interests in industrial physiology and industrial psychology in the form of a course on Human Factors in Industry, given in the University's Institute of Technology. I was happy that following his retirement from the University, with *Differentiation between Normal and Abnormal in Elecrocardiography* (1961) and *Cerebral Ischemia* (1964) in print, Ernst returned to what he visualized as a trilogy on fatigue: its physiology, psychology, and clinical aspects.

Early in his research career, Ernst carried out experimental investigations on the various aspects of this protean phenomena, including motor coordination (published in the journal *Arbeitsphysiologie, 7, 1934, 577-597*), and undertook a critical examination of the "Current Status of the Theory of Fatigue" (*Ergebnisse der Physiologie, 37, 1935, 299-365*). Thirty-odd years later he embarked on a comprehensive review of the newer literature which grew massive during the intervening years. The extensive bibliography (pp. 400-520) is an especially valuable feature of his *Physiology of Work Capacity and Fatigue* (Springfield, Ill.: Charles C Thomas, 1971), the first volume of the trilogy. The present work, seen through the publication process by Dr. P. C. Weiser, constitutes the second volume. It has been for me a source of regret that other responsibilities made it impossible to share in the preparation of *Work and Fatigue: Psychological Aspects and Physiological Correlates,* as I have intended to do. It is hoped that one of Ernst's former associates will bring forth an equivalent of the projected third volume, *Exercise and Fatigue in Disease,* and thus bring to completion Ernst's grand design.

JOSEF BROŽEK
Lehigh University
Bethlehem, Pennsylvania

Introduction

RELATIONSHIP TO PRECEDING VOLUME *PHYSIOLOGY OF WORK CAPACITY AND FATIGUE* AND GENERAL DESIGN

THE PRECEDING VOLUME, *Physiology of Work Capacity and Fatigue, (PWCF)* was concerned mainly with cardiovascular, respiratory, metabolic and biochemical processes. It was decided to include central nervous (CNS) functions in this subsequent volume because of their close relationship to psychomotor, sensory and mental functions. Structural (histological) changes of the CNS were included in the preceding volume, however, along with histological changes in other organs (Chap. 5), of cerebral blood flow with ischemic changes (Chap. 12) and pupillographic studies in connection with autonomic regulations (Chap. 9). Results of psychological tests were included in the discussion of external and internal stress situations. It is obvious that separation of physiological and psychological aspects of work and fatigue is to a large degree arbitrary. Thus, the first part of the present volume contains chapters with primarily physiological orientation followed by chapters with primarily psychological orientation. Therefore, the preceding volume and this volume are mutually supplemental.

Condensed physiological background information is provided here in the first chapter (P. Weiser). For the reader interested in greater detail, numerous references to the preceding volume are given.

Münsterberg (1912) had already recognized that the trend in industrial occupations can be characterized as a shift from the larger to the smaller muscle groups, i.e. a shift from muscular to CNS involvement, a trend which has continued since then. Unfortunately, the development of methods for measurement of CNS fatigue has lagged behind this trend. Measurement of the fusion frequency of flicker was proposed (Simonson and Enzer, 1941) for this purpose and has elicited a large and somewhat controversial literature. Use of other methods (visual thresholds, reaction times, pupil reflexes, etc.) for measurement of CNS fatigue is discussed in various chapters of this volume. These methods reflect changes related to the disturbance of central processes in fatigue, but the underlying processes within the CNS are not easily accessible for measurement. Therefore, psychological functions such as subjective sensation of effort and fatigue, motivation, etc. still play a major role in evaluation of human performance.

I was fortunate to have worked closely together with two psychologists,

Dr. Helmut von Bracken in Frankfurt (1927-1929, now Professor of Psychology emeritus, University of Marburg and editor of *Psychologische Beiträge*) and Dr. Josef Brozek at the Laboratory of Physiological Hygiene, University of Minnesota (1944-1962, now Professor of Psychology, Lehigh University, Bethlehem, Pa). I hope that these associations gave me the background for organizing this volume, selecting contributors and topics.

Five fundamental fatigue processes were discussed at length in *PWCF*: A. accumulation of substances producing fatigue, B. depletion of substances essential for activity, C. changes of the state of substance, D. disturbance of regulations and E. transmission of fatigue. Section D, with four chapters (pp. 97-204) took the greatest space). This does not necessarily mean that disturbance of regulations is the most important fatigue process. The relative importance of the various fatigue processes depends on the type, duration and intensity of work, and there is interaction between these five processes. However, the large space required for discussion of regulations reflects the ramifications and the volume of the large literature. In the design of the preceding volume, regulation of enzyme activity, of the support systems (respiration and circulation) and autonomic regulations were discussed in different chapters (6-9), so that the discussion of their interactions was somewhat shortchanged. In Chapter 1 (P. Weiser), synthesis of the various regulatory processes is attempted, together with some updating of the information since the publication of the *PWCF* (1971).

This volume contains five contributions from German authors, reflecting the extensive research in Germany on psychology of work and fatigue, which appears to be largely unknown to American psychologists, so far as can be judged from the literature, and would not be as easily accessible otherwise. While the coverage of the total field is not quite as comprehensive as the physiological literature reviewed in the preceding volume, the selected topics (some with novel approaches) are believed to be crucial and important for the further progress of the field.

INTERACTIONS AND REGULATIONS
The Central Command

It was Pavlov who proposed, on the basis of his work on conditioned reflexes, that the cortex regulates the activity of all internal organs. Pavlov's concept stimulated an enormous literature in the U.S.S.R., determining for nearly two decades the direction of Soviet biomedical research (Simonson, 1959). Pavlov's original work studied conditioned salivary and gastric secretion. The scope and experimental basis was considerably enlarged by elaboration of conditioned reflexes of various autonomic functions (diuresis, hypoglycemia, blood pressure, heart rate, Vo_2, etc.). The largest amount of work in this direction was carried out by Bykov and associates.[1]

Most of these investigations were concerned with application to different types of pathology, based on Pavlov's production of experimental neurosis by means of conflicting conditioned reflexes with secondary changes in various organs. For example, stable arterial hypertension and even myocardial infarction could be produced in dogs and monkeys by means of conflicting conditioned reflexes (reviewed by Simonson and Brozek, 1959). Conditioned reflexes changed in various types of pathology, and unconditioned reactions could be changed by stimulation of the cerebral cortex. Lesions of the cerebral cortex were found to affect the development of various types of pathology, which in turn affected conditioned reflexes. The view that the CNS had a dominant role in development of pathological states, of course, was not limited to the U.S.S.R., but in Western countries it was not in the mainstream of research. Most of the Russian work was concerned with the pathogenesis of various diseases, but this approach has also been applied to fatigue in several studies published in a volume edited by Folbort (1959), one of Pavlov's earliest and closest associates. However, this volume is concerned with side issues rather than the central problem.

The significance of cortical regulation of peripheral processes was undoubtedly exaggerated, and references to Pavlov are now rare in the Soviet biomedical literature. Nevertheless, the extensive Russian work has contributed to the information about cortico-visceral interactions. It may have some application to "visceral learning."

Experiments by Miller (1969) on learning of visceral and glandular responses are in line with Pavlov's concept, confirming cortical control of heart rate, blood pressure, and alpha waves in the EEG in rats. A reward technique was used that was similar to the elaboration of conditioned reflexes. As an interesting side observation, curarization facilitated the "learning" i.e. cerebral control of visceral functions, indicating that messages from muscle (i.e. muscle tension) are either not involved in the learning of visceral processes or only in an inhibitory role. Similar results have been reproduced in man. Human subjects can learn to initiate and terminate urination when completely paralyzed by curare or succinylcholine (Lapides, et al., 1957). Maslach, et al. (1972) and Roberts, et al. (1973) demonstrated that human subjects can produce a difference between the

---

1. Bykov (1959) was quite aware of the multiple interaction (which would be presently termed "feedback loops") involved in cortical control: "The cortex is the prime system for channelizing the host of external and internal signals and of integrating them into the integral complex of action called behavior. Information from the internal organs apparently reaches the cortical levels by sympathetic pathways." p. 335

temperature of two hands. The results were confirmed by N. E. Miller (1974, Personal Communication) in conditions eliminating any effect of respiration, emotional excitement or other general factors. Harris, et al. (1973) showed that baboons can learn to maintain over 30 mm Hg elevation of blood pressure over a 12 hour period. While these results show cortical control of visceral processes, these changes are quite modest in comparison with the effect of physical exertion.

In general, the interest has shifted from cortical to subcortical control (Lindsey, 1956). In fact, cortical control is largely mediated by the reticular activating system, as investigated by Magoun and Rhines (1946), Hess (1948), Bremer and Terzuolo (1954), Jasper (1949), Moruzzi and Magoun (1949), Lindsey (1956) and other authors. The role of a central inhibitory system was confirmed by Akert, et al. (1952), Caspers and Winkel (1954), and Monnier, et al. (1963) to quote but a few of the numerous contributions. Impulses from the reticular activating system spreading to the cortex produce arousal, and corticofugal impulses converging on the reticular formation may stimulate "the ascending reticular activating system which in turn maintains the cortex in a state of arousal and alertness" (Grandjean, 1970). All afferent sensory pathways send collaterals to the reticular formation and thus stimulate the ascending activating system. Stimulation of the activating system spreads to the autonomic centers, particularly the sympathetic centers with associated output of adrenal hormones, producing an ergotropic change such that the organism may activate itself for energy expenditure in all types of muscular activity (Grandjean). The complex hormonal feedback system involved in performance is illustrated in Figure 10 in *PWCF* (1971). The sympathetic stimulation is related to the Orbeli phenomenon, and a central sympathetic feedback mechanism was demonstrated in man by Lowenstein and Loewenfeld (1952), automatically and periodically counteracting CNS fatigue. Grandjean differentiated between active corticopetal inhibition from the thalamus and passive cortical inhibition as a result of lowered sensory input or "lowered corticofugal feedback" (sensory deprivation).

The involvement of this intracentral feedback mechanism in work and fatigue has been described by Haider (1962), Schmidtke (1965), Grandjean (1970) and is discussed in this volume in regard to reflex control by T. Easton, Chapter 3 "Reflexes and Fatigue: New Directions"; H. Wendt, Chapter 13 "Motivation"; H. Schmidtke, Chapter 8 "Vigilance"; and by Bartley and Simonson, Chapter 7 "Use of Visual Methods for Measurement of General Fatigue." H. Schaefer (1970, Fig. 7) has proposed a "Rück-Koppelung" (feedback) diagram for the interaction of supramedullary centers, the activation system in the reticular formation with regulation of blood pressure, hormones and peripheral motor control subordinated to the sensation of fatigue. The detailed diagrams of the multiple interactions in Chapter 1 (P. Weiser) include essential features of Schaefer's diagram. It appears that the central command is highly variable depending upon a multitude of internal and external environmental stimuli.

Peripheral Control

The literature of the peripheral control of movement is substantial. It has been reviewed in detail by P. O. Åstrand and Rodahl (1970), H. Schaefer (1970), most recently by Stein (1973), and in Chapter 1 (P. Weiser).

The ability of coordinated movements requires the interaction of central commands with sensory feedback, and several hypotheses of possible regulating mechanisms were discussed by Stein on the basis of recent information theory and systems analysis (Clark, 1962; D'Azzo and Houpis, 1966; Milsum, 1966). Merton's servo-mechanism (1953) is discussed also in Chapter 3 and 4. Merton proposed that most movements are produced by indirect actions on gamma motoneurons in the following sequence of interactions: 1. excitation of gamma motoneurons; 2. shortening of intrafusal fibers;[2] 3. excitation of spindle receptors; 4. excitation of extrafusal fibers[3] resulting in their contraction against the load. Thus, "sensory feedback would be prominently involved in generating movements as well as resulting from movements." The situation is quite complex because there are at least three major types of motor neurons (alpha plus "dynamic" and "static" gamma) as well as three types of sensory receptors (Golgi tendon organs, primary and secondary spindle afferents), resulting in multiple possible interactions for movement control. Stein (1974) broadened Merton's servo hypothesis in view of several weaknesses (involving gain, delays, noise and specificity) of Merton's original concept, by assuming that central commands activate primarily gamma-motoneurons. "There is considerable evidence for coactivation of alpha- and gamma-motoneurons in a way that produces a servo-assisted control of movement that can overcome many of these difficulties. There is also reason to assume three separate systems for control of force, length and velocity, consistent with the three major types of motor outputs and three types of sensory input." "Their combination would provide considerable flexibility in adaptive control of the wide range of movement animals require." For more details of peripheral feedback control, we refer to Stein's excellent review and to Chapter 1 (P. Weiser).

Thus, the functional variability of the central command, as discussed earlier, together with the functional variability of the peripheral control,

---
2. Intrafusal fibers are those located within muscle spindles.
3. Extrafusal fibers are those outside the muscle spindles and which compose the main muscle mass.

provide for the wide adaptability of behavior, movement and performance within the wide range of requirements for the preservation of life in various external and internal stress situations and for the various tasks of human performance.

Strictly isometric work is essentially an experimental laboratory situation, but every dynamic work has a static component (see *PWCF,* Chap. 10); thus, peripheral control involves both dynamic and static components. Peripheral control of movement is, of course, of primary importance in physical work, but movement is involved also in mental work (communication by speech or writing, use of eye muscles in visual perception). However, for the general stress of mental work, the control of movement plays a minor role. This has been shown for eye muscle involvement in mental work (arithmetic problems) with and without visual control (blindfolded, see Chap. 7). The stress of mental work or in tasks with minor muscular components, therefore, involves primarily the intracentral feedback processes briefly discussed above.

There are limitations of the control of movements at the peripheral end: the starting point of consideration is the All or None Law for contraction of the muscle fiber. Once the fiber is activated by one or more impulses, the complex enzyme processes associated with contraction are predetermined for the given condition of the muscle fiber. All experiments on peripheral feedback loops of enzyme processes (reviewed by Weiser in Chap. 6 in *PWCF* and in Chap. 1 of this volume) have been performed on isolated whole or minced muscle. The regulation of these enzyme processes in muscle is essentially automatic. There is no evidence for the existence of specialized sensors of any of the metabolic products in muscle for central regulation, such as ATP. Actually, none are needed. The autoregulation goes beyond the feedback loops of muscular enzyme processes and extends to fuel supply (glucose, FFA transport) via both autonomic nervous system control and hormonal regulation (Chap. 1).

Since the control of movement by feedback from specific metabolic products in the muscle can be dismissed, which are the regulatory processes for adaptation of force (tension) to the task? There are two main mechanisms of gradation of force (effort) in adaptation to load and the resulting energy expenditure: 1. recruitment of the number of motor units and 2. the firing rate of single motor units (Adrian and Bronk, 1929). Both mechanisms are consistent with, in fact, a consequence of the All or None Law. Thus, gradation of effort depends on the number and rate of acetylcholine (ACh) quanta liberated at the motor nerve endings. The considerable recent literature on these two major regulatory processes has been reviewed by Stein (1974), who concludes "recruitment appears to be the most desirable mechanism for grading force and is particularly prominent in very brief and very slow contractions. However, considering the entire physiological range, rate coding (impulse frequency) provides the majority of the force produced, at least for intermediate contraction speeds." Thus, peripheral control of movement terminates with the liberation of the transmitter ACh at the nerve endings. There is, at present, no evidence that ACh itself is involved in the regulating control of movement; it rather seems to be the end product, initiating the automatically controlled enzyme processes in muscular contraction.

It is in this context of sensory-intracentral-peripheral feedback control of the central command, as developed by numerous authors, that we have to visualize the regulation of motor and mental performance in various conditions of task demand and to view the resulting fatigue phenomena as a disturbance of these regulations. This is, of course, a major topic both of the preceding volume and this volume. In view of the importance of "cybernetic" regulation in work and fatigue, Otto H. Schmitt in Chapter 2 has presented an historical analysis of the theory of communication and feedback concept.

SOME GENERAL CONSIDERATIONS

We have defined fatigue as decrease of working capacity (not necessarily performance) due to preceding work, referring to the discussion of the term "fatigue" and related conditions (exhaustion, chronic fatigue, pathologic fatigue) in the Introduction of *PWCF* (E. Simonson) and the Closing Considerations (H. Bartley) in this volume.

While fatigue in man is a subjective phenomenon, it is obviously related to peripheral processes in the muscle or elsewhere. According to H. Schaefer (1959) "fatigue of the whole organism can be understood only on the basis of changes in active organs . . . only the active organ fatigues, and the whole organism only insofar as affected by chemical or neurological action of that organ." A good example is the close relationship between depletion of glycogen stores in active muscles and fatigue in hard, prolonged work, based on the recent work of Bergström and Hultmen (see Chap. 1). There is a high correlation between glycogen depletion and heart rate, which is, in its turn, related to subjective fatigue as discussed in Chapter 14 (R. Kinsman and P. Weiser). On the other hand, L. Rowell (1974) has suggested that muscular exertion is not limited by the metabolic capacity of the muscle, but by the ability to supply blood to the working muscles, enlarging the concept of "ischemic fatigue" (*PWCF,* Chap. 12). With these complex multiple interactions, however, it is often not easy to trace the relationship between subjective fatigue and changes in active organs. It is for this reason that in the preceding volume discussion of the site of fatigue was subordinated to the discussion of fundamental fatigue processes. The difficult differentiation between peripheral and central localization of fatigue was discussed in Chapter 10 and 11 in *PWCF*, and is discussed further in Chapter 3 of this volume (T. Easton). We conclude with a quotation from H. Schaefer (1970) "The problem 'Fatigue' is concerned with the central problems not only of the physiology and pathology of man, but also with social-political problems, as are not many other problems of medicine."

ERNST SIMONSON

Bibliography

Adrian, E. D., and D. W. Bronk: The discharge of impulses in motor nerves. Part II. The frequency of discharge in reflex and voluntary contractions. *J Physiol*, London *67*:119, 1929.

Akert, K., W. F. Koella, and R. Hess, Jr.: Sleep produced by electrical stimulation of the thalamus. *Am J Physiol, 168*:259, 1952.

Åstrand, I., P.-O. Åstrand, and K. Rodahl: Maximal heart rate during work in older men. *J Appl Physiol, 14*:562, 1959.

Åstrand, P.-O. and K. Rodahl: *Textbook of Work Physiology*. New York, McGraw-Hill, 1970.

Bremer, F., and C. Terzuolo: Contribution a l'etude des mécanismes physiologiques du maintien de l'activité vigile. *Arch Intern Physiol, 62*:157, 1954.

Bykov, K.: *The Cerebral Cortex and The Internal Organs*. Moscow, Foreign Language Publishing House, 1959, pp. 459.

Caspers, H., and K. Winkel: Die Beeinflussung der Grosshirnrindenrhythmik durch Reizungen im Zwischen- und Mittelhirn bei der Ratte. *Pflügers Arch Ges Physiol, 259*:334, 1954.

Clark, R. H.: *Introduction to Automatic Control-System*. London, Wiley, 1962.

D'Azzo, J. J., and C. H. Houpis: *Feedback Control System Analysis and Synthesis*. New York, McGraw-Hill, 1966.

Folbort, G. V. (Ed.): *Problems of the Physiology of the Processes of Fatigue and Recovery*. Kiev, The Academy of Sciences of the Ukrainian SSR, 1958. Translation from Office of Technical Services, U. S. Department of Commerce, 1960.

Grandjean, E. P.: Fatigue. *Am Industr Hyg Ass J, 31*:1, 1970.

Haider, M.: Ermüdung, Beansprunchung und Leistung. Eine Einführung in *die Ermüdung-und Monotonieforschung*. Wien, Franz Deuticke, 1962, p. 168.

Harris, A. M., W. D. Gilliam, J. D. Findley, and J. B. Brady: Instrumental conditioning of large-magnitude, daily, 12-hour blood pressure elevations in the baboon. *Science, 182*:175, 1973.

Hess, W. R.: *Die funktionelle Organisation des vegetativen Nervensystems*. Basel, Benno Schwabe, 1948.

Heymans, C.: Sur la regulation reflex du tonus de vasomotor et de la adrenaline secretion au rapport avec la pression arteriel. *C R Soc Biol, 100*:765, 1929.

Jasper, H. H.: Diffusion Projection Systems: The Integrative Action of the Thalamic Reticular System. *Electroenceph Clin Neurophysiol, 1*:405, 1949.

Lapides, J., R. B. Sweet, and L. W. Lewis: Role of striated muscle in urination. *J Urol, 77*:247, 1957.

Lindsey, D. B.: Physiological psychology. *Ann Rev Psychol, 7*:323, 1956.

Lowenstein, O., and I. E. Loewenfeld: Disintegration of central autonomic regulation during fatigue and its reintegration by psychosensory controlling mechanisms. II. Reintegration. Pupillographic studies. *J Nerv Ment Dis, 115:*121, 1952.

Magoun, H. W., and R. Rhines: An inhibitory mechanism in the bulbar reticular formation. *J Neurophysiol, 9:*165, 1946.

Maslach, C., G. E. Marshall, and P. G. Zimbardo: Hypnotic control of peripheral skin temperature: A case report. *Psychophysiology, 2:*600, 1972.

Merton, P. A.: Speculations on the servo-control of movement. In Wolstenholme, G. E. W. (Ed.): *Ciba Found Symp The Spinal Cord.* London, Churchill, 1953, pp. 247-255.

Miller, N. E.: Learning of visceral and glandular responses. *Science, 163:*434, 1969.

Milsum, J. H.: *Biological Control Systems Analysis.* New York, McGraw-Hill, 1966.

Monnier, M., Th. Koller, and S. Graber: Humoral influences of induced sleep and arousal upon electrical brain activity of animals with cross circulation. *Exp Neurol, 8:*264, 1963.

Moruzzi, G., and H. S. Magoun: Brain stem reticular formation and activation of the EEG. *Electroenceph Clin Neurophysiol, 1:*455, 1949.

Münsterberg, H.: *Psychologie und Wirtschaftsleben.* 4. Aufl. Leipzig, 1912.

Pavlov, I. P.: *Lektsii o rabote bol'skikh polusharii golovnogo mozga* (Lectures on the Function of the Big Hemispheres of the Brain). Moscow, Medgiz, 1949 (Posthum. Ed.).

Roberts, A., J. C. Kewman, and H. MacDonald: Voluntary control of skin temperature: Unilateral changes using hypnosis and feedback. *J Abnorm Psychol, 82:*163, 1973.

Rowell, L.: Human cardiovascular adjustments to exercise and thermal stress. *Physiol Rev, 54:*75, 1974.

Schaefer, H.: Physiologie der Ermüdung und Ershöpfung. *Med Klin, 54:*1109, 1959.

Schaefer, H.: Ermüdung und Müdigkeit. *Chapter 1* In Baust, K. (Ed.): *Ermüdung, Schlaf und Traum.* Stuttgart, Wissenschaftliche Verlagsgesellschaft MBH, 1970, pp. 1-25.

Schmidtke, H.: *Die Ermüdung,* Bern and Stuttgart, Verlag Hans Huber, 1965, p. 339.

Simonson, E.: Cardiovascular research in Russia. *Circulation, 19:*481, 1959.

Simonson, E., and J. Brozek: Russian research on arterial hypertension. *Ann Intern Med, 50:*129, 1959.

Simonson, E., and N. Enzer: Measurement of fusion frequency of flicker as test for fatigue of central nervous system; observations on latoratory technicians and office workers. *J Indust Hyg Toxicol, 23:*83, 1941.

Stein, R. B.: Peripheral control of movement. *Physiol Rev, 54:*215, 1974.

Acknowledgments

I WISH TO THANK Dr. Francisco Grande (Laboratory of Physiological Hygiene, University of Minnesota) for his critical advice on some of the physiological aspects involved in this volume.

I am also thankful to Mrs. Donna Rae Cintora and to Mrs. Eileen Ladd for librarian and technical assistance.

The preparation of the manuscript was supported in part by grant HD 02586, Institute of Child Health and Human Development, NIH, Bethesda, Maryland.

Contents

	Page
Contributors	v
In Memoriam	vii
Introduction	ix
Acknowledgments	xix

Chapter

SECTION ONE
BIOPHYSICAL MODELS AND PHYSIOLOGICAL BACKGROUND

1. INTERRELATIONSHIPS OF THE MOTOR AND METABOLIC SUPPORT SYSTEMS DURING WORK AND FATIGUE
   Philip C. Weiser 5
2. BIOPHYSICAL MODELS FOR STUDYING WORK AND FATIGUE
   Otto H. Schmitt 43

SECTION TWO
MOTOR ASPECTS

3. REFLEXES AND FATIGUE: NEW DIRECTIONS
   Thomas A. Easton 55
4. REACTION TIMES, REFLEX TIMES AND FATIGUE
   Keith C. Hayes 106
5. MOTOR COORDINATION
   Walter Rohmert 137

SECTION THREE
SENSORY ASPECTS: VISION

6. VISUAL FATIGUE
   S. Howard Bartley 155
7. USE OF VISUAL METHODS FOR MEASUREMENTS OF GENERAL FATIGUE
   S. Howard Bartley and Ernst Simonson 176

SECTION FOUR
ASPECTS OF CENTRAL PROCESSING

8. VIGILANCE
   Heinz Schmidtke 193
9. DISTURBANCE OF ACQUISITION OF INFORMATION
   Heinz Schmidtke 220
10. DISTURBANCE OF PROCESSING OF INFORMATION
    Heinz Schmidtke 238

SECTION FIVE
AGING

INTRODUCTION
Ernst Simonson 255

11 EFFECT OF AGE ON WORK, PSYCHOLOGICAL ASPECTS
Ursula Lehr and Hans Thomae 259

12 THE OLDER DRIVER
Ernst Simonson 272

SECTION SIX
INTROSPECTIVE ASPECTS OF WORK AND FATIGUE

13 MOTIVATION, VALUES, AND CHRONOBEHAVIORAL ASPECTS OF FATIGUE
Hans W. Wendt and Patricia R. Palmerton 285

14 SUBJECTIVE SYMPTOMATOLOGY DURING WORK AND FATIGUE
Robert A. Kinsman and Philip C. Weiser 336

SECTION SEVEN
CLOSING COMMENTS

15 WHAT DO WE CALL FATIGUE?
S. Howard Bartley 409

Epilogue—Hans Schaefer 415
Author Index 419
Subject Index 431

Psychological Aspects and Physiological Correlates of Work and Fatigue

SECTION ONE

BIOPHYSICAL MODELS AND PHYSIOLOGICAL BACKGROUND

Chapter 1

Interrelationships of the Motor and Metabolic Support Systems During Work and Fatigue

PHILIP C. WEISER

ORGANIZATION AND CONTROL OF THE MOTOR AND SUPPORT SYSTEMS

THE PURPOSE of this chapter is to describe the intricate system that governs motor activity and those systems that support motor performance. Furthermore, the regulation of physical activity by these systems during submaximal and intense muscular work will be examined.

In viewing man as a whole, performance is the product of two closed-loop control systems linked and regulated together. Figure 1-1 is a block diagram illustrating motor performance and the components of which it is comprised. First, the motoneuron and muscle contractile apparatus act as the *controlled system* whose function is motor action. Muscle spindles, tendon organs, and other mechanoreceptors detect changes in skeleto-muscular tension and position. They function as the detectors of the motor-*controlling system* and feed information back along the afferent pathways to the spinal cord and to the motor centers of the higher levels of the central nervous system (CNS). Second, information about the activity of numerous controlled systems supporting the motor-coordinating system is fed from chemoreceptors and other interoreceptors to support-controlling systems in the CNS and is also fed to hormonal controlling systems. Consequently, performance arises from the action of working muscles and is controlled by motor-coordinating and support-coordinating systems of the CNS which are shown much oversimplified in Figure 1-1 as motivational, personalogical, perceptual, and subjective influences.

The motor-metabolic aspects of performance (Fig. 1-2) result from the action of smaller subsystems that comprise each of the two fundamental control systems. Three interconnected subsystems make up the motor-coordinating system. Electrical information needed to initiate the motor unit response is transferred from the motoneuron to the muscle fibers innervated by it via chemical transmission resulting in *nerve-muscle action potential coupling* (A in Fig. 1-2). To provide the tension needed for physical activity, this electrical information is changed to mechanical energy by

---

This chapter was supported in part by NIH Grants HL14985-02 and MH24222-01.

excitation-contraction coupling (B). These two subsystems form the controlled components of the motor-coordinating system. Activating and coordinating these components are the functions of *contraction-coordination coupling* (C) which is comprised of detectors and of modifying centers in the CNS.

Supporting performance is another system that is likewise made up of two general subsystems. Linked directly to excitation-contraction coupling is a *contraction-energy regeneration coupling* (D) that uses muscle energy metabolism to replenish the ATP used during contraction. Muscle energy metabolism is further augmented by *energy regeneration-fuel supply coupling* (E). This provides for the mobilization and utilization of energy-supplying substrates like glucose, fatty acids, and oxygen.

The functional control of all the components involved in motor-metabolic processes, and consequently motor performance, occurs at all levels of biological organization, systemic to molecular. Through the interconnections and interactions of the molecular to systemic feedback controls, the motor and support activities are maintained within certain limits, i.e. are regulated as demanded and influenced by the behavior of the organism itself. The task in the next section is to describe how these systems are integrated and regulated to perform work, and how impairments in various components of the interrelated system may give rise to fatigue.

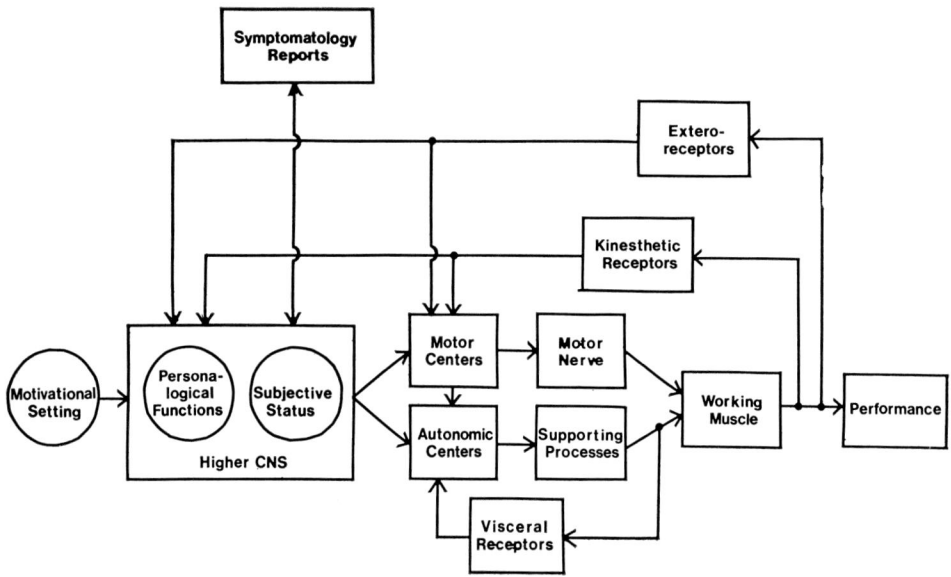

Figure 1-1. Schematic block diagram of motor performance with its control systems and feedback loops.

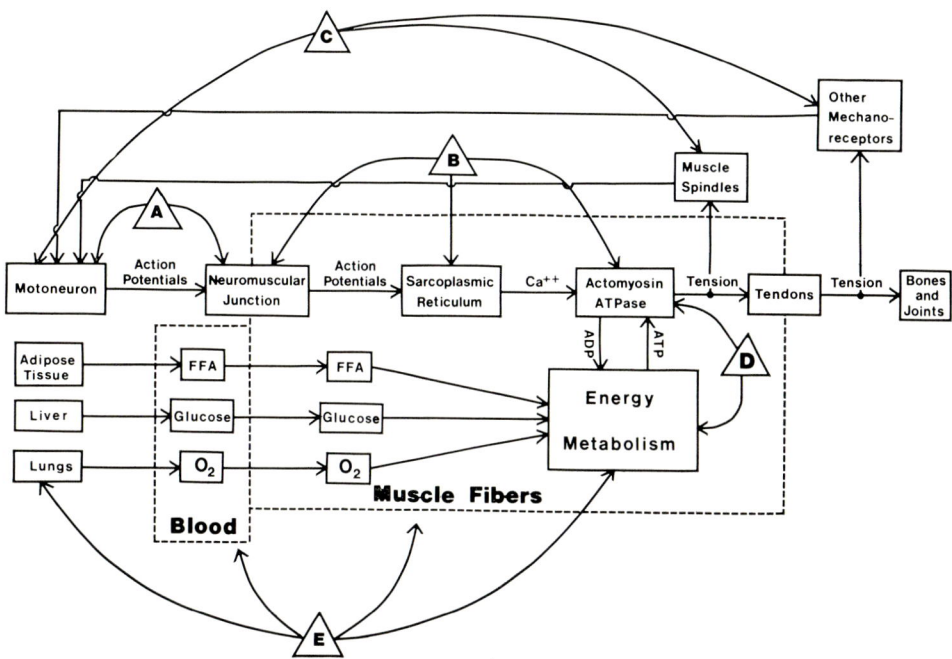

Figure 1-2. Block diagram of motor unit performance and the subsystems comprising it: A—coupling from the motoneuron to the muscle fiber; B—coupling from muscle excitation to contraction; C—coupling from muscle contraction to motor coordination; D—coupling from muscle contraction to muscle energy regeneration via adenosine di- and tri-phosphates (ADP and ATP); E—coupling from muscle energy regeneration to extramuscular sources of fuel.

Fatigue can be defined as a "reduction in working capacity" (Simonson and Enzer, 1942). Various manifestations of fatigue will appear when the task being performed varies from purely mental work to light industrial tasks to intense muscular exertion. In each situation the adaptations that take place will be analyzed for possible impairments that can or could be related to fatigue. These task-oriented analyses will be based on the hypothesis that fatigue occurs as the feedback regulation of the motor system and its support system become maladjusted. These maladjustments are apparent on a behavioral level as decrements in work capacity or reported as an increase in subjective symptomatology as described in the chapter on Subjective Fatigue.

Before addressing the questions concerning which feedback control processes could influence work capacity, the following section will discuss the adaptations the organism makes to an increased work load and will indicate how these adaptations forecast impairments that could lead to fatigue.

TRANSITION TO HIGHER WORK LEVELS

When one shifts from a standing to a walking activity during a job, for example, substantial adaptations of both the motor system and of its support system begin. Consequently, the concomitant transient phase of adaptations initiated by this change in activity represents an important regulatory situation. This transient phase will also be important in the analysis of work capacity and fatigue, since it initiates the adaptations which will become impaired or altered, thereby becoming the factors limiting physical performance. The shift from standing (energy cost about 1.6 kcal/min.) to rapid walking (abour 7 kcal/min.) will be used as an example to illustrate these adaptations.

Motor System Regulation

The neuro-motor adaptations quickly commence within seconds and involve all the components of the motor system. To begin the transition, the motor activity during standing must be changed and accelerated. To "get in step" will require at least a couple of steps. Figure 1-3 shows the basic components of the motor system, and details are reviewed in greater depth elsewhere (e.g. Åstrand and Rodahl, 1970; Henneman, 1968a,b; Houk and Henneman, 1968).

In general, when walking begins, each motor unit of the active muscles shifts from presumably infrequent to more frequent activity. The motor

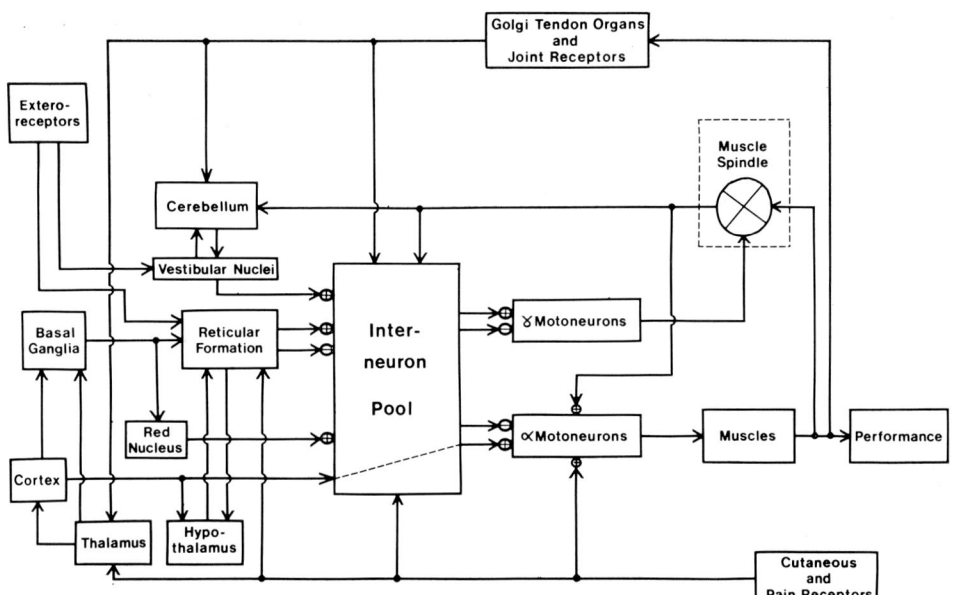

Figure 1-3. Block diagram of the feedback control of the entire motor system.

unit activity will primarily be equal to, but more likely be less than, once every step. In contrast to the motor-support systems, the fibers of a motor unit become active in an all-or-none manner in response to their alpha motoneuron activity. These muscle fibers operate by coupling with bursts of impulses from these nerves. Impairment of neuromuscular chemical transmission affecting this open-loop coupling must be considered as a factor which can influence voluntary work performance (see Simonson, 1971, Chap. 10).

Consequently, the transition of a motor unit from the inactive to the active state is essentially immediate. The presently suggested mechanism for coupling muscle excitation and contraction is shown in the upper half of Figure 1-4, and several recent reviews (Ebashi, et al., 1969; Sandow, 1970; Huxley, 1972; Taylor, 1972; Weber and Murray, 1973) give detailed descriptions. Briefly, it is thought that an action potential traveling along the muscle cell membrane releases Ca^{++} into the fiber. Ca^{++} acts to relieve the tropomyosin-troponin inhibition, allows actin to bind with myosin, and actomyosin binds and hydrolyzes ATP. With the hydrolysis of the bound ATP to ADP and the dissociation of actomyosin ADP into a complex of actin, myosin and ADP, a cycle of contractile events can recur. The tension developed is in large part regulated by the number and frequency of motoneuron impulses during contraction. Consequently, the length of Ca^{++} feed-forward control on actomyosin ATPase will define the period of that muscle fiber's active state.

Not all the fibers in a muscle have the same contractile properties (see Henneman, 1968b). However, all the fibers within a given motor unit seem to be functionally quite similar. Table 1-I lists the characteristics for the two extremes or types of mammalian muscle fibers. Small fibers are found having low actomyosin ATPase activity with only a slow build-up to peak twitch tension, and they have a capacity for a high rate of oxidative energy metabolism. At the other extreme are larger fibers that have a fast build-up to peak tension with a high level of actomyosin ATPase activity, and these fibers have a capacity for a high rate of anaerobic energy metabolism. In the continuum between these two extreme fiber types are muscle cells that have intermediate functional properties. Note that the high oxidative slow twitch fibers also have slow motoneuron conduction velocities (i.e. small axon diameters and cell bodies), low peak tensions, and a small number of fibers per motor unit. The opposite is true for the low oxidative fast twitch fibers. Finally, the contractility of slow fibers is maintained during prolonged work, whereas the tension developed by fast fibers begins to decrease soon after work begins.

As walking speed is increased faster and faster, more motor units will be

TABLE 1-I

A SUMMARY OF CHARACTERISTICS ASSOCIATED WITH MOTOR
UNITS WITH DIFFERENT FIBER TYPES*

Characteristc	Muscle Fiber Type†	
	High-Oxidative Slow Twitch (ST)	Low-Oxidative Fast Twitch (FT)
1. Fiber diameter	Small	Large
2. Actomyosin ATPase (pH 9.4)	Low	High
3. Motor nerve conduction velocity	About 40-60 m/sec (cat)	About 80-110 m/sec (cat)
4. Maximal tetanic tension (per motor unit)	About 0.5-10 g (cat)	About 40-120 g (cat)
5. Contraction time to peak tension	About 100-200 m/sec (cat)	About 10-40 m/sec (cat)
6. Number of fibers per motor unit	Small	Large
7. Number of mitochondria	Many	Few
8. Anaerobic glycolytic capacity	Poorly developed	Well developed
9. Oxidative phosphorylation capacity	High	Low
10. Number of capillaries	Greatest	Least
11. Fatigability (i.e. decreasing tension)	Highly resistant	Easily

* Compiled from J. A. Faulkner, "Muscle Fatigue," in E. J. Briskey, et al., eds., *The Physiology and Biochemistry of Muscle as a Food* (Madison, The University of Wisconsin Press, 1970) pp. 555-575; E. Henneman, "Peripheral Mechanisms Involved in the Control of Muscle," in V. B. Mountcastle, ed., *Medical Physiology* (St. Louis, C. V. Mosby Co., 1968) pp. 1697-1716; R. I. Close. "Dynamic Properties of Mammalian Skeletal Muscles," *Physiological Reviews*, 52:129, 1972; R. J. Barnard, et al., "Histochemical, Biochemical, and Contractile Properties of Red, White, and Intermediate Fibers," *American Journal of Physiology*, 220:410, 1971; and L. C. Maxwell, et al., "Histochemical Manifestations of Age and Endurance Training in Skeletal Muscle Fibers," *American Journal of Physiology*, 224:356, 1973.

† This classification of fiber types corresponds to types B and A of J. M. Stein, and H. A. Padykula, "Histochemical Classification of Individual Skeletal Muscle Fibers of the Rat," *American Journal of Anatomy*, 110:103, 1962; and E. Henneman, and C. B. Olson, "Relations Between Structure and Function in the Design of Skeletal Muscle," *Journal of Neurophysiology*, 28:581, 1965; and Intermediate and White of R. J. Barnard, et al., "Histochemical, Biochemical, and Contractile Properties of Red, White, and Intermediate Fibers," *American Journal of Physiology*, 220:410, 1971.

recruited (Bigland and Lippold, 1954; Grimby and Hannerz, 1968). According to Bigland and Lippold (1954), the degradations of contraction in the muscles are brought about mainly by motor unit recruitment and not by increased rate of impulse discharge, except at very low and high contraction strengths. This would correspond to the recruitment of slow twitch motor units and finally by fast twitch units (Henneman and Olson, 1965). However, this pattern for increasing motor strength and activity may differ depending on the velocity of the muscle contraction during task performance. A rapid contraction during the first step of walking may be initiated by some motor units setting up only a few discharges and then other units taking over at a constant rate of discharge. Some motor units, probably consisting of fast fibers, may be only active during extremely rapid and almost maximal efforts (Grimby and Hannerz, 1968; Warmolts and Engel, 1972).

Åstrand and Rodahl (1970) emphasize that "if the muscles are slaves of the motoneurons, then the motoneurons are slaves of spinal and supraspinal motor mechanisms." Furthermore, Eccles (1957) has stated "by establishing synaptic connections with [spinal] interneurons rather than with motoneurons the pyramidal and other descending tracts (from the cerebellum, the red nucleus, the reticular formation) are able to operate through the coordination [i.e. feedback] mechanisms at the segmental levels of the spinal cord" (our insertions). The interneurons (Fig. 1-3) in turn act in feedback loops to excite, facilitate, or inhibit the motoneurons during the transition to walking. It is the interneurons that provide for positive and negative input needed for reciprocal innervation and crossed (i.e. contralateral) innervation. However, the input of various receptors not only initiate action in that segment, but also they send collaterals to other segments along with those from interneurons. The segmental muscle spindle contraction-coordination system (Fig. 1-3) and its feedback control of nearby motor units has been excellently reviewed recently by Stein (1974) and by Easton (see Chap. on Reflexes). The closed loop from gamma motoneuron activity to increased muscle spindle afferent discharge to increased alpha motoneuron activity, is an excellent example of "follow-up-length-servo" control. This active motor feedback controlling system is a prime consideration when the mechanism is sought for impaired motor performance.

Presumably it is the higher motor centers that initiate the shift from standing to walking. The impulse activity down the pyramidal tracts would bring into action the motor units that power the first step. Simultaneously, and perhaps even before the first step, the neurons of the extrapyramidal tract become active (see Evarts, 1973). Some activate neurons within the basal ganglia which is thought by Grossman (1967) "to be the major integrative center for the extrapyramidal motor system." One of the next lower motor centers activated would be the subthalamic nuclei that may exert and maintain overall control of rhythmic movements of the limbs (Jung and Hassler, 1960) presumably via pathways through the reticular formation. The importance of the feedback role of the cerebellum in relaying information concerning joint position, limb velocity, and posture during the shift to walking is obvious.

Thus, the shifting of motor activity from standing to rapid walking alters muscular activity in a highly complex manner. It occurs through the action of a highly stratified motor-coordinating system whose operation is not well understood (see Chap. on Reflexes). The motor adaptation to a greater work load is essentially immediate and involves the recruitment of the appropriate motor units and their associated mechanoreceptors which provide the lowest level of motor feedback control. Intersegmental reflexes and higher motor center activity provide for the integration of segmental motor activity into the overall motor response.

The regulation of the motor system during this transition commences the coordinated, optimized patterns of locomotion. These regulatory changes during the onset of walking will be largely opposite to those that will subsequently occur as the limits of work capacity are reached. Mechanoreceptors will be able to detect imbalances between muscle tension development and desired activity, e.g. gamma-loop activity. Signals indicating errors from the motor units will be processed by the segmental reflex arcs or by input from higher centers. It is possible that these controlling components of the motor system could themselves become "fatigued." At the behavioral level, such "fatigue" may be observed as diminished motor coordination and would be of importance more in sedentary psychomotor tasks. For the maintenance of motor performance, then, the unimpaired operation of the overall motor system is crucial.

Metabolic Support System Regulation

ATP Regeneration

An active muscle's contractile response to walking is essentially immediate. It should be noted that ATP is also essential in the production of muscle fiber's active state. ATP quickly binds to myosin or actomyosin, facilitates the dissociation of actomyosin, and is energetically necessary for tension to be developed by muscle fibers. For the continuation of muscular contractions, the most vital support required is the regeneration of the ATP utilized to produce the muscle's active state. Obviously if the hydrolysis of ATP to ADP + P_i powers contraction, then the depletion of ATP in the muscle fiber will halt its ability to contract. The concentrations of ATP in human muscle is small, amounting to only 2.09 mmoles/100 g of dry weight (Hultman, et al., 1967). Some means of ATP regeneration must be provided for contractions to continue. In fact, the reaction product ADP does serve as a link to the cellular intermediary metabolic pathways that can regenerate ATP. These pathways of intermediary metabolism regenerating ATP are shown in the lower part of Figure 1-4. For details about the enzymatic steps for muscle energy metabolism, many recent reviews can be consulted (e.g. see Gollnick and King, 1969; Larner, 1971).

The following describes the three basic metabolic sources of ATP for the working muscle in the order of the rapidity with which ATP can be available. After the first step in walking, the regeneration of ATP must be essentially immediate so that further contractions can take place. This ap-

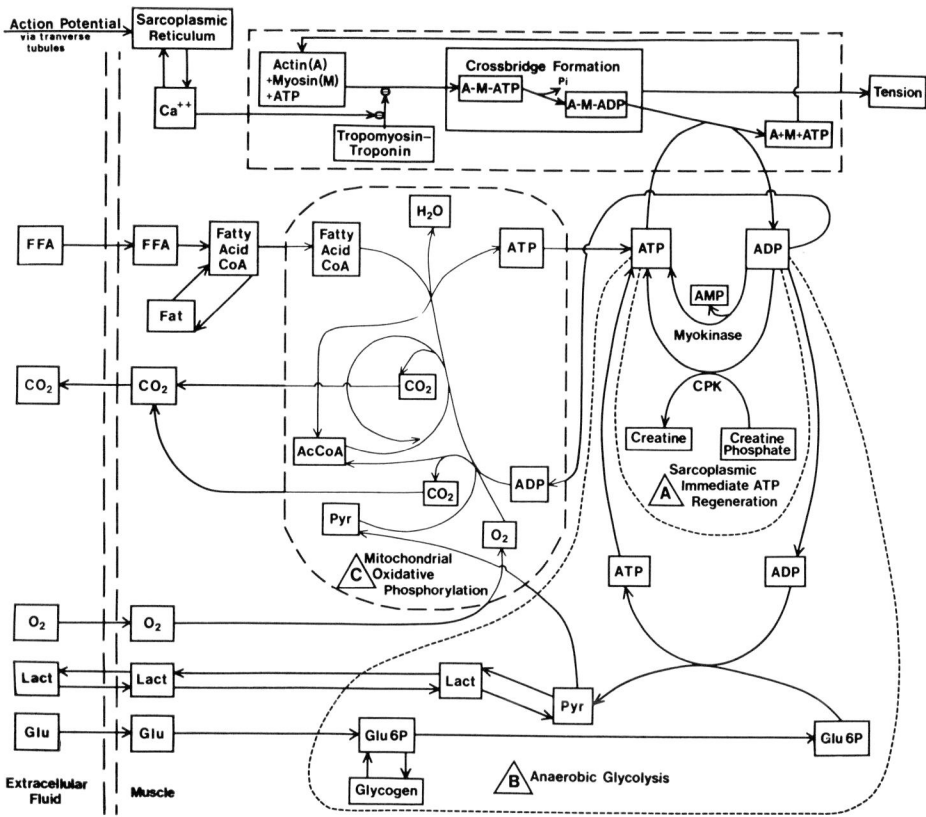

Figure 1-4. Block diagram of the feedback control of contraction-energy regeneration coupling. A—immediate adenosine triphosphate (ATP) regeneration using myokinase and creatine phosphokinase (CPK) enzymes. B—slower ATP regeneration from anaerobic glycolysis. C—slowest ATP regeneration from aerobic processes in mitochondria. Other abbreviations: AcCoA—acetyl coenzyme A; A—actin; ADP—adenosine diphosphate; AMP—adenosine monophosphate; Ca^{++}—calcium ion; CO_2—carbon dioxide; Fatty Acid CoA—fatty acid coenzyme A; FFA—free fatty acid; Glu—glucose; Glu-6-P—glucose-6-phosphate; H_2O—water; Lact—lactic acid; O_2—oxygen; Pyr—pyruvic acid.

pears to be true (see Weiser, 1971), since only at maximal or supramaximal work does muscle ATP concentration decrease (Helmreich, et al., 1965; Karlsson, et al., 1972). First, the most immediate energy sources for ATP regeneration (A in Fig. 1-4) are catalyzed by the cytoplasmic enzymes that shuffle a high-energy phosphate group from one ADP to another ADP (i.e. myokinase) and from creatine phosphate to ADP (i.e. creatine phosphotransferase). The concentration of creatine phosphate (CP) in muscle is also small, only three times that of ATP or 6.78 mmoles/100 g of dry muscle (Hultman, et al., 1967). CP breakdown appears to be highly coupled to

ADP production in all fiber groups. As a result, CP immediately begins to fall at the beginning of work (Hultman, et al., 1967; see Simonson, 1971, Chap. 2).

The second most available source of ATP regeneration during walking is anaerobic glycolysis (glucose breakdown to pyruvate) whose rate-limiting enzymes appear to be coupled to the contractile process by allosteric modifiers, perhaps ATP, ADP, and Ca^{++}. The concurrent allosteric activation of muscle glycogenolysis (glycogen breakdown to glucose units) provides most of the substrate for glycolysis (Hultman, 1967) and consequently lactate is produced (e.g. Karlsson, et al., 1972). This ATP regenerating process is slow, and it peaks about 30 to 40 sec. after starting to walk (see Keul, et al., 1972). This lag is partly due to the time necessary to convert phosphorylase-b to the -a form (see Weiser, 1971). During this time, net CP breakdown appears to stop and CP concentration remains constant after about 1 to 2 min. during submaximal work (Hultman, et al., 1967).

The third and least rapidly available source of ATP is the acceleration of the mitochondrial mechanisms via pyruvate and fatty acid oxidation. These lag times for these systems are 1 to 2 min. (see Keul, et al., 1972). Again this demonstrates that a complex enzymatic adaptation had commenced and shifted the active muscle fibers from one metabolic state to another. To increase oxygen consumption, the increased ADP diffusing to the mitochondria most likely "triggers" an increased activity of the electron transport systems within the mitochondria. The increased amount of oxidized hydrogen-ion carriers (e.g. NADH) then "turns on" the fatty acid β-oxidation and/or Kreb's cycle systems associated with electron transport. It is the interactions of this ADP "push" and β-oxidation/Kreb's cycle "pull" that produces the longer oxidative lag than is seen for glycolysis. Add to this lag in oxidative processes a further circulatory lag due to the time necessary to transport blood from the lungs to the working muscles, and one can understand a large part of the oxygen deficit observed during this transition. Pulmonary oxygen uptake reflect the energy cost of work only when this initial lag is over.

The relative contributions of FFA β-oxidation and glycolysis to the overall ATP regeneration is determined by three factors (see Simonson, 1971, Chaps. 2, 6, and 15). First, the time elapsed after starting to walk influences the proportional contribution of fat to glucose for ATP regeneration. During the initiation of walking, pyruvate from the accelerated glycolysis (and glycogenolysis) is utilized as the oxidative substrate. With time (2-5 min.), muscle FFA oxidation increases and is associated with a decrease in glycolysis. Just how this shift in oxidized substrate occurs is not well understood, but it may occur through allosteric interactions between the rate-limiting enzymes of the two pathways. Second, the work level to be performed will determine the proportion in substrate oxidation. With higher work loads, more carbohydrate oxidation will occur, while the proportion of FFA oxidation will be less (see Åstrand and Rodahl, 1970). Finally, the diet will influence the relative activities of the oxidative pathways: in general, the higher the carbohydrate content of the diet, the lower will be the proportion of FFA oxidation.

In summary, ATP regeneration goes through three phases during the transition to higher work levels. 1. The initial replacement of ATP (zero to about 45 sec.) via the local high-energy phosphate compounds such as creatine phosphate is critical for the possible depletion of substrates during maximal work. 2. A transient breakdown of muscle glycogen to lactate via anaerobic glycolysis (starting at 15 to 60 sec. or so) shows an accelerating ATP regeneration which peaks at about 45 sec. during submaximal work and will be importantly related to endurance capacity. 3. If glycolysis declines after 45 sec., mitochondrial oxidation of fatty acids and pyruvate for ATP regeneration becomes the critical, dominant supply of energy for contraction during prolonged work.

Substrate Supply

Much of the energy sources for ATP regeneration of course are not found in the muscle fiber itself. Substrates are transported to the working muscles from storage sites mainly in the adipose tissue and the liver.

Plasma FFA levels initially decrease as walking is begun and indicate that this early FFA utilization is greater than its mobilization (see Keul, et al., 1972; Simonson, 1971, Chap. 2 and 15; Weiser, 1971). FFA oxidation is proportional to plasma FFA concentration at rest and during light to moderate physical activity (see Paul, 1970). However, the proportionality constant relating FFA level to FFA oxidation increased during exercise in dogs so that at the same FFA level during work there is a greater turnover and oxidation of FFA. It is not well known just how fast this changes FFA entry into working muscle, but it probably occurs in less than 5 minutes (see Havel, et al., 1963). This increase of FFA entry into the muscle is rapid and remains constant thereafter, whereas the rate of FFA influx into the circulation is much slower and might not plateau until an hour after walking is begun. The mechanism and control of FFA entry and of the coordination of FFA influx to FFA oxidation are unknown. One factor involved might be the increased blood flow (Issekutz, et al., 1964) accompanying an increased volume and area for transport from the blood to the working muscles.

As described above, the increase in FFA mobilization appears to be a relatively slow process. The initial influx of FFA into the blood is probably due to increased sympathetic activity with additional humoral stimulation occurring later. The acceleration of the breakdown and release of FFA from adipose tissue appears to be greater in trained subjects with high endurance (Issekutz, et al., 1965). An enhanced capability to mobilize fat for fuel has been demonstrated especially well for trained dogs in studies by Issekutz, et al. (1965) and Paul (1970). These authors suggest that the increased lactate level of the "unfit" dogs acts on the fat cells to inhibit the lipolytic activity (i.e. ability to break down fat). Also, due to the inability of the working muscle fibers to be provided with FFA for fuel in these untrained subjects, their working muscles' ability to increase FFA oxidation for ATP regeneration is limited. The increased lipolytic activity of trained subjects could be partly due to a corresponding increase of sympathetic activity releasing norepinephrine in the vicinity of the fat cells (Havel, 1965) or due to a great response of triglyceride lipase to a given amount of norepinephrine (Gollnick, et al., 1970; Askew, et al., 1972).

Consequently, FFA mobilization could minimize the role of glycolysis in the working muscles. Thereby the potential energy source, muscle glycogen, would be conserved (see Weiser, 1971). Blood glucose utilization by working muscle shows a marked rate of increase within 15 min. in "unfit" dogs (Issekutz, et al., 1970). The mobilization of glucose from the liver at the beginning of walking must increase along with its utilization since no change or only a slight decrease in blood glucose is seen (Issekutz, et al., 1970; Keul, et al., 1972). However, the proportion of substrates being oxidized from blood glucose at the beginning of walking is small, less than 25 percent (Issekutz, et al., 1970).

Ventilation

The supply of oxygen to muscle fibers, plus the supply of the substrates described above, fulfills the fuel requirements for the ATP needed to support performance. A scheme illustrating oxygen supply is shown in Figure 1-5; detailed reviews can be found elsewhere (Dejours, 1965; Åstrand and Rodahl, 1970; Simonson, 1971, Chap. 8).

The increase in ventilation after the start of walking does not occur as fast as oxygen consumption by the working muscles. In support of this observation, alveolar pO_2 transiently decreases in the first two minutes and then increases to return to a value lower than at the previous steady-state (e.g. see Robinson, 1938; Balke, 1954; Craig, 1972). These transient changes indicate that oxygen uptake by the blood flowing through the pulmonary vascular bed temporarily increases faster than does alveolar ventilation.

As Dejours (1965) has reported for treadmill walking, there is an immediate increase in tidal volume during the first 40 sec. followed by a less rapid increase. Respiratory rate increases rapidly at first (0-60 sec.) although not as abruptly as tidal volume. However, after 40 sec., respiratory

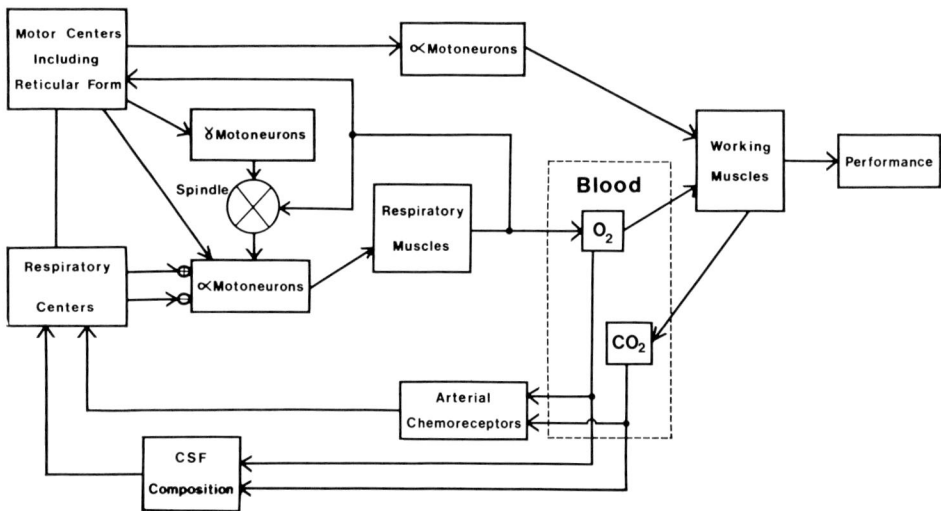

Figure 1-5. Block diagram of the feedback control of ventilation.

rate continues to increase slowly along with tidal volume for at least the next several minutes.

The respiratory changes can, therefore, be divided into an initial fast and a subsequent slow component (Dejours, 1965). Initially, ventilation is thought to change by an alteration in the neurogenic respiratory controlling system. In fact, the increased tidal volume commences on the breath during the first step, if one is in the phase of inspiration, or on the following breath, if one is expiring (Ingemann, et al., 1972). The input to the respiratory centers that initiates the fast component is presumably provided by higher motor centers. The changed output from these motor centers is an increase of impulse activity in respiratory motoneurons regulating the rapid acceleration of the depth and rate of breathing. Apparently the higher motor input to ventilatory control overrides the resting setting of ventilation by arterial pCO_2 and results in a transient increase of arterial pCO_2 (Ingemann, et al., 1972).

After 20 to 40 sec. of walking, the slow component of the ventilatory increase begins and lasts for at least several minutes (Dejours, 1965). Humoral modification of respiratory control seems to be the additional factor that stimulates the medullary control centers to increase ventilation even further and could become an important factor if dyspnea becomes a symptom (see Simonson, 1971, Chap. 8). This component is due in part to the increased arterial pCO_2 feeding back to the control centers. Also contributing could be an alteration in the chemosensitivity of the O_2 and CO_2 receptor cells (Weil, et al., 1972). The time course of the increased chemosensitivity is not well known, but it appears to commence within 3 min. after the start of walking (Weil, et al., 1972). Some intensification of the neurogenic feedback also appears to take place during the slow component (Dejours, 1965) which could become associated with the symptom of dyspnea reported to occur with the fatigue associated with prolonged work.

Blood Supply

Changes in circulation occur as rapidly as the changes in ventilation. The supply of FFA, glucose, O_2, and other substrates to muscle fibers is of course dependent on the supply of blood. The components of the muscle blood supply system are shown in Figure 1-6. Detailed reviews of the functioning and control of this system can be found elsewhere (Folkow, et al., 1965; Rowell, 1969, 1971, 1974; Åstrand and Rodahl, 1970; Guyton, et al., 1972).

Muscle blood flow can increase very fast to plateau in one minute (Barcroft and Dornhorst, 1949) or less (Kramer, et al., 1939). At the start of walking, impulses along sympathetic vasodilator nerves to the working muscles briefly dilate the arterioles in the working muscles. Soon afterward local factors, including the release of K+ from the working muscle fibers, in-

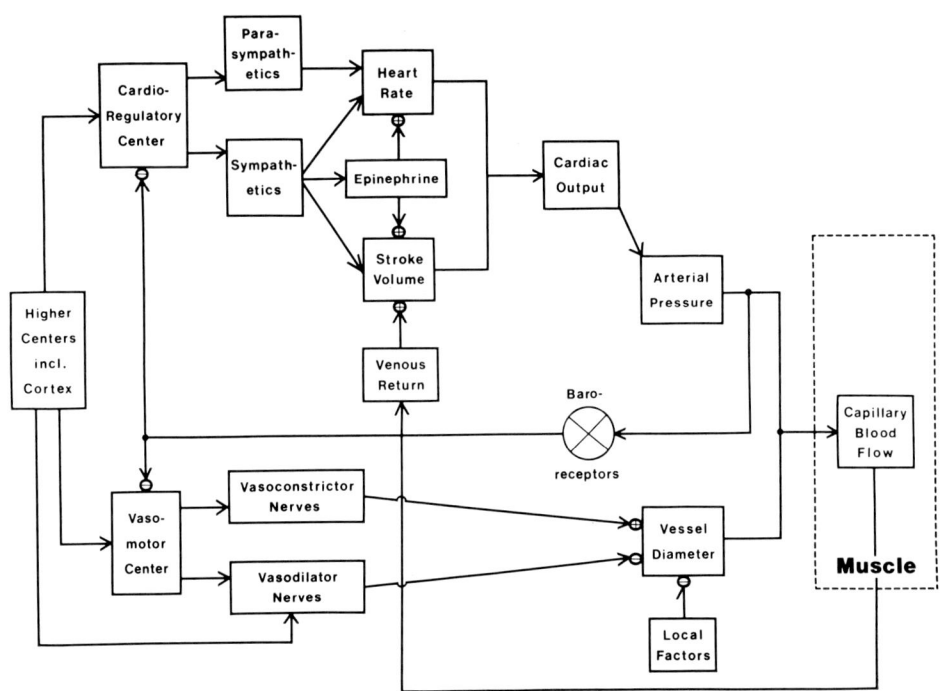

Figure 1-6. Block diagram of the feedback control of blood supply.

crease in the muscle interstitial fluid and assume the dilatating control of the arterioles (see Haddy and Scott, 1968).

Simultaneously, blood flow through the splanchnic and renal vascular bed presumably decreases (see Rowell, 1969, 1971). The time course of this reduction in visceral blood flow, in contrast to muscle blood flow, is not clearly understood. Most likely this change is initiated by increased sympathetic vasoconstrictor activity.

The central circulatory responses to walking are well known. These changes are very similar to those of ventilation. Stroke volume makes a rapid increase of 90 percent in the first 30 sec. of increased work to plateau by 1½ min. (Jones and Reeves, 1968). Like respiratory rate and tidal volume, heart rate increases rapidly but not as fast as stroke volume. The increase of heart rate is faster for higher walking speeds. Heart rate increases chiefly in response to increased sympathetic and decreased parasympathetic activity (see Åstrand and Rodahl, 1970; and Simonson, 1971, Chap. 9). Stroke volume increases due to increased sympathetic activity, but it could be influenced by the increased venous return from the working muscles (Bevegård and Shepherd, 1968).

When the working muscles limit the capacity to perform a task, this may be due to an inadequate supply of blood to the muscle fibers. First, local factors released from the muscle fibers could reduce blood flow. However, this impairment is not likely since most of these local factors known dilate muscle arterioles. Second, blood flow might be reduced due to redistribution of blood flow to other regions, e.g. to the skin for heat loss to take place. Such redistribution of blood flow could result from altered vasomotor center activity controlling the arteriolar tone in various regional vascular beds. Finally, in the case of maximal work, the heart might have reached a functioning level maximizing its ability to pump blood. Thus, the cardiovascular system and its feedback control is of considerable importance in the assessment of the factors that define work capacity and contribute to fatigue.

To summarize, during the transition to a greater work load, the role of both the motor and autonomic nervous system appears to be the main controllers of adaptation. But these two systems are primarily linked together by ATP/ADP in a contraction-energy regeneration coupling. Together, they all commence the motor and supporting responses. The adequacy of these adaptations to a new work task becomes readily apparent when one considers the possibility of fatigue in the response to maximal work.

MAXIMAL (AND SUPRAMAXIMAL) AEROBIC WORK

One of the most important factors determining work performance is the maximal aerobic work that one can do (Åstrand and Rodahl, 1970). First, a distinction must be drawn between maximal aerobic power and maximal aerobic endurance capacity. Since power is work done per unit time, then maximal aerobic power, i.e. max V_{O_2}, is the work level at which an individual attains his highest oxygen uptake. Traditionally, maximal work is taken as that which requires maximal aerobic power. Note that work loads greater than this require that the additional ATP regeneration come from purely anaerobic pathways. Endurance capacity, on the other hand, refers to the total duration of work that can be done. In addition to the question of what determines maximal aerobic power, there is also the question of what limits the capacity for prolonged (supra) maximal work.

In addition, another distinction should be made concerning the type of task under question. Tasks may partly or wholly involve the work of large muscle masses or of smaller muscle masses, or be dynamic or static in nature. The focus of this section will be on the factors that determine dynamic work performance involving a large muscle mass.

Maximal Aerobic Power

Maximal aerobic power can vary greatly from person to person depending on age, sex, and whether or not a pathological condition such as mitral stenosis exists. See Simonson (1971, Chaps. 7 and 16) and Åstrand and Rodahl (1970) for details. Max V_{O_2} is determined overall by two convective systems, i.e. pulmonary ventilation and blood circulation, and two diffusing systems, i.e. alveolar-capillary exchange and capillary-tissue-mitochondria exchange (see Holmgren, 1967).

In maximal dynamic work using large muscle masses, probably not all of the motor units in the working muscle groups are simultaneously active. Most likely it is only in supramaximal work near the maximal tensions developed by these muscles that all the motor units become active. At least this has been observed for EMG activity in static work (Lippold, 1952), in small muscle mass work (Bouisset and Goubel, 1973), and during cycling (Hendriksson and Bonde-Petersen, 1974; Bigland-Ritchie and Woods, 1974). During work at 100 percent max V_{O_2}, just what percent of the motor units are active and what proportion of fast twitch to slow twitch fiber activity exists has not yet been reported. Also, it should be noted that the transition to maximal dynamic work is fast and that muscle work is actually phasic, alternating between periods of contraction and relaxation.

The neuromuscular junction and the feedback loop involving mechanoreceptors are other possible components of the motor system that might limit maximal aerobic power. When the motor system has adapted to maximal work, most likely no impairment of either of these components has taken place (see Simonson, 1971, Chap. 10 and chapter on Reflexes). This implies that the limiting factor(s) must lie in the supporting systems of the working muscles.

The first two elements of O_2 delivery to the working muscles are pulmonary ventilation and alveolar-blood oxygen exchange. Neither of these processes seems to limit maximal oxygen uptake (Taylor, 1960). Physiological data, primarily from blood gases, indicate that the alveolar-blood oxygen exchange is not significantly altered except for some international class athletes at high altitude (see Buskirk, 1971).

The remaining two elements of O_2 delivery concern blood circulation and capillary tissue-mitochondria oxygen exchange. Many reports in the literature indicate that maximal cardiac output (i.e. max CO), and in particular maximal stroke volume (i.e. max SV), is a limiting factor for maximal aerobic power (see Rowell, 1971). For example, sedentary individuals, highly trained athletes, and patients with mitral stenosis have a tissue extraction of oxygen, i.e. maximal a-v oxygen difference, that are very nearly the same when work load is expressed as percent maximal aerobic power (see Simonson, 1972). Furthermore, the percentage of cardiac output distributed to the working muscles also appears to be about the same for all three groups. Finally, maximal heart rate is about the same in general for all groups. Rowell (1971) states that, "Stroke volume is then the circulatory parameter which most obviously separates those with very high and those with very low maximal oxygen uptake."

Although many experiments have been performed to eliminate muscle oxygen utilization as a determinant of max V_{O_2}, this factor still exists as a possibility. Rowell (1974) cites two key findings that seem to discount a metabolic limitation. First he notes that if leg muscle metabolic capacity is a limiting factor in leg work, then the addition of arm work should increase max V_{O_2}; such is not the case for most individuals. This suggests that max CO limits total muscle blood flow (MBF). The second observation cited by Rowell is that the addition of oxygen to the inspired air increases max V_{O_2} by an amount that is proportional to the increased arterial oxygen content. "Thus," he states, "muscle metabolism was not limited—it rose." This suggests again that maximal aerobic power is limited by the maximal amount of oxygen that can be delivered to the working muscles: arterial oxygen content × peak total MBF.

That MBF may not be maximal is demonstrated by experiments that investigated occlusion of the blood flow to one leg while cycling at max V_{O_2}. Clausen and Lassen (1971) and Pirnay, et al. (1972a) have shown that MBF can be increased approximately 15 percent when the MBF to the other leg is occluded. This indicates that MBF was not maximal. With the presumable increase in mean arterial blood pressure due to the occlusion, as Rowell (1974) has suggested, MBF can be increased. Whether or not MBF reaches its peak flow at max V_{O_2} is a controversial question. Black (1959), Tonnesen (1964), and Clausen and Lassen (1971) have reported that MBF peaks at about 70 percent maximal work performed. Grimby, et al. (1967) and Pirnay, et al. (1972a) have observed peak flow at maximal work load but with some subjects showing less of an increase in MBF between progressively increasing work loads near max V_{O_2} than between lower work loads.

Several studies have indicated that the capillary-tissue-mitochondria oxygen gradient may not be maximal during work at max V_{O_2}. First, in the *in situ* isolated dog skeletal muscle preparation, Stainsby and Otis (1964) have observed that the critical venous pO_2 level is about 10 mm Hg below which muscle V_{O_2} is depressed. During work at or above max V_{O_2} femoral vein pO_2 is decreased to no lower than 20 mm Hg (Hartley and Saltin, 1969; Keul, et al., 1972; Pirnay, et al., 1972b). Second, under β-adrenergic blockade that temporarily decreases maximal heart rate (about 40 beats/min.) and max CO (about 12-22%), max V_{O_2} can be maintained (Ekblom, et al., 1972) or decreases slightly about 6 percent (Epstein, et al., 1965; Pirnay, et al., 1972b). Consequently, the arterial-mixed venous oxygen difference must have been increased, and indeed a decrease in femoral venous pO_2 did take place (Pirnay, et al., 1972b). Since muscle oxygen extraction was increased, these studies suggest that the working motor units only incompletely extract the oxygen delivered to them under normal conditions.

In summary, maximal aerobic power is associated with the size of max SV, a peak but not maximal total MBF, a peak but not maximal muscle oxygen extraction, and possibly not all motor units recruited. With a similar line of reasoning, Rowell (1974) reached this summarization and has proposed that "perhaps a better expression . . . is max $\dot{V}_{O_2} = \frac{\text{max MP}}{\text{min TPR}} \times$ max A-V oxygen difference, where maximal CO is redefined as the ratio of maximal mean arterial pressure (max MP) and minimum total peripheral resistance (min TPR)." During arm work, Stenberg (1966) has shown that MP is higher than during leg work but max CO and peak V_{O_2} is less for arm work than for treadmill running. He suggests that "there is a smaller vascular bed dilated by (arm) exercise." The suggestion made by Rowell (1974) would imply that the limiting factor is the ability to perfuse the arm muscles. This arm work evaluation could be extended to explain the lower peak V_{O_2} observed during supine exercise, upright cycling, and β-adrenergic blockage.

Prolonged (Supra)Maximal Aerobic Endurance Capacity

Figure 9-7 of Åstrand and Rodahl (1970) illustrates the effect of training on work at 100 percent max V_{O_2}: an untrained individual is capable of running for less than 5 minutes whereas a well-trained subject may continue running for as long as 8 minutes (also see Saltin, 1973). That the metabolic supporting systems can limit maximal work is clearly seen when

TABLE 1-II

SOME FACTORS PRODUCING FATIGUE DURING PROLONGED
(SUPRA) MAXIMAL WORK

System	Impaired Component		Consequence
	Controlled System	Controlling System	
Motor	Fast twitch (?) muscle fibers excitation-contraction coupling giving less tension	Muscle Spindles (?)	Feedback error signal via muscle spindles; "weak legs"
ATP regeneration	Phosphocreatine depletion	Altered enzyme regulation	Reduced anaerobic capacity leading to motor impairment
Fuel supply	?	?	?
Blood supply	?	?	?
Ventilation	?	Altered activity of respiratory centers (?)	Hyperventilation; dyspnea

the factors determining prolonged maximal work are examined in Table 1-II.

Motor System Regulation

At the present moment, one can only speculate about possible changes in motor unit activity that could occur during prolonged maximal work. It is well-known that fast twitch motor units cannot maintain their initial developed tension for more than several minutes before the tension can no longer be developed. This suggests that during maximal work a time could be reached when fast motor units begin to exhibit impaired ability to develop tension. If this does take place, as it does in static work (Hirsch, et al., 1970), then this implies that information about the impaired contractile state would be fed back via muscle spindles and Golgi tendon organs to the spinal cord. Consequently, there might be at least two possibilities for the controlling elements of the motor system: 1. to inhibit the impaired motor units and recruit more fast units; or 2. to increase the impulse frequency of the motoneurons to the impaired fibers and perhaps to the other slower, and less fatigued, motor units.

With prolonged work of a dynamic type, impairment of the transmission across the neuromuscular junction is not thought to be likely (see Simonson, 1971, Chap. 10, p. 224). It is possible, however, that some impairment in the afferent feedback processes monitoring muscle functioning could take place (see chapter on Reflexes).

The question then arises as to the factor(s) responsible for the impairment of the working fiber's contractile state. As we shall see in the following section, the sites of possible impairment are primarily two-fold: 1. decreased O_2 transport to the working muscle groups, and 2. decreased ability to regenerate ATP by the working fibers and thereby maintain ATP levels.

Metabolic Support System Regulation

Dyspnea could be a factor limiting prolonged maximal work (see Simonson, 1971, Chap. 8), since one of the most common symptoms recalled is "too hard to breathe." Minute ventilation also does not plateau for untrained subjects. These observations suggest that the system controlling pulmonary ventilation might become impaired in individuals not trained for prolonged maximal work.

For prolonged (supra)maximal work, little emphasis has been placed upon changes in the processes that regulate oxygen delivery. Once oxygen uptake has increased and plateaued, it remains at this steady state for the duration of work (Robinson, 1938; Åstrand and Saltin, 1961). In well-trained subjects, heart rate also plateaus at its maximal rate and does not decline (Åstrand and Saltin, 1961). Dehydration decreases supramaximal work time but does not decrease max CO or max SV indicating that cardiac performance is maintained (Saltin, 1964). Perhaps during short-term heavy work, central circulatory function is not a limiting factor. Also changes in distribution of blood flow to the working muscles during prolonged maximal work has not been reported (see Rowell, 1971). This author has observed blanching of the skin in subjects at the end of performing max V_{O_2} tests at a constant work load. This is presumably due to cutaneous vasoconstriction, but no data apparently exists as to where the blood flow is redistributed from the skin. Perhaps this is an indication that muscle blood flow might be maintained.

During prolonged supramaximal work, the fundamental problem appears to be the establishment of a metabolic state that is not at a steady-state. As mentioned before, there is a full transition to a V_{O_2} plateau. Also rhythmic maximal ATP turnover should be reached in each active muscle fiber to meet the energy demands of contraction. But the fluxes of substances through the metabolic pathways regenerating ATP never seem to become steady. Creatine phosphate (CP) degradation initially is fast, but as maximal aerobic work continues CP breakdown does not stop (Hultman, 1967). The shift to oxidative metabolism is never complete especially in the low oxidative, high glycolytic, fast motor units. Consequently, during maximal work, there is always lactate production and possibly CP splitting (see Simonson, 1971, Chaps. 1 and 2). Associated with these conditions is metabolic acidosis, i.e. decreasing pH, and a reduced redox state, i.e. decreasing NAD/NADH ratio. More important is the decline in ATP concentration (Karlsson, 1971; Saltin and Essen, 1971; Knuttgen and Saltin, 1972, 1973). This decline in ATP level could well signal the decrease in contractile state in some motor units.

Thus, if the ATP regeneration-contraction coupling of the fast twitch motor units is impaired during a session of prolonged maximal work, then these changes should be detected by muscle spindles and Golgi tendon organs. Again it is tempting to speculate that via the feedback loops in the motor system, a. either more fast units would be recruited, and/or b. bursts of greater impulse frequency would be sent to the fast units (and perhaps to slow units), and/or c. more slow units would be recruited. Possibly these alterations continue to occur until no further motor feedback adjustments can be made to provide the necessary power required by the work task. The afferent signalling function of the mechanoreceptors could also be impaired. Consequently, the individual might stop and complain of an inability to develop leg power. These adjustments could also be very interrelated with the increased perceived effort reported (see Chap. on Subjective Fatigue), and they could be also associated with increased ventilation (see above) and reports of "hard to breathe."

SUBMAXIMAL AEROBIC WORK

Discussed so far has been the transition to walking fast which requires about 1.4 L/min. (7 kcal/min.) and (supra)maximal work requiring an energy expenditure of about 2 to 5 L O_2/min. depending on the age, sex, etc., factors that influence maximal aerobic power. This section is concerned with the regulatory changes in the motor and support systems during submaximal work, and how they affect the ability to maintain work involving large masses of working muscles at a given percent maximal aerobic power. Submaximal work will be defined as those tasks such as backpacking, heavy shoveling, and cycling that require an oxygen consumption somewhere between rest, about 7% max V_{O_2}, and 100% max V_{O_2}. Table 1-III indicates some of the factors that impair the performance of these tasks. In general, the adaptation of the motor and support systems involves an attempt to establish a "steady-state" at a higher level of functioning, and fatigue will be due to a particular set of components which do not adequately establish a steady-state.

Motor System Regulation

These examples of submaximal work (backpacking, heavy shoveling, and cycling) can involve a large proportion of the total skeletal muscle mass. Obviously, these tasks are very complex with respect to the neural controls used in regulating work output. Traditionally, steady-state work is consid-

TABLE 1-III

SOME FACTORS PRODUCING FATIGUE DURING PROLONGED SUBMAXIMAL WORK AT 50% MAX V_{O_2} OR GREATER

System	Impaired Component — Controlled System	Impaired Component — Controlling System	Consequence
Motor	α-motoneurons hyperpolarization (?); muscle fiber excitation-contraction coupling giving less tension	Muscle spindles (?)	Feedback error signal via muscle mechanoreceptors; "weak legs"
ATP regeneration	Increased enzyme degradation; Substrate depletion (glycogen & triglycerides); inadequate FFA oxidation	Altered enzyme regulations	Reduced contractility leading to motor impaired
Fuel supply	Inadequate enzyme concentration for FFA mobilization; liver glycogen depletion	Neurohormonal stimulation inadequate; regulation of liver glucose mobilization inadequate	Inadequate FFA supply for ATP regeneration; decreased blood glucose for CNS energy metabolism
Blood supply	Impaired myocardial contractility (?)	Altered cardiac control; altered regional blood flow for heat loss	Reduced stroke volume; increased heart rate
Ventilation	?	Altered activity of respiratory centers (?)	Hyperventilation

ered to be attained by 2 to 3 min. when V_{O_2} becomes steady. However, this steady-state occurs after a relatively long time compared to when one is "in stride." The regulation of the motor system can establish a steady, rhythmic pattern of movements within several strides. After some period of time, which is shorter for a task requiring a larger percent maximal aerobic power, the performer will voluntarily terminate work. A common complaint for prolonged submaximal work is that the working muscles had become "weaker and weaker" (Weiser, et al., 1973; and Chap. on Subjective Symptomatology).

At the beginning of submaximal work, developed power is sensed by muscle spindles, Golgi tendon organs, and other mechanoreceptors. Muscle spindles set the distance to be shortened by the extrafusal muscle fibers during each contraction via the gamma-loop, and spindle afferents relay information about the velocity and degree of actual shortening. Since the muscle spindle is thought to be linked to one or many motor units (Henneman, 1968c), it would signal any decrement in velocity or length of shortening coincident with the decrease in power generated by a motor unit. Similarly, Golgi tendon organs send information concerning the stretch exerted upon a tendon by several motor units of a given muscle (Henneman, 1968c). These signals, and the consequent alterations in motor unit performance, could be importantly related to the subjective experience, i.e. symptom, of "weak muscles." It remains to be shown that mechanoreceptor activity itself or spinal and supraspinal controls are impaired during prolonged submaximal work, but any distance runner or jogger will tell you that a key symptom of this form of fatigue is the loss of coordination (see Chap. on Reflexes).

Metabolic Support System Regulation

ATP Regeneration

The establishment of the steady-state, i.e. steady oxygen consumption, lags minutes behind the onset of this steady motor activity. For the oxidative ATP regenerating processes, the steady-state activity in the FFA and glycolytic pathways will be determined by the relative work load imposed, length of time on the task, and the diet (Christensen and Hansen, 1939b). Metabolic fuels calculated from the respiratory quotient and by other techniques indicate that after 5 minutes of 50 to 60% max V_{O_2} work, "the energy is supplied by fat and by carbohydrate, mainly glycogen, in about equal amounts" (Åstrand and Rodahl, 1970, Fig. 14-2). In heavier work loads, the glycolytic pathway provides a greater proportion of the increased energy requirement than does fat oxidation. Again the regulation of ATP regeneration for contraction acts by altering the metabolic control of the pathways. For example, the metabolites Ca^{++}, ATP, ADP, and fatty acyl CoA acting through allosteric mechanisms all influence the activity of phosphofructokinase, a key rate-limiting enzyme of glycolysis. This work load-energy supply relationship is altered by the composition of the diet, specifically the carbohydrate to fat ratio.

With the continuation of the submaximal work task, the contribution of fat oxidation increases and that of carbohydrate decreases. This is usually explained by an increased mobilization of FFA from adipose tissue resulting from increased sympathetic activity (Åstrand and Rodahl, 1970); consequently the elevated FFA levels increase muscle fat oxidation by mass action (Paul, 1970). In fact, this increase of fat oxidation, as indicated by a decrease of the respiratory quotient, also occurs when one is on a high-carbohydrate diet (Christensen and Hansen, 1939a; Bergström, et al., 1967).

Recently, the work of Bergström and co-workers has firmly established the possible limiting role of muscle glycogen in the regulation of ATP regeneration during submaximal prolonged bicycle exercise (see Simonson, 1971, Chap. 2). After running to exhaustion on a treadmill, the quadriceps glycogen level is not depleted nearly to the low levels as that observed with cycling (Costill, et al., 1971a,b). This indicates that the number of motor units active in the quadriceps is less during running and/or there is less glycogenolytic activity of the motor units utilized during running. The difference between running and cycling may be explained by the recruitment theory of Henneman and Olson (1965); running activates a certain population of slow twitch motor units along some fast twitch units, while cycling is powered by these fibers plus additional fast fibers. Since fast fibers are supported by high glycolytic, low oxidative energy metabolism, the larger depletion of muscle glycogen, sometimes almost complete emptying of stores, is due to glycogenolysis in these fast twitch fibers. This hypothesis based on motor unit recruitment is supported by the histochemical estimation of a reduced glycogen at first in slow twitch fibers, then later from fast twitch fibers during submaximal exhaustive cycling (Gollnick, 1973), and predominantly in slow fibers during prolonged running (Costill, et al., 1973).

Another source of energy implicit in the discussion above is FFA oxidation. Endurance trained subjects apparently can mobilize more FFA and also oxidize more FFA for ATP regeneration than do "unfit" subjects (Issekutz, et al., 1965; Paul, 1970). In experiments designed to block FFA mobilization and oxidation during prolonged submaximal work which seems to be a characteristic of endurance unfit subjects, muscle glycogen utilization was increased and the subjects reported that the work was "heavier and more fatiguing" (Bergström, et al., 1969). This suggests that increased fat oxidation might possibly be an important adaptation enhanced by endurance training which tends to reduce glycogen utilization.

Gollnick's (1973) interpretation of his histochemical observations as evidence that "slow twitch fibers were used preferentially in the early stages of moderately-intense exercise with fast twitch fibers being added as the slow twitch fibers became depleted of their glycogen reserves" is quite interesting. It is highly speculative in that it is solely based on the disappearance of glycogen from fibers and does not take into account the utilization of blood glucose or FFA (Faulkner, personal communication). Also, it does not prove or disprove the possibility that fast twitch fibers may have been active for the entire bout of exercise. Nevertheless, the idea has great merit. The questions arise, how does the feeling of "weak legs" take place, and how does the motor system compensate for "weak legs"? An explanation could begin with prolonged exercise altering the inhibitory state of the motoneurons involved. An altered input from muscle spindles could also contribute to this. If the actomyosin-ATPase functioning in the working fibers was impaired, for example, due to an inadequate ATP regeneration from glycogenolysis, etc. (see Weiser, 1971), then the shortening velocity and length relationships of the muscle fibers could become altered. These changes would then be detected by the muscle spindles and Golgi tendon organs. How this information is processed by the spinal reflex systems and the higher centers is unknown. One possibility is the motor units are recruited having more of the fast twitch characteristics than were previously activated which would fit Gollnick's suggested mechanism.

Substrate Supply

The importance of FFA mobilization for muscle energy metabolism has already been emphasized (see above). In fact, there is an overproduction of FFA in endurance trained subjects, and this results in an increasing plasma FFA concentration (Issekutz, et al., 1970). After the increase of FFA mobilization, probably brought about by increased sympathetic activity, the influx of FFA is most likely maintained by hormonal control (see Gollnick and King, 1969). During prolonged exercise, insulin decreases and norepinephrine, epinephrine, growth hormone, and cortisol increase (Hartley, et al., 1972), as does glucagon (Böttiger, et al., 1972; Felig, et al., 1972). In endurance untrained subjects blood lactate is also elevated and has been suggested to inhibit the fat cell lipase system mobilizing less FFA than does the trained individual (Issekutz, et al., 1965).

For submaximal work, the balance of the energy cost is primarily fueled by carbohydrate mobilization from muscle glycogen. Blood glucose will contribute to about 10 to 20 percent of the energy metabolism of dogs exercising at about 50% max V_{O_2}. For dogs, this is apparently independent of endurance conditioning (Paul and Issekutz, 1967; Issekutz, et al., 1970). However, Issekutz and his co-workers (1971) conclude from their research "that the duration of prolonged exercise mainly depends on the initial glycogen content of the liver." They also suggest that "the rate of gluconeogenesis during exercise from lactate and glycerol" is also a limiting factor. That is, those dogs who are unable to maintain hepatic glucose output tend to have a larger decline in blood glucose and do not work as long. This evidence corroborates the thesis that the energy supply to the CNS involved with the neural mechanisms for motor and supply system control can also be an important factor in determining prolonged performance. Further evidence is provided by Dill, et al. (1932) and of Christensen and Hansen (1939b) in that the oral administration of sugar both increases performance and temporarily decreases the subjective symptomatology associated with prolonged effort (Weiser, unpublished observations).

Ventilation

As submaximal work becomes prolonged, the ventilatory adaptations change. These changes in ventilatory control are apparently a function of endurance capacity. Minute ventilation increases with time at about 60 to 75% max V_{O_2} (Ekelund, 1967a), but it increases more for subjects who will perform for only a short duration than it does for longer performers (Rowan and Weiser, 1973). Respiratory rate tends to increase much more than tidal volume decreases for the "unfit" individually whereas respiratory rate increases only slightly and tidal volume shows a large decline for the "fit" person (Weiser and Rowan, unpublished observations). This implies that the "unfit" person does not regulate his ventilation in a steady-state, but that his ventilatory controlling system constantly stimulates more activity until termination of work. Since V_{O_2} stays constant or increases slightly, the respiratory oxygen utilization, sometimes called caloric ventilation quotient (minute volume in liters per min./V_{O_2} in ml per min.), also increases (see Simonson, 1971, Chap. 8). One may interpret this as an increased requirement for the minute volume to provide the same V_{O_2}, or that V_{O_2} remains independent of respiratory activity during prolonged work. Under endurance training, the factors tending to alter the control of ventilation obviously must be reduced.

The increase of ventilation appears to be controlled such that the elimination of CO_2 becomes regulated. During steady-state work, the humoral controlling systems are principally responsible for the increased ventilation. Neural controls also play a role as evidenced by the rapid changes in tidal volume immediately after work is started or stopped (Dejours, 1965; Fukuhari, et al., 1973a,b). The so-called anerobic threshold, at or above 60% max V_{O_2}, has been suggested to be a result of inadequate blood flow to the working muscle resulting in elevated anaerobic glycolysis (Wasserman, et al., 1973). Another contributing factor could be alterations in motor control leading to recruitment of fast twitch motor units with characteristically low oxidative, high glycolytic capacities.

Blood Supply

The role of the sympathetic nervous system in controlling the central circulatory response is obvious. Inputs to the medullary cardiovascular centers are from the visceral afferents, baroreceptors, and most importantly from higher integrative centers, probably the cerebral cortex, basal ganglia, and hypothalamus. One very interesting question is, how are the different parts of the cardiovascular system controlled during exercise so that a change in the work output, expressed as % max V_{O_2}, is met by a proportional change in heart rate and blood flow distribution? The fact that the subjective rating of effort exerted on a work task is proportional to the relative work load indicates that the higher centers are involved in this proportional control. The increase in the rating of perceived effort is also proportional to work heart rate (Borg, 1962; and see Chap. on subjective symptomatology).

Cardiovascular functions are also altered by prolonged work and are excellently discussed in detail by Rowell (1969; 1971; 1974). Briefly, the increased cardiac output is maintained nearly steady or increases less than 5 percent (Dill, et al., 1931; Cobb and Johnson, 1963; Saltin and Stenberg, 1964; Ekelund and Holmgren, 1964; Ekelund, 1966, 1967a). After 5 to 10 minutes, heart rate still continues to rise to reach 15 to 20 percent of the 10-minute value at the end of work (Ekelund, 1967b). The increase of heart rate between about 5 and 13 minutes tends to be greater for individuals with poorer endurance capacity (Weiser, et al., 1971). Stroke volume must be decreased and does so until at exhaustion it declined by 10 to 16 percent. Hartley, et al. (1970) have concluded from their studies using atropine parasympathetic blockade that this rise in heart rate must have been due to parasympathetic withdrawal.

Rowell (1971) suggests that another cause of the heart rate increase "has been thought to be the rise in body temperature with increased distribution to the skin." With increased skin blood flow it is possible that cutaneous venous tone has decreased and consequently the cutaneous venous volume would be increased. There is no literature directly supporting this suggestion; however, some indirect evidence is available from experiments involving cutaneous heating. With an increase in skin temperature during submaximal work, an elevated compliance, i.e. reduced wall-tension, occurs in the skin capacitance vessels with a sequestering of blood in that vascular bed (Bevegård and Shepherd, 1967; Rowell, et al., 1969). A reduction of blood flow and blood volume in the nonexercising regions would aid in the redistribution of blood flow to the skin (see Rowell, 1971, 1974). Rowell (1971) suggests that "certainly a progressive decline in sympathetic outflow to these vessels could largely be responsible" for the redistribution. As a consequence of this increased perfusion of the high-resistance cutaneous circulation, it could be that the baroreceptors feedback mechanisms acting to maintain aortic pressure reflexively increase heart rate but also decrease stroke volume. Thereby, cardiac output would be maintained.

Both Ekelund (1967b) and Saltin and Stenberg (1964), are noted by Rowell (1971) to "infer that functional changes in the myocardium itself may contribute to these effects—that is, aside from changes in ventricular filling pressure." In this case, and if cardiac output is regulated to be steady via baroreceptor reflexes, etc., then the heart rate would have to be increased. This appears to result from very severe exercise at 75 percent or greater max V_{O_2} (Rowell, 1974). The mechanism(s) of the impairments in the myocardium, if existent, are not clearly understood.

In summary, the factors that influence prolonged submaximal work performance are not only peripheral but are also central in nature. First, within the working muscle fibers, depletion of glycogen stores is highly correlated with the duration of prolonged work. In dogs untrained for prolonged running, an inadequate ability to mobilize free fatty acids from adipose tissue to be oxidized by working muscle appears to differ importantly from endurance trained dogs. These metabolic support impairments and their associated alterations in enzyme regulation would change muscle contraction characteristics; information of these changes would be fed back to the motor controlling circuits which have only been indirectly studied. Feedback to the CNS about recruitment of additional motor units or increased impulse burst activity to impaired motor units might result in the "legs tired" symptoms reported by fatigues subjects. Altered cardiovascular and ventilatory functioning also contribute to the symptoms of fatigue. Second, depletion of liver glycogen and altered enzyme regulatory processes supporting glucose mobilization and the maintenance of blood glucose presumably affect CNS and spinal reflex functioning. Also, hyperpolarization of spinal motoneurons might be affecting motor unit activity. These alterations could lead to disorganization of motor functioning and coordination and contribute to various symptoms of fatigue and affect the capacity to perform prolonged work.

SEDENTARY WORK

One may think of sedentary work as that which is done principally in either a sitting or standing position which requires an oxygen consumption of less than 0.500 l/min. Examples of this type of work could be the conceptualizing and writing of this chapter, washing dishes, or typing. Table 1-IV lists some of the possible alterations that might limit this type of performance.

TABLE 1-IV

SOME FACTORS PRODUCING FATIGUE DURING SEDENTARY WORK

System	Impaired Component		Consequence
	Controlled System	Controlling System	
Motor	?	Supraspinal inhibition (?); disorganization of information acquisition and processing	Performance errors of omission and accuracy

These tasks involve active participation of small groups of working muscles and of postural muscles. For a given muscle, a random selection of motoneurons is, presumably, activated to provide the number of motor units required for the particular performance pattern. The resulting activity for any muscle fiber is a random schedule of contractions, not often likely to occur at one movement cycle apart. Motor units would be recruited to make up the physical activity beginning with the smallest motoneuron since they have the lowest threshold for stimulation (Henneman and Olson, 1965). As the intensity of work increases, larger motoneurons would be recruited. In a muscle having a mixture of fiber types, this would correspond the activation of slow twitch fibers with quick movements specifically activating fast twitch motor units. For these light work levels no evidence for transmission or excitation-contraction impairments have ever been reported (see Simonson, 1971, Chap. 10).

To cover the low energy cost of these types of activities, only a small increase in ATP regenerating loops is required. The exact source will depend largely on how often a given motor unit is actively involved in the task. If the frequency of motor unit action is on the order of once every couple of minutes or more, ATP regeneration will probably occur during the fiber's recovery. Mitochondrial oxidative phosphorylation will reconvert ADP into ATP, and in the post-prandial nutritional condition on a mixed diet, fatty acid oxidation will reconvert most of the reduced hydrogen-carriers produced by ATP regeneration. The effects of meals and of diets high in carbohydrate, fat, or protein will by metabolic control adaptations shift energy regeneration toward the most abundant substrate available.

The supply of substrate and oxygen via the circulatory system will be altered insignificantly during sedentary work. Changes in ventilation, i.e. tidal volume and respiratory rate, will be principally influenced by factors due to activities such as speaking, etc.

A possible impairment of motor performance could arise from the misalignments of inputs to the contraction-coordinating system from supraspinal feedback loops. These could arise from errors in perceptual processes and in the processing of information such as that provoked by monotonous situations (see Chap. on Vigilance). Additionally, a disorganization of the activity within the spinal motor centers could occur.

As an example of fatigue associated with sedentary work, we can use the sensation of tiredness associated with prolonged automobile driving in monotonous surroundings (Schmidtke, Chap. 9). This form of fatigue has been termed "Stimmungsermüdung," i.e. fatigue of mood, by Schaefer (1959).

The concept of "Stimmungsermüdung" is based on the consideration (Schmidtke, 1960; Schaefer, 1970) that in man, the level of arousal originates from the fluctuating and circulating patterns of excitation between cerebral cortex and subcortical centers in the region of the reticular formation and the hypothalamus. Due to this mutual functional relationship, the mechanisms for circulatory regulation and those responsible for the actual

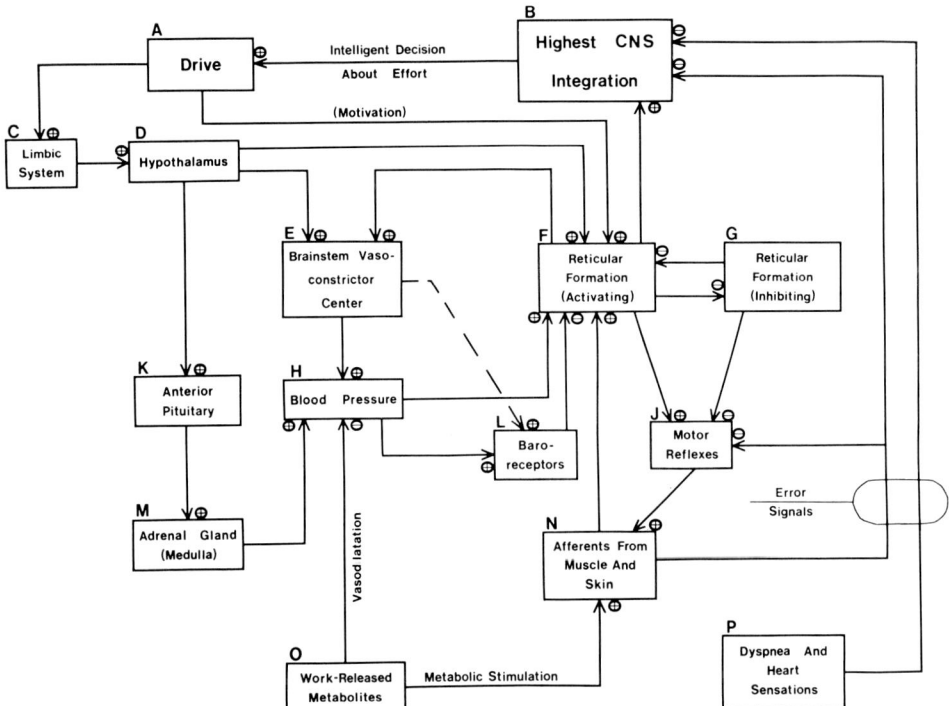

Figure 1-7. Schematic representation of the processes that interconnect the physiological and psychological effects of fatigue. In the medulla of the brain-stem lies the reticular formation that controls arousal level and contributes, along with the cortex, to the highest integration of the central nervous system (CNS, Block B). The drive to make decisions (Block A) develops from this integration to stimulate in turn the subconscious limbic system (Block C), which then activates the hypothalamus (Block D) as well as the sympathetic vasoconstrictor centers (Block E) and the reticular formation (Block F). From muscle and skin come sensory information which leads via reflexes to an elevation of drive and sympathetic tone. Metabolic products (Block O) arising from working muscle, etc., decrease blood pressure through their vasodilatating action. The hypothalamus stimulates the adrenal gland through the action of its hormones and in turn releases epinephrine and increases blood pressure. The reticular formation consists of two parts: an activating part (Block F) and an inhibiting part (Block G). Between both parts an antagonism exists which leads to rhythmic sleep-awake behavior. Drive itself effects not only the involuntary Blocks C and D but also communicates with the reticular formation. Error signals arise from work being sensed by the lungs and heart as well as muscle and skin to affect motor reflexes and to feed back to the highest level of CNS integration (From H. Schaefer, "Ermüdung und Müdigkeit," in W. Baust, ed., *Ermüdung, Schlaf und Traum* [Stuttgart, Wissenschaftliche Verlagsgesellschaft, 1970, pp. 1-25]).

state of consciousness are closely related. On the other hand, emotional processes affect autonomic innervation (pupil diameter, pulse rate, skin circulation, sweat secretion, etc.). The excitation extending into this system of feedback loops, therefore, will influence autonomic functions as well as consciousness. Although we do not have adequate information on how the subjective sensation of well being or mood corresponds to the objective neural processes, there is some indication that during the sensation of fatigue or tiredness the sympathetic nervous system is less activated than in fresh condition. The sympathetic tone drops during external stimulation. Thus, the disturbances of vigilance or the sensation of monotony in uniform working conditions are understandable. Due to the functional association of cortical, subcortical, and hypothalamic regions it is probable that motivation for work performance as well as other effects increase sympathetic tone, which includes, according to Schaefer's concept, all autonomic ergotropic functions (see Chap. on Motivation).

According to the block diagram (Fig. 1-7) illustrating the mutual psychosomatic effects, the sympathetic nervous system activates the cortical structures through a direct neural pathway and, therefore, the arousal level. This could be enhanced by humoral (increase of blood sugar) and hormonal (adrenal cortex) effects. These effects possibly could be mediated in part by changes in the activity of the reticular formation (Grandjean, 1970). For the psychological aspects the increased biological activation may result in subjective experience of success through a tendency toward positive motivation. On the other hand, lack of motivation or success may result in inhibition together with the subjective sensation of fatigue.

"Stimmungsermüdung," according to Schaefer, may develop after a physical stress. Similarly decreased enjoyment of work (such as in monotonous work) as well as anxiety, depressions, or hopelessness for the individual's situation may produce disturbance of motivation resulting in subjective tiredness without any apparent objective basis.

Although in this concept of Schaefer's, as condensed above, not all details are yet known, it affords a positive start for the understanding of the sensation of fatigue and tiredness and for the development of a theory of fatigue during sedentary work.

SUMMARY

This chapter illustrates the complexity in understanding the factors that lead to fatigue, i.e. decreased work capacity. However, a central role seems to be played by the feedback interrelations between the motor system and the other systems that support movement and work. Fatigue ultimately becomes manifest as the even more basic interrelations of the controlled and controlling components of these feedback systems and their subsystems become "misaligned." Several task-specific factors contribute importantly to this complexity. The intensity of the work task leads to differing degrees of adaptation for both the motor and support systems. Also the total muscle mass employed and the proportion of static to dynamic work will stress these systems to differing degrees. When one considers the adaptations taking place during the transition to higher work levels, it is apparent that the "adequacy" of these adaptations in establishing a steady state forecasts the impairments that initiate the onset of fatigue.

Maximal work can be defined as the work load that just elicits maximal oxygen consumption (max V_{O_2}). Any work load higher than the maximal aerobic power, consequently, is supramaximal and can only be done at the expense of anaerobic energy utilization. Thus, max V_{O_2} sets the upper limit for aerobic work. One's capacity for prolonged maximal work, and therefore for supramaximal work, is presently seen as limited 1. by impaired contraction and/or ATP regeneration of the working muscles leading to feedback error signaling of the reduced muscle tension developed and 2. by altered respiratory activity leading to hyperventilation. Subjectively, the symptoms frequently reported (supra)maximal work fatigue are 1. "weak muscles" and 2. "hard to breathe."

Fatigue at submaximal work levels relative to max V_{O_2} develops much more slowly but has some of the same types of impairments seen in maximal work. Above 50% max V_{O_2}, these are 1. reduced contraction and/or ATP regeneration with motor units derecruiting and 2. altered respiratory activity with hyperventilation, as well as 3. altered cardiovascular functions suggestive of cardiac decompensation and 4. decreased blood glucose level with altered CNS functioning. Commonly, symptoms such as "tired muscles," "heavy legs," and "uncoordinated" are reported. With tasks requiring less than 50% max V_{O_2} and especially below 30% max V_{O_2}, the factors giving rise to fatigue become much the same as those for sedentary work. It must be noted that at a given *absolute* work load, those individuals with lower max V_{O_2} must be working at a higher *relative* work intensity.

Prolonged sedentary work can be considered as that which requires less than 15% max V_{O_2} and which leads to a situation in which fatigue must be separated from monotony, if it can be. Thus, decreased capacity to do sedentary work commences with altered activity of the reticular activating system, etc., and with the disorganization of information processing.

It is hoped that this chapter sets the physiological framework for the following discussion of the roles that perception and information processing, reflexes and motor coordination, motivation, and subjective feeling states take in the development of fatigue in various work situations.

BIBLIOGRAPHY

Askew, E. W., G. L. Dohm, R. L. Huston, T. W. Sneed, and R. P. Dowdy: Response of rat tissue lipases to physical training and exercise. *Proc Soc Exp Biol Med, 141*:123, 1972.

Åstrand, P.-O., and K. Rodahl: *Textbook of Work Physiology*. New York, McGraw-Hill, 1970.

Åstrand, P.-O., and B. Saltin; Oxygen uptake during the first minutes of heavy muscular work. *J Appl Physiol, 16*:1971, 1961.

Balke, B.: Optimale körperliche Leistrungsfähigkeit, ihre Messung and Veränderung infolge Arbeitsermüdung. *Arbeitsphysiologie, 15*:311, 1954.

Barcroft, M., and A. C. Dornhorst: The blood flow through the human calf during rhythmic exercise. *J Physiol (London), 109*:402, 1949.

Barnard, R. J., V. R. Edgerton, T. Furakawa, and J. B. Peter: Histochemical, biochemical, and contractile properties of red, white, and intermediate fibers. *Ann J Physiol, 220*:410, 1971.

Bergström, J., L. Hermansen, E. Hultman, and B. Saltin: Diet, muscle glycogen and physical performance. *Acta Physiol Scand, 71*:140, 1967.

Bergström, J., E. Hultman, L. Jorfeldt, B. Pernow, and I. Wahren: Effect of nicotinic acid on physical working capacity and on metabolism of muscle glycogen in man. *J Appl Physiol, 26*:170, 1969.

Bevegård, B. G., and J. T. Shepherd: Regulation of the circulation during exercise in man. *Physiol Rev, 47*:178, 1967.

Bigland, B., and O. C. Lippold: Motor unit activity in the voluntary contraction of human muscle. *J Physiol, 125*:322, 1954.

Bigland-Ritchie, B., and J. J. Woods: Integrated EMG and oxygen uptake during dynamic contractions of human muscle. *J Appl Physiol, 36*:475, 1974.

Black, J. E.: Blood flow requirements of the human calf after walking and running. *Clin Sci, 18*:89, 1959.

Böttger, I., E. M. Schlein, G. R. Faloona, J. P. Knochel, and R. H. Unger: The effect of exercise on glucagon secretion. *J Clin Endocrinol Metab, 35*:117, 1972.

Bouisset, S., and F. Goubel: Integrated electromyographical activity and muscle work. *J Appl Physiol, 35*:695, 1973.

Buskirk, E.: Work and fatigue in high altitude. In Simonson, E. (Ed.): *Physiology of Work Capacity and Fatigue*. Springfield, Thomas, 1971, pp. 312-322.

Christensen, E. H., and O. Hansen: III. Arbeitsfähigkeit und Ernährung. *Scand Arch Physiol, 81*:160, 1939A.

Christensen, E. H., and O. Hansen: IV. Hypoglykamie, Arbeitsfähigkeit und Ermüdung. *Scand Arch Physiol, 81*:172, 1939B.

Clausen, J. P., and N. A. Lassen: Muscle blood flow during exercise in normal man studied by the ^{133}xenon clearance method. *Cardiovasc Res, 5*:245, 1971.

Close, R. I.: Dynamic properties of mammalian skeletal muscles. *Physiol Rev, 52*:129, 1972.

Cobb, L. A., and W. P. Johnson: Hemodynamic relationships of anaerobic metabolism and plasma free fatty acids during prolonged, strenuous exercise in trained and untrained subjects. *J Clin Invest, 42*:800, 1963.

Costill, D. L., R. Bowers, G. Branam, and K. Sparks: Muscle glycogen utilization during prolonged exercise on successive days. *J Appl Physiol, 31*:834, 1971B.

Costill, D. L., P. D. Gollnick, E. D. Jansson, B. Saltin, and E. M. Stein: Glycogen depletion patterns in human muscle fibres during distance running. *Acta Physiol Scand, 89*:374, 1973.
Costill, D. L., K. Sparks, R. Gregor, and C. Turner: Muscle glycogen utilization during exhaustive running. *J Appl Physiol, 31*:353, 1971A.
Craig, F. N.: Oxygen uptake at the beginning of work. *J Appl Physiol, 33*:611, 1972.
Dejours, P.: Control of respiration in muscular exercise. In *Handbook of Physiology*. Washington, American Physiological Society, 1965, Sec. 3, Vol. I, Chap. 25, pp. 631-648.
Dill, D. B., M. T. Edwards, P. S. Bauer, and E. J. Levinson: Physical performance in relation to external temperature. *Arbeitsphysiologie, 4*:508, 1931.
Dill, D. B., H. T. Edwards, and J. H. Talbott: Studies in muscular activity. VII. Factors limiting the capacity for work. *J Physiol (London), 77*:49, 1932.
Ebashi, S., M. Endo, and I. Ohtsuki: Control of muscle contraction. *Quart Rev Biophys, 2*:351, 1969.
Eccles, J. C.: *The Physiology of Nerve Cells*. Baltimore, Johns Hopkins Press, 1957.
Ekblom, B., A. N. Goldbarg, A. Kilborn, and P.-O. Astrand: Effects of atropine and propranolol on the oxygen transport system during exercise in man. *Scand J Clin Lab Invest, 30*:35, 1972.
Ekelund, L.-G.: Circulatory and respiratory adaptation during prolonged exercise in the supine position. *Acta Physiol Scand, 68*:382, 1966.
Ekelund, L.-G.: Circulatory and respiratory adaptation during prolonged exercise of moderate intensity in the sitting position. *Acta Physiol Scand, 69*:327, 1967A.
Ekelund, L.-G.: Circulatory and respiratory adaptation during prolonged work. *Acta Physiol Scand, 70 (Suppl 292)* 1, 1967B.
Ekelund, L.-G., and A. Holmgren: Circulatory and respiratory adaptation during long-term, non-steady state exercise, in the sitting position. *Acta Physiol Scand, 62*:240, 1964.
Epstein, S. E., B. F. Robinson, R. L. Kahler, and E. Braunwald: Effects of beta-adrenergic blockade on the cardiac response to maximal and submaximal exercise in man. *J Clin Invest, 44*:1745, 1965.
Everts, E. V.: Brain mechanisms in movement. *Sci Am, 229*:96, 1973.
Faulkner, J. A.: Muscle fatigue. In Briskey, E. J., et al. (Eds.): *The Physiology and Biochemistry of Muscle as a Food*. Madison, Wisconsin Pr, 1970, pp. 555-575.
Felig, P., J. Wahren, R. Hendler, and G. Ahlborg: Plasma glucagon levels in exercising man. *New Engl J Med, 287*:184, 1972.
Folkow, B., C. Heymans, and E. Neil. Integrated aspects of cardiovascular regulation. In *Handbook of Physiology*. Washington, American Physiological Society, 1965, Sec. 2, Vol. III, Chap. 49, pp. 1787-1823.
Fujihara, Y., J. Hildebrandt, and J. R. Hildebrandt: Cardiorespiratory transients in exercising man. I. Tests of superposition. *J Appl Physiol, 35*:58, 1973A.
Fujihara, Y., J. Hildebrandt, and J. R. Hildebrandt: Cardiorespiratory transients in exercising man. II. Linear models. *J Appl Physiol, 35*:68, 1973B.
Gollnick, P. D., R. B. Armstrong, W. L. Semrowich, R. E. Shepherd, and B. Saltin: Glycogen depletion patterns in human skeletal muscle fibers after heavy exercise. *J Appl Physiol, 34*:615, 1973.
Gollnick, P. D., and D. W. King: Energy release in the muscle cell. *Med Sci Sports, 1*:23, 1969.
Gollnick, P. D., R. G. Soule, A. W. Taylor, C. Williams, and C. D. Ianuzzo: Exercise-

induced glycogenolysis and lipolysis in the rat: hormonal influence. *Am J Physiol, 219:*729, 1970.

Grandjean, E. P.: Fatigue. *Am Ind Hyg Assoc J, 31:*401, 1970.

Grimby, G., E. Haggendal, and B. Saltin: Local xenon 133 clearance from the quadriceps during exercise in man. *J Appl Physiol, 22:*305, 1967.

Grimby, L., and J. Hannerz: Recruitment order of motor units on voluntary contraction: changes induced by proprioceptive afferent activity. *J Neurol Neurosurg Psychiat, 31:*565, 1968.

Grossman, S. P.: *A Textbook of Physiological Psychology.* New York, Wiley, 1967, pp. 265-80.

Guyton, A. C., T. G. Coleman, and H. J. Granger: Circulation: overall regulation. *Ann Rev Physiol, 34:*13, 1972.

Haddy, F. J., and J. B. Scott: Metabolically linked vasoactive chemicals in local regulation of blood flow. *Physiol Rev, 48:*708, 1968.

Hartley, L. H., J. W. Mason, R. P. Hogan, L. G. Jones, T. A. Kotchen, E. H. Mougey, F. E. Wherry, L. L. Pennington, and P. T. Ricketts: Multiple hormonal responses to prolonged exercise in relation to physical training. *J Appl Physiol, 33:*607, 1972.

Hartley, L. H., B. Pernow, H. Haggendal, J. Lacour, J. de Lattre, and B. Saltin: Central circulation during submaximal work preceded by heavy work. *J Appl Physiol, 29:*818, 1970.

Hartley, L. H., and B. Saltin: Blood gas tensions and pH in brachial artery, femoral vein, and brachial vein during maximal exercise. In Pourtsman, J. R. (Ed.): *Medicine and Sport Biochemistry of Exercise.* Basel, Karger, 1969, pp. 66-72.

Havel, R. J.: Autonomic nervous system and adipose tissue. In *Handbook of Physiology.* Washington, American Physiological Society, 1965, Sec. 5, Chap. 58, pp. 575-600.

Havel, R. J., A. Naimark, and C. F. Borchgrevink: Turnover rate and oxidation of free fatty acids of blood plasma in man during exercise: Studies during continuous infusion of palmitate-1-C^{14}. *J Clin Invest, 42:*1054, 1963.

Henneman, E.: Organization of the motor-system—a preview. In Mountcastle, V. B. (Ed.): *Medical Physiology.* St. Louis, Mosby, 1968A, Chap. 71, pp. 1675-1680.

Henneman, E.: Peripheral mechanisms involved in the control of muscle. In Mountcastle, V. B. (Ed.): *Medical Physiology.* St. Louis, Mosby, 1968B, Chap. 73, pp. 1697-1716.

Henneman, E., and C. B. Olson: Relations between structure and function in the design of skeletal muscle. *J Neurophysiol, 28:*581, 1965.

Helmreich, E., W. H. Danforth, and S. Karpatkin: The response of the glycolytic system of anaerobic frog sartorius muscle to electrical stimulation. In Chance, B., et al. (Eds.): *Control of Energy Metabolism.* New York, Acad Pr, 1965, pp. 299-312.

Henricksson, J., and F. Bonde-Peterson: Integrated electromyography of quadriceps femoris muscle at different exercise in intensities. *J Appl Physiol, 36:*218, 1974.

Hirsche, Hj., D. Grün, and W. Waller: Utilization of carbohydrate and free fatty acids by the gastrocnemius of the dog during long lasting rhythmical exercise. *Pflugers Arch, 321:*121, 1970.

Holmgren, A.: Cardiorespiratory determinants of cardiovascular fitness. *Canad Med J, 96:*697, 1967.

Houk, J., and E. Henneman: Feedback control of movement and posture. In Mountcastle, V. B. (Ed.): *Medical Physiology.* St. Louis, Mosby, 1968, Chap. 72, pp. 1681-1696.

Hultman, E.: Studies on muscle metabolism of glycogen and active phosphate in man with special reference to exercise and diet. *Scand J Clin Lab Invest 19 (Suppl 94):* 1, 1967.
Hultman, E., J. Bergström, and N. McL. Anderson: Breakdown and resynthesis of phosphorylcreatine and adenosine triphosphate in connection with muscular work in man. *Scand J Clin Lab Invest, 19:*56, 1967.
Huxley, H. E.: The mechanism of muscular contraction. *Science, 164:*1356, 1969.
Ingemann Jensen, J., H. Vejby-Christensen, and E. Strange Petersen: Ventilatory response to work initiated at various times during the respiratory cycle. *J Appl Physiol, 33:*744, 1972.
Issekutz, B., A. C. Issekutz, and D. Nash: Mobilization of energy sources in exercising dogs. *J Appl Physiol, 29:*691, 1970.
Issekutz, B., Jr., H. I. Miller, P. Paul, and K. Rodahl: Source of fat oxidation in exercising dogs. *Am J Physiol, 207:*583, 1964.
Issekutz, B., Jr., H. I. Miller, P. Paul, and K. Rodahl: Aerobic work capacity and plasma FFA turnover. *J Appl Physiol, 20:*293, 1965.
Karlsson, J.: Lactate and phosphagen concentrations in working muscles of man with special reference to oxygen deficit at the onset of work. *Acta Physiol Scand, 82 (Suppl 358):* 1, 1971.
Karlsson, J., L.-O. Nordesjö, L. Jorfeldt, and B. Saltin. Muscle lactate, ATP, and CP levels during exercise after training in man. *J Appl Physiol, 33:*199, 1972.
Keul, J., E. Doll, and D. Keppler: *Energy Metabolism of Human Muscle.* Baltimore, Univ Park, 1972.
Knuttgen, H. G., and B. Saltin: Muscle metabolites and oxygen uptake in short-term submaximal exercise in man. *J Appl Physiol, 32:*690, 1972.
Knuttgen, H. G., and B. Saltin: Oxygen uptake, muscle high-energy phosphates, and lactate in exercise under acute hypoxic conditions in man. *Acta Physiol Scand, 87:*368, 1973.
Kramer, K., F. Obal, and W. Quensel: Untersuchungen über den Muskelstoffwechsel des Warmblüters. III. Mitteilung. Die Saurestoffaufnahme des Muskels während rhythmischer Tätigkeit. *Pflügers Arch, 241:*717, 1939.
Jones, W. B., and T. J. Reeves: Total cardiac output response during four minutes of exercise. *Am Heart J, 76:*209, 1968.
Jung, R., and R. Hassler: The extrapyramidal motor system. In *Handbook of Physiology.* Washington, American Physiological Society, 169, Sec. 1, Vol. II, Chap. 35, pp. 863-927.
Larner, J.: *Intermediary Metabolism and Its Regulation.* Englewood Cliffs, Prentice-Hall, 1970.
Lippold, O. C. J.: The relation between integrated action potentials in a human muscle and its isometric tension. *J Physiol (London), 117:*492, 1952.
Maxwell, L. C., J. A. Faulkner, and D. A. Lieberman: Histochemical manifestations of age and endurance training in skeletal muscle fibers. *Am J Physiol, 224:*356, 1973.
Paul, P.: FFA metabolism of normal dogs during steady-state exercise at different work loads. *J Appl Physiol, 28:*127, 1970.
Paul, P., and B. Issekutz, Jr.: Role of extramuscular energy sources in the metabolism of the exercising dog. *J Appl Physiol, 22:*615, 1967.
Pirnay, F., M. Lamy, J. Dujardin, R. Deroanne, and J. M. Petit: Analysis of femoral venous blood during maximal muscular exercise. *J Appl Physiol, 33:*289, 1972b.

Pirnay, F., R. Marechal, R. Radermecker, and J. M. Petit: Muscle blood flow during submaximum and maximum exercise on a bicycle ergometer. *J Appl Physiol, 32*:210, 1972a.
Robinson, S.: Experimental studies of physical fitness in relation to age. *Arbeitsphysiologie, 10*:251, 1938.
Rowan, M. P., P. C. Weiser, and J. P. Hannon: Relationship of oxygen consumption and ventilation to the duration of heavy exercise. *Fed. Proc, 32*:436, 1973.
Rowell, L. B.: Circulation. *Med Sci Sports, 1*:15, 1969.
Rowell, L. B.: Cardiovascular limitation to work capacity. In Simonson, E. (Ed.): *Physiology of Work Capacity and Fatigue.* Springfield, Thomas, 1971, Chap. 7, pp. 132-169.
Rowell, L. B.: Human cardiovascular adjustments to exercise and thermal stress. *Physiol Rev, 54*:75, 1974.
Rowell, L. B., J. A. Murray, G. L. Brengelmann, and K. K. Kraning II: Human cardiovascular adjustments to rapid changes in skin temperature during exercise. *Circ Res, 24*:711, 1969.
Saltin, B.: Aerobic work capacity and circulation at exercise in man with special reference to the effect of prolonged exercise and/or heat exposure. *Acta Physiol Scand, 62 (Suppl 230)*:1, 1964.
Saltin, B.: Metabolic fundamentals in exercise. *Med Sci Sports, 5*:137, 1973.
Saltin, B., and B. Essen: Muscle glycogen, lactate, ATP and CP in intermittent exercise. In Pernow, B., and Saltin, B. (Eds.): *Muscle Metabolism During Exercise.* New York, Plenum Press, 1971, pp. 409-418.
Saltin, B., and J. Stenberg: Circulatory response to prolonged severe exercise. *J. Appl Physiol, 19*:833, 1964.
Sandow, A.: Skeletal muscle. *Ann Rev Physiol, 32*:87, 1970.
Schaefer, H.: Physiologie der Ermüdung und Erschöpfung. *Med Klin, 54*:1109, 1959.
Schaefer, H.: Ermüdung und Müdigkeit. In Baust, F. (Ed.): *Ermüdung, Schlaf und Traum.* Stuttgart, Wissenschaftliche Verlagsgesellschaft MBH, 1970, pp. 1-25.
Schmidtke, H.: *Die Ermüdung.* Stuttgart, Verlag Hans Huber, 160, pp. 31-36.
Simonson, E.: *Physiology of Work Capacity and Fatigue.* Springfield, Thomas, 1971.
Simonson, E.: Evaluation of cardiac performance in exercise. *Am J. Cardiol, 30*:722, 1972.
Simonson, E., and N. Enzer: Physiology of muscular exercise and fatigue in disease. *Medicine, 21*:345, 1942.
Stainsby, W. N., and A. B. Otis: Blood flow, blood oxygen tension, oxygen uptake, and oxygen transport in skeletal muscle. *Am J Physiol, 206*:858, 1964.
Stein, J. M., and H. A. Padykula: Histochemical classification of individual skeletal muscle fibers of the rat. *Am J Anat, 110*:103, 1962.
Stein, R. B.: Peripheral control of movement. *Physiol Rev, 54*:215, 1974.
Stenberg, J.: The significance of the central circulation for the aerobic work capacity under various conditions in young healthy persons. *Acta Physiol Scand, 68 (Suppl 273)*:1, 1966.
Taylor, E. W.: Chemistry of muscular contraction. *Ann Rev Biochem 41*:577, 1972.
Taylor, H. L.: Exercise and metabolism. In Johnson, W. R. (Ed.): *Science and Medicine of Exercise and Sports.* New York, Harper & Brothers, 1960, pp. 123-161.
Tonnesen, K. H.: Blood-flow through muscle during rhythmic contraction measured by ^{133}xenon. *Scand J Clin Lab Invest, 16*:646, 1964.
Warmolts, J. R., and W. K. Engel: Open-biopsy electromyography I. Correlation of

motor unit behavior with histochemical muscle fiber type in human limb muscle. *Arch Neurol, 27*:512, 1972.

Wasserman, K., B. J. Whipp, S. N. Koyal, and W. L. Beaver: Anaerobic threshold and respiratory gas exchange during exercise. *J Appl Physiol, 35*:236, 1973.

Weber, A., and J. M. Murray: Molecular control mechanisms in muscle contraction. *Physiol Rev., 53*:612, 1973.

Weil, J. V., E. Byrne-Quinn, I. E. Sodal, J. S. Kline, R. E. McCullough, and G. F. Filley: Augmentation of chemosensitivity during mild exercise in normal man. *J Appl Physiol, 33*:813, 1972.

Weiser, P. C.: Alternation in enzyme activity in work and fatigue. In Simonson, E. (Ed.): *Physiology of Work Capacity and Fatigue.* Springfield, Thomas, 1971, pp. 98-131.

Weiser, P. C., R. A. Kinsman, and D. A. Stamper: Task-specific symptomatology changes resulting from prolonged submaximal bicycle riding. *Med Sci Sports, 5*:79, 1973.

Weiser, P. C., D. A. Stamper, R. A. Kinsman, and J. P. Hannon: Relationship of heart rate increment during exercise to time of exhaustion. *Fed Proc, 30*:372, 1971.

Chapter 2

Biophysical Models for Studying Work and Fatigue

OTTO H. SCHMITT

ANY ATTEMPT to introduce the algorithmic, quantitative, modeling methods of the biophysical sciences into an examination of work and fatigue in the context of the extensive and good information to be found in the literature of psychology and physiology runs headlong into problems of definition. These are not the problems of tidying up and making exact and consistent the diverse and approximately compatible available definitions from various authors. A much more basic problem of definition is involved: we need to create a family of essentially new packages of old established facts and principles so organized as to constitute "Figures of Thought" that are readily manipulable by available or specially developed mathematical and computer processing and easily built into an image compatible with an organism that is not *homeostatic* only, but that is dynamic, and indeed dynamic not only parametrically but configurationally.

Let us start with a simple example. Work has one very firmly accepted and understood definition in the physical sciences where it is a precisely defined measure of energy as interpreted in mechanical terms, e.g. the expression $W = \int Fds$, or in words, work is the integral of force with respect to distance along its direction of action. This definition is so widely understood and accepted in the physical sciences, with which we must remain compatible, that it must not be disturbed or redefined for a study of this kind. Behind the term "work," as one can discover by context in studying psychological and physiological sources, there are, however, two other important aspects that will be lost if, for convenience, only this classical definition is admitted. First, there is the sense of "being in effective operation" that is attached to work in the sense of "The system is working hard" or "The system is working well." Second there is the subjectively familiar concept of work as embodied in the expression "This is hard work." Quantitating these concepts, especially the second, is not necessarily impossible or even extremely difficult once the task is defined and appropriate experimental data gathered.

Fatigue, in its turn, is also mostly a subjective concept, almost entirely without quantitative representation and basically unfamiliar as an algorithmic quantitative term—as a term that should be dimensioned, scaled and expressed in numbers. This does not mean that it cannot, or should not, be represented quantitatively, but rather that no model has been widely accepted for this purpose and, regrettably, that no great need for such a quantity has been felt.

One has only to go back to the much more familiar concept of *time* to discover a much worked-over example of this kind of duality and a resolution of the problem that has until recently nearly obliterated the very important intuitive subjective psychological and physiological aspects as they apply to biological organismic time and make it an internal entity that expands and contracts with respect to clock time and is perceived sharply defined or diffuse according to the individual's perceptual state.

We all know, if we stop and think about it, that time *is* basically a biological concept, a most fundamental experience on which we base almost all of our everyday actions and thinking. It is an internal metric of the scale along which our sequential experiences are strung. We know that biological time in our subjective experience may go quickly or slowly with reference to an external clock time. Yet, such is the dominance of the physical sciences that the universally acknowledged clock time that can be defined with great exactness and widespread consistency, sometimes even with relativistic corrections across physical phenomenology, has pushed back the parent biological time into apologetic acceptability at best. The source from which the axiomatic experience of time arose, the subjective experience of time passing by, has disappeared from current definitions.

The definition of a flexible, rubbery time metric that relates this internal measure of the passing stream of events in terms of universal external physical time provides a very useful concept that is subject to quantitation and that may prove exceedingly valuable in studying the trajectories of biological events within the timing structure of biological cells, organs, organisms and social systems of organisms, so that this duality, preferably differentiated by different names for biological times and physical time, appears to be one of extreme value currently.

Following this precedent it seems desirable to formulate similar measures relating to the intuitively familiar concepts of work and fatigue. Because the subjective quantities in work and fatigue must ultimately be tied dimensionally, and in scale, to the external physical correlates, we must certainly examine the transductive mechanisms by which the organism translates its interactions, both motor and sensory, with the external world, to the internal conscious and subconscious operative systems. We must use a somewhat wider interpretation of the powerful communication theory originally made useful quantitatively by the Shannon-Wiener efforts and their extensions during the past two or three decades.

We must incorporate into this theory the biological requirement that communication be a closed process topologically in the sense that a message, to be transducible, transmittable, processable and interpretable, must have a common or at least nearly matched code and scaling between the entering and leaving portals of the system under examination. This code link that may often depend on genetic commonality or community linguistic commonality is usually relegated to an implicitly understood assumption that generally escapes tight scientific examination for dimensional integrity. Any properly modeled communication system can always be examined in terms of this logical duality of code and message branches although these paired system elements be chosen arbitrarily at a modular, a very small, an organismic or even a cosmic scale.

As a crude illustration, it is evident that fatigue will, in my experience, have a scaling and an experiential set of dimensions which are presumed by me to match approximately those in any other human individual and by appropriate parametric adjustment should apply to any other human, to other higher vertebrates, or even beyond in the biological realm. Unless we are able to reach an agreement with some flexibility on the general dimensions, the rough scaling and the coupling of the several applicable parameters if more than a simple scale is developed in terms of externally accessible measures, this entry that we characterize as fatigue, we will continue to have only a qualitative discussion. Perhaps even the first order rough approximations that have molded the useful Phon or the Dol could by analogy get us started into better quantitation.

It is strange how the successful application of feedback theory in the physical sciences and technology originated well back in the middle of the nineteenth century but gained vast popularity and was made a part of the engineering education only after the successes of electronic feedback circuitry in the World War II era. These electronic and electromechanical successes have blinded even students in the life science areas to the essential coequality and coessentiality of the two parts of biological control and supervisory systems. This is the duality of the feed-forward, sometimes called the feed-ahead, systems with the feedback systems that have become so familiar.

It is perhaps useful to make a basic definition for distinguishing between these two fundamentally different and mutually supportive classes of control and supervision. The essential idea behind negative feedback theory is that the current status of a system should be compared with an ideal, target, or reference model of the system status, whereupon corrective action may be taken in terms of the discerned "error." The reference may be fixed as it is in the case of a simple regulator or homeostat, parametrically adjustable in its constancy as in a resettable thermostat or in an individual undertaking a set of physical exercises or suffering mild fever or, again, the target may be truly dynamic, in which case the system is often called a servo system. This error correcting procedure, contrary to simplistic modeling, need not be exclusively in terms of an addition to the input function related to the output state in terms of some data feedback scaling and modifying function (usually β). Similarly important are the modulatory feedback systems where we change the sensitivity or responsiveness of a system in terms of a comparison of the output with a standard—a set point in physiological terminology—for self-corrective adjustment of a system.

Feedback need not be *negative* feedback to be stable and useful, biologically or technologically. Positive feedback in controlled degree and form is very useful in enhancing sensitivity beyond the intrinsic sensitivity of the basically responsive components of a control or supervising system. Positive feedback systems must never be confused with feed-forward systems with which we will next be concerned.

In contrast to systems utilizing feedback, feed-forward systems compare at the outset a present status with an already known status from files of previous stored experience or with a status devised by extrapolation, interpolation or analysis based on such stored situations. In these systems, the performance of the system is modified, presumably toward an optimum, by comparing an initial input status or patterned sequence with an already stored and existing or *ad hoc* devised precedent model. A typical feed-forward system thus compares an existing situation, transduced through one or another physiological channel or channels, with a comparable situation drawn from short term, long term, or even race memory and takes optimal actions in terms of the comparison. This, it is easily seen, is vastly different from the feedback processes although the two may almost merge in special circumstances.

Anyone familiar with computer design and programming will see immediately in this duality the analog on the one hand of the preexisting logical "genetic" structure of the computer, which determines what operations it is capable of doing, of interpreting and even misinterpreting, and on the other hand the hierarchical building upon this genetic structure of a language of instructions and commands, a machine language built on these commands, a set of progressively higher level languages and subroutines, executable at chosen levels within this repertoire of operational languages. It is this class of solutions that I would like to see implemented in biophysical examination of problems, such as those in work and fatigue.

Let us trace this concept of a feed-forward and feedback duality historically back to its roots in the classical concepts of life systems. Every organism has at any given point of its existence, as is especially evident for a highly organized mammal in an early state of its development, a genetic package of experience and language or code with which it must carry out practically all of its interactions with internal and external environments.

While this concept must be interpreted carefully in the case of organisms that proliferate by other than the conventional egg-sperm fertilization and growth pattern, it is always possible to initialize a system in these terms distinguishing 1. a data bank of genetic information and 2. a set of scale- and dimension-specified transductions coupling the data base to the environment and determining, probabilistically at least, the organism's life trajectory.

The rules of these couplings and the interpretation of transactional logic are subject to strict analytic restraints, particularly those of dimensional and scaling closure. This principle may well be elaborated slightly to understand its applicability to a routine feedback case.

Let us suppose that we are examining one of the conceptually simplest biological systems of feedback—a coordinated hand-eye positioning task. If the objective of an experiment is to place a stylus tip on a designated dot on a piece of paper, we describe the feedback system in terms of the error signals transduced by the visual systems between the point of the hand held instrument and the target point. This is not enough. We must also define a family of response characteristics involving the voluntary as well as the autonomic systems that set in motion a series of self-corrective actions. It must be immediately obvious that these corrective actions are not strictly those of measurement of the error between point and point and initiation of a corrective muscle action, but strongly embody the feed-forward principles and data resulting from having done innumerable similar exercises before where this experience provides intermediate level language material for building in the feed-forward most likely trajectories that will lead to the target.

Now, in any such examination of a system, the specifier of the analysis may take his position anywhere he chooses within the system. He may be an external observer, he may take his observation post at reflex arc mechanism level, or he may be an empathetic psychological observer. But if he would apply the biophysical scaling and dimensioning rules that I recommend, he will acknowledge that he is at all times responsible for defining, authenticating and bringing back to a common referent each of the dimensioned measures he uses, and that he will be at fault if he assumes at any point that "everyone knows" what time is, what distance is, what fatigue is, without acknowledging that each of these has its dimensional relationships, which may be highly variable from one usage of the term to another.

Thus we must be free to use "work" in the terms of a subjective psychological, physiological experience as pointed out by H. C. Burger many years ago, without being denied the utilization of work as a measure of energy. We must identify which of the definitions is operative and must, on demand, verify dimensional closure.

This dimensional closure is a property that is widely recognized and used as an everyday tool in physical analysis. An equation, when it is written, is immediately examined for dimensional consistency and its scaling metric consistency, its units, to use the students' term. We must be able, around any feedback or feed-forward system, to provide a similar authentication or to declare arbitrariness in using a term that is not fully defined.

Let us take a simplistic view of this kind of dimensional analysis around the hand-eye coordinated motion previously mentioned. We may choose at our convenience the variables to be examined, for example the distance between the two points to be brought into contact. This distance will be transduced by the visual system into a pattern distance in the retinal system, which has a not very simple scaling system relating it to the physical separation of the points. Notice that this scaling system may very well be grossly modified by experiential scaling, such as in perspective. This is the basis of many optical illusions. The transduced visual distance now needs to be converted into a matching coordinated scaled instruction in terms of motor action resulting in hand movement where dimensioning and scaling will quickly bring to attention system incompatibilities such as those of defining muscular response in terms of grams of muscle tension per unit of stimulus frequency versus muscle shortening in centimeters. The muscular movement, however, has to go through a transformation involving the physiological response properties of the muscle and its inertial properties, and thus it is not immediately applicable to the corrective effort to reduce error by motion. When we have chosen the dimensions and scales of our system feedback model, then we can analyze safely.

The feedback, feed-forward system that I have proposed as a model thus far, is basically conceived of as stationary. It allows adaptive control only in the limited sense of a modulatory feedback or feed-forward that keeps the transducing system within an operative region, as with automatic gain control in a radio receiver or recorder, or the pupillary reflex control of brightness in the visual system. If we are to deal effectively with the fundamental but still unfamiliar biophysical realization of subjective experience as illustrated by work and fatigue, we must recognize a new and almost entirely unused modeling system, the principles of which are familiar but usually submerged into a set of psychological or behavioral terms not ordinarily reduced to quantitation.

This is the class of supervisory controls that I will call the "hierarchical feed-up, feed-down class of adaptive modifications." One could say that this class of control achieves orchestration of informational and control systems rather than simple feedback or feed-forward control.

Consider that the organism will have in operation at any one time a repertoire extending to between four and eight hierarchical levels, a resource of feed-forward and feedback techniques applicable to a problem. A "homeostatic" problem of temperature regulation may resolve itself into a cellular modification of an autonomous pseudoperiodic rhythm, cellular modification under hormonal or circulatory mechanical control, a neuromuscular response of shivering, a sweating reflex, or a high level conscious response leading to opening or closing a window or moving to a different home. The organism as a whole has a very elaborate and effective control system that brings into conscious, subconscious, and even more primitive level focus these alternative resources and blends them into an overall behavior pattern that is at least near-optimal and in many cases achieves an amazingly fine threading of a survival path through conflicting alternatives.

If the organism is to achieve a solution that avoids averaging a success strategy of avoidance by going to the left and avoidance by going to the right into a direct collision course, it must have a good inhibitory as well as a facilitatory feed-up, feed-down pattern of modulation. This type of modeling is relatively unfamiliar. While I might be able to illustrate these principles with many specific examples, it is perhaps sufficient here to recapitulate that these tools are offered as a biophysical basis for building an algorithmic system for examining work and fatigue.

We start by recognizing that biological systems have a dual but complementary information and control structure. It begins with a genetic or available status, an anatomical logical structure from which must stem all interaction with environment in development and learning. The quasi-stationary internal system has available to it at all times the techniques of feed-forward and feedback to perform the needed recognition and corrective operations. These occur through a family of transductions which could be legitimately considered quantitatively and must be scaled and dimensioned. Supervising this quasi-stationary system is the feed-up feed-down series of controls that governs the path of the organism from moment to moment, day to day, and ultimately from generation to generation. The increasing likelihood that even the macromolecular brain structure that is involved with memory and information processing is reconstituted over a relatively short period in days, suggests that this supervisory feed-up, feed-down strategy expresses itself as a time progressive episodal or perhaps mere periodic recycling of the logical machinery of control, thus offering facilities recently updated and purged of obsolete programs and ready for very rapid restructuring of function at a moment's notice, but still retaining the needed "old wisdom" for further advance and evolution of strategy and tactics.

It is this restructuring from moment to moment and day to day that gives us a model of great potential in examining physiological and psychological behavior and response of biological organisms. We begin to realize, as a valid and necessary consideration, that the organism has within it a wide repertoire of *internal* linguistic paths, and from this realization comes acceptance of the notion that we must define the level and assignment of weight to the several hierarchical levels of performance and internal language options at which a task can be performed before we can make a valid assessment of time, fatigue, work effort or remaining available effort resources.

If we are to bring these models to bear on real biological research problems, it is perhaps pertinent to review a few of the overall characteristics of behavior that accompany the several kinds of control communication and information processing that have been suggested. Classical closed loop negative feedback responding to a fixed sampling mechanism to give a continuous flow of sampled environmental data and a fixed "gain," within its range of stability, characteristically results in a conformity of the system to a desired model over a wide range of sensitivity and amplification. It is remarkable, when viewed in behavioral terms, to see how a system may lose 80, 90, or perhaps even 99 percent of its reserve capability of response without externally obvious modification of behavior across a feedback, input/output relationship.

Characteristically such systems, as they are pressed farther and farther into their fatigue regions, will suddenly break up and go into a quite unstable and/or saturated condition, often exhibiting limit cycle behavior. Provision against such catastrophic deterioration of an otherwise excellent strategy for preserving constant behavior with varying resource strength is one important feature that will certainly enter strongly into prospective studies of work and fatigue.

Second, we need to consider the transport delay, the always present time required for any measure of the present situation compared with a goal to be translated into instructions for a corrective action and the subsequent execution of those directions in terms of action, a muscular motion, a secretion or other motor response. So long as a feedback system is operating with substantial loop gain, it is subject to instability due, in effect, to the instructions being correct but out of date, so that in a dynamic process these correct instructions become completely incorrect and lead to oscillation, over-control and the familiar instabilities of too tight feedback control in terms of available margin of stability familiar to audio amplifier builders.

Feed-forward controls, except for the time needed to get program and language available, escape this problem of loop response time, and have therein a tremendous advantage. They rely on historical, retrospective genetic classes of information that may be internally compared with a current situation, and allow corrective action to be taken immediately.

Notice that while normal negative feedback procedures lead toward asymptomatic conformity with an ideal, feed-forward designs take as a target the ideal itself and may equally well overachieve or underachieve the goal. It is easy to confuse feed-forward control with positive feedback control in this sense. Positive feedback and negative feedback are widely used biologically but with opposite objectives. Negative feedback permits type conformity to an ideal over a wide range of system gain. Positive feedback permits, at the expense of stability, a sensitivity more than that intrinsically existing within the system. This positive feedback may usefully be built into a long loop feedback system with automatic stability. It is a common trick of the electronic designer to use positive feedback within a negative overall family of feedbacks to achieve superior control of an entire system. It is, however, fruitless to combine positive and negative feedback to exactly the same loop channel, unless these systems differ in their individual sampling and motor application, their β so to speak.

We have spoken next of feed-up, feed-down or supervisory control of the strategy and tactics of internal linguistics in meeting a problem. Identification of the levels at which a problem is being predominantly dealt with within the organism at a particular moment and determining the family of sub-routines by which its processing is being effectuated, is undoubtedly one of the highly fruitful approaches, one of the great hopes for reducing to quantitation the useful figures of thought that go into terms such as "fatigue." Without recognition of reassignment of level and weighting of component controls, we will find that we have no place to assign such concepts.

In my opinion, we will find that the experience of fatigue is largely associated with an internal assessment of the parametric status of the several systems serving the control being examined. A muscle may be fatigued in the sense of running out of energy substrate while the organism as a whole is not particularly "fatigued" at all. In contrast, the organism at a high level of unified action may be having difficulty in achieving sufficient loop sensitivity at high hierarchical levels to permit feed-up modality choice to allow it to include this feedback, feed-forward family effectively.

We may even find in this model a technique analogous to reading the S level of a radio receiver as a means of estimating its parametric control of sensitivity, hence the sensitivity at which it is operating and hence its reserve limits of available sensitivity. Implicitly we will sense how "hard" it is working.

To achieve biophysical modeling for analyzing work and fatigue, we will need to establish transduction, dimensions and scales. We must develop a family of measures where even the identity of the key variables is not currently available if we are to specify the level and modality of control algorithms that are currently in operation within the organism. We must recognize systems status measures of control loop parameters as a technique for nondestructive assessment of a system.

Finally, we should realize that covariance of real control parameters with other available but not directly involved variables gives a possible nondestructive access to psychological status. In one humble attempt now begun in our laboratory, we have observed, by our technique of voluntary cardio-respiratory synchronization, the day by day variation, in an individual, of the cardio-respiratory coupling coefficient along a regression trajectory characteristic of the individual. This could be a measure of internal system status variation readily accessible by this method, but only reachable by profound, possibly dangerous stressing by traditional techniques. We would hope that a whole family of nondestructive covariant tests like this will emerge by which we can examine the status of an individual and the margin of stability within his several feed-forward and feedback loops, both at one hierarchical level, and within the control of hierarchical level dominance and internal linguistic choice.

SECTION TWO
MOTOR ASPECTS

Chapter 3

Reflexes and Fatigue: New Directions

THOMAS A. EASTON

INTRODUCTION

While reflexes are apparently well suited for use as the language of motor control, few studies of normal coordination have been conducted with this suitability in mind. Of these few, most have been published in the literature of physical medicine. These studies have used as their primary tool of investigation the condition of *fatigue,* for when an animal is fatigued the motor patterns characteristic of the reflexes seem to appear most readily.

My own work has been toward elucidating the question of how normal, volitional movements are coordinated, a question that is the more urgent for the fact that the human body (for example) has over 200 bones and nearly that many joints. Over every joint there act at least two muscles and every muscle must be commanded to contract via a nerve issuing from the spinal cord and answering its own commands from the central nervous system (CNS), though it is rare indeed that a muscle contracts alone and in isolation. The central commands go rather to groups of muscles. How then does the brain orchestrate all the possible commands and all the possible muscular contractions and all the possible joint movements to produce the smoothly coordinated complex movements which we admire so much in the race horse or circus acrobat?

The answer to this question is hardly simple. No one, not even those simplistic souls who have claimed that the brain specifies the orders for every muscle, for every action of the multitudinous repertoire of which a man or animal is capable, has said so.

We know that, in general, movements are not composed by ordering singly all the muscles involved. That mode of control would be too complicated. The brain would have to calculate the present state of every muscle, the command necessary to change that state to the desired one, the effect of that change on all other muscles affected by it, the necessary corrections for those changes, and do all of these things, *for all the muscles involved,* within two tenths of a second (the average reaction time) from the decision to act. When we consider that *all the muscles involved* may, for reasons of balance, mean all or most of the muscles in the body, we can begin to see the immensity of the task. In fact, attempts to do similar things for very simple mechanical systems by using the best of modern computers have not been markedly successful.

How are movements composed? No one yet knows, though the Russians (Gelfand, et al., 1971, p. 331) are thinking in terms of *synergies*. To quote:

> In order for the higher levels of the central nervous system to solve effectively the problems of the organization of motor acts in the time required, it is essential that the number of controlled parameters not be too large and the afferentation requiring analysis not be too high. The so-called synergies play an important role in the establishment of such conditions of work. It is customary to call *synergies* those classes of movements which have similar kinematic characteristics, coinciding active muscle groups and conducting types of afferentation.
>
> For each synergy there are distinctive, specific connections imposed on certain muscle groups, a subdivision of all the muscles participating in a movement into a small number of connected groups. Because of this, for realization of a movement it is enough to control a small number of independent parameters, although the number of muscles participating in movement can be large.
>
> Although there are but a few synergies, they *make possible almost the whole variety of voluntary movements* to be included. We can distinguish relatively simple synergies of postural preservation (the stabilization synergy), cyclic locomotive synergies (walking, running, swimming, etc.), synergies of throwing, blowing, jumping, and a certain (small) number of others. (second italics added)

The word "synergy" is used here with a slightly different meaning from the common usage in the West, where it does indeed mean cooperation in action, as when several muscles work together to produce a complex act, but where it is not used as a noun meaning a class of movements using the same muscles for similar actions. To quote from another book, a popular basic text of neuroanatomy:

> The cerebellum is primarily concerned with synergy in the action of voluntary muscles, which implies widespread action at one time, since the mere shifting of the weight from one foot to the other necessitates adjustment of muscles in all parts of the body. This implies that proprioceptive information from the entire bodily musculature, as well as exteroceptive impulses giving details of the environment both near and at a distance, must be brought into use simultaneously by the cerebellum and that the action of the cerebral motor centers in setting off activity of voluntary muscles must be synchronized with the action of the cerebellum (Ranson and Clark, 1959, p. 274).

Such a definition of synergism in terms of cerebellar feedback and modification fails to lay adequate stress upon the cerebrally determined muscular composition of a movement. To the eyes of the Russian researchers, the basic synergies constitute a dictionary of movements, individual muscle contractions being, so to speak, the letters of the synergy-words and the synergies themselves forming both an external language of movements and an internal language of control. They allow the CNS to apply its efforts at calculation to a much smaller number of parameters.

These basic synergies may be regarded as essentially identical to the reflexes, for not only do single-limb movements resemble in kind the spinal reflexes of flexion and extension, and the limb-pair movements the more complex neck, vestibular, and long spinal reflexes, but each of these movements also involves a definite, restricted set of muscles which is controlled as a unit. Their similarity to reflexes, however, does require some explanation.

The idea of the reflex began with Descartes, who used it as the basis for regarding the animal nervous system as a machine whose activities were entirely involuntary responses to stimuli. Since then the term has come to refer to actions which are unlearned, based on genetically determined neural connections and pathways, predictable from the stimuli to which the animal is exposed, uniform, adaptive in function (e.g. protective), and involuntary, but which by no means comprise the whole of an animal's possible responses to a situation. Not requiring the highest levels of the CNS for their expression, true reflexes may still be seen in animals under anaesthesia and after removal of the higher centers. Other "reactions" which are often called reflexes, such as the placing response, *are* learned, at least in part, and disappear with damage or impairment of the cerebrum, but are so fixed in their expression that there is little *functional* difference between them and the true reflexes.

Over the years since Descartes, many reflexes have been discovered and described and they have often been used in attempted explications of such complex behaviors as locomotion. The commonest approach has been to speak of "chain reflexes," which, by the sensory situation produced by each of the component actions of a complex movement, lead one into the other. Chain reflexes do exist, but they are not common and they are not to be seen in most movements, which are now thought to be centrally patterned according to some template stored, in some sense, within the CNS. What is clear, though, is that the existence of a reflex implies the existence of a center within the CNS which can control it. Such centers are known to be controllable by the CNS as well as by peripheral stimuli, and their effects are known to be modifiable, as by sensory feedback.

It is therefore possible to say that all motor activities (involving the limbs) may be reduced to small, discrete components, the movements of a single limb, and their neural substrates. That much, indeed, seems obvious. One might even think that all that has been said so far has been a waste of time, but that thought itself would be needless. The value of the concept of reflexes as synergies lies in the way in which it points up the fact that all movements can indeed be reduced to small components and *can be controlled as such*.

For a demonstration of this important conceptual point, however, I will refer you to an earlier paper (Easton, 1972b). The purpose of this chapter is to list and describe the common motor reflexes, to review briefly their supraspinal control, to describe their interaction with the phenomenon of fatigue, and to indicate one or two ways in which fatigue might be used to throw more light upon the question of how reflexes are used in normal motor coordination.

THE REFLEXES

When an animal's neuraxis is sectioned at any level, that part of the CNS left connected, below the level of the section, to the animal's musculature displays a number of automatisms, or reflexes. Each reflex, furthermore, bears considerable resemblance to movements or fractions of movements seen in the intact animal; in fact, the principal difference appears to lie in their stereotyped nature. They are evoked by environmental stimuli, but they lack all the smoothly formed adaptiveness of normal "voluntary" movements. Even the decorticate cat, which is able to move about, eat, and defecate almost normally, does so only by means of its reflexes and displays a distinctly jerky, "movieola" character to its movements. Not only are its movements nonadaptive, but they seem segmented into definite components.

The decorticate cat's movements are, however, recognizable as the same, in kind and in rough form, as those an intact cat uses to achieve the same purposes. They lack only the smoothness, the facility, and the variability imparted by the motor mechanisms of the cerebral cortex. They may therefore be considered as "type" movements, at least conceptually.

However, because the reflexes do not resemble only normal movements, but also portions of other reflexes, those found when the neuraxial section is at a higher level of the CNS, the "type" movements seen in the decorticate cat may be further broken down. The reflexes of each level of the CNS appear to subsume those of the next lower level, until the lowest level of all is reached. There we see the spinal reflexes of flexion and extension, and from them we can see how all the others can be composed by concatenating these simplest reflexes.

The Stretch Reflex

The simplest reflex of them all is the *stretch reflex*, the muscular response to spindle primary discharge mediated by the synapse of the spindle afferent on the spinal motoneuron. It is most marked in extensor muscles, but it can readily be elicited in flexors as well. The monosynaptic relations are limited to the myotatic unit, those muscles acting together or in opposition about a single joint, but polysynaptic relations involve the muscles of other joints in the same and other limbs (Kots, 1969; Loofbourrow and Gellhorn, 1948, 1949; Pal'tsev, 1967). If the stretched muscle is, for instance, a biceps, then, as in the intact cat, facilitation may be observed in its own motoneurons and in those of the extensor carpi of the same limb and in the motoneurons of the triceps and flexor carpi of the opposite limb, while inhibition may be seen in the motoneurons of their antagonists.

The inhibitory effect upon the ipsilateral triceps illustrates the phenomenon of *reciprocal inhibition*, while that on this muscle *and* the contralateral biceps illustrates that of *double reciprocal inhibition*. Even though there are variations possible on this pattern, the same pattern of innervation may be seen in the motoneuronal response to motor cortex stimulation (Bosma and Gellhorn, 1947; Uemura and Preston, 1965) and in the other reflexes, where it underlies the patterns of locomotion, the flexion and crossed extension reflexes, and the righting and tonic neck reflexes.

Most often evoked in the laboratory by tapping a tendon (as in the classic, familiar knee-jerk reflex) or by exposing and stretching the muscle mechanically, the stretch reflex has been shown to increase in strength as the stimulus increases by increasing the number of contracting motor units, or active motoneurons, rather than the frequency of their contractions or firings, a phenomenon known as *motoneuronal recruitment*. As the amount of spindle discharge entering the spinal cord and playing upon the pool of motoneurons serving the stretched muscle increases, the motoneurons respond as the discharge they receive exceeds their individual thresholds.

The effect of the stretch reflex may best be described as *length control*, for it works to keep a muscle's length at some constant value set by the gamma fusimotor system, which controls the muscle spindle's sensitivity, or the length of the muscle beyond which the spindle begins to discharge. Thus, if the length of a muscle is increased, as by some outside force or the action of an antagonist, the stretch reflex evokes a contraction tending to restore the muscle to the "match point" of the spindle. It does not interfere with normal movement (except in spasticity, where it is hypersensitive), in which the muscle should lengthen to permit its antagonist's contraction, because alpha motoneuron activity is generally accompanied by gamma activity, changing the "match point" of the spindles of all muscles involved in a movement so that the contracting muscles will have their task facilitated (i.e. the "match point" may be set so low that the stretch reflex may appear before the muscle is actually ordered to contract by the alpha system) and their antagonists will be free to relax (i.e. their "match points" may be set so high that it is virtually impossible to evoke a stretch reflex in them) (see Granit, 1970, Chap. 7). As can be readily seen, the gamma system is thus entirely capable of evoking a movement by itself, and from this has come the notion of the "muscle servo," the notion that the feedback mechanisms acting upon the motoneuron serve to reinforce alpha commands by amplifying small gamma-mediated changes in the intrafusal fibers.

The muscle servo does not, however, include only those feedback mechanisms associated with the spindle. There are also the inhibitory effects of the Renshaw cells, which prevent the gain of the spindle loop from exceeding certain limits, and the tendon organs, which may serve as much to prevent damage to the muscle as to inform the central nervous system of muscle tension. The effect of the latter may be seen particularly clearly in the decerebrate animal, whose extensor stretch reflexes are hypersensitive, resulting in a continuous posture of limb extension. If one tries to flex the limb of a decerebrate animal, one will encounter an initial strong resistance due to the stretch reflex, but an increase in the flexing pressure, and hence an increase in the tension on the tendons of the extensor muscles, elicits a sudden "giving" of the joint as the tendon organ inhibition overcomes the stretch reflex and lets the extensors relax. The similarity of the investigator's sensations to those encountered in closing a clasp knife has not gone unremarked: the phenomenon is called the *clasp knife reaction*.

The various influences affecting the motoneuron and subsumed under the rubric of the muscle servo are schematized in Figure 3-1. The motoneuron pool receives a direct control, both inhibitory and facilitatory, from other levels of the CNS, a facilitatory influence from the primary spindle endings, and inhibitory ones from the tendon organ endings and the Renshaw cells. The output of the individual motoneuron depends upon its threshold and the interplay of these effects, and the effect of this output on the muscle depends upon the latter's physical state. In turn, the effect on the muscle determines the effect on the spindles and tendon organs (though the former are controlled by other sources as well), which feed back upon the motoneuron.

The stretch reflex, because of the possibility of its control by the gamma motor system, may be used to carry out movements or to assist in their execution (Gottlieb, Agarwal, and Stark, 1970), though the former is currently considered the less likely of the two uses (Stein, 1974). Shambes (1969) and Smith, et al. (1972) have found that blocking the gamma motor fibers with procaine or xylocaine results, in the case of the leg muscles (the sciatic nerve), in increased variability of postural sway and amplitude and timing errors in ankle movements, and, in the case of arm agonists and antagonists, in overshooting errors on the finger-to-nose placement task and slowing of rapid arm extension, suggesting that the alpha-gamma linkage is essential to the precise temporal patterning of normal motor coordination. It has also been suggested (Aizerman and Andrejeva, 1968) that the

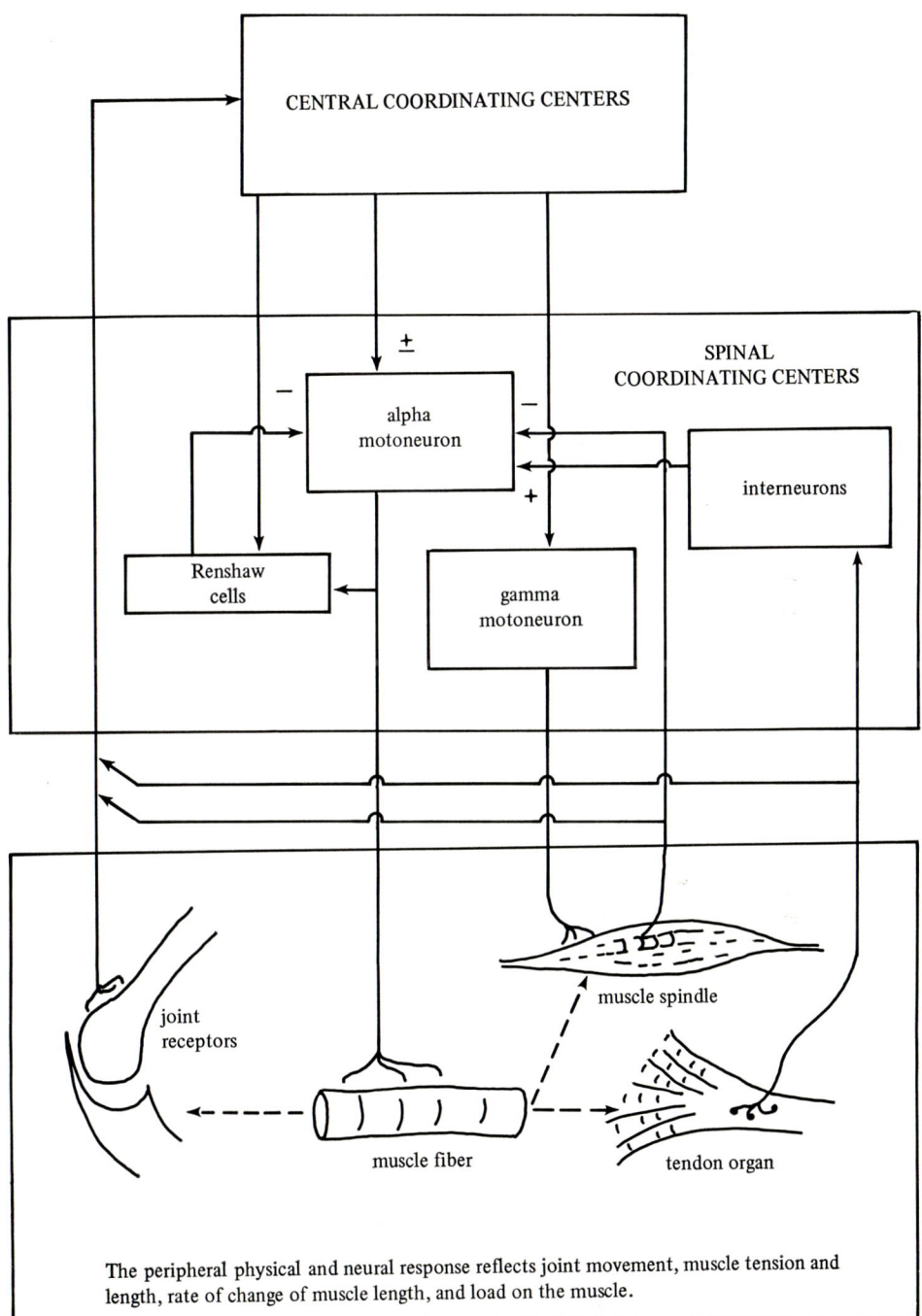

Figure 3-1

stretch reflex may lower the thresholds of motoneurons so that when a disequilibrium is sensed the cortex may send a simple command to all motoneurons which will fire only those serving stretched muscles.

The importance of the stretch reflex is great, and, even though it may be seen at the same level of CNS organization as few other reflexes, its chief importance does not lie in the area of motor organization, but rather in that of tuning, of adjusting the actions of muscles to smooth and ease their function, much as suggested by Lundberg (1969). By the very nature of the innervation in which it is realized, it imposes a certain form, a rule of synergistic action and reciprocal inhibition, on all movements. This form, this rule, can be overridden by the CNS, but it is nevertheless apparent throughout the animal's motor repertoire.

The Spinal Reflexes

The spinal reflexes are those relatively simple reflexes seen when the section of the neuraxis falls between the medulla oblongata and the lumbosacral enlargement of the spinal cord. Like other reflexes, they may also be seen in any other surgical preparation which leaves at least a few spinal segments linked to the musculature and in intact animals (though sometimes only under special conditions), as well as in the mammalian fetus, where they appear among the first organized movements (Windle, 1940). It is, however, the spinal preparation in which spinal reflexes, and the stretch reflex, have most often and most fruitfully been studied, often with a view to explaining locomotion in terms of them (see Easton, 1972b; Graham-Brown, 1911; Graham-Brown and Sherrington, 1912; McCouch, et al., 1971; Sherrington, 1910).

The stretch reflex, because it relies on neural mechanisms residing entirely in the spinal cord, falls into this category. It is intimately involved in the action of the motoneuron, and, because of its role in the muscle servo, plays some part as a modifier in all other reflexes.

The other spinal reflexes are both more complex and polysynaptic, being automatic responses to environmental stimuli as filtered by one or more interneurons. Foremost among them is the *flexion reflex,* consisting of flexion at all the joints of a limb in response to skin stimulation, usually noxious, or stimulation of other receptors lying in the muscles and tendons. It may be evoked from all skin areas of the limb except, apparently, those overlying the extensors (Hagbarth, 1952). It consists of excitation, or facilitation, of flexor motoneurons with inhibition of extensor ones. The opposite pattern has been shown to obtain if skin overlying an extensor muscle is stimulated.

One important feature of the flexion reflex is *local sign,* the phenomenon of differential response according to the area of the limb which is stimulated. This may be seen in the case of electrical stimulation of three hindlimb nerves, the internal saphenous, popliteal, and peroneal distal to the tibialis anticus, illustrated in Table 3-I. The response to stimulation of the saphenous is predominantly hip flexion (tensor fasciae femoris), then ankle (tibialis anticus) and knee (semitendinosus) flexion; for popliteal stimulation it is mainly ankle, then knee and hip flexion; while for peroneal the order is knee, ankle, and hip flexion (Creed, et al., 1932). Altogether, the response is such as to move the point of stimulation away from the stimulus without unnecessary or superfluous effort, and it indicates the existence of several alternative control centers for the flexion reflex, or more probably several interneurons, each serving the several motoneuronal pools to a different extent and able to be summed or separated to achieve a given result. This multiplicity of pathways or control centers may form one kind of tuning mechanism allowing the flexion reflex to be evoked from higher levels in a graded fashion. It is not, of course, a source of lability restricted to the flexion reflex, but may also be seen in most others.

The flexion reflex is usually accompanied by the *crossed extension reflex* so that the total response to a noxious stimulus to one limb is flexion of that limb with extension of the opposite one. Under prolonged or severe stimulation this response may become alternating so that it resembles stepping movements. Variations on this theme are contralateral extensor and flexor facilitation and, in the acute spinal preparation, extensor inhibition and flexor facilitation and inhibition of both extensors and flexors (Holmqvist, 1961).

The *extensor thrust reflex* is a response to a moving coarse contact from the ball of the foot onto the toes. Its significance is obvious: the stimulus is similar to that encountered in locomotion after a limb contacts the ground and while the body moves over it. This reflex would serve to propel the body forward. In a sensitive preparation this becomes the first phase of a gallop rhythm and also seems related to the jump reflex of the thalamic animal.

The *clasp knife reaction* is a spinal reflex hinging upon the nature of

TABLE 3-I

PATTERNS OF REFLEX FLEXION RESULTING FROM STIMULATION OF THREE HINDLIMB NERVES

Nerve	Hip Flexor (Tensor Fasciae Femoris)	Reflex Tensions (grams)	
		Knee Flexor (Semitendinosus)	Ankle Flexor (Tibialis Anticus)
Internal saphenous	100	56	87
Popliteal	3 or less	42	100
Peroneal distal to tibialis anticus nerve	14	100	69

From R. S. Creed, et al., *Reflex Activity of the Spinal Cord* (Oxford University Press, 1932).

the muscle servo and observable only when extensor tonus is high, as in the decerebrate preparation. It consists of a sudden decrease of extensor tonus and contraction of the flexors when the rigid limb is forcibly bent. There is often a concomitant contraction of the contralateral extensors, known as *Philippson's reflex*. This too is a local spinal reflex (Philippson, 1905) and is mediated by the stretch receptors in the muscle.

The *plantar reflex* is normally observable in man, as well as in dogs and monkeys (Philippson, 1905), although not in infants and certain pathological situations in which the *Babinski reflex*, a dorsiflexion of the hallux and fanning of the toes, is seen. The plantar reflex consists of a plantar flexion of the toes when the sole of the foot is scratched or stroked and is reminiscent of the primate grasp reflex, possibly harking back to an arboreal past.

Other observable reflexes are the *coitus reflex*, bilateral extension of the hindlimbs in response to appropriate stimulation of the perineum; the reflex posturings of defecation and micturition, which are, however, much better developed in the decerebrate and decorticate preparations; the *shake reflex*, a response to stimulation of broad areas of the back and thorax; and the *scratch*, or *scalptor, reflex*, focused on the area behind the ear, a response to nociceptive, especially moving, stimuli in any portion of a saddle-shaped zone covering the shoulders and neck. The latter two reflexes, together with the alternations of the flexion, crossed extension, and extensor thrust reflexes, demonstrate the existence in the spinal cord of rhythm generators, structures or functions capable of governing regularly repetitive movements in the intact and spinal animal. These rhythm generators also appear in the phenomenon of *reflex stepping*, in which the hindlimbs of the spinal animal, when dragged over the ground, respond by flexing and extending as in a step. When the dog's spinal cord is transected in the thoracic region, leaving the forelimbs able to drag the animal about, this reflex stepping may occasionally be seen as a natural consequence of movement, and when the animal is given strychnine, thus eliminating postsynaptic inhibition of the motoneuron, this reflex stepping can become reliable enough to deserve the name of *reflex walking* (Hart, 1971).

It should also be noted that there are apparently centers in the spinal cord which are involved in the control of other reflexes, such as the righting reflexes, or parts of them, for D-amphetamine releases fragmentary righting behavior in spinal cats (Maling and Acheson, 1946).

Each of these spinal reflexes may also be seen after neuraxial transections at higher levels and some of them become better coordinated (the scratch reflex becomes able to localize the point of stimulation quite accurately), well illustrating the observation that the more CNS tissue is left connected to the musculature, the more complex and accurate, as well as appropriate, is the motor repertoire elicitable from the animal.

This point may be clarified by considering a few observations from embryology and studies of the recovery of function after CNS damage. It was once thought that fetal movements similar to reflex movements such as the above were obtained by "individuation" from preexisting whole body movements (Coghill, 1929), but it was later effectively shown that, at least in mammals, stereotyped, invariable reflex-like movements appear first and are later integrated into more complex patterns (Barcroft, et al., 1963; Windle, 1937, 1940, 1950; but see Jacobs, 1967) as the CNS develops. In the fetal chick, on the other hand, it has been shown that the unformed, spontaneous motility observable from day 3.5 to day 17 is intrinsic to the spinal cord, independent of afferent data (Hamburger, et al., 1966). In contrast to Coghill's salamanders and to mammals, this activity lacks all apparent adaptiveness and is subject to integrative effects of higher centers only in its later stages. These observations led the investigators of the fetal chick's movements to posit two motor systems, one broad and diffuse, the second more specific and similar to the mammalian system, maturing at different times, and neither system identical to that of *Amblystoma* (Decker and Hamburger, 1967; Hamburger, et al., 1966). Bearing in mind that there is little reason to suppose that lower forms use control methods identical to those of mammals, it might fairly be said that in the mammals movement appears as if it were a house built of prefabricated components, while in lower forms the components emerge as if the house were carved from a single block of wood. How these lower forms use the components is difficult to say, though Riss (1969) has attempted to explain spinal organization and its embryonic development in a way that would permit the same answers to apply to all forms.

Such indications that reflexes are necessary prerequisites for voluntary movement are supported by observations on the recovery of function after mild to moderate hemiplegic paralysis due to cerebral hemisphere lesions (Denny-Brown, 1966, p. 113). Such damage may completely obviate voluntary movements for a time, but eventually and gradually control can be regained, often following a sequence similar to that followed by the maturing human infant. To quote:

> A few days before each recovered ability to make a "willed" movement appeared the same movement could first be demonstrated as a reflex effect to a specific stimulus. After recovery of a traction response that could activate all the flexors of the limb the patient soon found that by willed effort he could begin to initiate flexion of the limb as a whole. A few days after a grasp reflex first appeared the patient became able to flex all the fingers without flexing the elbow and shoulder. If instinctive grasping recovered and could activate individual fingers

the patient could rapidly learn to make such independent movements without a contactual stimulus.

That is, in the human infant, or adult human or monkey recovering from CNS damage, specific voluntary movements are not possible until *after* the reflexes using the same movement elements (e.g. grasping, flexion, extension, etc.) emerge or are recovered. This indeed suggests that the spinal, and other, reflexes may be regarded as the basic alphabet of movement.

Reflexes in the Decerebrate Preparation

The decerebrate preparations are those in which the neuraxis has been sectioned above the spinal cord, the level of section ranging from that of the bulbospinal preparation to that of the thalamic, or decorticate, in which the cerebral cortex, usually with its underlying white matter, has been removed. Simple reflexes observable in these preparations include the spinal reflexes and such others, equivalent to the spinal reflexes though mediated by low-level centers within the brain, as the lateral jaw movement reflex recently described by Lund, et al. (1971), a response to pressure on the teeth or electrical stimulation of the palatal mucosa or gum involving movement of the mandible to one side.

The most striking feature of both the bulbospinal (low decerebrate) and the mesencephalic (high decerebrate) preparations is the phenomenon of *decerebrate rigidity*, a condition of increased extensor tonus and stretch reflex sensitivity due to increased gamma motor activity, though after cerebellectomy the rigidity persists with hyperactivity of the alpha motor system. The condition is usually described as an extensor rigidity, but it might better be called a rigidity of the anti-gravity muscles, which support the animal in its normal posture against the drag of gravity, for in the decerebrate sloth, whose habitual posture is upside down, the rigidity appears in the anatomical flexors (Richter and Bartemeir, 1926).

Even though the subject of decerebrate rigidity is too complex to go into here in any detail, it does deserve the comment that it implies the existence, at intermediate levels of the CNS, of a mechanism capable of biasing the musculature of an animal, no matter what its current activity, toward its constant task, that of support. Such background biases are not uncommon and it is a frequent observation that a particular lesion in a particular preparation may release some function, just as ablation of the contralateral fastigial nucleus in the decerebrate animal may abolish the rigidity in one side of its body.

The so-called *long spinal reflexes*, observable in the spinal animal only under strychnine potentiation (Gernandt and Megirian, 1961), in the bulbospinal animal in which the level of the section passes through the calamus scriptorius, just rostral to the obex, and in intact humans if EMG responses are electronically averaged (Meier-Ewert, et al., 1972), involve a relay in the bulbar reticular formation, which has an apparent integrating effect on all ascending and descending interlimb reflexes, though medial brainstem reticular neurons also appear to be involved (Peterson and Felpel, 1971), and reentry into the spinal cord. They are modifiable by the tonic neck and stretch reflexes and are apparently mediated solely through the alpha motoneurons (Gernandt and Shimamura, 1961; Shimamura and Akert, 1965; Shimamura and Livingston, 1963).

The long spinal reflexes are responses to noxious stimulation of a foot, though they may also be elicited by electrical stimulation of a cutaneous nerve and similar effects may be obtained from muscle afferents. They consist of flexion of the stimulated limb and the one diagonally opposite, with extension of the other two limbs. The result is a withdrawal of the affected foot with preparation for movement away from the stimulus. It may be accompanied by head movement: if the right forepaw is stimulated (Fig. 3-2A) the head turns toward that foot while the right forelimb and left hindlimb flex and the other two extend. It may also be elicited by pinching the pinna (Fig. 3-2C): the head turns away from the affected side while the limbs respond as for the ipsilateral forepaw stimulus. In the intact animal the response is accompanied by a curving of the spine and neck (Fig. 3-2B) such that the center of gravity of the animal is shifted into the polygon of support formed when the affected foot is lifted from the ground. The pattern is very similar to that seen in diagonal progression.

The *tonic neck* (TNR) and *tonic labyrinthine* (TLR) *reflexes* are elicitable after neuraxial transections above the level of the second cervical roots and consist of postural responses to movement of the neck joints (TNR), especially of the atlanto-axial and atlanto-occipital joints (McCouch, et al., 1951), or to disturbances of the otoliths (TLR). The TNR afferentation has been shown to relay through spinal interneurons to reach forelimb motoneurons and there is no reason not to think that it also reaches hindlimb motoneurons in the same way since the TNR posture includes all four limbs (Mori and Matsumoto, 1972). The TLR, and the labyrinthine positional reflexes discussed below, are mediated by several interneuronal pathways linking the vestibulospinal tracts and the motoneuron (Aoyama, et al., 1971; Hongo, et al., 1971). These pathways have been shown to affect neck (Wilson and Yoshida, 1969a,b), back (Wilson, et al., 1970), and limb (Wilson and Yoshida, 1968, 1969b) alpha motoneurons and gamma motoneurons (Kato and Tanji, 1971).

The most common form of the TNR is as shown in Figure 3-2D: if the head and neck are turned to one side, the jaw limbs (those toward which the jaw points) extend while the skull limbs flex (in human infants the hand of the skull arm may be seen to flex also, as in a grasp [Pacella and

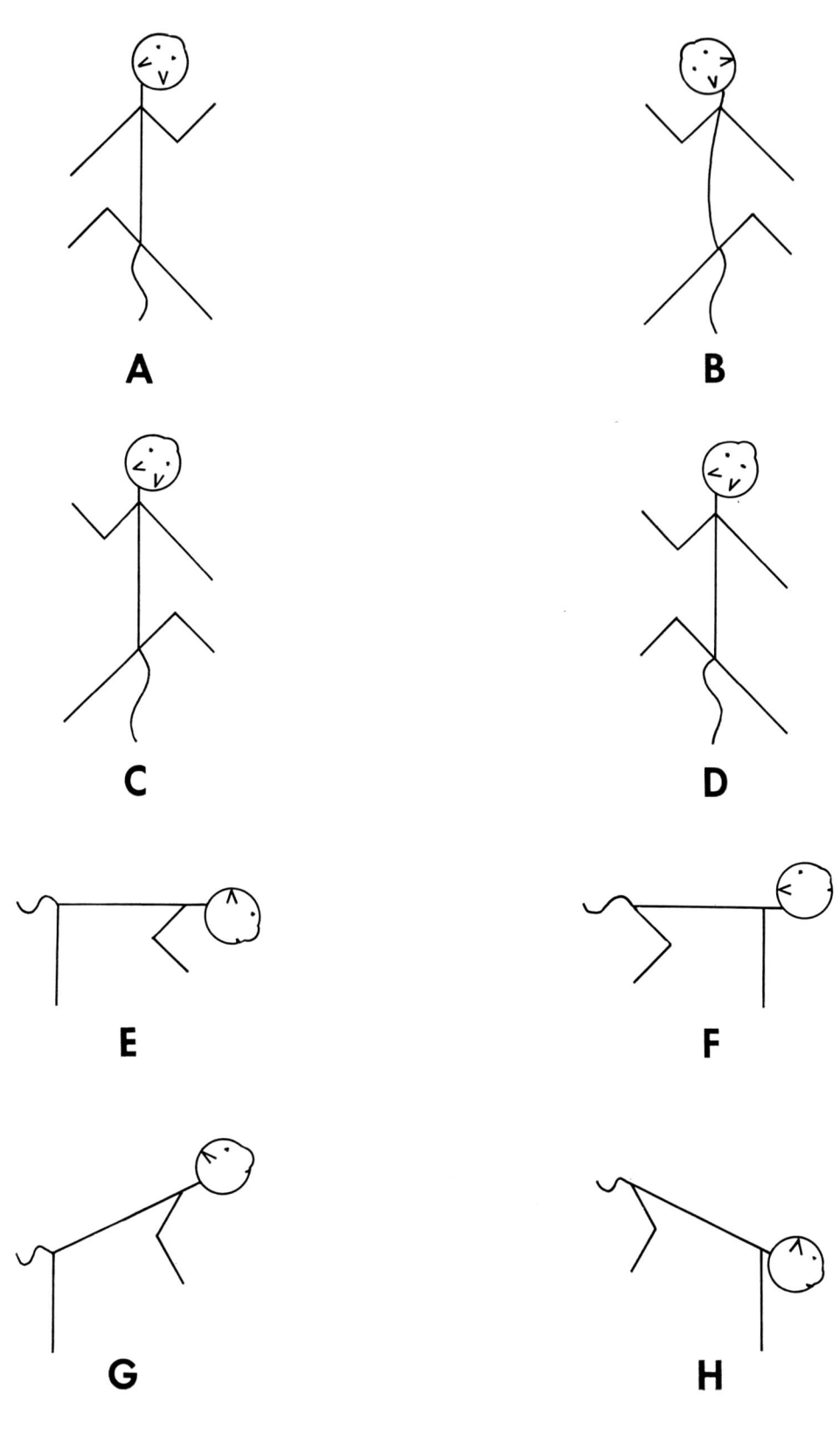

Barrera, 1940]); this postural pattern may also be obtained after fastigial stimulation (Manni, et al., 1964). The same pattern may be seen if the neck is bent to one side without rotation. Ventriflexion of the head (Fig. 3-2E) results in forelimb flexion and hindlimb extension, while dorsiflexion (Fig. 3-2F) has the opposite effect. The general effect of the TNR appears to be to prepare the animal for movement in the direction of gaze.

The TLR acts on all four limbs similarly and sums algebraically with the TNR when both are elicitable. The effect varies from a maximal extensor tonus seen in the supine animal with the mouth angled 45 degrees above the horizontal to a minimal extensor tonus seen in the prone animal with the mouth angled 45 degrees below the horizontal.

The mesencephalic preparation, unlike the bulbospinal, is capable of such behavior as standing and stepping and exhibits the righting reflexes, which are, however, much better developed in the thalamic preparation. The capacity to right, stand, and walk develops slowly after the neuraxial transection is performed. The thalamic animal may exhibit these capabilities immediately and even be able to run and climb, the major deficiencies being the lack of placing reactions and the high thresholds of the proprioceptive corrective reactions.

Locomotion is limited in the mesencephalic animal, but, in the cat, stimulation of certain midbrain regions may evoke locomotion, very similar to that seen in the intact cat, whose speed and gait may be controlled by varying the strength of stimulation (Orlovskii, 1969; Severin, et al., 1967; Shik, Orlovskii, and Severin, 1966, 1968; Shik, et al., 1966). The effects of midbrain and pons pyramid stimulation summate, the midbrain centers being essential, as is afferent input from the limbs, for both initiation and maintenance of locomotion, as well as for adjustments of the gait to the surface. The implication is that in and/or below the level of the midbrain there exist centers capable of organizing the complex arrangements of reflexes and synergies necessary for locomotion. Waller (1940), noting that electrical stimulation of the ventral thalamus dorsal to the mammillary

---

Figure 3-2. Reflex postural patterns of apparently adaptive significance. A: Long spinal reflex pattern evoked in the bulbospinal animal by pinch of the right forepaw. B: Long spinal pattern with back curvature evoked in the intact animal by pinch of the right hindpaw. C: Long spinal pattern evoked in the bulbospinal animal by pinch of the left pinna. D: Tonic neck reflex pattern evoked by rotation of the head to the right. E: Tonic neck reflex pattern evoked by head ventriflexion. F: Tonic neck reflex pattern evoked by head dorsiflexion. G: Labyrinthine positional reflex pattern evoked by tilt of the whole body with the head up. The neck is kept straight. H: Labyrinthine positional reflex pattern evoked by tilt of the whole body with the head down. The neck is kept straight.

bodies may elicit progression movements, thought that such a center might be found in the subthalamus.

It is thus certain that an animal's motor cortex need not organize so complex an act as locomotion from individual muscle contractions. In fact, it need do no more than issue a simple, steady command to lower centers in which concatenations of spinal reflexes may be coded for activation as a unit either pyramidally or extrapyramidally, via the midbrain.

In the hypothalamic cat, where the neuraxial section passes from the rostral border of the superior colliculi to the rostral border of the optic chiasm, the *jump reflex* may be evoked (Guzman and Del Pozo, 1953). If the animal is stood upon its hind paws with the thighs, legs, and feet in relative extension and the neck and head are moved through, first, neck extension and head flexion followed by, second, neck flexion and head extension, then after a short latency the hindlimbs flex and propel the cat by a sudden and energetic jump into the air while the forelimbs make a simultaneous jerk backward. This response is accompanied by a general rage reaction. The principal receptors for this reflex seem to be the deep proprioceptors of the neck and hindlimbs, and it appears to depend upon a facilitating influence from the hypothalamus.

The motor component of this reflex seems similar to the jump observable in both play and battle. As an integrated movement independent of the cortex it may be considered a suitable reflex for incorporation into volitional movements. The nature of the adequate stimulus suggests that it does not require any central command for its appearance, but may instead be evoked by an appropriate preceding movement, as in the chaining of the righting reflexes. It is interesting to note that the postural stimulus described above is similar to the postures a cat often takes before a jump.

The thalamic, or decorticate, preparation is capable of spontaneous standing, walking, and righting and is able to adjust its posture to the nature of the surface and to gravity. This last is due to the *labyrinthine positional reflexes:* if the neck is kept straight, or the TNR eliminated by dorsal rhizotomy, and the animal tilted so that the head is directed upwards (Fig. 3-2G), then the forelimbs flex and the hindlimbs extend, and vice versa if the head is directed downwards (Fig. 3-2H). The *labyrinthine acceleratory reflexes* may also be mentioned here: if the animal is dropped, subjected to linear acceleration, then all four limbs extend and the toes spread (a reflex of obvious utility for landing on the feet); if the animal is rotated, then nystagmic movements, tending to maintain visual and auditory fixation of the environment, of the eyes, ears (Meyer, et al., 1971, 1972; Schaefer, et al., 1971), and head occur while the limbs are influenced in such a way as to oppose, by either a counter-movement or bracing, the rotation.

There are four different and related *righting reflexes*. The *labyrinthine righting reflex* acts from the otoliths on the neck muscles to keep the head level. The *body-on-head righting reflex* is a response to asymmetry of pressure on the body of an animal lying on its side and may be prevented by placing a weighted board on the upper side of the body. It acts on the neck muscles to level the head. The *neck righting reflex* ensues from the head movement engendered by the first two reflexes and brings the thoracic, lumbar, and pelvic portions of the back upright by entraining limb movements. For example, if a horse is lying on one side, the head first bends upward, evoking by the TNR flexion of the lower limbs and extension of the upper. The head then rotates toward the level position, bringing into play the opposite TNR, extension of the lower limbs with flexion of the upper, which with the accompanying twist of the trunk following that of the neck lets the animal position its feet beneath itself and rise (Roberts, 1967). This chaining of the righting reflexes is fairly rigid in the horse, as is shown by the observation that if the head is kept from raising the horse cannot right; each reflex in the chain depends on the expression of the preceding one. In some animals, however, the fourth righting reflex, the *body-on-body righting reflex,* a response of the limb and back musculature to asymmetrical body stimulation and to distortion of mesenteric receptors (Ito and Sanada, 1965; Pollock, et al., 1955), may cause the body to right even when the head is held in the lateral position. It is this latter righting reflex whose prevention by pressure on body parts, inversion, and restraint may be involved in the so-called *immobility reflex* ("animal hypnosis") whose status was recently reviewed by Klemm (1971).

In the decorticate monkey (Bieber and Fulton, 1938), it has been noted that the body righting reflexes take the form, in the prone or supine animal, of the lower hindlimb flexing, the upper extending, when the pelvis is rotated by 15 degrees. The decorticate monkey also shows a *grasp reflex* in all four limbs in the seated or prone animal, but none in the supine animal and only in the upper limbs when the animal lies on one side. The authors described this as the basic subcortical prehension pattern on which the forced grasping phenomenon is built. They did not state that the grasping pattern was a part of the righting reflex, but the utility of such a linkage in any animal with the physical equipment to *pull* itself upright would seem obvious.

The labyrinthine righting reflex is at least partly dependent on the cerebral cortex, and the so-far-unmentioned *optical righting reflex,* for which the adequate stimulus is visual, depends entirely on the cortex. The controlling centers of the other righting reflexes lie chiefly in the medulla and mesencephalon.

It should be noted that in the progression of neuraxial transections from the spinal preparation to the decorticate there is a parallel progression of motor capability, suggesting that the hierarchical conceptualization of CNS function is not wholly misleading. The more nervous tissue is left connected to the musculature, the more complex the actions that may be evoked. This is what one might expect if the sections were cutting a functional tree at successively higher levels. It should also be noted that there is a phylogenetic progression: man has the reflexes, but they apparently depend more on cortical activation than in lower forms; the monkey is more capable than man when its higher levels have been separated from the rest, but less so than the cat or dog, which show spontaneous locomotion after decortication; and these are less capable than the rat, which, when decerebrated at the mesencephalic level, retains better righting and locomotor behavior as well as proprioceptive hopping reactions and will nibble at any object held against its snout, grasp a pipette with its forepaws, and drink, groom, and show typical rodent defensive behavior (Woods, 1964), which is, altogether, comparable, but superior, to the decorticate cat.

Reactions and Reflexes in the Intact Animal

As has already been mentioned, the reflexes are observable in the intact animal as well as in the animal with the higher levels of the CNS removed from any active part in its behavior. It should be clear by now that the reflexes as seen in such surgical preparations are suited for use as components of volitional movements, both because of their apparent adaptiveness and because of their resemblance to volitional movements and pieces of volitional movements. It is also true, however, that the reflexes play definite parts in volitional movement. Accordingly, this section is devoted to a brief description of those reflex-like reactions—the placing and hopping reactions—which require the integrity of the cerebral cortex, to a discussion of the TNR and TLR as seen in intact cats and humans, and to a brief discussion of the ontogeny and phylogeny of grasps and grips in primates.

The *hopping reactions* are those responses by which an animal keeps its legs beneath its body. If the animal is positioned with but one foot touching the ground, there appears the *positive supporting reaction,* the cocontraction of the limb flexors and extensors that turns the limb into a rigid pillar-like support for the body (the *negative supporting reaction* is a flexion response to ventriflexion or lateral compression of the toes). This reaction appears to be essential for walking (Denny-Brown, 1966) and is apparently mediated by the muscle spindles and muscle servo (Van Der Meulen and Gilman, 1965). If the animal is then dragged over the surface in any direction so that the leg bends at the hip or shoulder, the excursion of the limb steadily increasing, the muscle proprioceptors induce a hop of the limb, the positive supporting reaction melting away, to a new position beneath the body where support is reestablished. The hop is repeated so long as the animal is being dragged in order to maintain the support. The hopping reactions require the cerebral cortex for their most effective expression, but in the decorticate animal they may also be seen, though their thresholds are higher and they are much less accurate.

There are five *placing reactions*, all requiring the integrity of the cerebral cortex: 1. if the animal is supported freely and blindfolded or blinded to eliminate visual placing, and if the dorsum of the paw is allowed to contact lightly the edge of a table, then the foot is lifted and placed on the table, the opposite foot soon joining it; this particular placing reaction, if no other, appears to have a primitive, subcortical controlling center, subordinated in the adult to cortical control, involving the cerebellum, thalamus, and red nucleus (Amassian, Weiner, and Rosenblum, 1972); 2. if the chin is allowed to touch the table, both forefeet are instantly raised and placed beside the jaws; extension of the limbs usually follows so that a standing position is achieved; 3. if the animal is standing on a table and any leg is thrust over the edge, it is immediately brought back into the original position; 4. if any leg of the standing animal is passively abducted, it is immediately adducted and returned to its position; 5. if, instead of the chin, the vibrissae of a blindfolded or blinded cat are allowed to touch the table edge, the feet are promptly brought up onto the table. The one similar placing reaction which does not depend upon cortical control is the *proprioceptive placing reflex*, a less accurate response to contact so firm as to bend a joint.

How much of a part these hopping and placing reactions play in reflex walking, as of human neonates (Zelazo, et al., 1972), however, is not known. They would seem entirely capable of providing an animal with the capability of stepping when the standing posture is perturbed, but given the neonate's lack of time in which to learn placing, one might find more attractive the hypothesis that reflex walking depends more upon the spinal mechanisms described by Sherrington (1910) and sketched above as the spinal reflexes.

The TNR and TLR, as well as the righting and positional reflexes, may be seen, and have been described, in intact cats, dogs, horses, and man, among others, but it is chiefly in man that they have been studied and related to both normal and stylized activities. Fukuda (1961) has examined the sports of archery, baseball, dancing, diving, fencing, gymnastics, the high jump, judo, shot-putting, soccer, and sumo, and he has found many cases where the ideal or most efficient, or even the incidental, form follows the patterns of the TNR, TLR, and righting reflexes.

The TLR is best seen in certain idealized gymnastic postures such as the handstand, but it is also apparent where, as in certain sumo situations, the labyrinthine head righting reflex has brought the head (and labyrinths) into a position to evoke the TLR. The TNR is more common and a beautiful example may be seen in a ballplayer going after a fly ball: he looks toward the ball, the jaw arm is extended for the interception, the jaw leg is extended from the jump, but the skull limbs are both flexed, and for no apparent reason other than the TNR. The initial posture of a fencer is also in accord with the TNR, as are those postures of a soccer player heading a ball, an athlete putting the shot, an archer drawing a bow, and a tennis player awaiting the ball. The exceptions seem limited to occasions, as a fencer's lunge, when forward impetus is required and the skull limbs are suddenly and forcibly extended, resulting in a posture of extension in all four limbs. This is in accord with the earlier comment that the TNR posture prepares the animal for movement in the direction of gaze.

Involvement of the TNR in other movement sequences in other animals may be readily inferred if we but watch cats with a little care. They show many behavior patterns, of which two of the most prominent are stretching and washing. The former usually takes the form of forelimb hyperextension and hindlimb semiextension, with the head thrown back; the latter, whether of the forelimbs or of the hindlimbs and perineum, usually takes the form of head and neck flexion with either extension of one forelimb or extension of both hindlimbs and semiflexion of both forelimbs. They are distinct movement patterns, but washing may be begun from the stretching posture: if the stretching cat turns its head toward one forelimb, thus entering the washing posture, it may begin to lick. Perineal washing, though its typical posture bears no resemblance to that of a stretch, may also be begun if its posture is entered inadvertently, as when a supine cat arises by walking its forequarters back over its belly—as the neck flexes, the hindlimbs extend, and as the cat's mouth reaches the perineal region the animal begins to lick. This giving way of one movement pattern to another may be observed more often in kittens than in adult cats, an inconsistency which suggests that reflexes may indeed be the components of volitional movements. It is not unreasonable to expect that an immature CNS would have less complete control over its output and that it might hence not be able to maintain activation of only a fragment of a reflex pattern without occasionally losing its "grip" on the reflex circuitry and letting the peripheral stimulus pattern which can, alone, evoke the reflex take over or letting its activation of a fragment expand to the whole. Such behaviors may, of course, be due to no more than a simple reminder effect, but they are extremely suggestive of chain reflexes.

It would therefore seem that the TNR, TLR, and righting reflexes, and perhaps others, underlie volitional controls and may be called upon when a maximal muscular force or smoothly executed or patterned movement is desired. (Particularly illustrative of this point is the effect of fatigue on the patterning of movement, discussed below.) Movements are also apparently easier when patterned along the lines of these reflexes: it is the "natural" way of doing things. A good illustration of this may be obtained by listening to a coach instruct a novice diver in the art of a forward flip. "Keep your head down," he says and the TLR then produces, or fosters, an initial flexion of the limbs. As the diver comes out of the consequent roll, the angle of the head becomes such as to favor a posture of extension, and the effort of the movement is reduced by making at least part of its control automatic.

There is even some indication that this "naturalness" of the reflex patterns has affected the human aesthetic sense, for Fukuda (1961) observed that in much of Oriental and Western classical art the patterns of the TNR are followed.

As will be seen later, there is more concrete evidence that the TNR—and other reflexes—play an important role in the normal coordination of movement, but for now it is only necessary to note that the TNR has been shown to be *crucial* to normal coordination in monkeys and baboons. Cohen (1961) abolished the TNR in these animals by bilaterally anaesthetizing dorsal roots C1, C2, and C3, and observed severe disorientation, imbalance, and general motor incoordination in all his experimental animals, the symptoms resembling those of labyrinthectomized animals. This result implies that the TNR is a crucial underpinning of the ordinary movements of daily activity, serving to orient the animal's limbs to the requirements of intention as expressed, perhaps, by gaze, a point which finds some corroboration in Gazzaniga's work on split-brain monkeys (Gazzaniga, 1966, 1969a) and man (Gazzaniga, 1969b), whose seeing hemisphere can, or may, inform the other, acting one of a target location by moving the eyes, head, and neck so as to feed back reflex postural information.

Similarly, a postural reflex deriving from the activation of eye muscle stretch receptors during eye movement may be important for normal coordination of nystagmus, compensatory eye movements, eye-head coordination, and postural preparations for movement (Easton, 1971, 1972a). This reflex has been described in terms of changes in neck and limb muscle EMGs in response to eye muscle stretch in the intact cat. The changes consist of patterns of inhibition tending to support movements of the head and body in the direction opposite that of gaze.

Forced grasping, an involuntary response to palmar or plantar stimulation, may be seen in both man and monkey after cortical lesions which include the premotor cortex but not the motor cortex itself (Fulton, et al., 1932; Kennard, et al., 1934; Richter and Hines, 1932). It does not appear in the intact man or monkey, apparently being inhibited by some tonic action of the premotor cortex. In man it varies with changes of body position in space (Kennard, et al., 1934) similarly to the changes Bieber and Fulton (1938) reported in the thalamic monkey.

It is worth noting that the patterns of the grasp reflex and forced grasping seem to be the same and that the remark (Bieber and Fulton, 1938) that the grasp reflex represents the basic (subcortical) prehension pattern would seem to be supported by the observation (Bishop, 1962) that in primitive primates (Lorisiformes and Lemuriformes) there is only one pattern of reaching found in each species, with only whole-hand control with no separate control of the digits, as in the grasp reflex, and that in the human infant the whole-hand pattern of reaching and grasping is the first to develop (20-28 weeks) (Halverson, 1931). If reflexes are used as the basic components of movement, this implies that, in at least the initial stages of phylogeny and ontogeny, movement is limited to the patterns of the reflexes. Only later are other patterns of control added to the reflexes to produce variations of greater subtlety, these perhaps depending on the development of the motor cortex.

As the cortex develops, phylogenetically and ontogenetically, the grip does change, becoming more sophisticated: the advanced Ceboidea and Cercopithecoidea show good precision grips (Bishop, 1962), while grips similarly suited to picking up small objects and holding them gently appear in the human infant at ages of 28 to 52 weeks (Halverson, 1931). Power grips, suited to applying force to an object (e.g. the grip used in holding a baseball bat or golf club, or that used while moving along a branch), appear sharply differentiated from the precision grip in macaques and baboons (Bishop, 1962). Halverson (1931) did not test for any equivalent of the power grip in his study of prehension in the human infant, nor did he comment on it, but Shirley (1933) referred to abilities presumably requiring some equivalent of the power grip as occurring at ages of 32 to 60 weeks. Later, of course, the power grip is just as well differentiated in the human as in other primates.

The phylogeny and ontogeny of grips are an interesting sideline whose significance is not easy to understand in terms of the supraspinal control of reflexes, but it does lend some support to the contention that the motor capability of an animal is greater the more functioning CNS tissue is connected to its musculature. Of course, the same phylogenetic and developmental point may be made with reference to general motor behavior: adults and humans have, respectively, far more versatile motor repertoires than infants and the lower animals.

THE SUPRASPINAL CONTROL OF REFLEXES

To call the reflexes the elements of movement, it is necessary to do more than simply list them. There must also be some way of assembling them, of activating the neural centers that control them as reflexes, and of integrating them to produce complex, nonreflex movements. The latter will not be discussed at present, but the question of activation is the question of the supraspinal control of the reflexes, the facilitation and/or inhibition, originating in the cerebral cortex and brainstem, of the interneurons of the polysynaptic reflex arcs.

Volitional movement is mediated by the cerebral cortex, particularly the motor cortex, the axons of whose cells pass through the midbrain and brainstem as the pyramidal tract and enter the spinal cord. In the spinal cord, they synapse with interneurons solely, except in primates, where a few fast fibers synapse directly with the alpha motoneurons (Bernhard and Bohm, 1954; Kostyuk and Vasilenko, 1968; Lloyd, 1941; Nyberg-Hansen, 1966),[1] though apparently not with the gamma motoneurons (Granit, 1970, p. 211). These interneurons serve both gamma (Fidone and Preston, 1971; Grigg and Preston, 1971; Yokota and Voorhoeve, 1969) and alpha motoneurons (Grigg, 1972), both singly and together, as *alpha-gamma coactivation*, a phenomenon known to involve single, common interneurons in at least the case of the effect of the medullary respiratory centers on the motoneurons of the cat's intercostal muscles (Andersen and Sears, 1970). The importance of this effect is suggested by the observations that electrical stimulation of the cat's pyramid, which activates flexor muscles and inhibits extensors, affects both alpha and gamma motoneurons (Laursen and Wiesendanger, 1966a), and that, if one of the cat's pyramids is cut above the level of the pyramidal decussation, the contralateral flexor reflexes are subsequently diminished, indicating the existence, in the intact animal, of a flexor subsidy from the motor cortex (Laursen and Wiesendanger, 1966b). This represents part of the tonic function of the motor cortex, whereby tonic or phasic activity set in train at other levels may be moderated, steadied, reinforced, or facilitated, and whereby muscle tone is supported and thresholds are kept low (Tower, 1940). The phasic function of the motor cortex is concerned with maintaining posture and directing integrated movements of the body and limbs, similar to extrapyramidal systems, and confers adjustability in space, modifiability in the course of execution, the possibility of fractionation of movements as exemplified by individual finger movements, and a general accuracy and polish on the stereotyped extrapyramidal control (Lawrence and Kuypers, 1968a,b; Tower, 1940).

It has been observed in man that pyramidal system damage is accompanied by disturbances in the compensatory period of voluntary movement, that period during which the body adjusts to a new equilibrium, but not in the anticipatory period (Pal'tsev and El'ner, 1967), when the body carries

---

1. There is one recent study (Duffield, 1970), however, that suggests that in the dog some pyramidal fibers may synapse directly with thoracic motoneurons, but Duffield did not call his observation more than "apparent." There therefore remains no hard evidence for a direct pyramidal projection below the primates.

out adjustments of posture according to the disturbances expected to arise from the intended movement (Belenkii, et al., 1967). Cerebellar frontal lobe damage, on the other hand, is accompanied by disturbances in the anticipatory period but not in the compensatory period (Pal'tsev and El'ner, 1967), suggesting a predictive, or feed-forward, function for the cerebellar frontal lobe and a feedback function for the motor cortex. This fits well with the above observations that pyramidal control is responsible for the polish and lability of motor function.

It has been shown that the interneurons of the flexion reflex, tendon organ, spindle secondary, and cutaneous afferent arcs may be facilitated and inhibited by brainstem sources (Eccles and Lundberg, 1959; Holmqvist and Lundberg, 1959, 1961; Hongo and Jankowska, 1967; Kuno and Perl, 1960); that stimulation of the substantia nigra facilitates the spinal monosynaptic reflex (York, 1972); that mesencephalic stimulation can independently affect the static and dynamic gamma motoneurons of both flexors and extensors, without affecting the alpha motoneurons except reflexively (Appelberg and Emonet-Denand, 1965); that the cerebellum appears to have a tonic facilitatory effect on the spindle primary response, perhaps by raising the tonic level of the gamma activity, perhaps by facilitating the afferent interneurons (Gilman and McDonald, 1967); and that stimulation of the basal nuclei, reticular formation, and hypothalamus can have facilitatory, inhibitory, or reciprocal effects on gamma motoneurons, depending on the intensity of stimulation and depth of anaesthesia (Shimazu, et al., 1962), a result partially confirmed by Vedel and Mouillac-Baudevin (1969a,b). Further, it has also been shown that stimulation of sensorimotor cortex in the cat enhances spindle primary inhibitory, tendon organ reciprocal, flexion reflex afferent reciprocal and inhibitory-to-flexor, and cutaneous excitatory-to-extensory synaptic effects (Lundberg and Voorhoeve, 1962) and produces EPSPs (excitatory postsynaptic potentials) in interneurons receiving excitatory actions from muscle, flexion reflex, and cutaneous afferents (Lundberg, et al., 1962). These effects are mediated by the pyramidal tract (Lundberg and Voorhoeve, 1961), though similar effects may be obtained from the rubrospinal tract (Hongo, et al., 1965). Lundberg (1966), while reviewing some of the literature, even suggests that the facilitation of the interneurons of reflex pathways (such as the spindle primary and tendon organ afferent pathways) by impulses in the corticospinal, rubrospinal, and vestibulospinal tracts may be for the express purpose of mobilizing, from higher centers, particular reflexes, while inhibition by impulses in these tracts and the dorsal and ventral reticulospinal tracts must be involved in motor control in other ways. Perhaps the inhibitory control serves to turn off or prevent the appearance of unwanted reflexes or parts of reflexes.

It therefore seems reasonable to think that the higher levels of the CNS are able to activate the basic reflexes, as represented by the interneurons of the reflex arcs. If this could be shown to be true beyond question, then the notion that the higher levels of the CNS organize complex movements out of these components would be strongly supported.

That pyramidal activation of interneurons produces, or may produce, organized movements may be inferred from the finding (Bosma and Gellhorn, 1947) that suprathreshold stimulation of the monkey's motor cortex may produce both a progression pattern, characterized by hindleg flexion, retraction of the shoulder, extension of the elbow, and flexion of the wrist, and a prehension pattern, characterized by protraction of the shoulder, flexion of the elbow, and clenching of the fist, as well as combinations of these responses. The fact that different loci may produce the same movement, though with different relative involvements of the various muscles, suggests a cortical representation of local sign or some equivalent thereof. The stereotyped nature of these movements indicates that individual motoneurons are probably not being directly controlled, else greater variability of the response might be expected, and that very probably only the pyramidal pathway through the interneurons of the polysynaptic reflex arc is involved. The results of threshold stimulation of the motor cortex further support this notion, for it has been shown that the size of the EPSPs received by baboon motoneurons after cortical stimulation is associated with the size of the EPSPs received after reflex stimulation (Clough, et al., 1968), thus allowing the inference that the same interneurons are involved in each facilitatory pathway. In addition, it has been found that functionally interrelated groups of muscles respond as units to motor cortex stimulation, though the effects depend on the existence of afferentation from the limbs (Hyde and Gellhorn, 1949), suggesting that two or more facilitating influences may be necessary for a response; i.e. if a cortical command is set at a certain level, then reflex effects from the periphery may be needed to raise the membrane potential of a motoneuron beyond its threshold, and vice versa (see, for instance, the comments of Aizerman and Andrejeva [1968] on equilibrium, the muscle servo, and cortical commands). This conclusion is supported by the finding (Gellhorn, 1949; Gellhorn and Johnson, 1950) that stretch of a muscle by fixation of the joint increases the response to cortical facilitation of that muscle and its synergists, with reciprocal inhibition of their antagonists' responses. It is, of course, possible that the stimuli used in the studies cited above spread in the cortex to activate several, meaningfully related, cells, or that the cells are so interconnected within the cortex that a local stimulus results in the above apparently meaningful responses, but it is simpler to think, considering the evidence, that the cortical cells activated by Gellhorn and his colleagues connect with interneurons of reflex pathways. There is, however, another route to the motoneurons through interneurons not involved in the reciprocal relationships, those interneurons receiving the spindle secondary and cutaneous afferents (Asanuma, et al., 1971). This route may open the cortical effect to masking by peripheral events, but its existence does demonstrate that reflexes are not *necessary* elements of movement. It is true that many volitional movements seem to be accompanied by inhibition of antagonists (e.g. Kots, 1969), but there are interneurons through which this linkage may be bypassed.

It is obvious that pyramidal fine control might be achieved by direct control of single motoneurons, even though it would be unnecessarily complicated, but in animals lower than the primates something else must be used. The interposition of the interneurons of the reflex pathways into the motor pathway supports the notion that movements are composed from reflexes, but it necessitates some explanation of how reflexes may be composed to achieve the fine control so obviously attained by the animal; it is easy to see how gross control may be achieved. It is conceivable, and the CNS has the equipment to make it possible, that a logic is applied on the interneurons: if each interneuron either facilitates or inhibits a set of motoneurons, either within one motoneuronal pool or across several, and if these sets are not identical but do overlap, then by combining the activations of facilitatory and inhibitory interneurons sets of motoneurons both larger and smaller than any set controlled by a single interneuron may be made available as separate functional entities. This is illustrated, in principle, by Figure 3-3: if interneurons, or interneuronal pools, F_1 (facilitatory) and I_2 (inhibitory) are activated by higher levels, then only motoneuron sets A and B will fire, given appropriate threshold conditions, even though each interneuron controls more than two such sets; that is, both sets and their intersections may be controlled.

The existence of such paths and logics may cast some light on the problem of the progression of complexity of grips and grasps that may be observed in primates phylogenetically (Bishop, 1962) and in man ontogenetically (Halverson, 1931; Shirley, 1933). In animals without direct pyramidal projections to motoneurons, such as the cat and dog, the possible equivalent of the grasp reflex consists of simple plantar flexion (Philippson, 1905), corresponding perhaps to the activation of an interneuron or interneuronal pool. In the lower primates the nature of the pyramidal projection has not yet been determined, but it seems safe to assume that, if it reaches the motoneurons at all, it is probably less extensive than in higher forms, while the interneuronal organization controlling the form of the grasp is probably more complex than it is in the dog or cat and less so than in the higher primates. In the higher primates the interneuronal organization, however complex, has added to it a direct pyramidal projection to

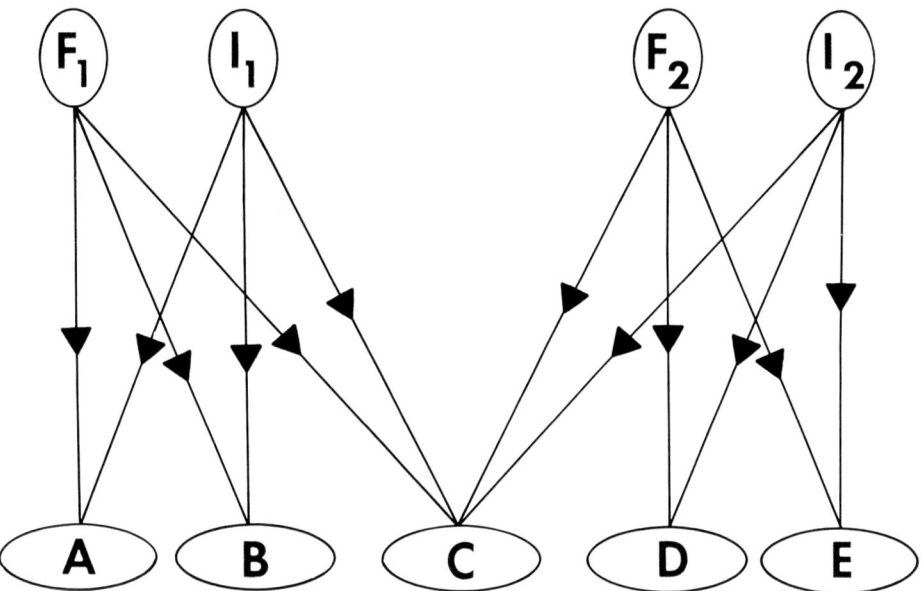

Figure 3-3. This schema represents an attempt to show how a logic might be applied to interneurons. Interneurons F_1 and I_1 either fire or keep from firing, respectively, motoneuron sets A, B, and C; F_2 and I_2 fire or keep from firing sets C, D, and E. By combining the active interneurons as F_1F_2, F_1I_2, I_1F_2, or I_1I_2, motoneuron sets ABCDE, AB, DE, and none, respectively, may be made to fire. A slight complication would provide even greater fractionation.

the motoneuron, which, though posing new problems of coordination by providing for activation of single muscles, provides the possibility of refining such a movement as a grip or grasp so that it becomes much more versatile. It also allows departures from the basic form of the reflex so that new, learned, forms of the grip or grasp become possible.

In man, the CNS does not complete its development, in the form of growth and proliferation of axons and dendrites, until long after birth. Since in the infant coordination develops parallel, to some extent, to the sequence seen in phylogeny, it may be inferred that the CNS develops in such a way as to realize the more primitive level of coordination first, the more complicated interneuronal organizations, or higher centers organizing more complicated reflexes than the spinal, and the pyramidal projection to the motoneurons developing later, much as suggested by Riss (1969). Human motor development is not, as was once thought, simply a matter of learning to use the equipment that we are born with.

There are, of course, modes of control other than modulation of motor activity at the levels of the interneurons of the reflex arcs and the motoneurons. The flow of afferent data may be affected presynaptically (Hongo and Jankowska, 1967) and at the interneuron (Tanaka, 1972), and its course to other levels, such as the cerebellum, where it would be used in the fine control of movements and posture, may be modulated as well (Holmqvist, et al., 1960a,b; Magni and Oscarsson, 1961; Oscarsson, 1960, 1965). It is well known, for example, that the unhampered working of the flexion reflex will cause a man to stagger if he steps on a tack while walking, but if footing becomes crucial, as in mountain climbing, he won't even flinch, while one recent study reports that, when a man or animal with cortical damage has a cutaneous nerve electrically stimulated while walking, the flexion reflex is replaced by an extension reflex; in the intact animal the flexion reflex only becomes weaker (Lisin, et al., 1973). Similarly, the facilitating effect of electrical vestibular stimulation on the gastrocnemius H-reflex (a version of the spinal monosynaptic reflex which can be obtained without surgical exposure of the spinal roots; it involves the stimulation of a sensory nerve through the skin and the direct recording of muscle response) is reduced or eliminated during the latent period of voluntary movements involving the gastrocnemius as agonist or antagonist (Kots and Mart'yanov, 1968), and the response of Deiters' nucleus neurons to tilt is diminished during locomotion (Orlovskii and Pavlova, 1972), thus minimizing the disruptive effects of vestibular disturbances on voluntary movements. The site of these inhibitory blocks, whether at the interneuron, the vestibular nuclei, the presynaptic terminals of afferent fibers, or elsewhere, is unknown.

Nor are alpha motoneurons necessarily the only ones affected by interneuronally mediated control. Gottlieb, et al. (1970) have found, in man, a mechanism for the regulation of the gain of the myotatic loop, i.e. the rate of firing of gamma motoneurons. Prior to the initiation of movement the agonist loop gain is turned up, allowing the intrinsic reflex mechanisms (the stretch reflex) to assist in activating the motoneuronal pool, while the antagonist loop gain is turned down to prevent reflex opposition to the movement. This effect may be mediated by interneurons, though it is so far unknown whether a similar process accompanies the reflexes, as there is reason to suspect (Grillner, et al., 1969).

A slightly different mode of control, probably operating together with the others, may be seen where the existence of several parallel reflex paths on the local level, as described by Holmqvist (1961), suggests that supraspinal control may be directed as much at suppressing or releasing one path as a modulating factor on other reflexes as at activating it for use as a reflex itself. Thus a pathway linking flexion of one limb with extension of the opposite one might be released for use in diagonal progression, but where the limbs work together, flexing or extending simultaneously as in a leap or certain postures and gaits, others might be released to support the desired action by specifying the form of the reflex interactions of the limbs obtainable from skin, muscle, and joint afferents.

Altogether, the data indicate the existence of neuronal circuitry apparently capable of mobilizing reflexes for use as components of volitional movements. Projections may be seen from the motor cortex and brainstem onto spinal interneurons which are apparently involved in local reflex arcs, if they are not the actual organizing centers for the local reflexes. These projections would seem to provide the various levels of the CNS with the capability of activating local reflexes, and the results of simple cortical stimuli suggest that they may activate complex movements which seem, from their stereotyped nature, to be organized at an interneuronal level.

The finding that there appear to be within the cerebral cortex separate excitatory and inhibitory zones for each muscle, with the possibility of coactivation of antagonists (Asanuma and Ward, 1971), but increases the number of movements available to the CNS. The probability that reflexes *can* be used in the composition of movements is not, however, to say that *only* reflexes are used. Whatever the level of versatility of the compositional method, there must be occasions where additional capabilities are needed. This may well be one role of the motor cortex.

THE EFFECT OF FATIGUE UPON REFLEXES

In general parlance, "fatigue" is understood as a subjective sensation of tiredness, but this is an entirely inadequate definition for the physiologist (the problem of defining fatigue is thoroughly discussed by Simonson [1971, pp. xiii–xvii]). To him, fatigue is a reversible loss of performance capability, or a condition in which increased effort is necessary to avoid a decrement in performance, and the development of this objectified fatigue has been localized as occurring at one or more of four sites: in the muscle; at the neuromuscular synapse; in the afferent fiber and its spinal synapses; and within the CNS itself, particularly within the spinal cord (Schwab and Pritchard, 1951). It is the last two of these sites with which I am concerned in this chapter.

The effects of exercise and fatigue on muscle directly spring from such factors as glycogen, creatine phosphate, and adrenal hormone depletion, deterioration of cardiac performance, ischemia, lactic acid accumulation, and temperature changes (see Simonson, 1971). Many investigators have credited these effects with the responsibility for the fatigue-induced performance decrement, and others have denied it, claiming that that responsibility is the CNS's, but the data discussed by Simonson (1971) would seem to indicate that, depending on circumstances, the dominant source of the performance decrement may be either physical or neural; it may lie in the chemical changes associated with the development of fatigue or it may lie in the less easily defined changes in the CNS. Under most conditions, both sources of decrement probably play a part, but this chapter is focused on that portion of the decrement for which the CNS may be thought responsible.

The CNS sites deserve attention because, while it is definitely possible to fatigue the muscle and the neuromuscular synapse, the fatigue encountered as a limitation of voluntary movement does not appear to reside entirely in these sites. Granted that a fatigued volitional movement may show lengthenings of both movement time and reaction time (muscle and neural effects, respectively) (Sheerer and Berger, 1972), an important source of the decrement can be shown to be neural in origin. As Simonson (1971, pp. 224-228) has discussed, if a person performs a movement to the point of exhaustion, i.e. to the point where he is unable to continue, he can still use the fatigued muscles for other movements and further contractions of the agonist may still be elicited by electrical stimulation of the muscle and its nerve and by evocation of the appropriate tendon reflex. The last of these, in particular, suggests that fatigue of voluntary movement must have at least one of its chief sources within the CNS, but in addition Rascano, et al. (1937) observed that while both the muscle and its nerve may show increases in threshold when fatigued by a voluntary movement, the changes are so irregular that fatigue can be explained only by putting its principal site of development in the CNS.

I have tried to show in the preceding pages that there is reason to regard the motor reflexes as the components of movement. By that token, the effect of fatigue upon volitional movement may perhaps be best understood by examining the effect of fatigue upon reflexes. Such an examination will not only help us localize more precisely the site of development of fatigue of volitional movement, but it will suggest one or two hypothetical answers to questions of fatigue and motor coordination and a way to determine whether reflexes are indeed the language of motor control.

Reflex Fatigue

Reflex fatigue, the fading of a reflex with repeated elicitation, is a phenomenon that has been studied remarkably little since Sherrington first described it at the beginning of this century. This lack of investigation may be because Sherrington described it so well or because few have seen how it could help our understanding of other questions, but it is not a deserved lack. The study of reflex fatigue has a great deal to say concerning the localization of fatigue of volitional movement, as exemplified recently only by Roberts' (1962) finding that *in the earthworm* fatigue of the giant fiber (withdrawal) reflex originates in neither the muscle, the neuromuscular junction, nor the intermotoneuronal junction, but in the junctions of the sensory neurons and the giant fiber and of the giant fiber and the motoneurons. This does not, of course, have any real bearing on fatigue or reflex fatigue in mammals, except to indicate that some of the conclusions that may be drawn for mammals may be general to synaptic nervous systems.

The phenomenon of mammalian reflex fatigue hinges upon Sherrington's (1947, p. 13) basic observation that conduction in the reflex arc is much more "fatiguable" than is conduction in the nerve fiber. Where an axon may fail to respond to an artificial stimulus after, say, 100 trials, a reflex becomes inelicitable after far fewer trials, and the more interneurons, or synapses, are involved in the reflex arc, the more quickly it may become fatigued. Characteristically, as fatigue of a spinal reflex develops under continuous or intermittent elicitation, the reflex's amplitude diminishes, often to zero. The rate of decrease of amplitude (or, rather, the rate of increase of threshold) for the cremasteric (testis elevation) reflex has been shown to depend on the time between successive stimulus presentations, where each stimulus is a brief series of electrical shocks (Fischgold and Bernard, 1935), and it has been observed that reflex fatigue develops more rapidly in spinal than in decerebrate cats (Forbes, 1912).

Sherrington (1947, p. 215) described the development of reflex fatigue for the flexion reflex in the following terms: as the duration of the reflex response increases, the originally steady muscle contraction declines in strength and becomes shaky, showing a tremor rhythm of about 10 per second (this is also a rhythm associated with volitional control; see Aizerman and Andrejeva, 1968); improved reflex contraction and tremor then alternate, with a progressive decline in the strength of the contraction, until the reflex contraction may cease completely, sometimes being replaced by extension; the final phase of flexion reflex fatigue is "an irregular phasic tremor of the muscles." That this fatigue resides neither in the muscles nor in the motoneuron is shown by the observation that muscles which can no longer contract in the service of the flexion reflex can contract in the service of another reflex, such as the scratch reflex.

The scratch reflex (Sherrington, 1947, p. 215-224), which is not a maintained contraction, but rather a rhythmic alternation of flexion and extension, responds to frequent or continuous elicitation by a weakening of the individual beats of its rhythm and a slowing of the rhythm, as well as with a growing irregularity, as indicated in Figure 3-4. Fatigue encroaches on this reflex much more rapidly than on the flexion reflex—there are more interneurons involved—but the scratch reflex can be fatigued for stimulation of only one point of the skin, perhaps for only one receptor, at a time, as illustrated by the observation that shifting the stimulus to a neighboring point two or more cm away renews the vigor of the reflex, though not to the level of the fresh reflex. This reinforces the conclusion from the flex-

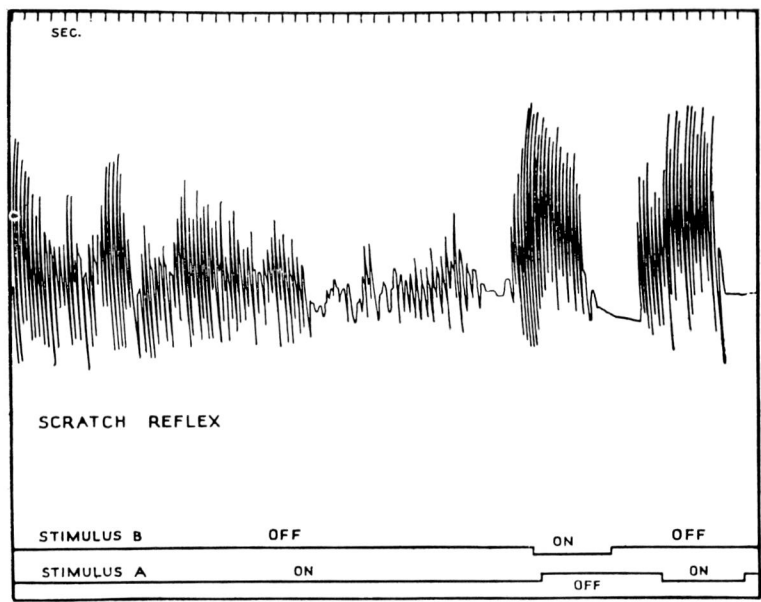

Figure 3-4. Fatigue and recovery of scratch-reflex (From C. S. Sherrington, "Flexion-Reflex of the Limb, Crossed Extension-Reflex, and Reflex Stepping and Standing," *Journal of Physiology, London*, 40:28-121).

ion reflex that fatigue does not reside in the muscles and further suggests that it may lie in the synapse of the afferent neuron with the first interneuron, perhaps in the exhaustion or depletion of neurotransmitter. The mechanism of reflex fatigue may thus be similar to that of neuromuscular fatigue in that it may be referrable to a decrease in the number of neurotransmitter quanta released at the synapse by each neural impulse (see Simonson, 1971, Chap. 10).

It is known that repetitive stimulation of an afferent nerve at frequencies of 1 to 2 Hz results in a fall-off of the motoneuronal response and that this fall-off occurs at the interneuronal level (Horn, 1970). However, although De Robertis (1958) has shown that the synapse is greatly depleted of its vesicles after prolonged intense stimulation, Eccles has discussed experiments indicating that, while the amount of neurotransmitter released by the arrival of an impulse at an afferent or interneuronal synapse on a motoneuron declines during long trains of impulses, the availability of neurotransmitter increases with synaptic activity; the amplitude of the EPSP generated in the motoneuron by a test stimulus following a prolonged synaptic activation shows a slow rise, great prolongation, and an increase in amplitude. Relatively shorter sequences of synaptic activations result chiefly in potentiation of the EPSP, and a question of interest is whether and at what point the rate of rise of the single, unsummated EPSP becomes insufficient, due to accommodation, to trigger an action potential in the motoneuron.

The fact that stimulation of a second receptor does not produce an entirely unfatigued scratch reflex indicates that some portion of the reflex fatigue may lie in the synapses of the interneurons of the reflex arc (see also Simonson, 1971, p. 226, Fig. 57), while the observation that as fatigue progresses other reflexes, such as the extensor thrust in the case of the flexion reflex, may become elicitable or appear spontaneously implies that both facilitatory and inhibitory synapses may become fatigued. In addition, the time to fatigue of a spinal reflex appears to depend upon the strength of stimulation, for increasing the strength of stimulation can revive a previously fatigued reflex, perhaps due to a spread of the stimulus to adjacent receptors and perhaps due to an increase in the number of neural impulses elicited by each stimulus and hence in the amount of neurotransmitter released at the synapse and consequent summation of EPSPs.

It was, however, reported in 1912 that elicitation of a flexion reflex by electrical stimulation of one sensory nerve (saphenous or peroneal) may sometimes impair and sometimes actually facilitate the flexion reflex elicited by stimulation of a second sensory nerve (sciatic or popliteal), the facilitatory effect disappearing above a certain strength of stimulation (Forbes, 1912). Forbes also demonstrated that the crossed inhibitory pathway involved in the flexion reflex could be fatigued and remarked that "The reflex centre is not fatigued as a whole, but merely the particular [interneuronal or synaptic] channel of approach employed." The state of knowledge at that time hardly permitted him to offer a complete explanation of his observations, but it is now possible to suggest that while the fatiguing of a reflex elicited from one nerve by stimulation of another may be due to the synaptic fatigue discussed above, the facilitatory effect may be due to the minutes-long duration of the EPSP elicited after a long train of synaptic activations (Eccles, 1964, p. 98). This thought, however, must not be taken as any more than highly tentative.

The further observation of Sherrington (1947, p. 220) that if several points on the skin are stimulated in rotation then the scratch reflex can be elicited for a much longer period of time without apparent fatigue, though it tends eventually to cease abruptly, suggests a "cascade hypothesis" of reflex—and volitional—fatigue. If we assume that reflex fatigue is indeed due to a failure of transmission at the spinal synapses, to a decrease in the number of quanta of neurotransmitter released by each neural impulse to the point where the consequent EPSP is insufficient to discharge the target neuron, then we can see that a reflex is "fatigued" whenever one synapse in the reflex arc fails to pass on the signal or to maintain the signal's strength. A reflex such as the scratch reflex, which involves several interneurons, only a few of which would be common to the paths from several receptors, will then show precisely the behavior described by Sherrington. As the stimulus point rotates, each receptor and the non-common interneurons will have time to recover, to regenerate completely the neurotransmitter used up in passing one impulse or brief series of impulses, and will not show fatigue. The common interneurons, on the other hand, will be in continuous use, and, since the signal is attenuated at each target cell after many synaptic activations, the smaller number of successive attenuations represented by the common interneurons will mean a longer life for the reflex; the abruptness of the eventual failure of transmission is less easy to explain.

This hypothesis would also, of course, apply to fatigue of volitional movements, for the same convergence of motor pathways onto the interneuron and the motoneuron exists then; if reflexes are the components of volitional movements, the same interneurons may be involved. Furthermore, where several converging pathways each contribute to the threshold depolarization of a target neuron, the failure of transmission in only one pathway or in only one synapse may be all that is needed to prevent firing of the target neuron.

Fatigue and Reflexes

The study of reflex fatigue is not, however, the study of the effect of fatigue upon reflexes, for where the former is a readily definable phenomenon, the latter encompasses many poorly understood situations. Not only is it difficult to define and quantify the entity *fatigue,* but the same term is used to encompass both physical—or neuromuscular—and mental fatigue, the one resulting from muscular effort and at least rudely quantifiable and the other from long-continued attention or wakefulness and hardly at all quantifiable. Cherepakhin's (1968) observation that a converse of fatigue, prolonged bed rest, has no apparent effect upon proprioceptive reflexes, though it does decrease muscle tone, is not entirely atypical of the less sophisticated studies in this area. A number of studies have attempted to deal with the problem, but most have suffered from such drawbacks as a tendency to include physical and mental fatigue in the same investigation, a lack of consistency in their methods of measuring fatigue, and a narrowness of vision that has restricted them largely to investigations of the effects of fatigue upon stretch reflexes, as also discussed by Dr. K. C. Hayes in this volume.

Early reports included the observations of Burge, et al. (1938), that the threshold of the patellar tendon reflex rises with exercise and the development of fatigue, and of Quo (1949), that the thresholds of both patellar and Achilles tendon reflexes rise with the development of physical and mental fatigue (where fatigue was defined as the condition obtaining after a "day's work" of physical or mental labor). Quo felt that this increase of reflex thresholds offered a valuable means of evaluating fatigue, and later investigators have continued the study, often with an eye toward such applications of their findings as evaluating neuromuscular condition (Kroll, 1974)—Lipak (1961), in fact, described a device for registering reflex thresholds and stressed its cheapness and simplicity. There is also some interest in various temporal parameters of the reflexes (e.g. contraction time and half-relaxation time) as indicators of such things as thyroid function (Verdy, et al., 1968).

Tipton and Karpovich (1966), exercising their subjects until they could no longer maintain a cadence on the friction bicycle or continue quadriceps contractions against a 25 pound load, reported that fatigue of either ipsilateral or contralateral quadriceps has the effect of lengthening the patellar reflex time, although reflex facilitation by the Jendrassik maneuver (fist clenching) can reverse the effect. Kroll (1974) confirms these findings in a report that a bench stepping exercise, performed to the point of a 17.4 percent decrement in maximum voluntary quadriceps contraction, results in a small but significant increase in the latency of the patellar tendon reflex and also adds that the Jendrassik maneuver tends to reverse the effect. Henane (1968a,b), using the Harvard step test, has reported that unspecified levels of fatigue have the effect of decreasing the size of the EMG response of the Achilles tendon reflex and the H-reflex (in one of his 12 subjects, the Achilles reflex was inhibited while the H-reflex was facilitated; in another subject, the Achilles reflex was facilitated while the H-reflex was inhibited [Henane, 1968a,c]). Macarez and Henane, using both the Harvard step test and the "cyclo-ergometer," later showed that fatigue increases the thresholds of the Achilles tendon reflex (Macarez and Henane, 1970a) and of the H-reflex (Macarez and Henane, 1970b). One of their control experiments, a test of the muscular response to electrical stimulation after fatigue, indicated that at least part of the effect is attributable to spinal mechanisms (Macarez and Henane, 1970b). Most recently, Henane and Macarez (1972) confirmed these results in a larger study; they again found that discordant tendon and H-reflex responses to fatigue are rare and added that they disappear in any event when exercise is maximal, i.e. when fatigue is extreme; they also reported that after about five minutes the increase of threshold and decrease of amplitude are reversed.

Each of the above findings can be understood in terms of synaptic fatigue, for if reflex stimuli affect the motoneuron less efficiently, thresholds will be raised and latencies will be increased. Even the effect of mental fatigue can be understood in these terms, for it is common experience that mental fatigue is accompanied by increased muscular tension, or increased activity of the synapses in the motor pathway. It is less easy to understand the observation of Tipton and Karpovich (1966) that fatigue of one quadriceps increases the latency of the tendon reflex in the other; perhaps the key may be found in fatigue of the quadriceps' antagonist and of the synapses of the crossed reflex pathway.

It is, however, difficult to explain in the same way the report of Hayes (1973) that when the triceps surae is fatigued by nearly isometric exercise to the point of a 36 percent decrement in the maximal voluntary contraction the latency of the Achilles tendon reflex is possibly shortened, rather than increased, as reported by Tipton and Karpovich (1966) and by Kroll (1974) for the patellar reflex, and the force exerted by the reflex is actually and definitely increased, rather than decreased, as suggested by Henane's (1968b) finding of a diminished Achilles reflex EMG response. Hayes' positing of a compensatory increase in the gamma loop gain may clarify the conflict of his results with those obtained on the patellar reflex, for the triceps surae has a larger population of muscle spindles than the quadriceps, but it cannot do the same for the other observations on the Achilles tendon reflex unless, perhaps, the observed difference in the effects of fatigue induced by isometric exercise and by isotonic exercise (Kroll, 1965a, b) can be attributed in some way to a difference in the effects of this increased gain in the two conditions. One could wish that Hayes had included observations of reflex threshold in his study for the sake of further comparisons, for the conflicts are not entirely resolvable at this point.

No work to speak of has been done on the effect of fatigue on other reflexes other than the study of how fatigue is reflected in the Babinski-Weil test (in which the subject walks forward and backward for six steps; a normal subject changes his direction by no more than 45 degrees), possibly expressing the functioning of the vestibular reflexes, by Rougier, et al. (1961); no effect of fatigue was found. It is, however, apparent that extreme mental fatigue increases the amplitude of several reflexes used in neurological diagnosis, such as the balancing and tendon reflexes (informal, personal observation), and there have been a number of studies of the effect of fatigue upon normal movement with strong implications concerning reflexes. Much of this work has been carried out by F. A. Hellebrandt and her colleagues, most recently at the Motor Learning Research Laboratory of the University of Wisconsin; the bulk of it has been reviewed by Joan Waterland (1967). Their findings are highly interesting, but some skepticism should be reserved for their frequent use of a "functional decortication" to eliminate any interference of cortical activity in their subjects' reflexes and spontaneous patterns of movement; this condition is claimed to obtain when their subjects achieve a "mindless set," perhaps akin to self-hypnosis, either as a willed state of consciousness or as an involuntary concomitant of physical fatigue.

Early studies of the phenomenon of "indirect learning" or "cross education," known since the 1890s, showed that fatigue induced by flexion of a finger of one hand may result, depending on the subject, in either facilitation or inhibition of flexion of the same finger of the opposite hand (Joteyko, 1900) and that repetitive pronation-supination of one arm "as fast and as hard as possible" results in decreased rate of movement and increased amplitude of movement of the opposite arm, effects possibly of central origin (Collier, 1938). More recent studies have shown that isotonic exercise of one muscle is reflected in increased strength and endurance of that muscle, its antagonist, and their contralateral homonyms, and that as stress, or fatigue, mounts, other movements appear besides the one being exercised (Hellebrandt, et al., 1947; Hellebrandt and Waterland, 1962a). It was also found that if two limbs are exercised alternately until the weaker one can go on no more, and that if both limbs are then exercised synchronously, the weaker, fatigued limb then revives and can function in the exercise for a while longer (Hellebrandt, et al., 1950). Since the effects of exercise appear only as fatigue mounts, as the effort exerted by the subject becomes "all out" and he exercises in the "overload zone," it was thought that these effects are the visible results of widespread synergistic cocontractions, perhaps consequent upon reflexes arising in the exercising limb during fatigue.

Kroll (1965a,b), using isometric rather than isotonic exercise (though his fatigue levels were distinctly less than those obtained by Hellebrandt, et al. [1950, 1962a]), sought similar bilateral effects after unilateral fatigue and failed to find them, suggesting that isometric exercise may not activate the muscle receptors responsible for the crossed reflexes which may reverse the effects of fatigue. Thus the responsible receptors almost must be the muscle spindles, which are not stretched by isometric contractions, and it may be that Hayes' (1973) proposed fatigue-compensatory mechanism of gamma loop gain increase may come into play only near the level of fatigue he imposed on his subjects, for if that mechanism does indeed exist, one would expect it to be apparent in conditions of both isometric and isotonic exercise.

The effect of "active pauses," a variable facilitation of recovery from fatigue by exercise of nonfatigued muscles, was discovered by Sechenov (1901) and discussed by Simonson (1971, pp. 456-458). The observation that when the exercising muscles are antagonistic to the fatigued muscles the facilitation is more marked (Foltz, et al., 1942) suggests some relationship of the phenomenon to "indirect learning." It may perhaps indicate that neuronal fatigue may be reversed by reciprocal inhibition, or it may only indicate that the increased muscular blood flow sustained by exercise hastens recovery from muscular fatigue.

The idea expressed earlier in this chapter that the TNR may lend a facilitatory influence to volitional effort gains further support from the work of Hellebrandt, et al. (1956) and Hellebrandt and Waterland (1962b), who described the TNR in normal human subjects together with some methods of evoking it (Hellebrandt, et al., 1962). They found that when a subject, attached to an ergograph, was lifting a load either by extension or by flexion of the wrist, the work output could be either increased or decreased by voluntary rotation or flexion of the head so as to evoke a TNR supporting or opposing the action needed to do the work, i.e. if the load were lifted by wrist flexion, then more work could be obtained with the head ventriflexed or rotated away from the exercising arm; if by extension, then more work could be obtained with dorsiflexion or rotation toward the exercising arm. If the exercise were prolonged to the point of stress, i.e. to the point where fatigue was so great that the subject was using maximal effort, then not only were the above effects more pronounced, but spontaneous posturing was observed as well. The assumed postures included the TNR pattern and movement of the other limbs, especially the opposite arm, and seemed to be such that, alone, they would tend to produce or facilitate reflexively movements of the same kind as those involved in the exercise.

Later studies (Waterland, Doudlah, and Shambes, 1966; Waterland and Hellebrandt, 1964; Waterland and Munson, 1964b; Waterland and Shambes, 1970) indicated the possibility that the tonic neck pattern may include definite shoulder girdle postures. The observed postures, in conditions of fatigue and deliberate "functional decortication," included an association with volitional ventriflexion of shoulder girdle protraction and spinal flexion; with volitional dorsiflexion, of retraction and extension; with bending of the head to one side, of shoulder depression on that side and elevation on the other; and with rotation of the head to one side, of shoulder retraction and elevation on that side, with arm abduction. There was also reason to think that the pelvic girdle was involved in these reflex responses to movement of the head and neck, and there were indications that the effects were two-way; that is, movements of the shoulder girdle and arms seemed to be causally associated with changes in head position. Indeed, their work, together with that of Hellebrandt and Waterland (1962a), has suggested the possible identification of a hitherto unsuspected reflex linking neck, shoulder girdle, and arm musculature, including a possible link of forearm pronation and supination with shoulder protraction and depression and head and neck ventriflexion and contralateral rotation, and with shoulder protraction and elevation, head dorsiflexion and contralateral rotation, and vertebral extension, respectively (Waterland and Munson, 1964a). It is not, however, necessary to conclude from these observations that reflexes arising in a fatigued arm regulate the posture of the head, evoking the TNR which in turn expedites the performance of the exercise, as suggested by these authors.

The observation that bimanual exercise can counter unimanual fatigue (Hellebrandt, et al., 1950) suggests that if the CNS does compose volitional movements out of reflexes and complex reflexes out of simpler ones, then when the command lines to the component reflexes of a movement, or to their controlling centers, are saturated by effort or fatigue, and more effort is required, the appropriate level of the CNS may call upon other reflexes using the same component reflexes but with additional command lines to them. According to the above results, the consequent increase in strength and endurance, and in motor patterning, in the involvement of additional muscles, is the same whether the complex reflex is called upon volitionally or spontaneously, and it matters little whether the reinforcement so obtained is applied to a movement composed of reflexes or to one composed of some other basic units. There is little or no evidence in the literature for the conclusion of Hellebrandt and her colleagues that complex reinforcing reflexes arise from exercising muscles, while there is some reason to believe the alternative possibility.

This calling up of additional reflexes to strengthen a movement might, as I have suggested before (Easton, 1972b), perhaps be termed *reflex recruitment,* in analogy with motoneuronal recruitment. The observation that bimanual exercise makes it possible to use again a muscle fatigued to exhaustion in unimanual exercise certainly suggests that synapses other than those whose capabilities have been fatigued can be activated by the reciprocal concomitants of activation of contralateral muscles (perhaps according to the schemes described by Holmqvist [1961]). That additional reflexes do indeed make it possible to contract a muscle fatigued to the point where it may no longer be contracted volitionally is also indicated by the observation of Schwab and Prichard (1951) that a "vigorous patellar reflex" can then still be elicited, and by the observations of Tipton and Karpovich (1966) and of Kroll (1974) that the Jendrassik maneuver reverses the fatigue-induced lengthening of the patellar reflex latency and of Hayes (1973) that this maneuver can increase the force exerted by the Achilles tendon reflex.

Reflex recruitment could work because a motoneuron is influenced by many interneurons, each one of which has its own synapses with the motoneuron, and because each reflex must use different interneurons, if not at the pre-motoneuronal stage, then at some earlier one. Thus, because the site of the kind of fatigue involved in the above cases would seem to lie in the synapses which transmit the commands to movement, the effects of fatigue may be circumvented by using different synapses, different interneurons, and different reflexes. Denny-Brown's (1966) report of reflex availability preceding voluntary motor abilities suggests that, indeed, either reflexes are summoned as necessary aids to movement—are *recruited,* in other words—or their control centers and command lines must exist before voluntary movement can occur, implying that the various reflexes and their interneurons can and do act as additional pathways that may be used to add strength to a command.

Thus stretch reflexes may be called upon to reinforce muscle contractions weakened by fatigue, as suggested by Hayes (1973), and the TNR and crossed flexion and extension reflexes may be summoned to the aid of a fatigue-weakened movement. The observation of Schaffer (1954) that when a person is fatigued or stressed his movements take on a stereotyped air may be due not to any shift in motor control from cortical to subcortical centers, as he suggested, but to the recruitment of more reflexes than are used in the composition of the basic movement, and hence to a fixed expansion of motor patterning along the lines dictated by the additional, recruited reflexes. It is also possible, of course, that the appearance of movements and movement patterns other than that one being exercised is due to a lessened inhibition of the extraneous portions of the reflexes that are used, but the effect of fatigue remains such that the effect of fatigue upon voluntary movement must be understood as a matter of slowing, weakening, and compensatory expansion of the motor pattern, much as we can all see from personal experience.

Suggestions for Research

It is apparent that the topics of reflex fatigue and fatigue effects on reflexes have serious implications both for each other and for the study of how volitional movement is controlled. Before these implications can be adequately explored, however, the precise mechanisms of reflex fatigue must be ascertained. If synaptic fatigue, a depletion of the synaptic vesicles and the neurotransmitter they carry, indeed plays a part, then we have an immediate and strong hypothesis that synaptic fatigue may underlie the central component of fatigue of volitional movement. That volitional fatigue has been reported to be associated with fading of reflex EMG response (Henane, 1968b), raising of reflex thresholds (Macarez and Henane, 1970a), and lengthening of reflex times (Tipton and Karpovich, 1966) certainly suggests some phenomenological similarity of the two processes. They are not identical, of course, for volitional fatigue does not provoke an entirely parallel reflex fatigue; when a muscle cannot be contracted volitionally, it can be contracted reflexively. The conflicts in the presently available data mean principally that the effect of volitional fatigue on tendon reflexes—and on other reflexes—needs more precise determination, more consistent definitions and measurements of fatigue, greater consistency of the tendon reflex characteristics observed, and more consistent use of comparable levels of fatigue.

It is much more significant, however, that investigators of this problem have studied only the effect of volitional fatigue on reflexes. No one has yet fatigued a reflex and examined consequent changes, if any, in a volitional movement, although it would be relatively simple to invert Hayes' (1975) experiment, elicit repetitively the Achilles tendon reflex until it is fatigued, and ask whether there is then any change in the force of the maximum voluntary contraction of the triceps surae, or in the latency, speed, or smoothness of the voluntary contraction. It would also be useful to observe the function of the muscle in such normal activities as walking after reflex fatigue. Similarly, other reflexes, such as the flexion and scratch reflexes, as well as—if possible—the tonic neck, long spinal, and vestibular reflexes, could be fatigued in animals or man and consequent changes in volitional movements using the same synergic groups of muscles could be observed. The results of such experiments could well reveal not only whether reflexes and volitional movements use the same, fatiguable interneurons, but also whether and which reflexes are components of volitional movements and at which interneuronal level volitional movements are composed from reflexes.

SUMMARY AND CONCLUSIONS

There is a wealth of simple movements—the reflexes—which have obvious purpose, or adaptiveness, and are available for the CNS to use in the construction of more complex volitional movements. These reflexes are not entities appearing only when isolated portions of the CNS are examined—they exist, as reflexes, in the normal, healthy, intact animal, though they are sometimes demonstrable only with special techniques (as in Easton, 1971, 1972a; Hellebrandt, Schade, and Carns, 1962), and patterns coincident with the patterns of these reflexes may be seen in normal motor activities. Furthermore, these reflexes—or the interneurons that control them—may be facilitated and inhibited by the higher centers of the CNS and may well be subject to flexible organization into more complex movements through ordering, summing, fragmentation, and their "local sign" properties. It may thus be hypothesized that the reflexes do underlie normal motor function, though it should also be kept in mind very carefully that this does not mean that normal motor function may not be achieved without the reflexes.

It is possible, as I have shown elsewhere (Easton, 1972b), to construct a functional tree, as in Figure 3-5, consisting of an executive function which may specify a movement in broad terms and lower levels which may suc-

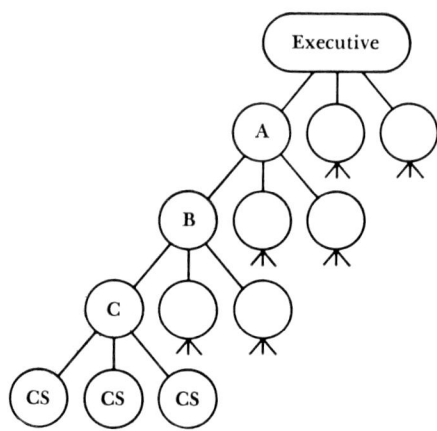

Figure 3-5. The central nervous system schematized as a hierarchy. The "tree" may be considered to pertain to either CNS function or its anatomy (From Easton, 1972b, Copyright © 1972 by The Society of the Sigma Xi).

cessively elaborate the broad instruction until a specific set of reflexes, or "coordinative structures" (CSs), is activated, with the elements of this set in the appropriate order. It is also possible to attribute the anatomy and reflexes to the levels of this tree, as in Table 3-II, to reveal parallel hierarchies of complexity whose regularity and order leave little to be desired: local spinal reflexes, such as the flexion reflex, appear to be subsumed by re-

TABLE 3-II

Tree Level	CNS Equivalent	Attributed Reflexes
Executive	Cerebral cortex	Command decisions; conditioned reflexes; placing and supporting reactions
A	Midbrain	Proprioceptive placing; hopping reaction; grasp reflex; jump reflex; locomotion; positional, acceleratory, and righting reflexes
B	Pons and medulla	Tonic neck and labyrinthine reflexes; long spinal reflexes
C	Spinal cord, extended	Long spinal reflexes (under strychnine); shake and scratch reflexes
CS	Spinal cord, local	Flexion, crossed extension, extensor thrust, clasp knife, Philippson's, and stretch reflexes

Attributions of anatomy and reflexes to the hierarchy tree of Figure 3-5. The labels in the left-hand column correspond to the labels on the levels of the tree in Figure 3-5. Copyright © 1972 by The Society of the Sigma Xi. From T. A. Easton, "On the Normal Use of Reflexes," *American Scientist, 60*:591-599, 1972.

flexes requiring an intact spinal cord, such as the scratch and long spinal reflexes, and these in turn are subsumed by pontine and medullary reflexes such as the tonic neck and vestibular reflexes, and, at still higher levels, by locomotion and righting.

The crucial point of this chapter, however, is not the hierarchical organization of motor coordination, but the use of reflexes in normal coordination revealed by several studies of fatigue effects. The implication is strong that reflexes play an important role, at least in the reinforcement of fatigued movements and possibly in the strengthening and patterning of unfatigued movements. This in turn leads to hypotheses of *reflex recruitment* and of reflexes as components of movement that may be supportable or disprovable by experiments extending some of the recent work on the effect of fatigue upon reflexes. The study of the central nervous system component of fatigue may thus be crucial to a modern understanding of motor coordination.

BIBLIOGRAPHY

Amassian, V. E., H. Weiner, and M. Rosenblum: Neural systems subserving the tactile placing reaction: A model for the study of higher level control of movement, *Brain Res, 40*:171-178, 1972.

Aizerman, M. A., and E. A. Andrejeva: *On Some Control Mechanisms of Skeletal Muscles,* Institute of Automation and Telemechanics, Moscow, USSR, 1968.

Andersen, P., and T. A. Sears: Medullary activation of intercostal fusimotor and alpha motoneurones. *J Physiol London, 209*:739-755, 1970.

Aoyama, M., T. Hongo, N. Kudo, and R. Tanaka: Convergent effects from bilateral vestibulospinal tracts on spinal interneurons. *Brain Res, 35*:250-253, 1971.

Appelberg, B., and F. Emonet-Denand: Central control of static and dynamic sensitivities of muscle spindle primary endings. *Acta Physiol Scand, 63*:487-494, 1965.

Asanuma, H., S. D. Stoney, Jr., and W. D. Thompson: Characteristics of cervical interneurones which mediate cortical motor outflow to distal forelimb muscles of cats. *Brain Res, 27*:79-95, 1971.

―――, and J. E. Ward: Patterns of contraction of distal forelimb muscles produced by intracortical stimulation in cats. *Brain Res 27*:97-109, 1971.

Barcroft, J., D. H. Barron, and W. F. Windle: Some observations on genesis of somatic movements in sheep embryos. *J Physiol London, 87*:73-78, 1936.

Belenkii, V. Ye., V. S. Gurfinkel', and Ye. I. Pal'tsev: Elements of control of voluntary movements. *Biofizika, 12*:154-161, 1967.

Bernhard, C. G., and E. Bohm: Cortical representation and functional significance of the corticomotoneuronal system. *A.M.A. Arch Neurol Psychiat, 72*:473-502, 1954.

Bieber, I., and J. F. Fulton: Relation of the cerebral cortex to the grasp reflex and to postural and righting reflexes. *A.M.A. Arch Neurol Psychiat, 39*:433-454, 1938.

Bishop, A.: Control of the hand in lower primates. *Ann NY Acad Sci, 102*:316-337, 1962.

Bosma, J. F., and E. Gellhorn; The organization of the motor cortex of the monkey based on electromyographic studies. *Brain, 70*:127-144, 1947.

Burge, W. E., R. Krouse, H. L. Terry, and E. L. Burge: The effect of exercise, fatigue, and exhaustion on the electrical potential of the brain cortex and threshold of the knee jerk. *Res Quart, 9,* No. *3*:45-53, 1938.

Cherepakhin, M. A.: Effect of prolonged bed rest on the muscle tone and proprioceptive reflexes of a healthy man. *Kosm Biol Med, 2*:43-47, 1968.

Clough, J. F. M., D. Kernell, and C. G. Phillips: The distribution of monosynaptic excitation from the pyramidal tract and from primary spindle afferents to motoneurones of the baboon's hand and forearm. *J Physiol London, 198*:145-166, 1968.

Coghill, G. E.: *Anatomy and the Problem of Behavior*. New York, Macmillan, 1929.

Cohen, L. A.: Role of eye and neck proprioceptive mechanisms in body orientation and motor coordination. *J. Neurophysiol, 24*:1-11, 1961.

Collier, R. M.: The crossed effects upon voluntary movement of a unilaterally induced fatigue. *J Exp Psychol, 23*:26-44, 1938.

Creed, R. S., D. E. Denny-Brown, J. C. Eccles, E. G. T. Liddell, and C. S. Sherrington: *Reflex Activity of the Spinal Cord*. Fair Lawn, Oxford Pr, 1932.

Decker, J. D., and V. Hamburger: The influence of different brain regions on periodic motility of the chick embryo. *J Exp Zool, 165*:371-384, 1967.

Denny-Brown, D. E.: *The Cerebral Control of Movement*. Springfield, Thomas, 1966.

De Robertis, E.: Submicroscopic morphology and function of the synapse. *Exp Cell Res*, Suppl., *5*:347-369, 1958.

Duffield, D. W.: A study of the effects of direct pyramidal stimulation on some thoracic spinal cord reflexes in the dog, Ph.D. dissertation, University of Missouri, 1970.

Easton, T. A.: Patterned inhibition from horizontal eye movement in the cat. *Exp Neurol, 31*:419-430, 1971.

———: Patterned inhibition from single eye muscle stretch in the cat. *Exp Neurol, 34*:497-510, 1972a.

———: On the normal use of reflexes. *Am Sci, 60*:591-599, 1972b.

Eccles, J. C.: *The Physiology of Synapses*. New York, Acad Pr, 1964.

Eccles, R. M., and A. Lundberg: Supraspinal control of interneurones mediating spinal reflexes. *J Physiol London, 147*:565-584, 1959.

Fidone, S. J., and J. B. Preston: Inhibitory resetting of resting discharges of fusimotor neurons. *J Neurophysiol, 34*:217-227, 1971.

Fischgold, H., and J. Bernard: Mesure de la fatigue des centres réflexes medullaires. *Comptes Rendus Soc Biol, 120*:710-712, 1935.

Foltz, E., A. C. Ivy, and C. J. Barborka: Use of double work periods in study of fatigue and influence of caffeine on recovery. *Am J Physiol, 136*:79, 1942.

Forbes, A.: The place of incidence of reflex fatigue. *Am J Physiol, 31*:102-124, 1912.

Fukuda, T.: Studies on human dynamic postures from the viewpoint of postural reflexes. *Acta Oto-Laryngologica, suppl. 161,* 1961.

Fulton, J. F., C. F. Jacobsen, and M. A. Kennard: A note concerning the relation of the frontal lobes to posture and forced grasping in monkeys. *Brain, 55*:524-536, 1932.

Gazzaniga, M. S.: Visumotor integration in split-brain monkeys with other cerebral lesions. *Exp. Neurol, 16*:289-298, 1966.

———: Cross-cuing mechanisms and ipsilateral eye-hand control in split-brain monkeys. *Exp Neurol, 23*:11-17, 1969a.

———: Eye position and visual motor coordination. *Neuropsychologia, 7*:379-382, 1969b.

Gelfand, I. M., V. S. Gurfinkel, S. V. Fomin, and M. L. Tsetlin (eds.): *Models of the Structural-Functional Organization of Certain Biological Systems*. Translated by Carol R. Beard. Cambridge, MIT Press, 1971.

Gellhorn, E.: Proprioception and the motor cortex. *Brain, 72:*35-62, 1949.

―――, and D. A. Johnson: Further studies on the role of proprioception in cortically induced movements of the foreleg in the monkey. *Brain, 73:*513-531, 1950.

Gernandt, B. E., and D. Megirian: Ascending proprio-spinal mechanisms. *J Neurophysiol, 24:*364-376, 1961.

―――, and M. Shimamura: Mechanisms of interlimb reflexes in cat. *J Neurophysiol, 24:*665-676, 1961.

Gilman, S., and W. I. McDonald: Cerebellar facilitation of muscle spindle activity. *J Neurophysiol, 30:*1494-1512, 1967.

Gottlieb, G. L., G. C. Agarwal, and L. Stark: Interactions between voluntary and postural mechanisms of the human motor system. *J Neurophysiol, 33:*365-381, 1970.

Graham-Brown, T.: The intrinsic factors in the act of progression in the mammal. *Proc Roy Soc Lond Biol, 84:*308-319, 1911.

―――, and C. S. Sherrington: The rule of reflex response in the limb reflexes of the mammal and its exceptions. *J Physiol London, 44:*125-130, 1912.

Granit, R.: *The Basis of Motor Control.* New York, Acad Pr, 1970.

Grigg, P.: Motor cortex modulation of knee flexor and extensor fusimotor neurons in the "pyramidal" cat. *Brain Res, 48:*390-393, 1972.

―――, and J. B. Preston: Baboon flexor and extensor fusimotor neurons and their modulation by motor cortex. *J Neurophysiol, 34:*428-436, 1971.

Grillner, S., T. Hongo, and S. Lund: Descending monosynaptic and reflex control of γ-motoneurones. *Acta Physiol Scand, 75:*592-613, 1969.

Guzman, F. C., and E. C. Del Pozo: "Jump reflex" in hypothalamic cat. *J Neurophysiol, 16:*376-380. 1953.

Hagbarth, K.-E.: Excitatory and inhibitory skin areas for flexor and extensor motoneurones. *Acta Physiol Scand, 26: suppl 94,* 1952.

Halverson, H. M.: An experimental study of prehension in infants by means of systematic cinema records. *Genet Psychol Monogr, 10:*107-284, 1931.

Hamburger, V.: Some aspects of the embryology of behaviour. *Quart Rev Biol, 38:*342-365, 1963.

―――, E. Wenger and R. Oppenheim: Motility in the chick embryo in the absence of sensory input. *J Exp Zool, 162:*133-160, 1966.

Hart, B. L.: Facilitation by strychnine of reflex walking in spinal dogs. *Physiol Behav, 6:*627-628, 1971.

Hayes, K. C.: Effect of serial isometric contractions with varied rest intervals upon reaction and reflex time components, Ph.D. dissertation, University of Massachusetts at Amherst, 1973.

Hellebrandt, F. A., S. J. Houtz, and A. M. Krikorian: Influence of bimanual exercise on unilateral work capacity. *J Appl Physiol, 2:*446-452, 1950.

―――, ―――, M. J. Partridge, and C. E. Walters: Tonic neck reflexes in exercises of stress in man. *Am J Phys Med, 35:*144-159, 1956.

―――, A. M. Parrish, and S. J. Houtz: Cross education: The influence of unilateral exercise on the contralateral limb. *Arch Phys Med, 28:*76-85, 1947.

―――, M. Schade, and M. L. Carns: Methods of evoking the tonic neck reflexes in normal human subjects. *Am J Phys Med, 41:*90-139, 1962.

―――, and J. C. Waterland: Indirect learning: The influence of unimanual exercise on related muscle groups of the same and the opposite side. *Am J Phys Med, 41:*45-55, 1962a.

———, and ———: Expansion of motor patterning under exercise stress. *Am J Phys Med, 41*:56-66, 1962b.

Henane, R.: Exercice musculaire et réflectivité spinale chez l'Homme. *J Physiol (Paris), 60*:457-458, 1968a.

———: Exercice musculaire sous-maximal et réflectivité spinale chez l'Homme. I. Variations concordantes des réponses tendineuse et de Hoffman. *Comptes Rendus Soc Biol, 162*:698-702, 1968b.

———: Exercice musculaire et réflectivité spinale chez l'Homme. II. Variations discordantes des réponses tendineuses et de Hoffman. *Comptes Rendus Soc Biol, 162*: 1354-1358, 1968c.

———, and J. A. Macarez: Effets de l'exercice physique sur la réflectivité spinale chez l'Homme. *Internat Z angew Physiol, 30*:315-334, 1972.

Holmqvist, B.: Crossed spinal reflex actions evoked by volleys in somatic afferents. *Acta Physiol Scand, 52: suppl 181,* 1961.

———, and A. Lundberg: On the organization of the supraspinal inhibitory control of interneurones of various spinal reflex arcs. *Arch ital Biol, 97*:340-356, 1959.

———, and ———: Differential supraspinal control of synaptic actions evoked by volleys in the flexion reflex afferents in alpha motoneurones. *Acta Physiol Scand, 54: suppl 186,* 1961.

———, ———, and O. Oscarsson: Supraspinal inhibitory control of transmission to 3 ascending spinal pathways influenced by the flexion reflex afferents. *Arch ital Biol, 98:* 60-80, 1960a.

———, ———, and ———: A supraspinal control system monosynaptically connected with an ascending spinal pathway. *Arch ital Biol, 98*:402-422, 1960b.

Hongo, T., and E. Jankowska: Effects from the sensorimotor cortex on the spinal cord in cats with transected pyramids. *Exp Brain Res, 3*:117-134, 1967.

———, ———, and A. Lundberg: Effects evoked from the rubrospinal tract in cats. *Experientia, 21*:525-526, 1965.

———, N. Kudo, and R. Tanaka: Effects from the vestibulospinal tract on the contralateral hindlimb motoneurones in the cat. *Brain Res, 31*:220-223, 1971.

Horn, G.: Changes in neuronal activity and their relationship to behavior. In Horn, G., and Hinde, R. A. (Eds.): *Short-Term Changes in Neural Activity and Behavior.* Cambridge, Cambridge University Press, 1970, pp. 567-606.

Hyde, J., and E. Gellhorn: Influence of deafferentation on stimulation of motor cortex. *Am J Physiol, 156*:311-316, 1949.

Ito, T., and Y. Sanada: Location of receptors for righting reflexes acting upon the body in primates. *Jap J Physiol, 15*:235-242, 1965.

Jacobs, M. J.: Development of normal motor behavior. *Am J Phys Med, 46*:41-51, 1967.

Joteyko, J.: Participation des centres nerveux dans les phenomenes de fatigue musculaire. *Annee Psychol, 7*:161-165, 1900.

Kato, M., and J. Tanji: The effects of electrical stimulation of Deiter's nucleus upon hindlimb γ-motoneurons in the cat. *Brain Res, 30*:385-395, 1971.

Kennard, M. A., H. R. Viets, and J. F. Fulton: The syndrome of the premotor cortex in man: impairment of skilled movements, forced grasping, spasticity, and vasomotor disturbance. *Brain, 57*:69-84, 1934.

Klemm, W. R.: Neurophysiologic studies of the immobility reflex ('animal hypnosis'). In Ehrenpreis, S., and Solnitzky, O. C. (Eds.): *Neurosciences Research.* New York, Acad Pr, 1971, Vol. 4, pp. 165-212.

Kostyuk, P. G., and D. Vasilenko: Transformation of cortical motor signals in spinal cord. *Proc IEEE, 56*:1049-1958, 1968.

Kots, Ya. M.: Supraspinal control of spinal centers for antagonist muscles in man. 1. Reflex excitability of motoneurones to antagonist muscles during voluntary movement. *Biofizika, 14*:167-172, 1969.

———, and V. A. Mart'yanov: Cutting out the vestibulo-spinal influences in the period of organization of voluntary movement. *Biofizika, 13*:958-967, 1968.

Kroll, W.: Central facilitation in bilateral *versus* unilateral isometric contractions. *Am J Phys Med, 44*:218-223, 1965a.

———: Isometric cross-transfer effects under conditions of central facilitation. *J Appl Physiol, 20*:297-300, 1965b.

———: Fractionated reaction and reflex time before and after fatiguing isotonic exercise. In press, 1974.

Kuno, M., and E. R. Perl: Alteration of spinal reflexes by interaction with suprasegmental and dorsal root activity. *J Physiol London, 151*:103-122, 1960.

Laursen, A. M., and M. Wiesendanger: Pyramidal effect on alpha and gamma motoneurons. *Acta Physiol Scand, 67*:165-172, 1966a.

———, and ———: Motor deficits after transection of a bulbar pyramid in the cat. *Acta Physiol Scand, 68*:118-126, 1966b.

Lawrence, D. G., and H. G. J. M. Kuypers: The functional organization of the motor system in the monkey. I. The effects of bilateral pyramidal lesions. *Brain, 91*:1-14, 1968a.

———, and ———: The functional organization of the motor system in the monkey. II. The effects of lesions of the descending brainstem pathways. *Brain, 91*:15-36, 1968b.

Lipak, J.: A reflexometric method for the study of fatigue. *Ideggyogyaszati Szemle, 14*:300-304, 1961.

Lisin, V. V., S. I. Frankstein, and M. B. Rechtmann: The influence of locomotion on flexor reflex of the hind limb in cat and man. *Exp Neurol, 38*:180-183, 1973.

Lloyd, D. P. C.: The spinal mechanism of the pyramidal system in cats. *J Neurophysiol, 4*:525-546, 1941.

Loofbourrow, G. N., and E. Gellhorn: Proprioceptively induced reflex patterns. *Am J Physiol, 154*:433-438, 1948.

———, and ———: Proprioceptive modifications of reflex patterns. *J Neurophysiol, 12*:435-446, 1949.

Lund, J. P., R. S. McLachlan, and P. G. Dellow: A lateral jaw movement reflex. *Exp Neurol, 31*:189-199, 1971.

Lundberg, A.: Integration in the reflex pathway. In Granit, R. (Ed.): *Muscular Afferents and Motor Control*, New York, Wiley, pp. 275-305, 1966.

———: *Reflex Control of Stepping*. Oslo, Universitetsforlaget, 1969.

———, U. Norrsell, and P. Voorhoeve: Pyramidal effects on lumbo-sacral interneurones activated by somatic afferents. *Acta Physiol Scand, 56*:220-229, 1962.

———, and P. Voorhoeve: Pyramidal activation of interneurones of various reflex arcs in the cat. *Experientia, 17*:46-47, 1961.

———, and ———: Effects from the pyramidal tract on spinal reflex arcs. *Acta Physiol Scand, 56*:201-219, 1962.

Macarez, J. A., and R. Henane: Influence d'un exercice musculaire sous-maximal sur les seuils des réflexes monosynaptiques chez l'Homme. I. Effets sur les seuils des réponses tendineuses. *Comptes Rendus Soc Biol, 164*:1524-1528, 1970a.

———, and ———: Influence d'un exercice musculaire sous-maximal sur les seuils des réflexes monosynaptiques chez l'Homme. II. Effets sur les seuils du réflexe de Hoffman. *Comptes Rendus Soc Biol, 164*:1743-1747, 1970b.

McCouch, G. P., I. D. Deering, and T. H. Ling: Location of receptors for tonic neck reflexes. *J Neurophysiol, 14*:191-195, 1951.

———, C. N. Liu, W. W. Chambers and R. Tarnecki: The early phase of reflex activity after spinal cord transection. *Exp Neurol, 33*:88-92, 1971.

Magni, F., and O. Oscarsson: Cerebral control of transmission to the ventral spino-cerebellar tract. *Arch ital Biol, 99*:369-396, 1961.

Maling, H. M., and G. H. Acheson: Righting and other postural activity in low-decerebrate and in spinal cats after D-amphetamine. *J Neurophysiol, 9*:379-386, 1946.

Manni, E., H. D. Henatsch, Eva-M. Henatsch, and R. S. Dow: Localization of facilitatory and inhibitory sites in and around the cerebellar nuclei affecting limb posture, alpha and gamma motoneurons. *J Neurophysiol, 27*:210-228, 1964.

Meier-Ewert, K., U. Huemme, and J. Dahm: New evidence favoring long loop reflexes in man. *Arch Psychiatr Nervenkr, 215*:121-128, 1972.

Meyer, D. L., K.-P. Schaefer, and A. Winkelmann: Interaction of acoustic and vestibular afferent activity observed in ear muscles. *Z Neurol, 200*:213-218, 1971.

———, ———, and ———: Single unit responses of rabbit ear-muscles to postural and accelerative stimulation. *Exp Brain Res, 14*:118-126, 1972.

Mori, S., and A. Matsumoto: The effects of stimulation of nerves to neck muscle upon flexor reflex in the forelimb. *Brain Res, 43*:645-648, 1972.

Nyberg-Hansen, R.: Functional organization of descending supraspinal fibre systems to the spinal cord. Anatomical observations and physiological correlations. *Ergebnisse der Anatomie und Entwicklungsgeschichte,* Band 39, Heft 2, 1966.

Orlovskii, G. N.: Spontaneous and induced locomotion of the thalamic cat. *Biofizika, 14*: 1154-1162, 1969.

———, and G. A. Pavlova: Response of Deiters' neurons to tilt during locomotion. *Brain Res, 42*:212-214, 1972.

Oscarsson, O.: Functional organization of the ventral spino-cerebellar tract in the cat. III. Supraspinal control of VSCT units of I-type. *Acta Physiol Scand, 49*:171-183, 1960.

———: Functional organization of the spino- and cuneo-cerebellar tracts. *Physiol Rev, 45*:495-522, 1965.

Pacella, B. L., and S. E. Barrera: Postural reflexes and grasp phenomena in infants. *J Neurophysiol, 3*:213-218, 1940.

Pal'tsev, Ye. I.: Interaction of the tendon reflex arcs in the lower limbs in man as a reflexion of locomotor synergism. *Biofizika, 12*:1048-1059, 1967.

———, and A. M. El'ner: Preparatory and compensatory period during voluntary movement in patients with involvement of the brain of different localization. *Biofizika, 12*:161-168, 1967.

Peterson, B. W., and L. P. Felpel: Excitation and inhibition of reticulospinal neurons by vestibular, cortical and cutaneous stimulation. *Brain Res, 27*:373-376, 1971.

Philippson, M.: L'autonomie et la centralisation dans le systéme nerveux des animaux. *Trav Lab Physiol Inst Solvay (Bruxelles), 7*:5-208, 1905.

Pollock, L. J., B. Boshes, I. Zivin, S. W. Pyzik, J. R. Finkle, E. L. Tigay, B. H. Kesert, A. J. Arieff, I. Finkelman, M. Brown, and N. B. Dobin: Body reflexes acting on the body. *AMA Arch Neurol Psychiat, 74*:527-533, 1955.

Quo, Sung-Ken: A new method of measuring fatigue by the threshold stimulus of the Achilles tendon reflex. *J Appl Physiol, 2:*148-154, 1949.

Ranson, S. W., and S. L. Clark: *The Anatomy of the Nervous System,* 10th ed. Philadelphia, Saunders, 1959.

Rascano, V., M. Kapri, and V. Busila: Variation de l'excitabilite neuro-musculaire sous l'influence de la fatigue musculaire chez l'Homme. *Comptes Rendus Soc Biol, 126:* 824-826, 1937.

Richter, C. P., and L. H. Bartemeir: Decerebrate rigidity in the sloth. *Brain, 49:*207-225, 1926.

———, and M. Hines: Experimental production of the grasp reflex in adult monkeys by lesions of the frontal lobes. *Am J Physiol, 101:*87-88, 1932.

Riss, W.: Introduction to a general theory of spinal organization. *Brain Behav Evol, 2:* 51-82, 1969.

Roberts, M. B. V.: The giant fibre reflex of the earthworm Lumbricus terrestris L. II. Fatigue. *J Exp Biol, 39:*229-237, 1962.

Roberts, T. D. M.: *Neurophysiology of Postural Mechanism.* Reading, Maine, Butterworth, 1967.

Rougier, G., Y. Linquette, and R. Joly: L'epreuve de Babinski-Weil peut-elle servir de test d'entrainement et de fatigue. *Arch Mal Prof, 22:*783-784, 1961.

Schaefer, K.-P., D. L. Meyer, and D. Schott: Optic and vestibular influences on ear movements. *Brain Behav Evol, 4:*323-333, 1971.

Schaffer, H. R.: Behavior under stress: A neurophysiological hypothesis. *Psychol Rev, 61:*323-333, 1954.

Schwab, R. S., and J. S. Prichard: Neurologic aspects of fatigue. *Neurol, 1:*133-135, 1951.

Sechenov, I. M.: *Ocherk Rabochikh Dvizhenii Cheloveka* (Outline of the Working Movements of Man), 1901 (Russ.)

Severin, F. V., M. L. Shik, and G. N. Orlovskii: Work of the muscles and single motor neurones during controlled locomotion. *Biofizika, 12:*762-772, 1967.

Shambes, G. M.: Influence of the fusimotor system on stance and volitional movement in normal man. *Am J Phys Med, 48:*225-236, 1969.

Sheerer, N., and R. A. Berger: Effects of various levels of fatigue on reaction time and movement time. *Am Corr Ther J, 26:*146-147, 1972.

Sherrington, C. S.: Flexion-reflex of the limb, crossed extension-reflex, and reflex stepping and standing. *J Physiol London, 40:*28-121, 1910.

———: *The Integrated Action of the Nervous System.* New Haven, Yale U Pr, 1947.

Shik, M. L., G. N. Orlovskii, and F. V. Severin: Organization of locomotor synergism. *Biofizika, 11:*1011-1019, 1966.

———, ———, and ———: Locomotion of the mesencephalic cat elicited by stimulation of the pyramids. *Biofizika, 13:*143-152, 1968.

———, F. V. Severin, and G. N. Orlovskii: Control of walking and running by means of electrical stimulation of the mid-brain. *Biofizika, 11:*756-765, 1966.

Shimamura, M., and K. Akert: Peripheral nervous relations of propriospinal and spinobulbo-spinal reflex systems. *Jap J Physiol, 15:*638-647, 1965.

———, and R. B. Livingston: Longitudinal conduction systems serving spinal and brain-stem coordination. *J Neurophysiol, 26:*258-272, 1963.

Shimazu, H., T. Hongo, and K. Kubota: Two types of central influences on gamma motor system. *J Neurophysiol, 25:*309-323, 1962.

Shirley, M. M.: *The First Two Years: A Study of Twenty-Five Babies.* Minneapolis, U of Minn Pr, 1933, vol II, pp. 14-33.

Simonson, E.: *Physiology of Work Capacity and Fatigue.* Springfield, Thomas, 1971.

Smith, J. L., E. M. Roberts, and E. Atkins: Fusimotor neuron block and voluntary arm movement in man. *Am J Phys Med, 51:*225-239, 1972.

Stein, R. B.: Peripheral control of movements. *Physiol Rev, 54:*215-243, 1974.

Tanaka, R.: Activation of reciprocal Ia inhibitory pathway during voluntary motor performance in man. *Brain Res, 43:*649-652, 1972.

Tipton, C. M., and P. V. Karpovich: Exercise and the patellar reflex. *J Appl Physiol, 21:*15-18, 1966.

Tower, S. S.: Pyramidal lesions in the monkey. *Brain, 63:*36-90, 1940.

Uemura, K., and J. B. Preston: Comparison of motor cortex influences upon various hind-limb motoneurones in pyramidal cats and primates. *J Neurophysiol, 28:*398-412, 1965.

Van Der Meulen, J. P., and S. Gilman: Recovery of muscle spindle activity in cats after cerebellar ablation. *J Neurophysiol, 28:*943-957, 1965.

Vedel, J. P., and J. Mouillac-Baudevin: Contrôle de l'activité des fibres fusimotrices dynamiques et statiques par la formation réticulée mésencéphalique dans le chat. *Exp Brain Res, 9:*307-324, 1969a.

———, and ———: Étude fonctionelle du contrôle de l'activité dés fibres fusimotrices dynamiques et statiques par les formations réticulèes mésencéphalique, pontique et bulbaire chez le chat. *Exp Brain Res, 9:*325-345, 1969b.

Verdy, M., J. Lapierre, H. Sansoucy, and R. Lefebvre: Shortening of Achilles reflex time after exercise. *JAMA, 204,* No. 1, 71-73, 1968.

Waller, W. H.: Progression movements elicited by subthalamic stimulation. *J Neurophysiol, 3:*300-307, 1940.

Waterland, J. C.: The supportive framework for willed movement. *Am J Phys Med, 46:* 266-278, 1967.

———, A. M. Doudlah, and G. M. Shambes: The influence of the tonic neck reflex: Vertical writing. *Acta Oto-laryngol, 61:*313-322, 1966.

———, and F. A. Hellebrandt: Involuntary patterning associated with willed movement performed against progressively increasing resistance. *Am J Phys Med, 43:*13-30, 1964.

———, and N. Munson: Involuntary patterning evoked by exercise stress. *J Am Phys Ther Assoc, 44:*91-97, 1964a.

———, and ———: Reflex association of head and shoulder girdle in nonstressful movements of man. *Am J Phys Med, 43:*98-108, 1964b.

———, and G. M. Shambes: Head and shoulder girdle linkage. *Am J Phys Med, 49:*279-289, 1970.

Wilson, V. J., and M. Yoshida: Vestibulospinal and recticulospinal effects on hindlimb, forelimb, and neck alpha motoneurons of the cat. *Proc Nat Acad Sci, 60:*836-840, 1968.

———, and ———; Monosynaptic inhibition of neck motoneurons by the medial vestibular nucleus. *Exp Brain Res, 9:*365-380, 1969a.

———, and ———: Comparison of effects of stimulation of Deiter's nucleus and medial longitudinal fasciculus on neck, forelimb, and hindlimb motoneurons. *J Neurophysiol, 32:*743-758, 1969b.

———, ———, and R. H. Schor: Supraspinal monosynaptic excitation and inhibition of thoracic back motoneurons. *Exp Brain Res, 11*:282-295, 1970.

Windle, W. F.: On the nature of the first forelimb movements of mammalian embryos. *Proc Soc Exp Biol Med, 36*:640-642, 1937.

———: *Physiology of the Fetus*. Philadelphia, Saunders, Chap. 12, 1940.

———: Reflexes of mammalian embryos and fetuses. In Weiss (Ed.): *Genetic Neurology*. Chicago, U Chicago Pr, 1950, pp. 214-222.

Woods, J. N.: Behavior of chronic decerebrate rats. *J Neurophysiol, 27*:635-644, 1964.

Yokota, T., and P. E. Voorhoeve: Pyramidal control of fusimotor neurons supplying extensor muscles in the cat's forelimb. *Exp Brain Res, 9*:96-115, 1969.

York, D. H.: Potentiation of lumbo-sacral monosynaptic reflexes by the substantia nigra. *Exp Neurol, 36*:437-448, 1972.

Zelazo, P. R., N. A. Zelazo, and S. Kolb: 'Walking' in the newborn. *Science, 176*:314-315, 1972.

Chapter 4

Reaction Times, Reflex Times and Fatigue

KEITH C. HAYES

IN THE PRECEDING CHAPTER, Dr. Easton has described, in fine detail, a very plausible view of the role that cerebrospinal reflexes play in motor coordination. At the most fundamental level of the scheme that has been presented is the role of the tendon reflex; for not only is this myotatic reflex held to be important in the "tuning," or as a "modifier" of all other reflexes but also is *sine qua non* in the current views of peripheral motor control viz. alpha-gamma linkage (Granit, 1955) and Merton's servo-theory (Merton, 1953) (see also Stein, 1974). The effect of reflex fatigue, as manifest in increased thresholds and delayed latencies, may thus be expected to have dire consequences upon the execution of skilled motor acts and as we are well aware skilled performances are frequently disrupted with the onset of fatigue.

Another element of motor control that has been considered of paramount importance for the successful execution of skilled acts is the ability to voluntarily respond, with a minimum of delay, to some form of predetermined stimulus. This ability is usually reflected in the popular experimental measure of reaction time; a measure which is familiar to all psychologists and which should not be confused in any way with the involuntary reactions (hopping, placing, etc.) referred to in the previous chapter. In much the same way that skilled motor performance is held dependent upon the integrity of the tendon reflexes, so too, a similar argument exists for reaction times.

It is generally acknowledged that the appropriate timing of constituent elements of a skilled motor performance is a prerequisite to successful execution of the task. This timing may be considered in terms of the latency of onset of different components of the motor act, the sequential ordering of the components, or simply to the duration of individual or group muscular contractions. While the ability to react rapidly and appropriately to an antecedent event necessarily constitutes only one of the temporal factors that may be identified in this context, its significance is evident especially in tasks involving some form of tracking behavior.

Sir Frederic Bartlett (1953), in discussing the leading psychological criteria of fatigue, has commented,

> Evidence is accumulating from many directions to show that the earliest and by far the most delicate criterion of change in activity due to the continuance of

that activity is increasing irregularity in the internal timing lay-out of the successive items of the performance which must be repeated.

Although, as we have mentioned, reaction time constitutes only one of the major components of the internal timing it may, as Bartlett contends, be lengthened under some circumstances. Quoting again from Bartlett (1947):

> Nothing in the whole course of the total reaction time is rigidly set. Like every other measure of human function this turns out to be a measure of range. There are limits, upper and lower, within which the timing can rapidly fluctuate and the essential adaptive spacing of actions still be maintained. Outside these limits only the skill breaks down.

Reaction time (RT) lags attributable to fatigue are thus held to be of some importance when considering the disruption of skilled motor performance.

The present chapter is devoted exclusively to a consideration of the effects of muscular work and fatigue upon tendon reflexes and upon reaction times. While some of the information concerning tendon reflex fatigue has been presented in Chapter 3, much remains to be told, particularly with respect to the evidence for reflex augmentation following fatiguing work. Similarly, man's information processing capabilities under conditions of fatigue have been discussed elsewhere (Schmidtke, Chap. 10), but in view of the fact that the bulk of experimental evidence suggests that acute fatiguing exercise does not, contrary to popular expectation, produce elongation of RT, it is appropriate to consider this phenomenon further.

While both reaction times and tendon reflexes have been studied independently, under a variety of neuromuscular fatigue conditions (Henane, 1968; Tipton and Karpovich, 1966; Sheerer and Berger, 1972) only a few investigations have looked at the two responses concurrently (Asami, 1971; Hayes, 1975 and Kroll, 1974). It is not immediately obvious from the available literature whether the apparent resistance to disruption by neuromuscular fatigue exhibited by reaction times, is attributable to the volitional element (not present in tendon reflex times), to basic differences in the neural pathways subserving the two responses, or, alternatively, to the different experimental conditions under which the reaction and tendon reflex times have been studied. If, as many studies suggest, reaction times are resistent to change under conditions of fatigue induced by strenuous muscular activity, while tendon reflexes are changeable, this differential effect may have some implications for understanding the mechanisms involved in the control of skilled movement as well as the mechanisms involved in one of the basic physiological processes underlying fatigue, that of disturbance of regulation and coordination (in the neuromuscular system) (Simonson, 1971, p. 5-6).

SIMPLE REACTION TIMES AND FATIGUE

Helmholtz is credited with some of the earliest investigations of simple reaction time (RT) performed as long ago as 1850, and, since that time, psychologists and physiologists alike have continued to work toward understanding the processes involved in the organization of a rapid, voluntary motor response. Reviews of the literature by Woodworth (1938) and later by Teichner (1954) revealed a wealth of information pertaining to the effects of numerous environmental, physiological and psychological factors upon reaction times. It was noticeable, however, that even in such comprehensive reviews as these, little mention was made of the effect of fatiguing physical work upon the time lag between stimulus presentation and initiation of the voluntary response. The experimental evidence that is available suggests that, under conditions of fatigue resulting from extreme muscular exertion, RT remains essentially unaltered.

Man's information processing capability in the fatigued state provided the focus for a number of studies concerned with reaction times. As might be expected, the work of psychologists has been primarily devoted toward understanding the central nervous system's role in the organization of a response and how this role is affected under adverse conditions. The type of fatigue situation typically studied has involved long, boring, and monotonous work producing decrements in performance on vigilance or cognitive-perceptual tasks (Wojtczak-Jarosz and Maciaszek, 1971). The influence of fatigue, induced by strenuous muscular activity, upon reaction time, has been relatively neglected. Notable exceptions do exist, however, and the present section is devoted to consideration of the work of these investigators.

In 1940 Elbel investigated the effects of muscular exertion upon RT in one hundred and twenty-nine subjects who participated in strenuous activities including bench-stepping and push-ups and a number of competitive sports such as basketball and boxing (Elbel, 1940). Following exercise, simple RT of the finger, hand, and total body, were measured and compared to RTs under resting conditions. No change in RT was witnessed following push-ups and bench-stepping, but a slight decrease in RT was noted following the competitive activities. This faster RT was evident despite reports from the subjects of marked feelings of fatigue.

Elbel suggested that in competitive exercises an emotional component arises which may be an influencing factor in the reduction of response times. The fact that RT *before* competitive exercise was faster than *before* bench-stepping and push-ups added credence to this view. However, in later reports, a similar speeding up of RT, only this time following bench-stepping, has been reported (Sorge, 1960 and by Malomsoki and Szmodis, 1970).

Phillips (1963) continued this line of inquiry by recording arm RT following two types of exercise continued to the point of fatigue. One exercise involved arm movements, designed to induce a local muscular type of fatigue, and the other involved a more general fatiguing activity of sit-ups. The principal finding was that RT was unchanged following both forms of fatiguing exercise. Meyers, Zimmerli, Farr and Baschnagel (1969) later confirmed this view based on their findings of no change in finger RT or foot RT following a bench-stepping exercise.

Also concerned with the influence of physical effort upon reaction time were Malomsoki and Szmodis (1970) who investigated the trend of changes in nervous activity seen actually during the participation in work on a bicycle ergometer (see Fig. 4-1). This investigation differed from the earlier

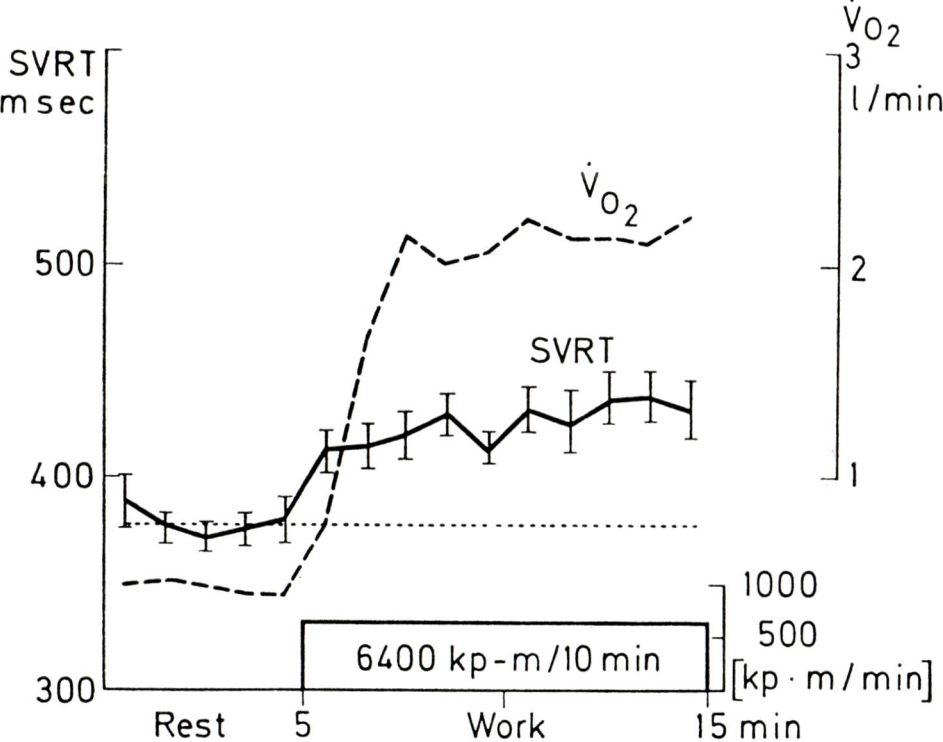

Figure 4-1. Change of response time in steady state bicycle ergometer exercise. Dotted line: pre-exercise mean of SVRT (Simple Visual Response Time) (From J. Malomsoki, and I. Szmodis, "Visual Response Time Changes in Athletes During Physical Effort," *Internationale Zeitschrift fur angewandte Physiologie einschlieblich Arbeitsphysiologie,* 29:65, 1970).

studies which all looked at RT before and after exercise. It was noted that a hand response to a visual stimulus was markedly delayed during work and this elongation of RT was attributed primarily to biochemical changes influencing the functioning of the central nervous system. Furthermore, it was reported that changes in RT were proportional to the work load imposed and to the excess oxygen consumption. An observation made by Malomsoki and Szmodis effectively countered the argument that division of attention between cycling and attending to the stimulus might have been responsible for the lengthened RTs. They argued that step increases in work load would not impose additional attention demands and therefore the RT changes that were noted must have been related to the intensity of work (see Fig. 4-2).

Evident from the majority of foregoing studies was the principal concern with gross bodily activities and that little objective quantification of the extent of fatigue and in particular the extent of local neuromuscular

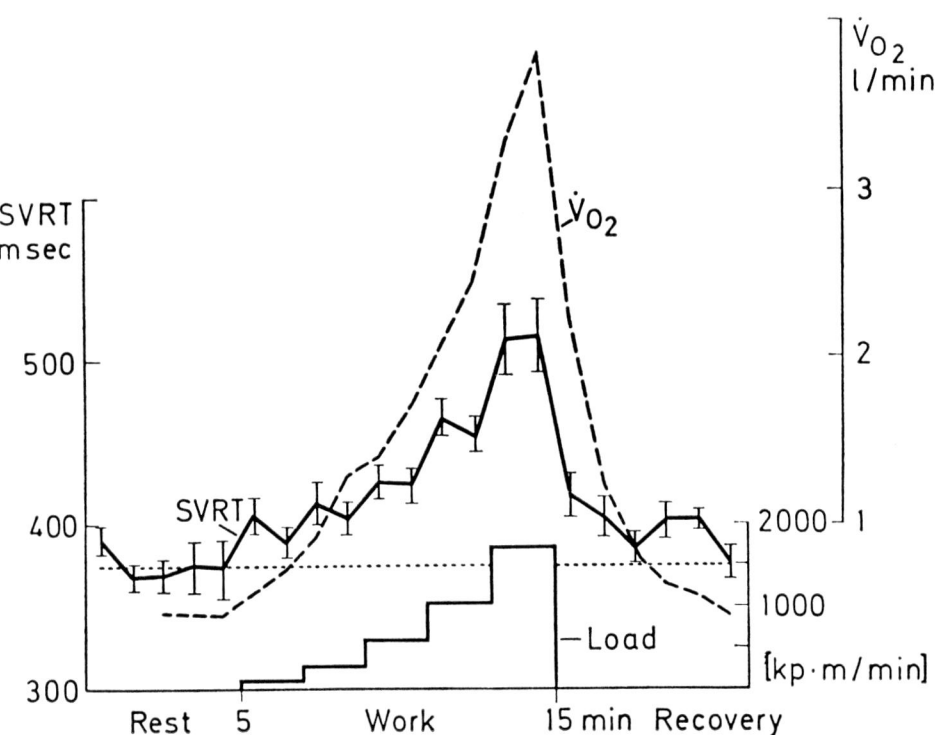

Figure 4-2. Change of response time in graded bicycle ergometer exercise; load increased in every second minute. Dotted line: pre-exercise mean of SVRT (Simple Visual Response Time) (From J. Malomsoki, and I. Szmodis, "Visual Response Time Changes in Athletes During Physical Effort," *Internationale Zeitschrift fur angewandte Physiologie einschlieblich Arbeitsphysiologie*, 29:65, 1970).

impairment, had been attempted. The lack of complete agreement in the results obtained by Elbel, Phillips, Meyers, et al., Sorge and various European investigators cited by Malomsoki and Szmodis (1970) (Babadjanian, et al., 1965; Nemessuri, et al., 1965 and 1969, and Fruktov, 1953) suggested that the extent of local neuromuscular impairment of the responding member might be responsible for any changes seen in RT. Adding to this suggestion was the observation by Kroll (1973) that even in the studies where local muscular fatigue may have been present, the reaction task frequently involved a body part not directly involved in the fatiguing activity.

An unpublished study by Babin (1966) looked specifically at RT following local muscular exercise. Babin's subjects performed ergometer work with their arms and legs. Following light exercise, RTs recorded from arms and legs, were faster than during pre-exercise conditions but following heavy work RTs were slower than the RTs measured during resting conditions. Work by Sheerer and Berger (1972) also appeared to provide evidence to support the view that fatiguing local muscular work may cause slowing of reaction time. Sheerer and Berger's (1972) 16 male subjects performed three different shoulder flexion exercises. Each exercise condition varied in the load to be moved and decrements of 15, 30, and 45 percent of maximal voluntary strength were indicated. A lengthening of the elbow flexion RT by approximately 8 to 10 milliseconds was noted and was rather speculatively attributed to metabolic changes within the responding musculature.

More recent work has failed to find support for the view that significant amounts of local muscular fatigue are reflected in slower reaction time. In one study by Kroll (1973), subjects who were required to perform isotonic (bench-stepping) and isometric (knee extension) exercises, showed no lengthening of their knee extension RT despite decrements in quadriceps maximum voluntary contraction (MVC) of 24 percent. A similar finding was reported for subjects required to complete a series of 30 isometric plantar flexions (Hayes, 1975). The extent of fatigue induced under these conditions was of the order of 36 percent MVC and even with this considerable local muscular impairment no RT changes were observed.

It appears from the information presently available that in the few studies where changes in RT have been noted following fatiguing muscular activity, the changes are small and virtually unpredictable. In fact, the scant evidence for a slight speeding up of reaction time and that for a slowing of reaction time tend to balance each other and one is left with the overall impression that, perhaps, no obvious or meaningful alteration in reaction time really does exist following strenuous exercise. A similar lack of uniformity of results pertaining to the effects of fatigue on RT exists in the work of the East European and Soviet investigators cited by Wojtczak-Jarosz and Maciaszek (1971) (Vassilev, et al., 1957; Carstocea, et al., 1966; Gawrilescu, et al., 1966; Yurchenko, 1967; Witte and Okhrimenko, 1968; Angeleri, et al., 1969; Calapay and Bellia, 1969).

To briefly summarize the relationship between fatigue and RT, there are indications that reaction times may be altered *during* work and, under some circumstances, following work. In particular, the implication is that prolonged work of either a physical or mental nature may cause some elongation of RT. For brief bouts of strenuous exercise, however, evidence suggests that if any changes are observed, they tend toward a shortening of RT. Various authors have interpreted information of this nature in terms of an inverted U relationship between the stress associated with physical exertion and mental performance (Gutin, 1972; Welford, 1973; Davey, 1973). Studies related to electroencephalographic correlates of arousal (Moruzzi and Magoun, 1949) and autonomic system changes accompanying activation and muscular exertion (Vendsalu, 1960; Haggendal and Werdinius, 1966) are typically cited in this context. However, as Cooper (1973) points out, the evidence relating cortical correlates of activation and autonomic function is not at all well established and one would appear to have to await further developments in this area for the situation concerning the complex relationships between arousal, RT and muscular exertion, to be clarified.

FRACTIONATED REACTION TIME

Even though it would seem that reaction times are not lengthened by fatigue induced by brief bouts of strenuous work, this does not preclude the possibility that component latencies of RT undergo change. If this is the case, then alterations of the temporal parameters of movement organization may still be instrumental in the disruption of skilled motor behavior; much as Bartlett (1953) contended. Moreover, if any one component in the chain of events occurring prior to the overt response does undergo alteration, one might assume a compensatory or reciprocal change in another component to maintain the witnessed constancy of reaction time under fatigue conditions. The possibility of adjustments of this nature was explored in a series of recent investigations into the behavior of individual components of reaction time under fatigue conditions (Wojtczak-Jarosz and Maciaszek, 1971; Kroll, 1973, 1974; Hayes, 1975 and Wood, 1974).

Donders (1865) developed the idea of partitioning reaction times into component latencies about a century ago. Later investigators have built on this approach and various experimental techniques have been developed (Monnier, 1952; Vaughan, Costa, Gilden and Schimmel, 1965; Weiss, 1965; Haider, Ganglberger and Groll-Knapp, 1969). Monnier (1952), for example, partitioned reaction time into several different components corresponding to retinal time, opto-motor integration time, cortical time, and motor reaction time. By simultaneously recording the electroretinogram, electroencephalogram, and electromyogram of the overt response, Monnier (1952) was able to demonstrate delays in the cortical integration time and, as a consequence, in the time delay before onset of the electromyogram (see Fig. 4-3). Unfortunately for the present discussion, the nature of the fatiguing activity was not specified by Monnier, but a rather similar approach of partitioning reaction time into various cortical latencies has been employed in studying the effects of locally fatiguing isotonic contractions of the dorsiflexors of the foot (Wood, 1974).

Another experimental method for partitioning RT into its component latencies was presented by Weiss (1965), who monitored the onset of electromyographic (EMG) activity in the responding musculature as well as recording the first signs of overt movement. In this way he was able to fractionate total reaction time (TRT) into a central nervous system compo-

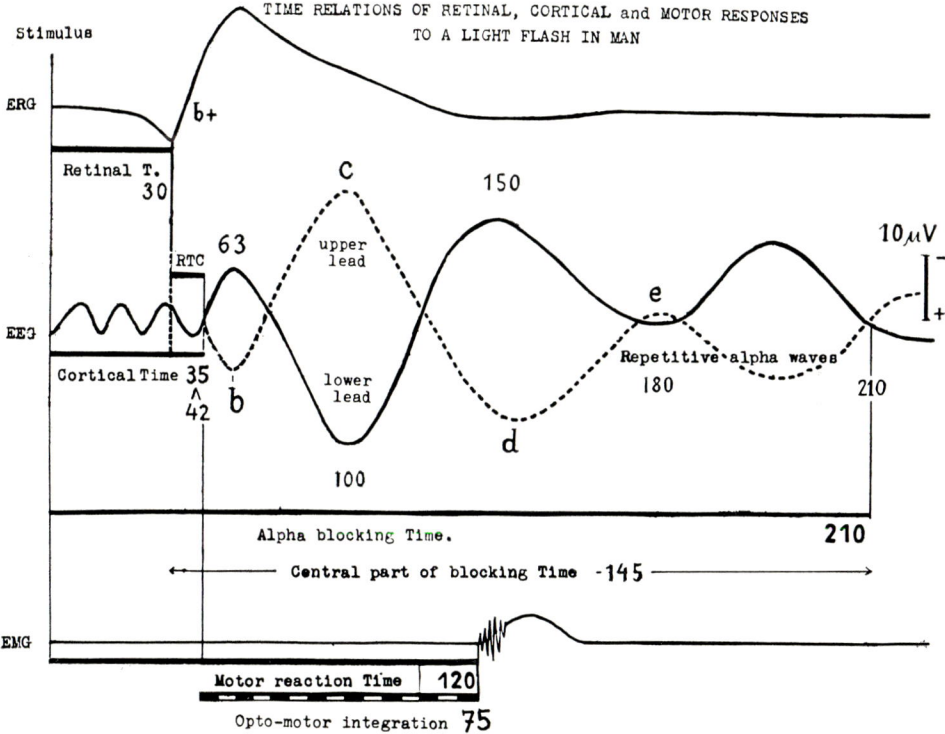

Figure 4-3. Relations between retinal time, cortical time, blocking time with its central period and motor reaction time. Fatigue was shown to lengthen the cortical integration time and the motor reaction time (from 115-125 msec) for the thenar muscle (From M. Monnier, "Retinal Cortical and Motor Responses to Photic Stimulation in Man," *Journal of Neurophysiology*, 15:469, 1952).

nent, which he designated premotor time (PMT) and a peripheral muscular component, which he termed motor time (MT). Expressed in equation form:

$$TRT = PMT + MT$$

Somewhat similar techniques had been employed earlier by Hathaway (1932, 1935), but Weiss was the first to formally consider the behavior of the motor time (MT) component. Weiss investigated the effects of set, motivation, and age upon the components of TRT, and since then, the technique of fractionating reaction times has been employed in the study of numerous other phenomena (Botwinick and Thompson, 1966a,b; Schmidt and Stull, 1970; Santa Maria, 1970).

The preoccupation of psychologists with central nervous system mechanisms for a long time overshadowed the fact that RT also comprises a peripheral muscular component which represents between 16 percent (Botwinick and Thompson, 1966a,b) and 47.5 percent (Kroll, 1973) of the time lag between presentation of the stimulus and overt movement. The percentage contribution of MT to TRT appears to be dependent upon the mass of the responding body part and the reaction time task characteristics (Kroll, 1973). A customarily held view, that RT reflects central nervous system delays, appeared to be supported by observations of a high correlation between PMT and TRT ($r = .89$) reported by Lagasse and Hayes (1973). However, it was evident from the works of others (Schmidt and Stull, 1970 and Weisendanger, Schneider, and Villoz, 1969) that the implicit acceptance of invariant temporal characteristics of muscle contraction, in other words, a constant MT, did not hold true for all situations. The possibility that changes in the muscle's contractile properties could influence TRT can not easily be dismissed.

Weiss's (1965) procedure of differentiating central from peripheral components of TRT has provided a simple experimental strategy for determining the locus of any component latency change associated with fatigue. Wojtczak-Jarosz and Maciaszek (1971) were among the first to recognize the advantages that this procedure might have for understanding some of the phenomena associated with fatigue. Simonson (1971, p. 225-232) has noted that for many years authorities have been divided as to the locus of fatigue; with proponents for a primarily CNS locus (Reid, 1928; Mateev, 1961) being opposed by those contending a peripheral or muscular locus (Merton, 1954, 1956) and it appeared to Wojtczak-Jarosz and Maciaszek (1971) that partitioning TRT into central and peripheral elements and studying the individual component responses under fatigue conditions may help to shed some light on the issue of the locus of impairment.

Wojtczak-Jarosz and Maciaszek (1971) were concerned with RT changes accompanying a prolonged task. The serial RT responses that the subjects were required to make, were considered as an experimental model of work with an automatized course of movements and requiring a constant concentration of attention. However, their results are of interest to the present discussion of fatigue induced by muscular work as one of their observations was that in some trials "abortive" responses occurred. An abortive response was a trial where EMG activity in the responding muscle was present but the mechanical response was not generated (see Fig. 4-4).

The problem of the origin of abortive reactions was left for further study; however, the authors did implicate the role of fatigue connected with muscular work. In particular, they suggested that the effort manifested by bioelectric activity of the muscles may be, during fatigue, not transformed into mechanical work at all. The work of Merton (1954) and Lippold, et al. (1960) was cited in an attempt to explain this phenomenon in terms of decreased contractility of muscle fibers without a concomitant decrease in the amplitude of EMG potentials. With respect to the components of RT, Wojtczak-Jarosz and Maciaszek (1971) noted a slight length-

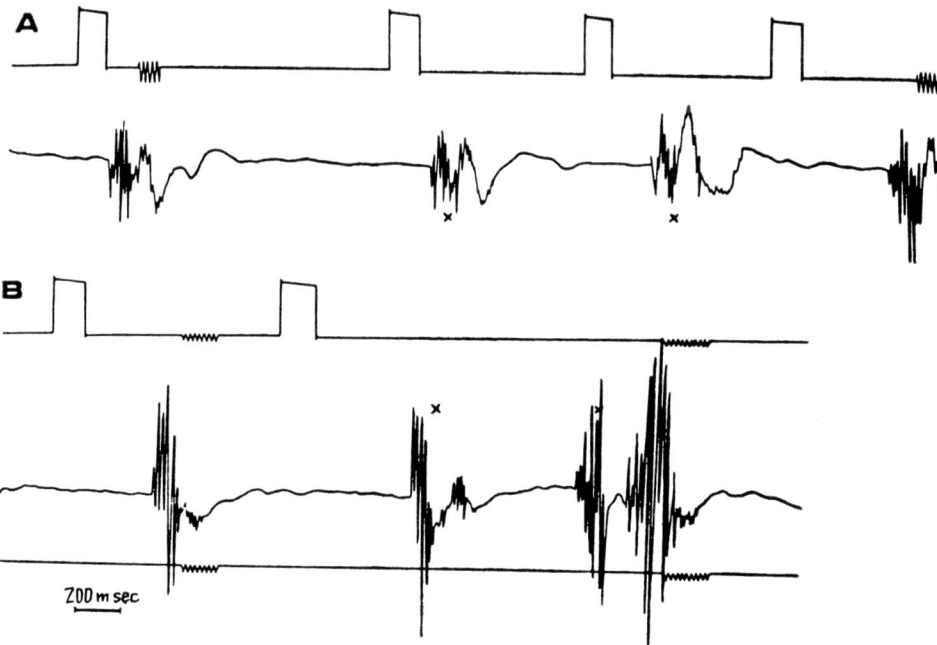

Figure 4-4. Abortive reactions (marked by crosses), that is, those without a mechanical effect. A: Single abortive reactions as a response to two stimuli in succession; B: Three reactions following each other as a response to a single stimulus (two abortive reactions, the third with a mechanical effect). A mechanical effect is shown in the upper trace of A following the first square wave (which indicates the stimulus) (From J. Wojtczack-Jarosz, J., and Z. Maciaszek, "Electromyographical Analysis of Reaction Time," *Acta Neurobiological Experimentalis, 31*:141, 1971).

ening of PMT during prolonged work but no alteration in MT. This latter observation was a little difficult to reconcile with their arguments for a muscular type of fatigue through impairment of the action potential-contractile mechanism coupling and one might question whether their task really was sufficient to produce muscular fatigue.

Local muscular fatigue effects upon fractionated RT components were studied by Kroll (1973). An isotonic exercise involving bench stepping (in which subjects performed 10,000 ft-lb and 15,000 ft-lb of work) induced a 24 percent decrement in knee extension MVC of the eight male and eight female subjects. However, even with this substantial local muscular impairment no lengthening in either the central component, PMT, or the peripheral muscular component, MT, was noted. A similar observation was made following two different isometric knee-extension exercise regimes (Kroll, 1973).

Essentially similar results of a null effect of local muscular fatigue upon fractionated RT components were reported for subjects required to perform three different series of maximal isometric plantar flexions (Hayes, 1975). The subjects were examined for any changes in ankle extension PMT, MT, and TRT, following the exercise conditions which varied in the rest interval between successive MVCs. Despite average decrements in plantar flexion MVC of 36 percent, no changes were seen in either the PMT or MT components of TRT or in the TRT itself.

Measurement of PMT and MT components has enabled some insight into the composition of TRT under various fatigue conditions. Although changes in the PMT component were noted following prolonged work (Wojtczak-Jarosz and Maciaszek, 1971) which some authorities might maintain was indicative of a central or "mental" type of fatigue (Hartson, 1932), no differences in either the PMT or MT component were noted following strenuous bouts of local muscular exercise. In essence, these results confirm the TRT literature and provide some evidence to suggest that, at least with gross partitioning of central from peripheral factors, no obvious compensatory temporal adjustments are being made to retain the constancy of TRT following strenuous work.

Several implications concerning the breakdown of skilled performance or of the role of fatigue in motor learning situations may be drawn from the fractionated RT literature. The breakdown in motor skills under conditions of fatigue may be attributed to reaction time changes, primarily due to PMT variation, only when the fatigue inducing activity is of a prolonged attention demanding nature. Bartlett's (1953) observation of internal timing changes being instrumental in skill disruption is seen to be quite appropriate in this case. When the skilled performance under study has a large dependence upon central nervous system processing time (analogous to PMT) detrimental effects of fatigue-induced temporal delays may be quite considerable. Conversely, when the performance is contingent upon the properties of muscular contraction, the performance is unlikely to be disrupted by a prolonged vigilance task.

In the case where fatigue is induced by strenuous muscular activity and evidenced in performance decrements such as reduced MVC, RT and its components PMT and MT do not demonstrate any change. It seems, therefore, that disruption of skilled tasks cannot be attributed simply to a RT lag. If skilled motor performance suffers when the involved musculature becomes "too weak to make the necessary movements" (Merton, 1956) then the impaired contractile properties of the muscles would presumably be reflected in lengthened MT. Such lengthening of MT has not been shown, despite decrements in MVC of responding muscle groups of 24 and 36 percent and the view that skilled performance disruption may be due to RT changes associated with muscular impairment is, therefore, still open to further question. As Kroll (1973) has commented "consideration of the actual strength losses present when skilled performance breaks down as well as an assessment of fractionated RT components for the involved muscles seems prudent to test the interaction of local muscular fatigue, RT, and skilled performance."

TENDON REFLEXES

We now turn our attention to the question of tendon reflexes, the involuntary muscular contractions occurring in response to stretching of a muscle. Tendon reflexes, frequently termed myotatic or stretch reflexes, are familiar to all when manifest in the popular, though rather artificial, phasic muscular response to deformation of a tendon by means of a percussion hammer.

Wilhelm Henrich Erb and Carl Friedrich Otto Westphal independently described, in 1875, the phenomenon now known as the patellar reflex. Since then, this particular tendon reflex and others have been used extensively as diagnostic and research tools. Tendon reflexes provide convenient and noninvasive indications of the status of the nervous system at a given point in time and, as such, have found wide application in both clinical and laboratory settings. Some measure of the popularity of this index of central nervous system functioning is evident in the large number of articles pertaining to tendon reflexes (over 500) cited by Sternberg (1893) in a monograph published a mere twenty years after the initial reports by Erb and Westphal. Subsequent investigators have tended to maintain interest in the behavior of reflexes and impetus has recently been given to study in this area by establishing the dependence of volitional motor control upon the mechanisms subserving the myotatic reflex. Further interest may be generated as a result of Easton's discourse on the role of the myotatic reflex in coordination.

With the technological advancement of recent decades, greater sophistication of measurement has been introduced into the recording of reflex parameters. Measurement of limb movement or muscle thickening, registered by wooden leverage systems, has been substituted by decidedly more accurate electromyographic techniques used in conjunction with electronic transducers for measuring the isometric force of contraction or the limb's kinematic properties, viz displacement and velocity. Derived from records obtained in this way have been innumerable different indices of the involuntary response. The magnitude of the reflex has been described in terms of peak amplitude of EMG activity, or the mechanical response of the muscle has been measured directly and reported either as maximum displacement, or as isometric force. Similarly, the temporal parameters of a large number of different phases of the response have been described. One unfortunate outcome of all this has been the rather indiscriminate use of the term "reflex time," variously describing the onset of EMG activity in the responding limb, the onset of muscle thickening, the beginning of the overt response, and a number of other measures of the duration of muscular contraction and relaxation phases of the reflex response. When interpreting the information on reflex times and their behavior under various experimental conditions, one is thus obliged to look closely at the method of recording and the exact temporal parameters in question.

With respect to the effects of fatiguing muscular activity upon tendon reflexes, the experimental evidence must be considered equivocal. A number of investigators have established that tendon reflexes become depressed (reflex fatigue) following arduous (Quo, 1949), or very strenuous muscular activity (Tuttle, 1930; Tipton and Karpovich, 1966 and Henane, 1968) and in Chapter 3, some of the mechanisms which may underlie such an effect have been identified. Lombard's (1887) investigation of the patellar reflex was one of the earliest to demonstrate a reduction in the amplitude of the muscular response following strenuous activity and confirmation of reflex fatigue following work was later provided in evidence of reductions in the amplitude of the reflex response (Tuttle, 1930), increased thresholds for elicitation of the reflex (Henane, 1968) and delays in the onset of EMG (Kroll, 1974) and the overt response (Tipton and Karpovich, 1966).

Contrasting with this evidence is a substantial amount of experimental support for the view that tendon reflexes may be maintained or even potentiated following severe muscular exertion. For every report of reflex depression in subjects who have been fatigued, it is also possible to find another study in which the muscular contraction associated with the reflex has been potentiated. Sternberg (1887) provided evidence of an enhancement of reflex contraction following work and more recent studies have confirmed this view (Cheah and Tan, 1970; Petajan and Eagan, 1968; Westerman and Gerbrandy, 1969; Verdy, et al., 1968; Hayes, 1975). Other investigators whose principal concern has been with the neural elements of the reflex arc have reported no change in the latency of tendon reflexes following strenuous exercise (Margaria, et al., 1956, 1961, and Nystrom, 1933).[1] As Schwab and Prichard (1949, 1951) reported, after complete voluntary fatigue of the quadriceps muscles, a vigorous patellar relex can still be elicited (see also Simonson, 1971, p. 226).

Unlike the situation in voluntary reaction times where small and relatively insignificant variability of response was noted, the involuntary reflex changes are relatively large and no doubt remains that meaningful changes can and do occur. The questions that do exist, however, are why and under what conditions do reflexes demonstrate potentiation and what are the conditions that have to be satisfied to cause reflexes to be depressed.

When attempting to determine the conditions under which reflexes are depressed, one is confronted with several possibilities, among the more obvious being the degree of neuromuscular fatigue experienced by subjects. Tuttle (1930) appeared to have settled the differences in opinion resulting from Lombard and Steinberg's conflicting observation of the effect of muscular work upon reflex activity, by implicating the fitness level of the individual. Trained subjects demonstrated an early augmentation of the achilles tendon reflex following a series of deep knee bends but as work continued this augmentation was followed by a depression of the response. In untrained subjects there was no evidence for potentiation but instead an early depression of reflex amplitude occurred. Tuttle suggested that the degree of fitness of the subjects determined whether reflexes were initially potentiated or depressed and put this forward as an explanation for the conflicting findings of earlier investigators.

Tipton and Karpovich (1966) later questioned this interpretation by Tuttle, based on their evidence of longer reflex times (measured as the onset of movement). Tipton and Karpovich argued that in the course of work (knee extension exercises) an early augmentation of the patellar reflex was later followed by depression, and this was attributed to the extent of local muscular fatigue. Impaired contractile properties of the muscle were deemed responsible for the slower reflex times, a hypothesis based on the observation that studies of reflexes in which only the neural conduction times were measured (Margaria, et al., 1958, 1961) did not reveal any such

---

1. Although Margaria, et al. (1958, 1961) reported no change in the latency of onset of the reflex muscle contraction, sensory and motor nerve conduction velocities were reported to change. Sensory conduction velocities increased by 12 percent and motoneuron conduction velocities decreased by the same amount.

changes. The reflex measures taken by Tipton and Karpovich did include the time taken for muscular contraction.

The extent of local muscular fatigue, which is contingent upon a subject's fitness, assuming a constant work load, appears as an important factor in determining whether reflexes become potentiated or depressed following exercise. The problem, however, is not quite this simple, for in a study in which subjects performed several isometric contractions of the plantar flexor muscle group, decrement in maximal voluntary contraction of up to 39 percent MVC were noted and yet the achilles tendon reflex showed no signs of depression; to the contrary, the tendon reflex appeared potentiated (Hayes, 1975). It is unlikely that local muscular fatigue greater than 39 percent of MVC was evident in Tuttle's subjects following their bench-stepping exercise.

Finding potentiated achilles tendon reflexes at a time when local neuromuscular fatigue was evident prompts closer scrutiny of some of the earlier studies in which this particular tendon reflex had been examined. Nystrom (1933) found no change in the onset of EMG activity in the achilles tendon reflex following plantar flexion to exhaustion, similarly Margaria, et al. (1958, 1961) noted no change in the latency of onset of EMG following bicycle ergometer work and treadmill running to exhaustion. Later studies (Cheah and Tan, 1970; Reinfrank, et al., 1967; Verdy, et al., 1968; Johnson, et al., 1963; Petajan and Eagan, 1968 and Kawamura, 1971) all of which examined the temporal characteristics of muscular contraction and relaxation phases following various types of exercise, all confirmed the view that the achilles tendon reflex becomes potentiated rather than depressed following strenuous work; potentiation here being reflected in increased force of contraction, and reduced contraction and half relaxation times. A word of caution is pertinent perhaps, for in these studies no assessment of local muscular fatigue was made. As in the previously mentioned studies of reaction time, concern with gross bodily activities such as treadmill running, bicycle ergometer work, and bench-stepping has dominated this area of study and local muscular fatigue effects have rarely been considered. Acknowledging this, it is still difficult to reconcile augmentation of achilles tendon reflexes following the maximal exertion of a Masters two-step exercise (Masters, 1935) continued for as long as possible (Cheah and Tan, 1970), with the observation that the patellar reflex becomes depressed following a brief walk (Lombard, 1887) or following a one mile run (Wickwire, et al., 1938).

One is tempted to look toward the characteristics of the different tendon reflexes to help explain some of the exercise-induced changes that have been reported. Differences may exist for example between the muscle group involved in the patellar reflex and the muscle group involved in the achilles tendon reflex. The rectus femoris, a "phasic" muscle (Person and Kudina, 1972) might be considered to have a preponderance of fast-twitch, glycolytic muscle fibers, whereas the triceps surae is generally considered to be more "tonic" with a mixture of both glycolytic and slow-twitch oxidative fibers. The morphological composition of the two muscle groups and the well recognized differential fatiguability of the fiber types (Kugelberg and Edstrom, 1965) may provide some clue as to why patellar reflexes appear depressed following even moderate exercise whereas achilles tendon reflexes show little evidence of such changes. Also related to the morphological composition of the two muscle groups is the number of muscle spindles present. If we can be permitted to extrapolate from animal studies, we find the number of muscle spindle capsules per gram of muscle to be less in the rectus femoris (12 spindle capsules/gram) than in the soleus muscle (23 spindle capsules/gram) (Mountcastle, 1968; Barker and Chin, 1960 and Chin, et al., 1962).

If the fiber type composition of the two muscle groups is sufficiently different to be a factor influencing the observed differences in reflex changes under fatigue conditions, then the type of fatigue-inducing activity, in terms of its glycolytic and oxidative requirements may also be a factor. It is worth noting here that an underlying assumption in this line of reasoning is that fatigue, as reflected in decrements in MVC, is associated primarily with impairment of the muscle's contractile apparatus. As Easton has argued in Chapter 3, and other authorities have noted (Simonson, 1971, p. 232), this may not necessarily be the case.

So far, the primary factor which has been implicated as influencing the tendon reflex response to exercise has been the degree of local muscular impairment. This is, of course, contingent upon the fitness of the subject and the type of exercise performed, as well as the characteristics of the muscle involved in the reflex (i.e. associated with the choice of tendon reflex being studied). To this list might be added other factors worthy of consideration, for example, that of the stimulation technique and the measurement employed. Henane and Macarez (1972) noted that achilles tendon H reflex and M response thresholds were elevated after a submaximal step-test. However, they also remarked that at higher intensities of electrical stimulation, the H reflex amplitude was not diminished. In fact, their graph (Fig. 4, page 322 in Henane and Macarez, 1972) indicates the converse, a slight increase in amplitude of H response. One might interpret this as indicating that where sufficient stimulus has been given, the H reflex amplitude is not adversely affected by fatigue, and the question for further research then turns to the cause of the elevated thresholds.

The mechanisms underlying reflex depression (reflex fatigue) have been considered in Chapter 3 but the mechanisms of augmentation have yet to be discussed. We now focus attention on this aspect of the tendon reflex changes associated with fatigue. Perhaps the most plausible explanation for augmentation of the achilles tendon reflex following strenuous work is the known potentiating effect of increased intramuscular temperature. Temperature effects, produced by elevated metabolic levels and increased local blood supply, have been invoked as explanations for enhanced reflexes following treadmill running (Petajan and Eagan, 1968) and work on a bicycle ergometer (Westerman and Gerbrandy, 1969). Johnson, Jokl and Jokl (1968) may well have considered this as part of an "ergotropic" shift; that is, a sympathetic nervous system response to exercise, which they claimed was responsible for the observed reflex changes following a 1.1 mile run. Westerman and Gerbrandy (1969) and Petajan and Eagan (1968) looked specifically at the temperature effects induced by passive heating and by exercise and postulated that increased intramuscular temperatures, mediated by increased local circulation, provided the most plausible explanation for enhanced tendon reflexes. The rise in muscle temperature was thought to accelerate the chemical reactions occurring during muscle contraction and relaxation.

FRACTIONATED REFLEX TIMES

In the preceding section on tendon reflexes, brief mention was made of the problems associated with the term "reflex times." The problems revolved around exactly what part of the reflex activity was being timed. Some recent studies have utilized a technique defining and partitioning reflex times in a manner analogous to that developed by Weiss (1965) for reaction time and since these particular studies are germane to the present discussion it is worthwhile to consider these in some detail.

Asami (1971) and Kroll (1974) both studied the effects of various forms of exercise upon patellar reflexes and selected as their criteria of reflex activity the time delay from tendon percussion to the onset of EMG and the time from tendon percussion to beginning of the overt movement. By subtracting the EMG latency from the overt movement time, a third measure was obtained, corresponding to muscle contraction time. In the equation form total reflex time (TRfT) is thus seen as the sum of reflex latency (LAT) and reflex motor time (RfMT).

$$TRfT = LAT + RfMT$$

The importance of this fractionation of total reflex time into component latencies lies in its applicability to the problem of the locus of fatigue-induced changes in the reflex response and its provision for some form of comparison with similarly partitioned voluntary response times when these are measured concurrently. Kroll (1974) noted that the elongation of total reflex time was attributable to the lengthening of the motor

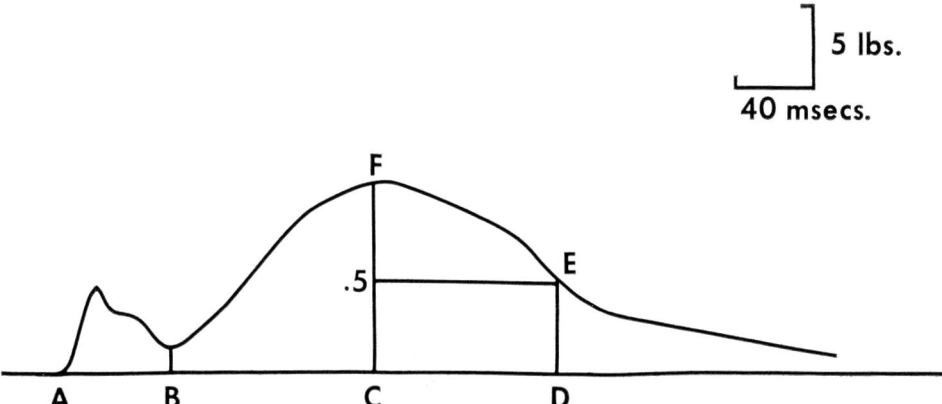

Figure 4-5. Conventional clinical indices of the Achilles tendon reflex when measured by the strain gauge technique. Following exercise, most investigators have reported shortened HRT and CT and increased Force values (see for example, Kawamura, 1971) (From K. C. Hayes, "Effect of Serial Isometric Contractions with Varied Rest Intervals upon Reaction and Reflex Time Components," Ph.D. dissertation, University of Massachusetts, Amherst, 1973).

time component (RfMT) i.e. the time taken for the responding muscle (s) to generate sufficient tension to overcome the inertia of the limb (Hayes, 1972). This observation confirmed earlier speculation by Tipton and Karpovich (1966).

By virtue of the fact that a voluntary knee-extension RT motor time was unaltered at the time when reflex motor times were significantly longer, Kroll reasoned that the depletion of neuromuscular transmitter substance (myoneural junction failure) could not be the cause of the reflex changes. Instead he argued the case for a compensatory adjustment of the central nervous system (effective only for the voluntary reaction time) to overcome impairment of the muscle's contractile apparatus. Macarez and Henane (1970) had reached similar conclusions of a muscular site for reflex fatigue.

The technique of fractionating reflex times and concurrently recording fractionated voluntary reaction time components, has also been applied to studying the effects of exercise upon the achilles tendon reflex. Just before moving on to this, however, it is worthwhile to briefly outline the conventional assessment of this reflex. Clinical interest has been mainly focused upon the duration of the muscular contraction and the time to half-relaxation period. Lambert, et al. (1951), Kimura (1971) and Kawamura (1971) all used these parameters derived from isometric force-time curves[2] ob-

---

2. A slightly different procedure of extracting contraction times, half-relaxation times, etc. from a photomotograph is also widely used (Gilson, 1959 and Cheah and Tan, 1970).

tained from strain gauge. Figure 4-5 shows some of the conventional parameters of the duration of the reflex while Figure 4-6 shows the reflexly elicited muscle action potentials of the soleus muscle. Subtraction of the time delay between hammer impact and onset of EMG from the independently monitored time interval A-B in Figure 4-5 defines the RfMT component.

Following a series of thirty maximal isometric voluntary contractions of the plantar flexors, sufficient to induce 36 percent decrement in the strength of plantar flexion, achilles tendon reflexes were found to be potentiated (Hayes, 1975). Contraction times and half-relaxation times were markedly reduced while the force of the involuntary response was definitely augmented. At the same time that the achilles tendon reflexes were potentiated, voluntary reaction time components PMT and MT were unal-

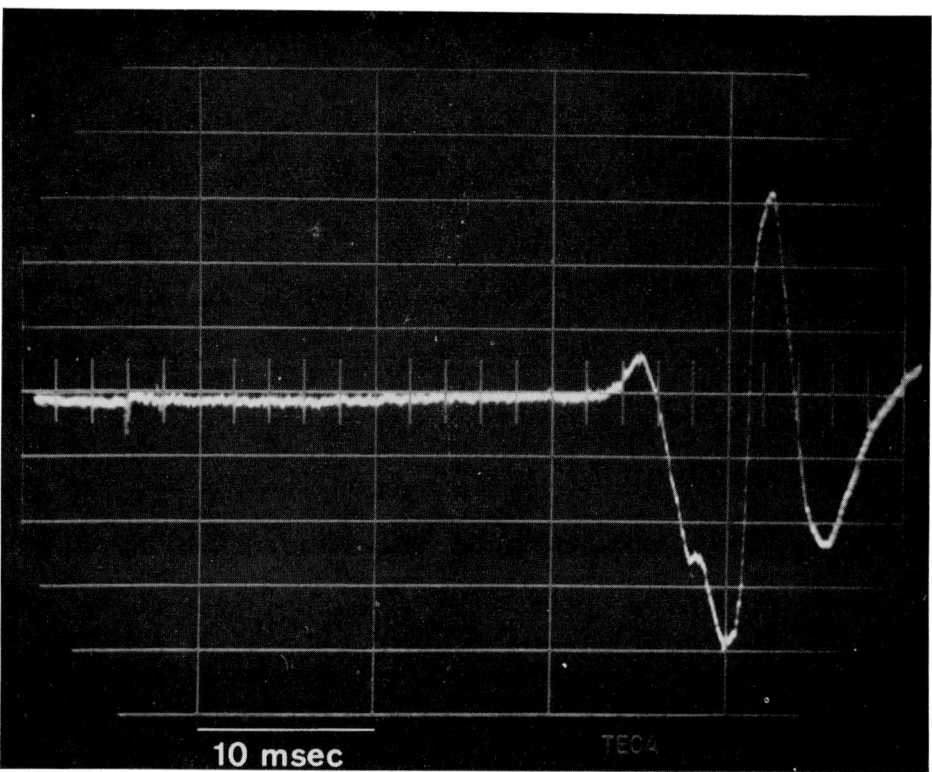

Figure 4-6. The synchronous muscle action potentials of soleus following percussion of the achilles tendon. Reflex latency is measured from the hammer impact to the beginning of the electromyographic activity (32.5 milliseconds) (From K. C. Hayes, "Effect of Serial Isometric Contractions with Varied Rest Intervals upon Reaction and Reflex Time Components," Ph.D. dissertation, University of Massachusetts, Amherst, 1973).

tered. A paradoxical situation was thus present in which strength loss was not associated with any lengthening of the motor time components of either the voluntary or an involuntary response. Indeed, the latter, the contractile properties of the involuntary response, appeared definitely enhanced.

It was suggested that the MVC, the RT and the reflex contractions differed in their respective dependence upon phasic and tonic motor units (Hayes, 1975). The differential fatiguability associated with the motor units (Kugelberg and Edstrom, 1968) could account for the rapid decrements associated with MVC, presumably utilizing phasic (glycolytic) motor units, and the reaction time and reflex responses, presumably using a greater percentage of tonic motor units (oxidative), were relatively unaffected.

The interpretation given above may satisfactorily explain the relative amounts of impairment associated with MVC, RT and the achilles tendon reflex but it does not account for the augmentation of the reflex response. As we have noted earlier, increased temperature effects may have served to augment the reflex contraction, but if this were the case, the voluntary motor time component would have been expected to similarly demonstrate a speeding up of the muscle contraction processes. Furthermore, the finding that the force of the reflex contraction was augmented simultaneously with a shortening of the contraction time might be considered indicative of the recruitment of additional, "faster," motor units—the *motoneuron recruitment* referred to by Easton (Chap. 3) and suggested from the work of Buchtal and Schmalbruch, 1970. The possibility of a spinal mechanism compensating for fatigued muscle fibers, inducing the recruitment of additional motoneurons by increased reflex loop gain, should be explored.

REFLEX LOOP GAIN COMPENSATION FOR FATIGUE

Associated with the myotatic apparatus is a means for adjusting the sensitivity of the muscle spindles to stretch. This is accomplished by the small gamma motoneurons which comprise the fusimotor system. As we have seen earlier (Easton, p. 59) this system may be considered as adjusting the "match point" of the muscle spindles. The sensitivity of the muscle spindle's discharge in response to stretch, together with the degree of amplification given to the signal coming from the spindles is frequently expressed, in engineering terms, as the "gain" of the stretch servomechanism. The fusimotor system, with its own higher level control, and certain other segmental influences, can thus be seen to have a large influence on the amplitude and temporal parameters of the reflex response.

Adjustment of the "gain" of the myotatic reflex, as a mechanism of compensation for muscular fatigue, has been conjectured by several different authorities and, in fact, constituted one of the original arguments in favor of the follow-up servomechanism model of peripheral motor control (Merton, 1953). Experimental evidence in support of this compensatory mechanism, in fact, for the follow-up servomechanism mode of control itself, is hardly robust, but nonetheless is worthy of review.

The idea of increased muscle spindle sensitivity to stretch, as a means of increasing reflex loop gain under conditions of fatigue, was put forward by Lippold, Redfearn and Vuco (1960). The idea was advanced as an explanation for electromyographic evidence of increased amplitude and synchronization of muscle action potentials suggestive of motoneuron recruitment under fatigue conditions. More recently, Chaffin (1973) has presented a similar interpretation of his electromyographic evidence of frequency spectra shifts.

Marsden, Morton and Merton (1972), from whom much of the "servo-theory" has been generated, have presented tension records of the flexor pollicis longus which are suggestive first of all of the existence of the servo control in humans, but also of increased stretch reflex loop gain under conditions of muscular fatigue (see Fig. 4-7).

They used a low inertia electric motor to provide a constant force opposing flexion of the top joint of the thumb. Perturbations of the opposing force were introduced by the motor, under rested and fatigue conditions, and unpredictably caused "release," "halt" or "stretch" of the thumb muscle. Records of the resulting change in muscle tension and integrated electromyographic activity disclosed latencies indicating stretch reflex activity.[3] By changing the initial resistance offered to movement, a proportional change in degree of muscle activation in release, halt and stretch trials was shown which was constant regardless of the initial force. The muscle activation (reflex activity) turned on by a given misalignment (the gain) was thus proportional to the initial force.

Marsden, et al. (1972) also showed reflex loop gain changes under fatigue conditions. Fatigue in this study was induced by muscular work while the circulation was occluded by a blood pressure cuff on the upper arm (ischemic fatigue). They speculated that the loop gain adjustments compensated for fatigued muscle fibers and, furthermore, argued that cutaneous receptors could not be controlling the mechanism that boosts the gain.

Most of the discussion about loop gain changes has emanated from interpretation of electromyographic records. To this we might now add evidence presented earlier on the augmenting effect of exercise on achilles tendon re-

---

3. The Halt and Release responses had the same latency as the Stretch response and were considered as manifestations of the same mechanism. Since the Release response was the "negative" of the stretch reflex, it demonstrated that the muscle must have been receiving excitation via the stretch reflex arc at the moment of release. A similar argument exists for the widely studied "silent period" phenomenon.

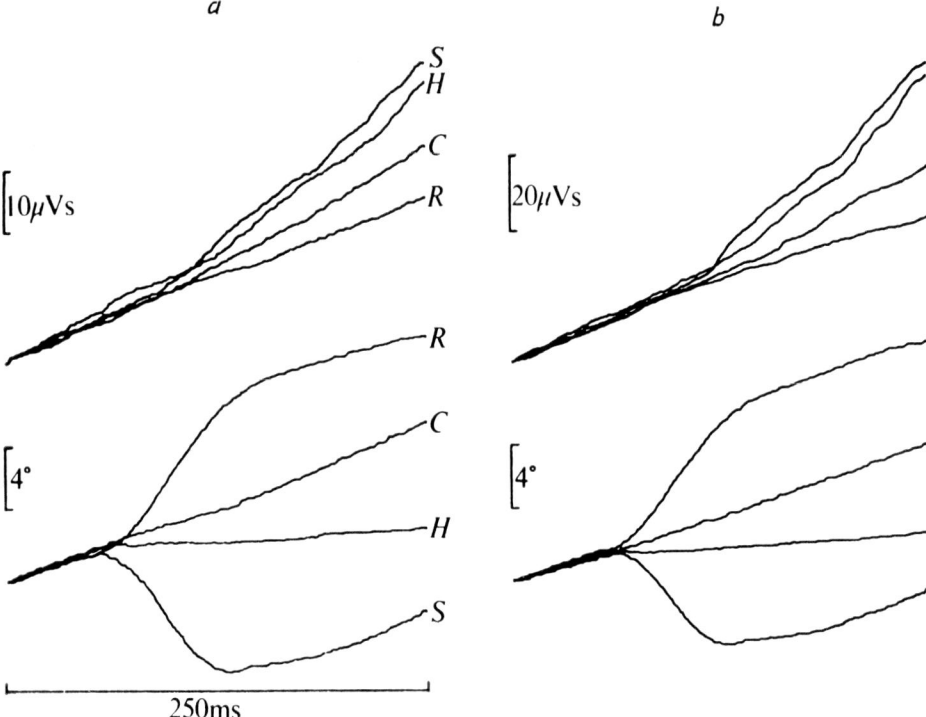

Figure 4-7. Gain compensation during fatigue. The initial resistance to movement (a torque of 150 gcm) was low. A: Fresh muscle. The muscle was then fatigued by applying maximal shocks to the median nerve at the elbow at 50s^{-1} for 60s. Recovery was prevented by a blood pressure cuff on the upper arm, arresting the circulation. B: Muscle fatigued. The electrical responses, upper records, (integrated emg of thumb flexor muscle) are of the same form as before fatigue, but scaled up by a factor of roughly 2, as shown by the calibrations. Force records (not illustrated) showed that the forces developed in the halt and in the other responses were the same as before fatigue. Bottom records indicate angular position of the terminal phalanx of the thumb. The initials S, H, R, C describe the perturbations to muscular contraction introduced by the torque motor.
S = stretch
H = hold
R = release
C = control
(From C. D. Marsden, P. A. Merton, and H. B. Morton, "Servo Action in Human Voluntary Movement," *Nature*, 238:140, 1972.

flexes (Reinfrank, et al., 1967; Verdy, et al., 1968; Petajan and Eagan, 1968; Cheah and Tan, 1970; Westerman and Gerbrandy, 1969 and Hayes, 1975). All of these studies reported shortened contraction times for the reflex response; findings which may reflect the recruitment of greater numbers of motoneurons as a result of increased loop gain. Caution must be exercised, however, not to preclude the possibility of concurrent intramuscular temperature effects.

From a very different line of inquiry comes other data which is not too far removed from implicating changes in reflex loop gain. Sympathetic nervous system concomitants of strenuous exercise are well documented and, as Johnson, Jokl and Jokl (1963) indicated, are reflective of a heterostatic shift of the automatic nervous system. With this in mind, Hunt's (1960) observation that stimulation of a sympathetic tract lowers the threshold of muscle spindle's response to stretch, may be likened to the sympathetic nervous system changing the loop gain. The presence of unmyelinated fibers entering mammalian muscle spindles has been known for several years but their functional significance has remained obscure. The fibers are known to degenerate on removal of the appropriate sympathetic ganglia. Hunt reported that with muscle (gastrocnemius, soleus and tenuissimus muscles of cat) held under constant tension, sympathetic stimulation produced on initial rise followed by a fall in discharge frequency in muscle spindle afferents. This effect paralleled the change in stretch threshold of the spindle receptors. As the effect was also demonstrated in the tenuissimus muscle deprived of its circulation, the changes in muscle spindle sensitivity to fusimotor stimulation could not be attributed to alterations in blood flow.

Golgi tendon organ influence on muscle contraction may also have an important bearing on the postulated compensatory mechanism. Houk and Henneman (1968) have described the role that tension feedback, and in particular the inhibitory action of Golgi tendon organs, is presumed to play in automatically compensating for muscle fatigue.

Although the gain of tension feedback is characteristically rather small compared to length feedback (Houk, et al., 1971) the tension servo-loop has been considered capable of up to 40 percent compensation for fatigue of muscle fibers (Houk, et al., 1971; see Fig. 4-8). Furthermore, the gain of this reflex pathway is not constant but is subject to control from various supraspinal influences (for example, the red nucleus) which appear to exert an influence over the internuncial neurons (see Fig. 4-9). It is quite conceivable, therefore, that alterations in the gain of either the length (muscle spindle) or tension (muscle spindle and Golgi tendon organ) servo-loops may serve to compensate against peripheral fatigue.

As with most speculations, the loop gain model does not explain all of the facts that are known. The work of Henane, et al. (1968a,b,c and 1972) on the effects of a step test on the achilles tendon reflex appears at first sight to conflict directly with the postulated mechanism. Henane and Macarez (1972) concluded that elevated thresholds of the achilles tendon reflex were attributable to peripheral inhibition (muscle excitability)

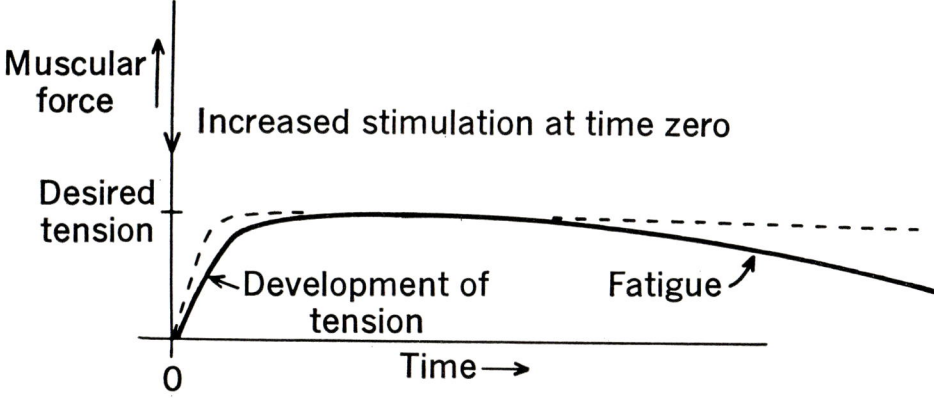

Figure 4-8. Dependence of muscular force on variables other than efferent nerve signals. Temporal factors influence development and maintenance of tension. Rise of muscular forces is not instantaneous; also, prolonged excitation results in fatigue, which reduces the force produced. Dashed trace indicates how tension feedback may compensate for these effects (modified from J. C. Houk, and E. Henneman, "Feedback Control of Movement and Posture," in V. Mountcastle, ed., *Medical Physiology II*, 12th ed. (1968) Chap. 72.

and a central inhibition mechanism. However, inspection of some of the graphs of Henane and Macarez (1972) shows that, once elicited, the H reflex does appear slightly augmented whereas the M response is depressed even at high stimulation intensities. This observation is not inconsistent with the idea of increased loop gain compensation for peripheral muscular fatigue and furthermore it suggests that the mechanism might well be operational within the spinal cord. (The H reflex may be thought of as bypassing the muscle spindle in the reflex.) The question then is posed, "What determines the higher thresholds for reflex elicitation?" Whether this will turn out to be the more pertinent question or not awaits further research.

The notion of increased proprioceptive reflex loop gain, however accomplished, is appealing from a teleological viewpoint, as well as providing some form of an explanation for conflicting experimental data. Animals able to postpone fatigue temporarily, by increasing the gain of their reflex arcs, would stand a greater change of survival from preditors, and hence, reproductivity, than animals without such a compensatory mechanism.

Concluding the discussion on reflex gain adjustments, we might note that the evidence to date is far from conclusive. The possibility does exist that the postulated changes in gain may explain why, under some circumstances, reflexes appear augmented and voluntary contractions are maintained despite some muscular impairment. As Marsden, et al. (1972) have stated:

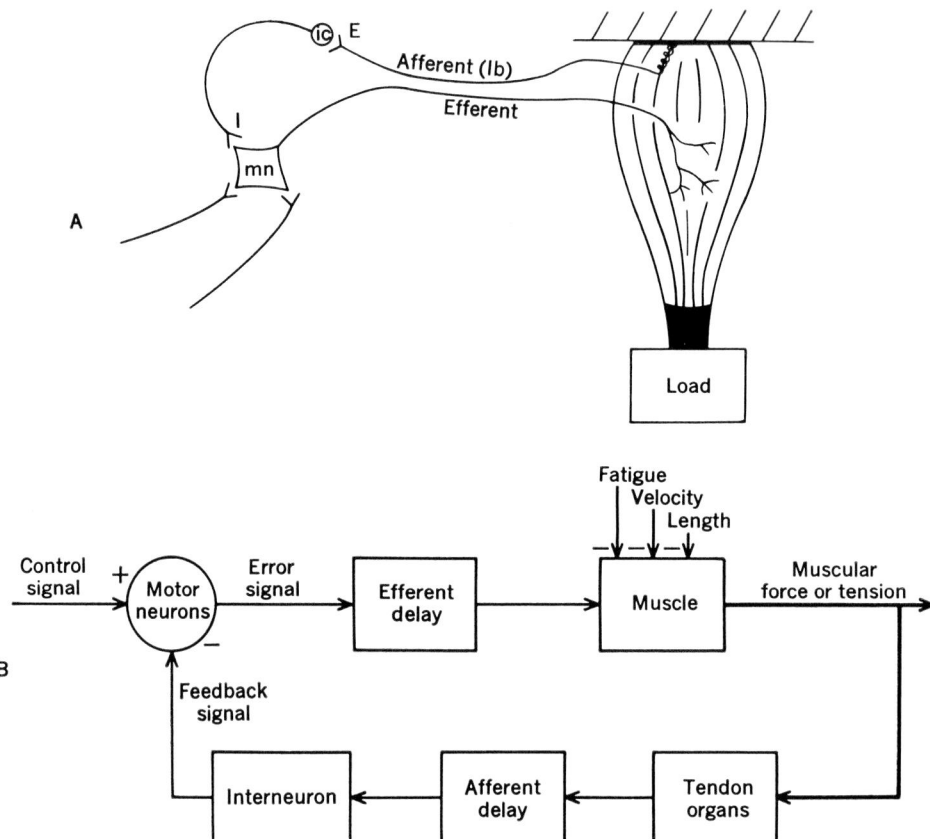

Figure 4-9. Tension Control System. A: Schematic diagram of the physiologic system responsible for tension control. Action potentials from Golgi tendon organs in muscle are transmitted to the spinal cord in Ib afferent fibers. Those signals excite, E, internuncial cells, i.e. which in turn inhibit I, motor neurons. B: Block diagram of tension control system, showing that the system counteracts the disturbing effects of fatigue (muscle velocity and length) (From J. C. Houk, and E. Henneman, "Feedback Control of Movement and Posture," in V. Mountcastle, ed., *Medical Physiology II*, 12th ed. (1968) Chap. 72.

Automatic compensation for load and fatigue have always been numbered among the supposed advantages of the muscle servo but the original theory (Merton, 1953) did not predict that the compensation would take the form or show the effectiveness that it does. Even at that time, however, it was noted that, contrary to expectation, when skilled finger actions, such as writing or playing musical instruments, are carried out during circulatory arrest, there is little falling off in performance almost until the muscles become so weak that they are unable to execute the necessary movements at all (Merton, 1956). This now becomes intelligible.

If this is the case then future research might be directed toward identifying the circumstances under which this postulated phenomenon operates. From the mechanistic viewpoint, it may prove profitable to explore motor unit recruitment patterns (see for example the work of Ashworth, Grimby and Kugelberg, 1967 and Grimby and Hannerz, 1968) under conditions of neuromuscular fatigue aimed at differentially fatiguing phasic and tonic motor units. Such an approach could bring together information concerning voluntary and involuntary mechanisms and deal with the problems of motor control and of the effects of fatigue upon control and organization at a very fundamental level, that of motor integration.

SUMMARY

In this chapter, the relationships between tendon reflexes, reaction times and fatigue induced by strenuous muscular exertion have been examined. On the pessimistic side, one can identify many studies lacking in attention to detail (for example, those discussing fatigue but not providing any criterion of the extent of impairment), and those which have failed to make any differentiation between fatigue induced by local muscular activity, general body exercise, or prolonged and monotonous work tasks. The diverse and sometimes less than sophisticated methods of recording various reflex measurements have also contributed to the lack of congruity in both the design and results of investigation in this area.

On the optimistic side, however, one can find technological and methodological advances that appear capable of providing greater insight into the problems at hand. In particular, the development of electroencephalic techniques for further fractionation of reaction times into component cortical latencies may prove beneficial in unravelling the complex relationships between exercise induced activation, work, stress, and the locus of any RT changes associated with central nervous system delays. Additionally, the concurrent assessment of fractionated voluntary (RT) and involuntary (tendon reflex) response times, particularly one might note, the motor times, under similar experimental conditions, in the same subjects and with similar degrees of precision, would appear to be capable of shedding further light on the mechanisms of fatigue-induced impairment of peripheral motor control. Furthermore, some insight may be permitted into some of the basic fatigue processes themselves.

Also on the optimistic side, one now finds several plausible theories related to the interaction of voluntary and involuntary responses under conditions of fatigue. The activation-work-stress approach provides one avenue for psychological-physiological investigation while on more purely physiological grounds, the effects of temperature variation, and the characteristics of different motor units under fatigue conditions as well as the postulated reflex loop-gain compensatory mechanism may provide investigators with some guidelines for future research.

BIBLIOGRAPHY

Angeleri, F. A., A. Granati, R. Lenzi, and A. Ferroni: Studio polifisiografico e psicologico sugli effetti della fatica indotta dal lavaro industriale monotono. *Med Lav, 60:* 528-542, 1969.

Ashworth, B., L. Grimby, and E. Kugelberg: Comparison of voluntary and reflex activation of motor units. *J Neurol Neurosurg Psychiatr, 30:*91-98, 1967.

Asami, T.: Basic Experiment on Reflex Time and Reaction Time. *Bulletin of Institute of Sports Medicine.* The Faculty of Physical Education. Tokyo University of Education, *9:*31-42, 1971.

Babadjanian, M. G., V. N. Sokolova, J. I. Kostina, M. I. Mamazashuili, and V. J. Tchirkov: Research on the causes of fatiguability of train dispatchers. (Russ.) In H. Schmidtke: *Die Ermudung.* Bern-Stuttgart, Huber, 183, 1965.

Babin, W. L.: The effects of various work loads on simple reaction latency as related to selected physical parameters, Ph.D. dissertation. University of Southern Mississippi, 1966.

Barker, D., and N. K. Chin: The number and distribution of muscle-spindles in certain muscles of the cat. *J Anat* (Lond.) *94:*473-486, 1960.

Bartlett, F. C.: The measurement of human skill. *Journal of Occupational Psychology, 22:*31-38, 1947.

———: Psychological criteria of fatigue. In Floyd, W. F., and Welford, A. T. (Eds.): *Fatigue.* London, H. K. Lewis, 1953.

Botwinick, J., and L. W. Thompson: Premotor and motor components of reaction time. *J Exp Psychol, 71:*9-15, 1966.

———: Components of reaction time in relation to age and sex. *J Gen Psychol, 108:* 175-183, 1966.

Buchthal, F., and H. Schmalbruch: Contraction times of twitches evoked by H-Reflexes. *Acta Physiol Scand, 80:*378-382, November, 1970.

Calapay, G. G., and G. Bellia: Valutazioni psicometriche su soggetti exposti al rumori di motori a reazione. *Med Lav 60:*43-52, 1969.

Carstocea, L., R. Elias, R. Mateescu, and Cristescu: Some peculiarities of fatigue in shift work in an automatised section. Prox XV *Int Congr Med Travail* (Vien), *4:*99-102, 1966.

Chaffin, D. B.: Localized muscle fatigue—definition and measurement. *J Occup Med, 15:* 346-354, 1973.

Cheah, J. S., and B. Y. Tan: The effect of exercise on the Achilles tendon reflex time. *Med J Aust, 1:*1050-1051, 1970.

Chin, N. K., M. Cope, and M. Pang: Number and distribution of spindle capsules in seven hindlimb muscles of the cat. In Barker, D. (Ed.): *Symposium on Muscle Receptors.* Hong Kong University Press, 1962.

Cooper, C. J.: Anatomical and physiological mechanisms of arousal, with special reference to the effects of exercise. *Ergonomics, 16:*601-609, 1973.

Davey, C. P.: Physical exertion and mental performance. *Ergonomics, 16:*595-599, 1973.

Donders, F. C.: Official report of the ordinary meeting of the royal academy of sciences. 1865. In Koster, W. G. (Ed.): *Acta Psychologica 30. Attention and Performance II.* 409, 411, 1969.

Elbel, E. R.: A study of response times before and after strenuous exercise. *Res Quart, 11:*86-95, 1940.

Erb, W.: Uber sehnenreflexe bei gesunden und bei ruckenmarkskranken. *Arch Psychiatr Nervenkr, 5:*792-802, 1875.

Fruktov, J. M.: On the reaction time of competition starts (Russ). *Teoriya Praktica fizitcheskoi Kulturi, 4:*279-299, 1943.

Gawrilescu, N., M. Pafnote, I. Vaida, I. Mihaila, L. Carstocea, O. Luchian and P. Popesco: Control-board shift work turning every two days. *Proc XV Int Cong Med Travail* (Vien), *4:*103-106, 1966.

Gilson, W. E.: Achilles Reflex Recording with a simple photomotograph. *N Engl J Med, 260:*1027-1028, 1959.

Granit, R.: *Receptors and Sensory Perception.* New Haven, Yale University Press, 1955.

Grimby, L., and J. Hannerz: Recruitment order of motor units on voluntary contraction: changes induced by proprioceptive afferent activity. *J Neurol Neurosurg Psychiatry, 31:*565-573, 1968.

Gutin, B.: Exercise Induced Activation and Human Performance: A Review, Paper presented at the Scientific Congress in conjunction with Olympic Games, Munich, 1972.

Haggendal, J., and B. Werdinius: Dopamine in human urine during muscular work. *Acta Physiol Scand, 66:*223-225, 1966.

Haider, M., J. A. Gangleberger, and E. Groll-Knapp: Thalamo-cortical components of reaction time. *Acta Psychologicá 30 Attention and Performance II,* 378-381, 1969.

Hartson, L. D.: Analysis of skilled movements. *Personnel Journal, 11:*28-43, 1932.

Hathaway, S.: Some characteristics of the electromyograms of quick voluntary muscle contractions. *Proc Soc Exp Biol Med, 30:*280-281, 1932.

Hathaway, S.: An action potential study of neuromuscular relations. *J Exp Psychol, 18:*285-298, 1935.

Hayes, K. C.: Jendrassik maneuver facilitation and fractionated patellar reflex times. *J Appl Physiol, 32:*290-295, 1972.

Hayes, K. C.: Effects of fatiguing isometric exercise upon Achilles tendon reflex and plantar flexion reaction time components in man. *Eur J Appl Physiol, 34:*69, 1975.

Helmholtz, H. von: On the rate of transmission of the nerve impulse. Translated in Dennis, W. (Ed.): *Readings in the History of Psychology.* New York, Appleton-Crofts, 1948.

Henane, R.: Exercice musculaire et reflectivite spinale chez l'homme. *J Physiol, 60:*457-458, 1968.

Henane, R., and R. Flandrois: Exercice Musculaire et Reflectivite Sous-Maximal Et Reflectivite Spinale Chez l'Homme. 1. Variations Concordantes des Reponses Tendineuse et de Hoffmann. *Comptes Rendus Societe Biologie, 162:*698-702, 1968.

———: Exercice musculaire et reflectivite spinale chez l'homme. 2. Variations discordantes des reponses tendineuse et de Hoffmann. *Comptes Rendus Societe Biologie, 162:*1354-1358, 1968.

Henane, R., and J. A. Macarez: Effets de l'exercice Physique sur la Reflectivite Spinale Chez l'Homme. *Internationale Zeitschrift fur angewandte Physiologie einschlieblich Arbeitsphysiologie, 30:*315-334, 1972.

Houk, J. C., J. J. Singer, and M. R. Goldman: An evaluation of length and force feedback to soleus muscles of decerebrate cats. *J Neurophysiol, 33:*784-811, 1970.

Houk, J. C., and E. Henneman: Feedback control of movement and posture. In Mountcastle, V. (Ed.): *Medical Physiology II,* 12th Ed. 1968, pp. 1681-1696.

Hunt, C. C.: The effect of sympathetic stimulation on mammalian muscle spindles. *J Physiol, 151:*332-341, 1960.

Johnson, B. L., E. Jokl, and P. Jokl: The effect of exercise upon the duration of the triceps surae stretch reflex. *J Assoc Phys Ment Rehab, 17*:172-176, 1963.

Kawamura, T.: Studies on the Achilles tendon reflex for the application to the physical fitness. *Hiroshima J Med Sci, 20*:1-18, 1971.

Kimura, N.: On the Achilles tendon reflex recorded by new strain gauge method. *Hiroshima J. Med Sci, 16*:139-151, 1967.

Kroll, W.: Effects of local muscular fatigue due to isotonic and isometric exercise upon fractionated reaction time components. *Journal of Motor Behavior, 5*:81-93, 1973.

Kroll, W.: Fractionated reaction and reflex time before and after fatiguing isotonic exercise. *Medicine and Science in Sports, 6*:260-266, 1974.

Kugelberg, E., and L. Edstrom: Differential histochemical effects of muscle contractions on phosphorylase and glycogen in various types of fibres: Relation to fatigue. *J Neurol Neurosurg Psychiatry, 31*:415-423, 1968.

Lagasse, P. P., and K. C. Hayes: Premotor and motor reaction time as a function of movement extent. *Journal of Motor Behavior, 5*:25-32, 1973.

Lambert, E. H., L. O. Underdahl, S. Beckett, and L. O. Mederos: A study of the ankle jerk in myxedema. *J Clin Endocrinol, 11*:1186-1205, 1951.

Lippold, O. C. J., J. W. T. Redfearn, and J. Vuco: The electromyography of fatigue. *Ergonomics, 3*:121-131, 1960.

Lombard, W. P.: The variations of the normal knee jerk and their relation to the activity of the central nervous system. *Am J Psychol, 1*:2-17, 1887.

Macarez, J. A., and R. Henane: Influence d'un exercice musculaire sous-maximal sur les seuils des reflexes monosynaptique chez l'homme. 1. Effets sur les seuils des reponses tendineuses. *Comptes Rendus Societe Biologie, 163*:1743-1747, 1970.

———: Influence d'un exercice musculaire sous-maximal sur les seuils des reflexes monosynaptique chez l'homme. 2. Effets sur les seuils du reflexe de Hoffmann. *Comptes Rendus Societe Biologie, 163*:1743-1747, 1970.

Malomsoki, J., and I. Szmodis: Visual response time changes in athletes during physical effort. *Internationale Zeitschrift fur angewandte Physiologie einschlieblich Arbeitsphysiologie, 29*:65-72, 1970.

Margaria, R., and T. Gualtierotti: Functional fundamental characteristics of the nervous system in athletes and the effects of performance. In *Health and Fitness in the Modern World.* Chicago, Athletic Institute, 1961.

Margaria, R., T. Gualtierotti, and D. Spinelli: Effect of stress on lower neuron activity. *Exp Med Surg, 16*:166-176, 1958.

Marsden, C. D., P. A. Merton and H. B. Morton: Servo action in human voluntary movement. *Nature, 238*:140-143, 1972.

Masters, A. M.: Two-step test of myocardial function. *Am Heart J, 10*:495, 1935.

Mateev, D.: Muscle fatigue. *Sechenov Physiological Journal of U.S.S.R., 47*:75-78, 1961.

Merton, P. A.: Speculations on the servo-control of movement. In J. L. Malcolm, J. A. B. Gray and G. E. Wolstenhome (Eds.): *Ciba Found Symp The Spinal Cord,* London, Churchill, 1953, 247-255.

Merton, P. A.: Voluntary strength and fatigue. *J Physiol, 123*:553-564, 1954.

Merton, P. A.: Problems of muscular fatigue. *Br Med Bull, 12*:219-221, 1956.

Meyers, C. R., W. Zimmerli, S. D. Farr, and N. A. Baschnagel: Effect of strenuous physical activity upon reaction time. *Res Quart, 40*:332-337, 1969.

Monnier, M.: Retinal cortical and motor responses to photic stimulation in man. *J Neurophysiol, 15*:469-486, 1952.

Moruzzi, G., and H. W. Magoun: Brain stem reticular formation and activation of the EEG. *Electroenceph Clin Neurophysiol, 1*:455-473, 1949.
Mountcastle, V. B.: *Medical Physiology*, 12th ed., St. Louis, Mosby, 1968, vol. II.
Nemessuri, M., and J. Malomsoki: The role of medical gymnastics in rehabilitation (Hungarian). *Rheum Baln Allerg, 1*:47-49, 1965.
Nemessuri, M., I. Szmodis, and M. Szaszne: Relationship of response time and effort. (Hungarian) *Testnev Sproteu Szle, 10*:13-18, 1969.
Nystrom, C. L.: A comparative study of the Achilles and the patellar response latencies as measured by the action current and the muscle thickening methods. *Psychol Monogr, 44*:61-82, 1933.
Person, R. S., and L. P. Kudina: Discharge frequency and discharge pattern of human motor units during voluntary contraction of muscle. *Electroencephalog Clin Neurophysiol, 32*:471-483, 1972.
Petajan, J. A., and C. J. Eagan: Effect of temperature, exercise and physical fitness on the triceps surae reflex. *J Appl Physiol, 25*:16-20, 1968.
Phillips, W. H.: Influence of fatiguing warm-up exercises on speed of movement and reaction latency. *Res Quart, 34*:370-378, 1963.
Quo, Sung-Ken: A new method of measuring fatigue by the threshold stimulus of the Achilles tendon reflex. *Journal of Applied Physiology, 2*:148-154, 1949.
Reid, C.: The mechanism of voluntary muscular fatigue. *Quart J Exp Physiol, 19*:17-42, 1928.
Reinfrank, R. F., R. P. Kaufman, H. J. Wetstone, and J. A. Glennon: Observations of the Achilles reflex test. *JAMA, 199*:59-62, 1967.
Santa Maria, D. L.: Pre-motor and motor reaction time differences associated with stretching of the hamstring muscles. *J Mot Behav, 2*:163-173, 1970.
Schmidt, R. A., and G. A. Stull: Premotor and motor reaction time as a function of preliminary muscular tension. *J Mot Behav, 2*:96-110, 1970.
Sheerer, N., and R. A. Berger: Effects of various levels of fatigue on reaction time and movement time. *Am Correct Ther J, 26*:146-147, 1972.
Schwab, R. S.: Research of reviews. Office of Naval Research, June, 1949, p. 17.
Schwab, R. S., and J. S. Prichard: Neurologic aspects of fatigue. *Neurology, 1*:133-135, 1951.
Simonson, E.: *Physiology of Work Capacity and Fatigue*. Springfield, Thomas, 1971.
Sorge, R. W.: The effects of levels of intense activity on total body reaction time, Ph.D. dissertation, Colorado State College, 1960.
Stein, R. B., Peripheral control of movement. *Physiol Rev, 54*:215-243, 1974.
Sternberg, M.: Sehnenreflexe bei Ermüdung. *Centralbl f Phys*, 1887.
Sternberg, M.: *Die Sehnenreflexe ünd ihre Bedeutung fur die pathologie des Nervensystems*. Leipzig, 1893.
Teichner, W. H.: Recent studies of simple reaction time. *Psychol Bull, 51*:128-149, 1954.
Tipton, C. M., and P. V. Karpovich: Exercise and the patellar reflex. *J Appl Physiol, 21*:15-18, 1966.
Tuttle, W. W.: The effect of exercise on the Achilles jerk. *Arbeitsphysiologie, 2*:367-371, 1930.
Vassilev, I. G., L. P. Zimnitzkaya, E. L. Skyarchik, K. M. Smirnov, B. G. Filippov, S. A. Khitum, and A. M. Shatolov: On the daily rhythmicity of human efficiency. (In Russian) *Fizjol Zh SSSR, 43*:817-824, 1957.
Vaughan, H. G., L. D. Costa, L. Gilden, and H. Schimmel: Identification of sensory

and motor components of cerebral activity in simple reaction-time tasks. *Proc 73rd Conf Am Psychol Assoc, 1:*179-180, 1965.

Vendsalu, A.: Studies on adrenaline and noradrenaline in human plasma. *Acta Physiol Scand, 49,* Suppl. 173, Ch. VI, 1960.

Verdy, M., J. Lapierre, H. Sansoucy, and R. Lefebvre: Shortening of Achilles reflex time after exercise. *JAMA, 204:*169-171, 1968.

Weisendanger, M., P. Schneider, and J. P. Villoz: Electromyographic analysis of a rapid volitional movement. *Am J Phys Med, 48:*17-24, 1969.

Weiss, A. D.: The locus of reaction time change with set, motivation and age. *J Gerontol, 20:*60-64, 1965.

Welford, A. T.: Stress and performance. *Ergonomics, 16:*567-599, 1973.

Westerman, R. F., and J. Gerbrandy: Muscle temperature and ankle jerk. *Folia medica Neerlandica, 12:*51-57, 1969.

Westphal, C. I. O.: Ueber einige durch mechanische kinwirkung auf sehnen und muskeln hervorgebrachte bewegungs-erscheinungen. *Arch psychiat nervenkr, 5:*803-834, 1875.

Wickwire, G. C., H. L. Terry, R. Krouse, W. E. Burge, and C. D. Monsson: Further study on threshold of knee jerk—an index to physical fitness. *Am J Physiol, 123:* 213-214, 1938.

Witte, N. K., and A. P. Okhrimenko. Physiological peculiarities of female labor in sewing industry. (In Russian) *Gig Tr Prof Zabol, 12:*45-47, 1968.

Wojtczak-Jarosz, J., and Z. Maciaszek: Electromyographical analysis of reaction time. *Acta Neurobiologicae Experimentalis, 31:*141-150, 1971.

Wood, G. A.: Neuromuscular correlates of sensori motor performance in normal and fatigued states, Ph.D. dissertation, University of Massachusetts at Amherst, 1974.

Woodworth, R. S.: *Experimental Psychology.* New York, Holt, 1938.

Yurchenko, A. S.: Evaluation of the higher nervous system activity in performing work of different complexity at control desks of industrial enterprises. (In Russian) *Gig Tr Prof Zabol, 11:*35-39, 1967.

Chapter 5

Motor Coordination

WALTER ROHMERT

THE COURSE OF HUMAN movements through time and space are to some extent the connecting link between the single "stationary" events within a human movement and therefore are important components of all human activities. The study of these connecting links is very diversified. Many disciplines are interested in the study of motor coordination of human motions.

Anatomy studies the limits of all movements due to the type and shape of joint surfaces (passive motion analysis). *Physiology of motion,* in contrast to anatomy, directly studies motion and speed (active motion analysis) that are carried out by the living body. While the physiology of motion primarily investigates the factors of controlling flow and stress of energy balance and circulation, the *psychology of motion* tackles the interpretation of functional motion flow as an external expression in the form of motion. A variety of studies in this field can be classified into studies of a *common theory of human motions,* i.e. wholly theoretical studies, analysis of variance in motions and studies of information theory, and studies of kinesthetic and coordination theory. In *biomechanics and sports* the flow of motions by limb-links will be analysed; the human body is regarded as a mechanical form, to which rules of mechanics can be applied in principle. In *choreography* at least the phenomenon of motion will be pursued from the beginning to the end states. A static description describes the posture, a dynamic description proceedings and events. In practical *time and motion studies,* a time analysis follows a motion analysis with a splitting up of the motion elements and the time factors (predetermined motion time systems) with the aim of predetermining time and designing motion at definite work locations.

We will confine our considerations of motor coordination during the course of manual aimed movements to three essential aspects:
1. mechanics of movements
2. control of movements
3. trainability of movements

The most often considered types of motions are called psychomotor skills (Rohmert, Rutenfranz, and Ulich, 1971). By skills we mean (Ulich, 1967) human motor capacities that are adapted to stressors of a relatively stereotyped type and flow. Psychomotor skills are those skills which enable voluntary performance of partial or complex movements with different sensory and motor portions. The sensory aspects may consist in perception from each sensory modality, but most often these are visual, acoustical, and tactile perceptions. The motor aspects consist in performing a simple or complex controlled movement, the kind, extent, accuracy, and speed of which depend on information fed back from the perceptual areas. The motor action (or reaction, respectively) can be accompanied by sensory (perceptual) activities which send information about the accuracy of the movement and which lead in turn to its correction.

In comparing aimed human motions with a control process, Mayne (1951) found two different control loops working with each other: the internal control loop has its receptor elements in muscle and other locations of deep sensibility, and its governor in the central nervous system, which manipulates information over the motor nerves to the muscles; the external control loop has its receptor elements in the external sensory organs, while the remaining components of the control loop are similar to the internal control loop. Küpfmüller and Poklekowsky (1956) found that the internal control loop is involved in the beginning of the movement for a quick and rough approach to the point of aim, while the external control loop is employed later in the aim and provides exact corrections.

By training a movement, the external control loop becomes involved later and later. In the ideal situation, the eye only gives information about the space coordinates while the internal control loop alone controls the aiming movement. The relief of higher nervous control systems facilitates the realization of complex adaption, which can be described as skill. In this stage total skill can be represented by one "signal" only, which is connected closely to the imagination of the aim of this portion of movement.

MECHANICAL FUNCTIONING SYSTEM OF THE ARM

The organizing principle for the various forms of mechanical behavior of the human body is the relation between load (stress) and strain (Rohmert, 1971). This relation corresponds to the correlation between the cause and its consequence, between the action and its effect, between input and output. Regarding human motions, there are different kinds of loads to which the corresponding kinds of strain correlate. Mechanical load factors in human motions can be classified (Jenik, 1972) into kinematic and dynamic factors as well as into qualitative and quantitative factors (see Fig. 5-1). By combining the qualitative mechanical load factors in various ways, it is possible to define the kind of movements together with the kind of mechanical load as a movement form. Individual quantitative data about the size of movement and the size of load determine an individual movement type. It should be emphasized that the individual different body type (physical somatotype) could be inserted into this model (of Fig. 5-1) as a load factor with the corresponding effect on the strain variables.

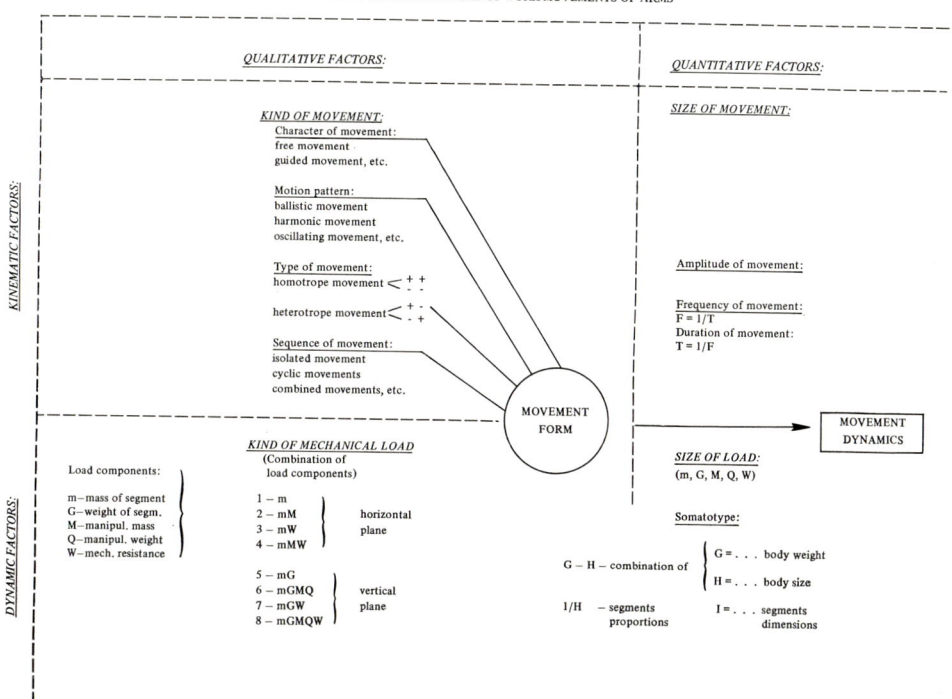

Figure 5-1. Factors of mechanical load of work movements of arms.

By using the model, many useful results have been obtained. The computer can be used for a biomechanical analysis of individual types of arm movements. For all these individual types of movements described in literature or studied in our own research, the course of mechanical strain variables during a movement cycle can be calculated by the computer: angular velocity and acceleration, static and driving movements in the shoulder and elbow joint, mechanical power, and static and dynamic work.

It is interesting to note that during the dynamic motion process a static component of strain is also produced simultaneously as a product of the force and moving time in contrast to the dynamic component of strain as a product of force and distance. With some difficulty the results of both the mechanical as well as the physiological functioning cycles can be compared on the output side, meaning that mechanical power and physiological energy production (or consumption) can be compared. The problems of correlating the static work produced during the dynamic action of a motion to the corresponding component of energy expenditure could not yet be solved in the past. The addition of the static and dynamic work in the mechanical work had to be excluded.

The biomechanical computer calculations allow the formulation of a

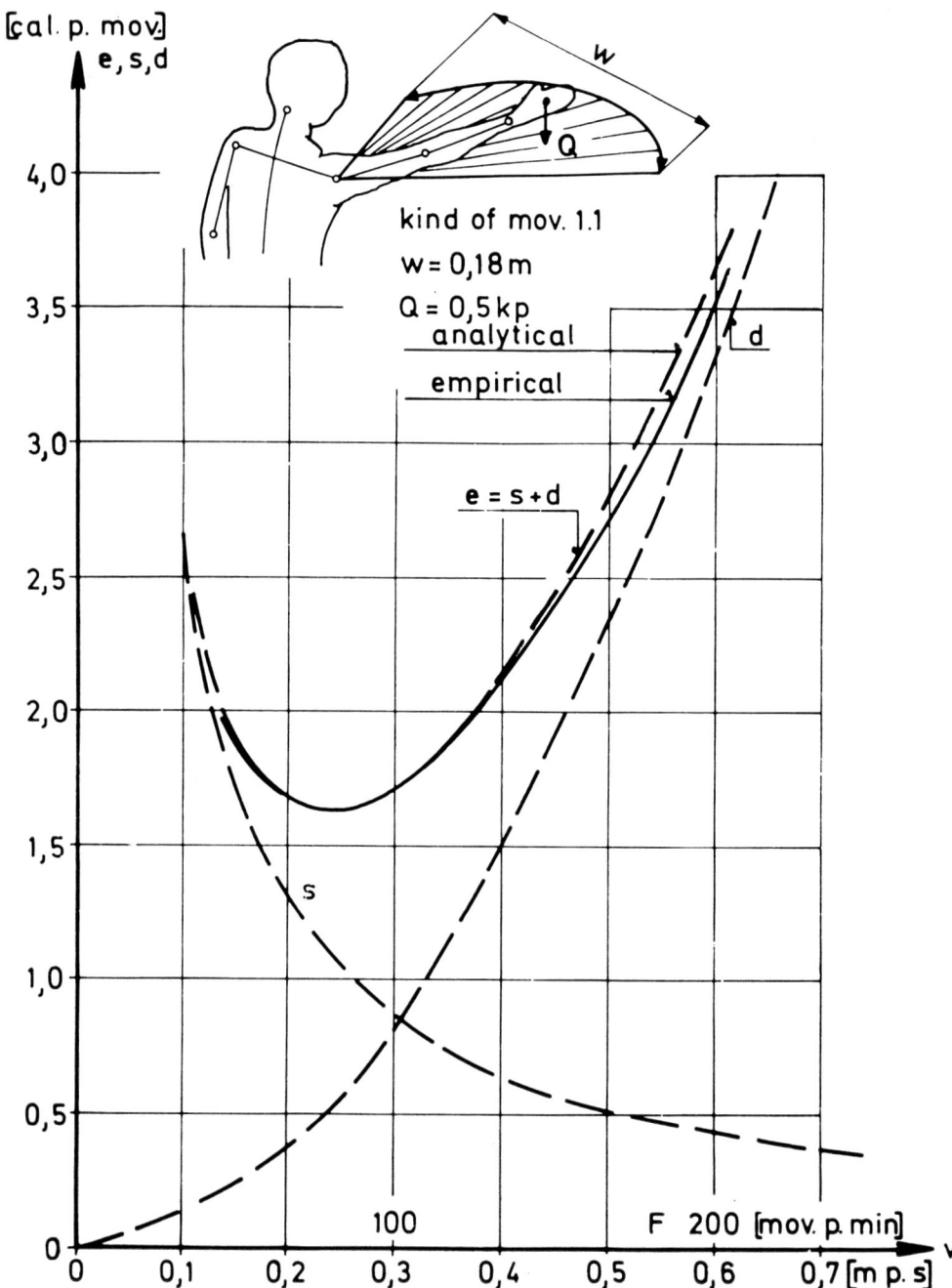

Figure 5-2. Correlation between the empirical and analytical specific energy consumption.

quantitative relation between energy consumption and movement frequency. Simple expressions which include factors that explain the causality of the mechanical processes allow a satisfactorily reliable prediction of the energy expenditure for any individual type of movement. The biomechanical analysis enables the formulation of a logically and causally based a priori hypothesis before beginning any laboratory experiment as well as selecting load factors to diminish expensive and extensive laboratory experiments. Experiments can be planned, projected and arranged much more easily and reliably. Any discussion of empirical data can be supported by objective facts, and incorrect results obtained by measuring, e.g. energy expenditure, can be easily identified. Multiple measuring of fewer variables guarantees a higher accuracy of results than does a greater number of measures in more types of movements.

Figure 5-2 gives an example for the biomechanical procedure and its advantages. The case of movement was studied by Stier (1959): free horizontal swinging movements of the straight arm in manipulating an additional weight of 0.5 kp over a distance of 18 cm with frequencies between 25 and 250 movements per minute. The static load by the additional weight was eliminated. The results of these experiments are well known: the total energy consumption increases with increasing frequency of movement in an exponential manner. The specific energy consumption (related to one

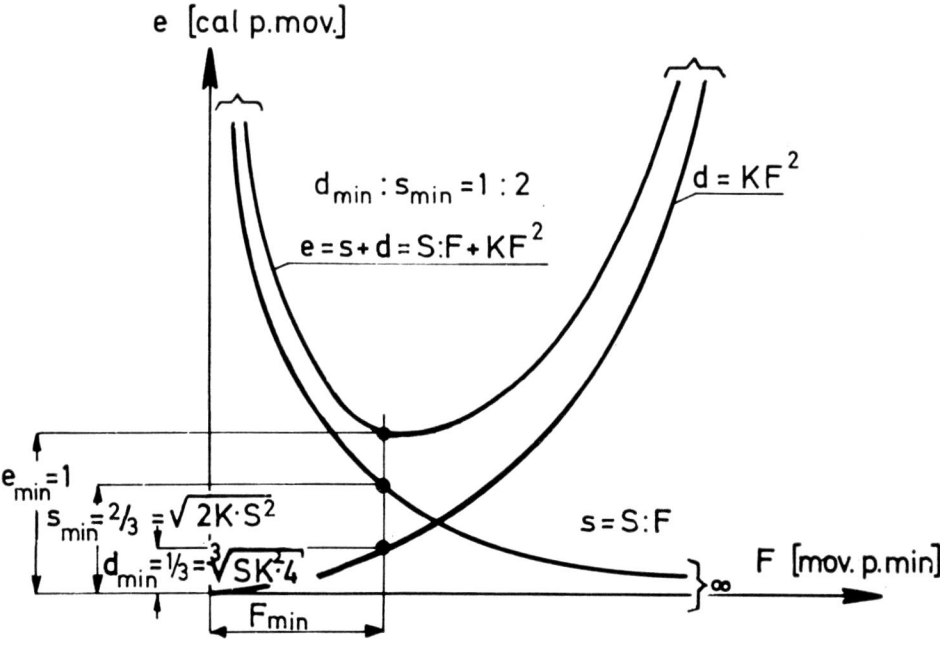

Figure 5-3. Specific energy consumption (schematically).

movement cycle) shows an evident minimum as also seen in Figure 5-3. The dynamic component, d, increases exponentially; the static one, s, decreases hyperbolically. For movements with sinusoidal moving patterns (with weights manipulated between 0 to 1.5 kp and moving distances between 10 and 50 cm), the dynamic work produced during a movement is proportional to the square of the frequency and the power to its cube. The position of the minimum specific energy consumption, e, is determined by the proportion $d_{min} : s_{min} = 1 : 2$ (see Fig. 5-3). Figure 5-2 shows good agreement between measured (Stier, 1959) and calculated (Jenik, 1972) results. (Small deviations for higher movement frequencies are due to different considerations of the movement distances, which were measured in the experiments as a straight line but in the calculations as a ballistic arc.)

MOTOR COORDINATION IN SPACE AND TIME

In an early fundamental study, Simonson, et al. (1934) investigated the spatial and temporal coordination of sequential movements. Simonson classified different components of motor coordination:

1. Spatial Coordination
   a. motion pattern

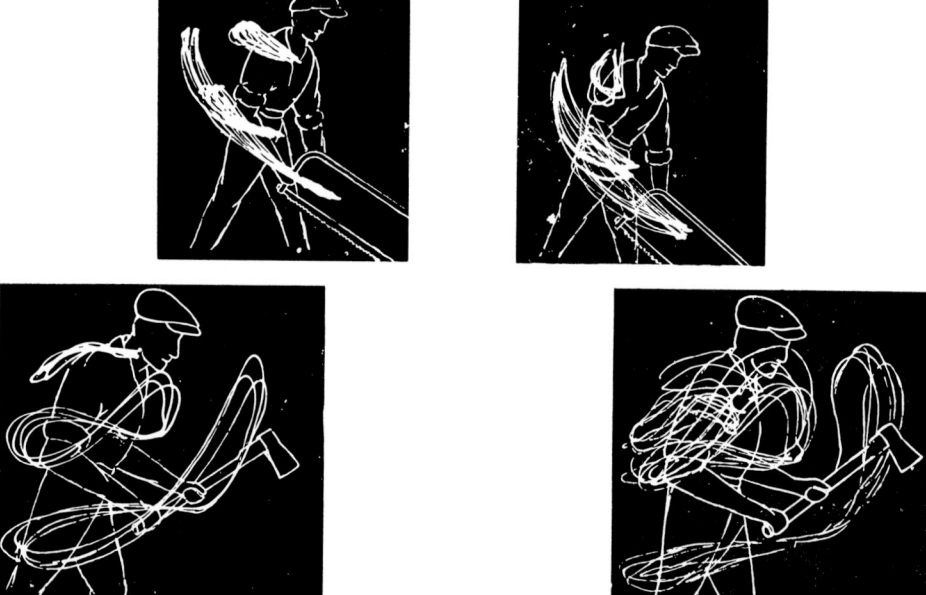

Figure 5-4. Cyclographic pictures of working movements with the subject drawn (Foto G. KAMINSKY).

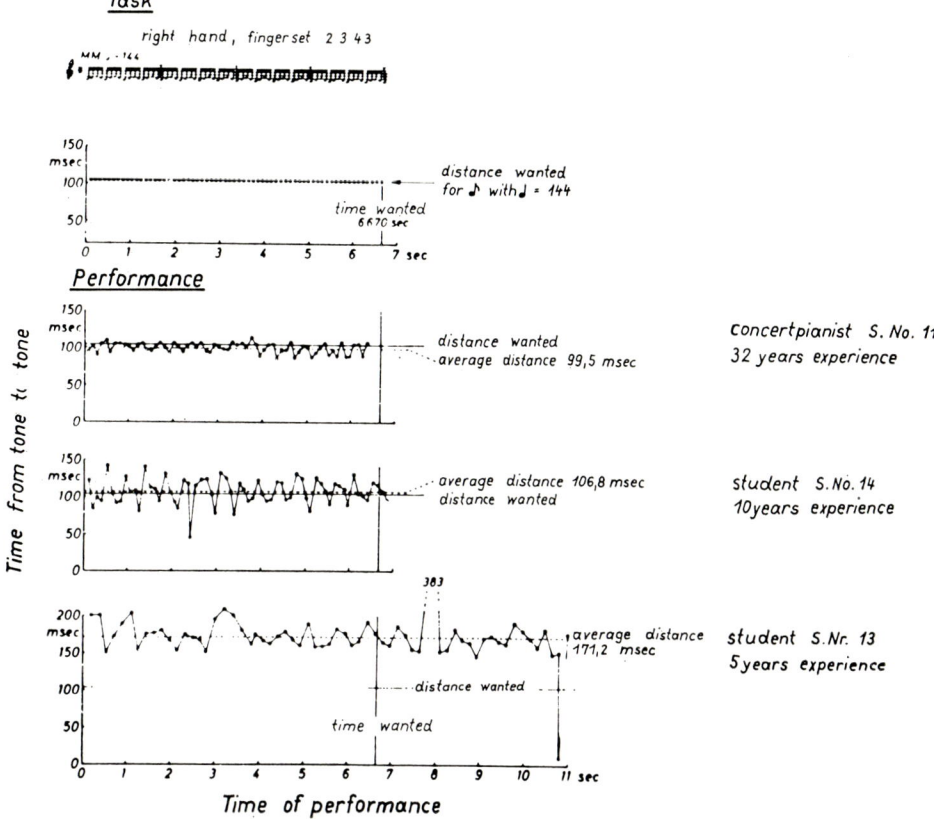

Figure 5-5. Performing a distinguished piano playing task by three different skilled subjects (From Ch. Wagner, "Untersuchungen zur Ergonomie des Klavierspiels," In *Biomechanics 1, First Int. Seminar Zurich, 1967* (Karger, Basel, New York) 1968.

    b. coordination of sequential movements
  2. Time Coordination
    a. time of motion
    b. structure of motion elements (proportion of motion to rest times)
  3. Spatial and Time Coordination
    a. flow of velocity
    b. flow of acceleration
    c. integral of mechanical power and dynamic work
  4. Coordination of different body limbs and muscle groups.

A gain of coordination was found in the beginning of sequential arm movements with a loss at the end. Figure 5-4 (Kaminsky, 1960) shows the typical result of those studies using a cyclographic analysis of working movements. The left panels demonstrate favorable motion patterns where in a highly skilled and unfatigued subject all movements are repeated quite exactly, while the right panels demonstrate the opposite for nonskilled, fatigued subjects. Wagner (1968) measured the improvement in coordination as piano players became experienced: at first a speed coordination seems to occur and later an accuracy coordination of movements develops (see Fig. 5-5). The student with five years experience was not able to perform an experimental task in time or accurately. The task was to play the following tones c - d - e - d - c -, etc., with the fingers of the right hand. The ten years experienced student performed well in time but with insufficient accuracy, while only the highest experienced master player performed the task as well in time as in accuracy.

The studies of the type mentioned use output capacity criteria to evaluate motor coordination. Evaluation of motor coordination, however, should not be made only in terms of objective assessments of movement variables which affect man's motions. This type of stressor analysis should be extended also by a strain analysis (Rohmert, 1973) that required the determination of the effects of stressors put on man called strain. Only subject-related methods, i.e. mainly peripheral and central physiological measures, are suitable to evaluate strain. Those measures used in laboratory as well as in field studies are, for example, heart rate, heart rate variability, and electromyogram of muscles involved or the electrical eye movement activity (i.e. electrooculogram). These measures together with output measures of the performance should be determined as a time series. Correlations between those time series enable a deeper look into the problems of motor coordination. This model of research in motor coordination evaluates different degrees of coordination (see Table 5-I). Motor coordination will be better if performance increases while the strain remains constant; or the strain de-

			Strain measures (average)			
			peripheral		central	
			constant	increasing	constant	increasing
Performance measures	Variability	constant	4	3	3	2
		increasing	2	2	2	2
	MEAN	constant	2	2	2	2
		decreasing	1	1	1	1

Table 5-I: Classification for evaluating the degree in motor coordination

creases while performance remains constant; or there are variations in time of sequential movements within some performance and strain measures. The different measures are expressed primarily as means, secondly as variability. Combinations of these, however, are not equal in the evaluation of the degree of motor coordination. We propose the following scale of degrees of motor coordination:

a. Motor coordination shows effects indicating improvement when movements are sequentially repeated (degree 4).

b. Motor coordination shows slight disturbances while work is in progress, mainly measurable in those areas of functions which are primarily involved in the performance. At first one may expect reactions in the areas of the convergence in functional pathways (area of bottleneck); peripheral physiological measures of strain deteriorate (degree 3).

c. Motor coordination is altered to the extent that the deterioration reaches the self-observation of the individual. Also the means of performance measures still remain constant, but the variability of these measures

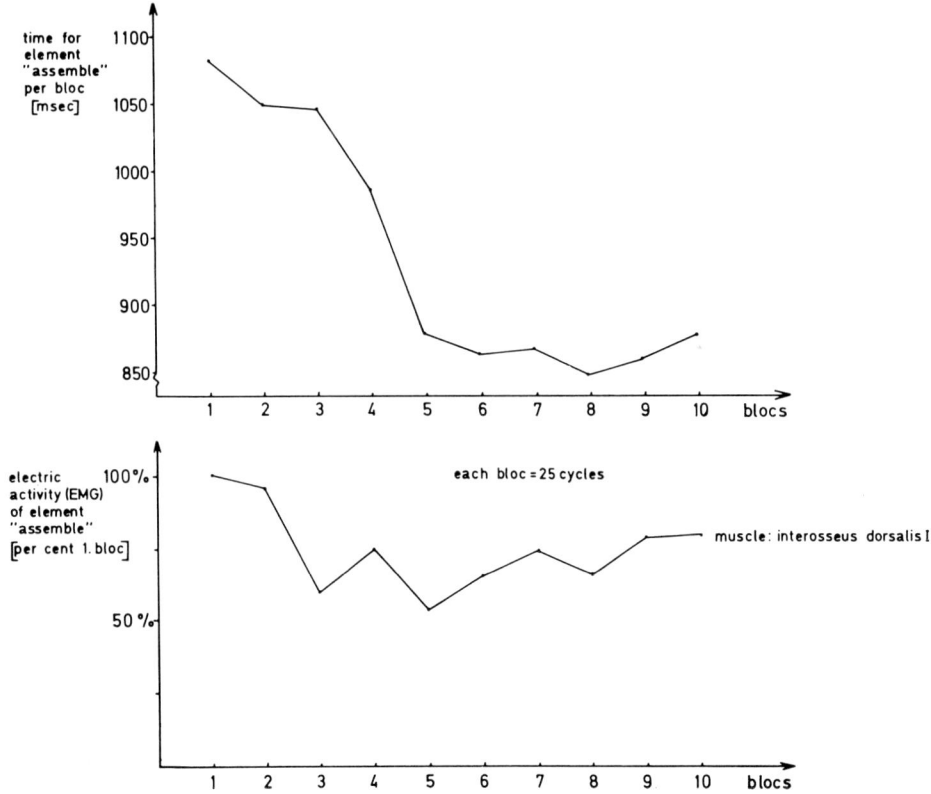

Figure 5-6. Correlation between surface-EMG and motion time in a simple assembling task.

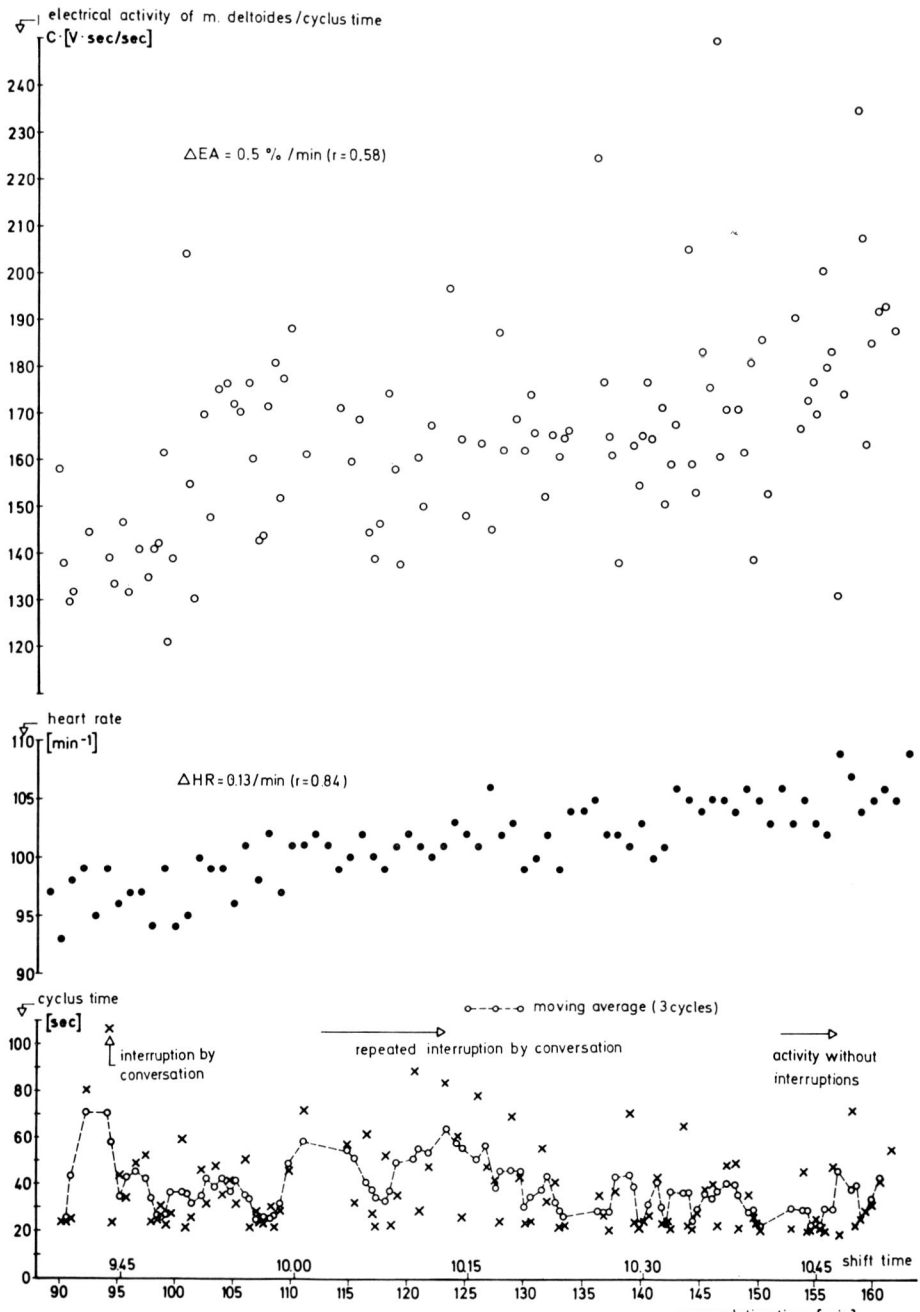

Figure 5-7. Time series of heart rate and electrical activity of a subject operating a hand lever repetitively (pressing soldering-tags).

increases. The individual tries to perform to his best by activating greater levels of motivation. Strain reactions of central nervous activity should be expected (degree 2).

d. Motor coordination is worse. The individual does not succeed in performing well, when repeating visible movements. Personality disturbances occur and individuals tend to withdraw from performance (degree 1).

Related to this 4-step scale, degree 3 may be evaluated by peripheral strain measure deterioration. Measures of higher variability as well as unchanged mean strain measures may indicate degree 2. Absolute figures of mean performance explain degree 1. Table 5-I explains this in more detail.

Figure 5-6 (Rohmert and Laurig, 1971) represents an example of the model. With the aid of an electrophysiological technique we get close to the true muscular actions used in motor coordination during a simple assembling task. At the beginning of the task (up to bloc no. 5) a clear relationship is shown between average performance time and the electromyogram (with surface-electrodes, representing an integrated EMG, calculated by electronic summation technique). This illustrates degree 4 of the model. Beginning with bloc no. 6 performance remains constant, however, peripheral strain is increasing which means degree 2 of the model. One may interpret this as a definite balance between training processes and fatigue. Also, in field studies covering a total shift, we obtained the same results as shown in Figure 5-7. In this case, the peripheral as well as the central physiological measures are increasing while performance time remains constant.

Hand-eye-movement coordination (evaluated with electromyogram and electrooculogram) also shows a more sensitive relationship for motor coordination than the limited evaluation using performance measures only (an extensive publication is in preparation by Rosenbrock).

TRAINABILITY OF MOTOR COORDINATION

Motor coordination can be learned and improved by a. sequential repetitions of the performance (active training), b. observation of the performance of other subjects (observational training), or c. mental practice through repeated imagination of the performance to be trained (mental training) (Rohmert, Rutenfranz, and Ulich, 1971). In all studies the effects of these three types of training on motor coordination can be ranked as follows: active, mental and observative training. Mental training performances were better retained than others (Ulich, 1967). Alternating periods of active and mental training are, in general, more successful for motor coordination than interrupted active training only. Interrupted training (training with breaks) is better than massed training. Already, af-

ter a very short time, the performance limit of massed training will be reached (Rohmert, Rutenfranz, and Ulich, 1971; Iskander, 1968). The positive effects of organized breaks in the training of motor skills are:
—psychological effect of awaiting a break
—recovery from central fatigue
—recovery from muscular fatigue
—possibility for mental or observative training.

The length of the break will also influence forgetting.

Rohmert and Schlaich (1966) found that there was no performance limit in repeating a very simple assembling task (assemble a washer on a plug) even after four months of repetitions of ca 1 hour per day (= 1296 assemblings) in 4 subjects (see Fig. 5-8). A longer weekend is clearly distinguished (circles in Fig. 5-8) by a lower mean performance even in the state of high motor skill. Increasing a financial incentive improves performance about 10 percent even if a high degree of motor coordination was reached, while performance decreases despite financial incentive as a consequence of fatigue (broken line in Fig. 5-8 and long arrow which means experiments with very short cycles over small distances of reaching). Figure 5-9 shows that all improvement in performance shown in Figure 5-8 for the 4

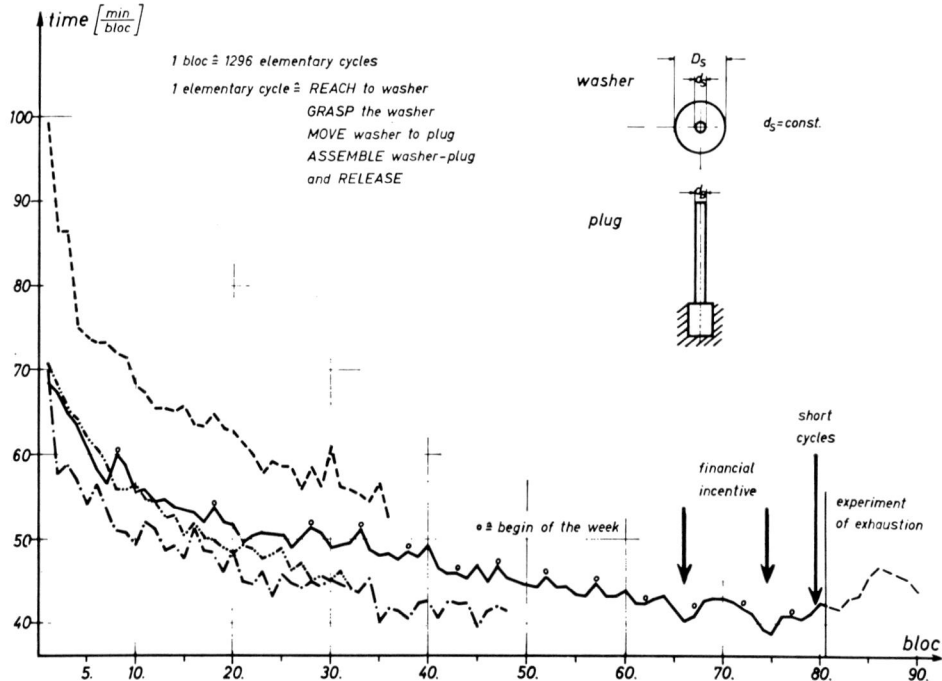

Figure 5-8. Learning-curves for assembling-work (washer-plug).

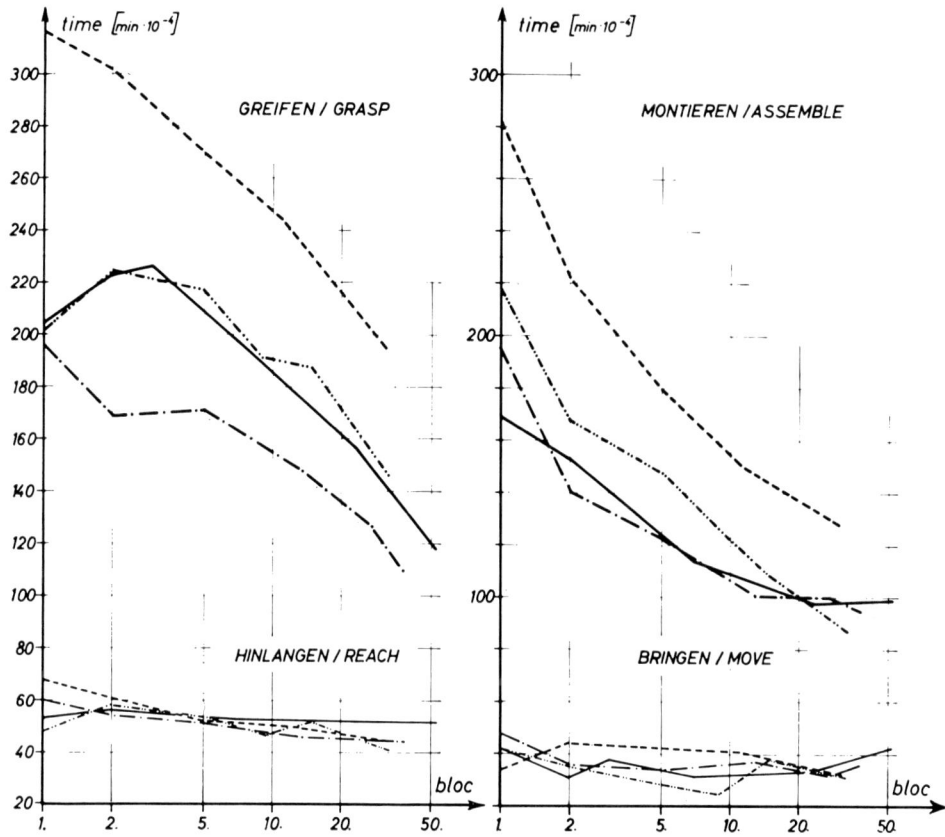

Figure 5-9. Learning-curves of the single motion-elements.

subjects is gained exclusively in the more sensory oriented motion elements of grasping and assembling and not at all in the motor-oriented elements of reaching and transporting. Also, all individual differences in performance are found only in grasping and assembling and not, however, in the motor functions of reaching and transporting.

In different tracking experiments, Rutenfranz, Rohmert, and Iskander (1971) studied the changes in heart rate that were in relationship to the conditions of massed or distributed training. Figure 5-10 shows heart rate under these conditions while subjects were performing a 60-minute Rotary Pursuit Apparatus Tracking Task. Heart rate is divided into physical and nonphysical portions. There is an increasing heart rate due to static load (SA), while the fraction of heart rate due to dynamic work (DA) remains small and constant. A nonphysical fraction as the result of psychogenic, mainly emotional reactions (B), disappears during the experiments. Also

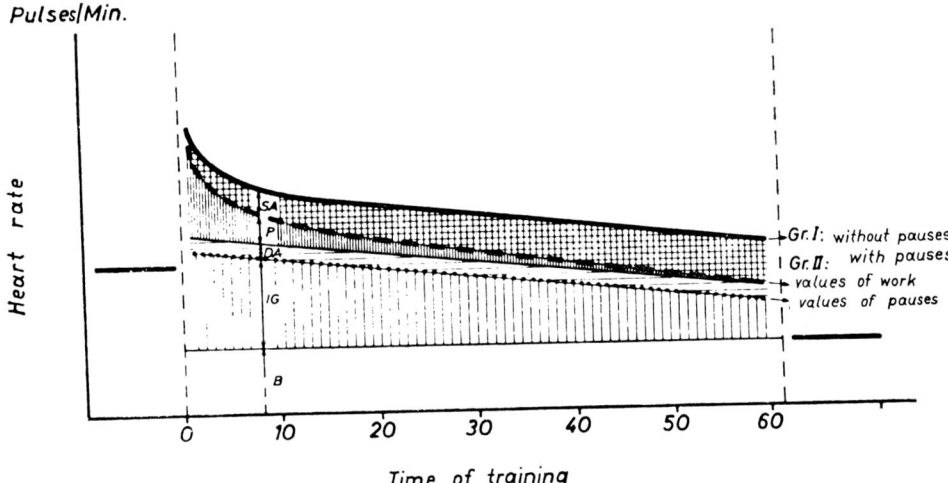

Figure 5-10. Schematic diagram of the changes of pulse frequency "fractions" on practicing a tracking task after different kinds of practice. B: Basic pulse frequency at repose while sitting (working position) after the trial. IG: Raise of pulse frequency as the result of the intentional basic tension. DA: Raise of pulse frequency as the result of dynamic work. P: Raise of pulse frequency as the result of psychogenic, mostly emotional reactions. SA: Raise of pulse frequency as the result of static muscle work.

another nonphysical fraction is explained as the result of an intentional basic tension (IG) that decreases but does not disappear completely.

These are preliminary but promising first results. The studies are to be continued.

BIBLIOGRAPHY

Iskander, A.: *Über den Einfluss von Pausen auf das Anlernen sensumotorischer Fertigkeiten.* Berlin-Köln-Frankfurt, Beuth-Vertrieb, 1968.

Jenik, P.: *Biomechanische Analyse ausgewählter Arbeitsbewegungen des Armes.* Berlin-Köln-Frankfurt, Beuth-Vertrieb, 1972.

Kaminsky, G., and H. Schmidtke: *Arbeitsablauf und Bewegungsstudien.* München, Verlag C. Hanser, 1960.

Küpfmüller, K., and G. Poklekowsky: Der Regelmechanismus willkürlicher Bewegungen. *Z Naturforsch, 11b:*1, 1956.

Mayne, R.: Some engineering aspects of the mechanism of body control. *Electr Eng, 70:*207, 1951.

Rohmert, W.: An international symposium on objective assessment of work load in air traffic control task: Introduction. *Ergonomics, 14:*545, 1971.

Rohmert, W.: *Psychophysische Belastung und Beanspruchung von Fluglotsen.* Berlin-Köln-Frankfurt, Beuth-Vertrieb, 1973.

Rohmert, W., and K. Schlaich: Learning of complex manual tasks. *Int J. Production Res, 5:*137, 1966.

Rohmert, W., and W. Laurig: Work measurement. Psychological and physiological techniques for assessing operator and work load. *Int J Production Res, 9:*157, 1971.

Rohmert, W., J. Rutenfranz, and E. Ulich: *Das Anlernen sensumotorischer Fertigkeiten.* Frankfurt, Europäische Verlagsanstalt, 1971.

Rutenfranz, J., W. Rohmert, and A. Iskander: Über das Verhalten der Pulsfrequenz während des Erlernens sensumotorischer Fertigkeiten unter besonderer Berücksichtigung der Pausenwirking. *Int Z Angew Physiol, 29:*101, 1971.

Simonson, E., S. Simonson, and A. Sokolow: Beiträge zur Physiologie der motorischen Koordination. 1. Mitt.: Die räumliche Koordination aufeinanderfolgender Bewegungen. *Arbeitsphysiologie, 7:*577, 1934.

Simonson, E., and S. Simonson: Beiträge zur Physiologie der motorischen Koordination. II. Mitt.: Über die Koordination der Bewegungszeit. *Arbeitsphysiologie, 7:*598, 1934.

Stier, F.: Die Geschwindigkeit von Armbewegungen. *Int Z Angew Physiol, 18:*82, 1959.

Ulich, E.: Some experiments on the function of mental training in the acquisition of motor skills. *Ergonomics, 10,* 4:411, 1967.

Wagner, Ch.: Untersuchungen zur Ergonomie des Klavierspiels. In *Biomechanics I, First Int. Seminar Zurich, 1967,* New York, Karger, Basel, 1968, pp. 264-270.

SECTION THREE

SENSORY ASPECTS: VISION

Chapter 6

Visual Fatigue

S. HOWARD BARTLEY

In 1939, The National Research Council held a conference on visual fatigue (National Research Council Conference on Visual Fatigue, May 20-21, Washington, D.C., 1939).

At this conference were many of the nation's best informed workers in visual fatigue. Curiously, however, it was agreed that despite extensive research on vision, no suitable method had been devised up to that time for measuring visual fatigue. In fact, they admitted that no precise and usable definition of visual fatigue, itself, existed. So George Wald suggested that the more feasible procedure would be to devote attention to the optimal conditions for visual performance. It seemed to some that this endeavor would be no simpler than dealing with the question of what visual fatigue is. Walter Miles summarized the conclusion of the meeting by saying that the several methods for studying the general topic should be combined into a test battery. This battery could then be used in connection with the study of any work task. He said we needed comparative findings on the different subtests applied to the same subjects in connection with various kinds of work, and that experimentation should not neglect the subjective findings obtainable under the conditions used. Here he brought in the concept of "motivation" as a factor in determining performance.

These suggestions seem to be exemplified to some degree or other in the studies of others that have been classified as fatigue studies. Part of the time the efforts are simply devoted to determining the most efficient conditions for given sorts of performance as, for example, those performances critically involving the use of the eyes. At other times, the question of what sorts of work situations evoke the feelings of tiredness are studied. At still other times the intent is to determine the way a given aspect of ocular function tallies with work output, or to determine how ocular processes tally with feelings of tiredness and discomfort. As a result, a material fraction of all studies of human physiology and overt performance becomes labelled as fatigue studies. What fatigue is, is bypassed or loosely assumed.

The psychology of fatigue includes, of course, the consideration of visual fatigue, the topic of this chapter. Vision is a direct mode of gaining information from the environment. Since vision is mediated by body mechanisms, they, too, are sometimes called vision but, strictly speaking, vision is only the end result—the expression of the organism as a person. Visual fatigue is often the label for local phenomena *within* the vision-producing body mechanisms themselves as a function of their activity. Since various authors' conclusions which imply widely different concepts of fatigue will be quoted, the reader is asked to keep in mind the implied differences.

The term fatigue arose originally to designate a human condition, an experienced self-evaluation, a feeling of discomfort or inability to continue the activity presently engaged in. The notion became prevalent that this feeling was produced by the expenditure of energy. So the processes in the body that had to do with metabolism and the like came into focal attention. Further observation disclosed that this same feeling syndrome would arise when an individual was merely faced with performing some task that was odious to him. The emergence of fatigue prior to exertion failed to be commonly seen as showing that fatigue was the product of the organism as a person, a system that evaluated situations and its own capacities. Early studies attempting to connect fatigue feelings with selected activities failed (for reasons we shall not go into here). This was a major basis for abandoning feelings (sensations) as studiable and thus as objects of fatigue investigations. Fatigue was largely ignored by psychologists and was relegated to the domain of physiology, and it has become the label for several classes of bodily change brought about by body-process activity.

Since so many varieties of task performance involve vision, it is easy for most any study to be called a visual fatigue study under views commonly held.

In this chapter several kinds of information will be dealt with. Bartley and Chute (1947) state that there are five major ways in which visual fatigue has been studied. These, of course, reflect the concept the various investigators have of fatigue before they begin to study it. These five classes of study are: 1. sensory, 2. ergographic, 3. symptomatic, 4. ease of seeing, and 5. conflict.

In examining the literature, I find no way to classify fatigue studies into a small number of categories. The best I can do is to use the five categories already mentioned and add two additional ones, namely: 6. studies of visual task performance, and 7. studies of nonvisual functions related to vision.

In making the classification, the categories have had to be rather loose, so that in some cases they include a heterogeneity of topics. Ergographic studies have had to include not only accommodation and convergence studied by the ergographic method but in other ways. Symptomatic studies are those in which, although some of the phenomena or processes studied could be classified elsewhere, the experiences of the subjects are of material concern. Ease of seeing studies stem from the supposition that environmental conditions have a material influence on the ease and effectiveness of performing visual tasks. In conflict studies, the possible conflict or disorganization

SENSORY STUDIES

McFarland, Holway and Hurvich (1942) studied decline in visual sensitivity (reciprocal of threshold) over a 30-minute period. The subjects were confined to steady posture during this period. These periods were repeated with 10-minute intervals between. During these intervals, some subjects were maintained in fixed posture; some were allowed to move about.

During the test periods sensitivity dropped. For those kept immobile during the intervals between, no recovery occurred. For those allowed to move about, recovery occurred. This was true whether the room was dark or the test level of illumination was maintained. The explanation given to these results was that decline in alertness involved in maintaining fixed posture and decrease in cerebral circulation precluded recovery. The degree to which the subjects became experientially tired of their task was not specifically dealt with. The study did show, at least, that there is more to the question of visual thresholds than the photochemical processes in the retina.

Another of the older findings relative to reduction in visual performance with time (thus "fatigue") was the fact that a small target viewed steadily blurs and finally disappears. Geldard (1928) photometrically matched two halves of a disk-target, following exposure of the eye to the one half for various lengths of time. The second half, in some experiments, was imaged on the adjacent area of the same eye; in others, the image was placed on the appropriate area of the other eye. Following a 20-minute pre-exposure of the first half-disk, only 55 percent of the intensity was required for the second half-disk to look as bright as the first when the images were on separate eyes. When the images were adjacent on the same eye, only 28 percent of the intensity for the first image was required. This was taken to mean that not only the imaged area but those adjacent to it underwent change in sensitivity. This I would suppose was due to scattered (stray) illumination (see Bartley, 1935; Bartley and Fry, 1934; Fry and Bartley, 1935). However, the area adjacent to the first half-disk image was made more sensitive than the equal area in the second eye when tested.

Not all shifts in outcome upon retinal exposure are changes in sensed intensity (brightness). Some have to do with hue and saturation in perceived color. Cogan and Cogan (1938) studied what was commonly called color fatigue. This took three forms: 1. a colored target desaturating and becoming similar to background; 2. the sudden disappearing of the target and adjacent background, followed by a "granular form of blackness"; 3. the disappearing of the background before the colored target.

Cogan and Cogan found a progressive drop in disappearance time from fovea to periphery. The lower temporal quadrant displayed the longest disappearance times, while the shortest was in the upper vertical field. The disappearance times for red were the longest, and green the shortest. And, usually, the larger the retinal area the longer the time required for disappearance. Dark adaptation shortened the disappearance time for red and blue. The time of disappearance was a function of stimulus intensity. Binocular and monocular disappearance times were about equal.

The same authors (1939) studied recovery times. Recovery time was found to be shorter at 30 degrees than at 10 degrees from the fovea and eye movements seemed to have no effect on recovery time.

Hartridge (1947) investigated what he called fatigue effects produced by using one part of the spectrum for the pre-exposure and then testing vision when stimulating other parts of the spectrum. Desaturation effects were produced and these did not shift toward gray. Accordingly, he did not classify his effects as color adaptation, but fatigue. There is a rather large and controversial literature on the application of the critical (or fusion) frequency of flicker (CFF or FFF) as a fatigue test. Since it was used, as originally proposed by Simonson and Enzer (1941), in the large majority of studies as a test of general fatigue in tasks not involving appreciable visual effort, the bulk of the literature will be reviewed in the chapter "Use of Visual Methods for Measurement of General Fatigue."

The effect of two hours strenuous visual work (task described on p. 167) on the CFF was studied by Simonson and Brozek together with other visual functions and performance trends. Involvement of accommodation and eye muscles was minimal; therefore, the task involved nearly exclusively visual receptors and pathways. There was a small, but statistically highly significant drop of the CFF which was nearly identical at the grossly inadequate illumination level of 2 F.C. and the adequate illumination levels of 100 and 300 F.C. It was suggested that the drop of the CFF is related to the general fatigue in this type of work rather than to the visual stress per se.

Schmidtke (1951) found a similar significant drop of the CFF in types of work involving visual effort (fine assembly, linotype, microscopy) as in mental calculations (with open eyes and blindfolded), and concluded that the depression of the CFF is related to general fatigue rather than to strictly visual fatigue. However, Brozek, et al. (1944) and Busch and Wachholder (1953) found no consistent changes of FFF in microscopic work, although there was a depression of the CFF in the majority of subjects (Busch and Wachholder). In general, the results in laboratory conditions were more consistent than determination of the CFF at the start and end of occupational work as will be discussed later.

Florek (1969) compared the performance of stereoplanigraphers and workers in a TV factory with control subjects on certain tests used as indicators (intermittent photic stimuli). It may be assumed that the work involved recognition of fine details. Brightness rather than frequency was the variable used for the intermittent stimuli. 1. Brightness at critical flicker frequency, 2. brightness when the intermittent light was perceived "adequately," and the difference in brightness between the two (1 and 2) were used as indicators. The tests were performed after dark adaptation of the subjects. None of the indicators resulted in a performance difference between the beginning and the end of a single work shift, which were unlike those of the control subjects. There was, however, evidence of long-term effects: the CFF of the workers in the TV plant was consistently lower than that of the controls. Florek concluded that the CFF may be used as index of chronic visual fatigue. However, his results may not apply to the conventional technique of CFF measurement.

ERGOGRAPHIC STUDIES

Ergographic techniques represent one way of studying certain motor mechanisms in the eye. The three motor processes within the eye are accommodation, convergence and pupillary reflex adjustments (change in pupillary diameter). In viewing visual targets, the two eyes must converge, the amount depending upon target distance. The accommodative reflex which adjusts lens thickness to change in optical power (to focus) is coupled in certain ways to accommodation. As a visual target is moved alternately toward and away from the eyes, this process simulates the ergographic process used in causing a muscle system to contract and relax.

The visual ergograph is a device consisting of a bar positioned in the line of regard. On this bar is a carrier which can be slid back and forth. It carries a card containing test material. Several different authors have applied the ergographic method: Lancaster and Williams (1914), Howe (1916a, 1916b, 1917), Blatt (1931), Berens and Stark (1932), Hofstetter (1943), and Berens and Sells (1950).

Hofstetter's investigation will serve to show some of the kinds of results obtained with an accommodative ergograph. *Sustained effort*—in this case, the smallest letter seen at a remote distance was used as the origin. While he steadily fixated it, the target was brought toward the subject till blur was reported. Then it was taken further away to the point at which the letters on the target cleared again. Continued effort to keep the target clear was required. Another experiment called for *repeated efforts*. In this case, the target was brought in closer till blur occurred. Then the target was abruptly taken back to the original starting place. Another type of experiment called for *an almost complete relaxation of accommodation* between trials. This was obtained by having the observer fixate upon a chart of letters 5 meters away while the target was being returned to the starting position.

From his experiments, Hofstetter found 1. that diminution of amplitude was obtained more readily by repeated than by sustained effort. He had expected the opposite, and concluded that the results showed that diminution of amplitude is not dependent upon the ciliary muscle alone. He found 2. a discrepancy between discomfort symptoms and amplitudes of accommodation expected to provide for satisfactory seeing at close range. Amplitude was unpredictable, disappearing suddenly, with added or resumed effort, a shift in attitude or following distraction. He also found 3. that reduction in amplitude during his tests was the exception rather than the rule. He was unable to assign any diagnostic significance to the results.

McFarland (1937) showed that the amplitude of the excursion between blurring and clearing diminished during 10 minutes of repetition. The curves showing this were called "fatigue curves." As altitude above sea level was increased, the decreases in amplitude came on progressively earlier and its rate was more rapid. In fact, at the higher altitudes, a full 10-minute test period was not possible. Changes in performance were viewed as indicators of fatigue. Convergence was found to deteriorate in much the same manner as accommodation.

Krivohlavy, et al. (1969) studied six female machinists, four times a shift for one week on convergence and accommodation, blink rate and "usual information transfer efficiency." The authors found that both convergence and accommodation were affected, blink rate was increased, and so were number of errors in visual information transfer.

Narasaki, et al. (1969) studied fatigue in civil air transportation crews using certain visual functions as indicators. Five 25 to 29-year-old flight engineers were tested before and during the first, second and third days of continuous training flights for effects in accommodative near-point, depth perception, vertical and horizontal phorias, visual acuity and night vision. Prolonged accommodation at near-point was the first evidence of fatigue found. Night vision was not affected, but there were vertical phoria and diminished visual acuity. In this study, the criteria for fatigue were, of course, nonexperiential.

SYMPTOMATIC STUDIES

It is supposed that exercising the eyes (eye muscles) will disclose in individuals with ocular complaints behavior not characteristic of normal subjects. Phorias are, for example, one of the conditions that will produce complaints and these complaints are interpreted as fatigue or signs of fatigue by some investigators. From this point, some investigators start their search for concrete physiological processes which would be the explicit factors involved.

For example, Kurtz (1937) used the task of 30 minutes' reading before and after which he tested his subjects with an ophthalmograph (an eye movement camera). Only one out of his seven subjects manifested a considerable decrement in amplitude of accommodation. The others showed virtually no decrement but, nevertheless, reported the unfavorable symptoms of experientially defined fatigue such as a "tired feeling of the eyes," difficulty in holding the eyes open, eye ache, "drawing" of the eyes, and a feeling that suggested nystagmus, periodic disappearance of the print being read, difficulty in reading, and double vision. Some included reports of general feeling of tiredness.

This study, of course, failed to show a correspondence between fatigue feelings and the accommodation factor studied.

Carmichael and Dearborn (1947) studied the possible development of fatigue in reading, the very task which would most likely produce process inadequacy. They had subjects read for a number of hours. From the results, they concluded that reading did not produce fatigue according to the criteria used.

Despite the findings in such studies, one of the most common complaints that optometrists and ophthalmologists hear is visual fatigue.

EASE OF SEEING STUDIES

Ease of seeing is another nebulous term, like fatigue itself. That is to say, it has more than one meaning. Whereas ease of seeing might be the experienced ease with which a target is seen, it may also be defined in terms of maintenance of a given visual process during continued activity or in terms of overt performance. Indistinctness or blurring of a target is a criterion. Rate of blinking is another common indicator.

Blinking is an involuntary activity, and it is generally thought that a subject's attention to such processes influences them very little. Thus using this as an indicator precludes the traditional distrust in dealing with measures that are voluntary expressions of the individual.

Luckiesh and Moss (1935) found that what they called "convergence reserve" diminishes as reading continues over an extended period. They report that one hour's reading under an illumination of 1 ft-c produces three times as much diminution as reading under 100 ft-c. In another study, this time on key punch operators, the diminution was four times as great at 10 ft-c as at 60 ft-c. These subjects were measured daily for six weeks.

Ponder and Kennedy (1927-1928) found no variation in blink rate under a range of intensities including complete darkness. Similar results were obtained by Blount (1928) when he studied eyelid movements in animals.

McFarland, Holway and Hurvich (1942) obtained no consistent results when attempting to study blink rate as a possible index of fatigue. In contrast, they considered the possibility that blinking was a factor in helping prevent fatigue.

Luckiesh (1944) reporting some earlier work of Luckiesh and Moss told of consistent results in testing blink rate in 5000 reading periods in 81 subjects with normal or corrected-to-normal vision. The conclusions stated were that blink rate and fatigue can be expected: 1. to increase as reading continues, 2. to be greater while reading small print than large, 3. to be greater under uncorrected vision, and 4. to be greater under glare.

They found a differentiation between illumination levels. So did Simonson and Brozek (1948), but the changes in blink rate as a function of work duration were not consistent and could not be used as a fatigue index. Strangely enough, the rate decreased (showing improvement) under the extreme conditions of stress (2 ft-c). This change may have been compensatory (see McFarland, Holway and Hurvich, 1942).

A still different kind of result was found by Tinker (1943) in which blink rate was the same under two conditions of illumination (2 and 100 ft-c), but deterioration set in during a performance period of 55 minutes. The discrepancy was explained, however, by Simonson and Brozek (1951) in their remarks bearing on the statistics of the two investigations.

Blink rate has proven to be a controversial matter. Brozek, Simonson and Franklin (1948) found that blink rate could not be used as a reliable indicator for fatigue in the experiments they performed.

Bitterman and Solway (1946) and Bitterman (1947) have studied blink rate. Luckiesh (1947) defended blink rate as an indicator and such workers as Bitterman (1947) attacked it.

Luckiesh and Moss (1938) tested office workers with reference to *pupil area* and found that it increased about 15 percent during the day. The investigation lasted four weeks. From week to week the reversal over the weekends became less and less.

The basal metabolism and pulse rate of subjects were compared for periods up to an hour under illuminations of 1 ft-c and 50 ft-c. The study was made in an air-conditioned room with temperature and humidity under control. Under these conditions, McFarland, Knehr and Berens (1939) found no relation between the basal metabolic rate and level of illumination.

Ferree and Rand (1927, 1931, 1934, 1935, 1937, 1940) studied various features of visual performance under various levels of illumination.

Tinker (1939) used tests to determine the illumination beyond which no increase in efficiency of reading would occur. He also was concerned with the critical illumination for fatigue in reading. Speed of reading was the test of efficiency, disturbance to clear seeing was the criterion for fatigue. Earlier, Tinker and Paterson (1928) found that subjects could read lower case type 13 percent faster than capitals. Later, they (1939) found through eye movement photographs that the advantage was connected with the need for more fixations in reading all capital type, and a decreasing number of words per fixation. There were the same number of regressions in reading lower case letters as in reading capitals, so it was concluded that the difficulties in reading capitals were no greater than in reading the lower case letters.

Luckiesh, et al. (1921) studied the rate of reading letters on a revolving drum under illuminations ranging from 0.39 to 25.0 ft-c and found an increase in rate with increase in illumination up to approximately 11 ft-c or a little higher. Above 7 ft-c the rate of increase was not very marked.

Atkins (1927) used the clerical task of crossing out numbers, a coordination test and a chain association test performed under five intensities of illumination ranging from 916 ft-c to 118 ft-c, working one hour per day. The conclusion was drawn that 34 ft-c gave the greatest efficiency, but Carmichael and Dearborn (1947) in examining the data conclude that there was no change in efficiency over the whole range.

Chernilovskaya (1966) compared results of human working efficiency with illumination constant and with increasing illumination at the onsets of visual fatigue (defined in reduction in speed of discrimination of fine detail). It was found that illumination step-ups at such points decreased this "fatigue"—increased the working efficiency.

Simonson and Brozek (1948a) studied the effects of illumination on visual task performance, fatigue, and upon certain other activities such as blink rate. They tested their subjects with a 2-hour visual task at three levels of illumination: 5, 100, and 300 ft-c. A significant drop in performance at all levels was found. This, of course, was taken to be a measure of fatigue. Blink rate, however, did not change significantly at any of the levels of illumination and thus was not considered a fatigue index. The questionnaire that was used to denote feeling of well-being did not show distinct deterioration in it except at a grossly low level of illumination, 2 ft-c (in a supplemental experiment). At 100 ft-c, however, optimal scores did result. Results of testing recognition time showed that it became progressively greater with lowering of illumination. Critical flicker frequency manifested the same significant progressive deterioration at all levels of illumination. Tests of brightness discrimination showed no significant changes as the task progressed.

Various ophthalmological tests were also given, and only the adduction test was changed significantly by the task. Adduction improved. The other tests showed at least a tendency in this direction.

One of the important demonstrations of this investigation was that under a chosen set of conditions, the function tested may fail to tally with task performance. Since these selected functions involved different structures and in different ways to different degrees, it is not surprising that they do not all tally equally with the degree of work decrement in the task. In fact, some may even improve during the task performance.

Simonson and Brozek (1948b) studied the possible effect of qualitative features of illumination on visual performance and fatigue. In this study differences in illumination intensity were eliminated when sources of different spectral distributions were used. These sources were: 1. ordinary inside frosted tungsten lamps, 2. natural white lamps, and 3. Verd-A-Ray lamps (each at three levels of illumination—5, 100, and 300 ft-c). The adjustments in luminous output for the targets were made by diaphragms with multiple perforations and by variations of the distance between lamps and the target screen. They found that comparatively few of the functions tested (average performance, performance drop, blink rate, recognition time for threshold, size stimuli, CFF and questionnaire score) were affected by the task. The same functions which did not respond to the variables in the preceding investigation (1948a) were found to be less likely affected by the variations in the spectral distributions in the three illuminations used. At the 100 and 300 ft-c levels no significant differences in the task performance scores resulted. A work decrement showed up for all three. This was designated as the fatigue effect, and an index of *visual strain*. The blink rate did not vary appreciably as a function of the task performance, nor as a function of the illuminants. The ophthalmological tests did not show any differences between illuminants.

In 1951 Simonson and Brozek summarized the understandings up to that point regarding the relation of work, vision and illumination. Various codes had existed with reference to the illumination levels needed for various kinds of visual tasks. The major finding in this respect is that the levels suggested then were considerably higher than those indicated thirty years earlier. For instance, for general reading a level of 30 ft-c was recommended then whereas thirty years before only 3 to 6 ft-c were considered sufficient (Lighting for School Buildings, Illuminating Engineering Society, 1917; American Standard Code of Lighting, 1922; American Recommended Practice of Industrial Lighting, 1942; American Standard Practice for School Lighting, 1948).

Simonson and Brozek suggest, among other things, that the increase in the levels of suggested illumination over the period represented here is due to a compromise between ideal and attainable levels, attainable levels having risen during the period.

Troland (1931) reviewed the results from many tasks using vision. He concluded that for gross industrial task, as little as 1 ft-c is likely sufficient, but fine detailed work may require as much as 200 to 300 ft-c.

Tinker (1940) improved upon this by preadapting his subjects and found that the preferred intensity reported by his subjects was closely related to the level of preadaptation. He used two preadaptation levels, namely, 8 and 52 ft-c. He (1942) also determined the affect of changes in illumination level on the speed of reading under intensities ranging from 0.1 to 53.3 ft-c. In one case he used two minutes of preadaptation to the intensity used. The conclusion from using eighty-two university students was that when the preadaptation period was only two minutes, the speed of reading increases as intensity is increased in the range of 3.1 to 10.3 ft-c where a plateau seems to be reached.

In another case, the preadaptation period was 15 minutes. Under these conditions reading rate increases as intensity level is increased from 0.1 to 3.1 ft-c where increases in rate cease.

In some studies on the effect of level of illumination, it was found that raising illumination improved performance. A control or return to original illumination sometimes failed to impoverish performance. Two things are plausible: practice may have been involved in improving performance, or increased motivation entered into the situation. That motivation is sometimes involved was dramatically shown in the Hawthorne studies (Fatigue of Workers, 1941) and those of Ives (1925) and White, et al. (1929).

CONFLICT STUDIES

Another class of studies having to do with visual performance involved the study of conflict. Several visual mechanisms are muscular, and these muscular systems consist of opposing sets of muscles, whose contraction and relaxation may get into inefficient opposition with each other.

Studies of eye movement sometimes turn out to be cases of this sort. Dodge (1917) used a series of repeated horizontal ocular excursions. These excursions were photographed by using a luminous spot reflected from the cornea. The eye movements were looked upon as a product of the action of the extrinsic eye muscles, and thus it was muscular organization that was being studied. He showed that the overall coordination in contraction and relaxation in this muscle group became less exact in successive repetitions of fixation. There were also evidences of central nervous involvement in the deterioration of ocular performance.

Disorganization (conflict) has been shown to occur in pupillary reflexes. Bartley (1942) found that slowly repeated flashes (pulses) produced a definite form of discomfort. This led him to photograph pupillary reflexes in response to intermittent photic stimulation and record at the same time degrees of discomfort. Varying the rate of intermittency enabled him to show the relation of amplitude in the constricting and dilating to rate. The supposition was that the feeling of ocular discomfort would occur when the amplitude of constricting and dilating would be at a maximum.

He found that the contracting and dilating phases occupied unequal amounts of time and that this led to a kind of conflict between the two phases so that at rates in which amplitude of excursion between the two phases was at a minimum, the maximum of discomfort occurred. A muscular tug-of-war was substituted for the usual reciprocal innervation and activity. His notion that tensions, if not active pupillary contractions, are productive of ocular discomfort was further substantiated by Halstead (1941) who showed that when the pupillary mechanism was immobilized by drugs, the discomfort such as found by Bartley did not occur in experiments with intermittent photic stimulation.

Lowenstein and Givener (1943) showed that a pupillary *dark* reflex survives the elimination of the *light* reflex in the subjects they studied. The discovery of a *dark* reflex and the fact that it works somewhat differently than the traditional *light* reflex was in line with the conflict activity just described. Bartley (1943) included the ocular mechanism activity as an example of conflict in his conflict theory of fatigue.

In another investigation, Bartley (1942) had his subjects gaze as steadily as possible midway between two lights in a dark field for five minutes, with no fixation point provided. The eye movements of the subjects were observed, and the subjects asked to report at the end of the period on their effort to hold fixation and the discomfort that accrued. It was found that steady fixation was impossible, and the effort and discomfort was considerable. Despite the eye movements, including nystagmus, the subjects were not always aware of them. They only felt some kind of ocular discomfort along with a general bodily tension.

Luckiesh and Moss (1938) also observed ocular motor conflict in some of their investigations.

STUDIES OF VISUAL TASK PERFORMANCE, ETC.

Shek (1963) tested eight subjects in a scanning test, before and following visual and auditory work tasks. Index of efficiency was the information loss. His subjects showed greater auditory than visual loss, and greater information loss in the evening than in the morning. Subjects performing routine laboratory work in the interval between tests did better in the evening than in the morning.

Collins and Pruen (1962) had subjects view Landolt rings at two different distances for two hours. They concluded that the time required to perceive accurately the rings at the two distances is worth considering as a visual fatigue index.

Brozek, Simonson and Keys (1947, 1950) developed a test for the experimental investigation of visual performance and fatigue. The test was designed to simulate the essential features of an industrial conveyor inspection-operation and thus serve as a "miniature job situation." It consisted of recognizing single letters as they pass a slit. The visual angle of the letters as viewed was 10 minutes. The letters were viewed at illumination levels of 2 to 5 and 50 ft-c. The overall exposure time for a letter was .573 sec. Performance scores were taken at the beginning, midpoint and at the end of a 2-hour session to discover possible performance decrements for each of the three levels of illumination mentioned above. It was found that performance decrement resulted for all three illumination levels. Other factors were variable, and it was concluded that the test was quite applicable as a testing technique since it produced visual "strain" and could be used as a means of studying the effect of a variety of variables.

The problem of the transfer of decrement in one performance to another was studied by Bitterman (1946). The main thing concluded was that a kind of interference in going from one ocular task to another did appear but the author refrained from calling this fatigue.

Short photic pulses of various durations were compared with photic stimuli of extended durations ("continuous" stimulation). In such a task, Rudolph (1951) found random shifts in the difference in brightness the two produced. These were attributed to fatigue in the visual system. However, no fatigue of the experienced sort was produced.

Recordings of change in eye position, speed and acceleration of eye movement were made by Lion (1952) at intervals during a "jump" fixation task. The changes in performance during the task were called fatigue by the author and attributed to central nervous function.

In connection with the idea of fatigue being a work decrement, the concepts of cost of performance and efficiency have also appeared. Cost is defined by Ryan (1947) as equivalent to *input* which is "any adverse effect of work done, or anything which the individual expends in carrying on the activity under study." This brings in the question of *energy* and *effort*. Energy is that which can be expressed in terms of physical units such as calories, footpounds, watts, etc. Ryan defines *effort* as describing the *relationship between actual rate of performance and the capacity of the individual at a given time*. Efficiency is the relation between the cost of doing work and the outcome (i.e. amount or quality of work performed). Travis, et al. (1951) also have dealt with the cost of seeing via recording muscle action potentials. Allphin (1951) also studied cost.

Lybrand, et al. (1954) used performance on Kohs Block Designs, the Müller-Lyer Illusion and Hidden Figures as indices of perceptual organization. Supposed fatigue was induced by loss of one night's sleep, or by a 5-

mile march with a 40-lb pack. Since the results varied with the task, the authors concluded that "perceptual organization is more efficient after mild physical activity and less efficient after sleep deprivation." They believe that this supports the supposition that perceptual organization is sensitive to systemic fatigue.

Florek (1965) found small changes (microchanges) in the binocular visual field in connection with work shifts.

Several classes of workers were exposed to a visual field 2-mm in diameter and found small changes, particularly at the beginning and end of the work shifts.

Friedman, et al. (1970) observed the visual responses of newborn humans to repeated presentations of two checkerboard targets. Visual regard decremented for both targets. To ascertain whether this was to be interpreted as habituation or sensory fatigue, new targets were substituted after the infants showed the decrement. Preliminary tests resulted in increased visual regard in 15 out of 21 subjects. Accordingly, the decrement was taken to be due to a central process rather than a peripheral one. I should say it showed that the decrement was not a result of impairment ("fatigue") of a peripheral mechanism. This investigation brings up the inappropriateness of using infants in a fatigue study when fatigue is defined as an experimentally expressed self-assessment of inability or discomfort (negative stance toward a task).

Brozek and Simonson (1952) varied both length of work time and illumination but found it difficult to draw any valid conclusions.

NONVISUAL FUNCTIONS

In studying such things as visual fatigue, it is important to realize that they are not isolated phenomena. Nonvisual body-processes are involved in some way. Vision, for example, involves the body as a whole. This point was made by Luckiesh and Moss (1938). This supposition would provide for the expectation that changes in "nonvisual" functions would occur in prolonged visual performance. If so, some of these would provide the investigator looking for fatigue indexes, some usable data. Muscle tension outside the visual system is one of the functions in question. Bitterman, et al. (1948) and Ryan, et al. (1950) found that work performed at the performer's own pace did not result in increased tension, whereas activities that were paced (performed at a predetermined rate) resulted in a significant increase of muscle tension. At various times, the muscle behavior measured was misinterpreted. Luckiesh and Moss (1935) found lower heart rates at poorer illumination which, apparently, was taken to be fatigue rather than improvement.

Weston (1952) lays fatigue in visual tasks to eye position in looking down. This posture is said to produce neck pains. The same author in other studies (1953a, 1953b) attributes visual fatigue to muscular exertion that lies outside the visual system, and to "mental exertion" as well. Not all other difficulties which ensue are classed as fatigue. For example, some of it is called boredom and some, sleepiness. This he blames on room lighting. We can take this as another example of the strange variation in what is called fatigue. Some workers class all decremental or unpleasant effects from activity as fatigue; others pick out certain results to be given the fatigue label and exclude others.

The effect of meals on visual performance and fatigue has also been studied (Simonson, Brozek and Keys, 1948). This task consisted of the recognition of small letters presented in random order behind a narrow slit. The letters subtended a visual angle of 10 minutes for 0.56 seconds. These letters were copied by the subject on a band of paper. The illumination level was only 5 ft-c. The task was performed continuously for two hours and was scored in terms of the number of letters correctly recognized out of samples of 200 letters requiring six minutes each, the first sample being obtained five minutes after beginning the task; a second at the end of an hour; and a third sample near the end of the two hours. The subjects had the impression that their work was being continuouly evaluated. The investigation reports the effects of meals in a miniature job situation demanding constant attention and which produces performance decrement but little energy expenditure. The visual functions tested were blink rate, recognition time of threshold targets, critical flicker frequency, the ophthalmological tests used in the studies just mentioned, and brightness discrimination. In addition to these, a discomfort questionnaire was given. The meals were: 1. standard meal (carbohydrate 50%, protein 12%, and fat 38%) totalling 1300 calories; 2. high fat meal (fat 83%, carbohydrate 14% and protein 3%), total calories 1400; 3. a high carbohydrate meal (carbohydrate 80%, protein 10% and fat 10%), a total of about 1300 calories; and 4. no meal.

The results showed the average performance was lowest with the high carbohydrate meal. This type of meal produced the greatest variability of performance. However, the performance decrement was lowest. This may have been due to the average being the lowest. Moreover, the discomfort was least pronounced after the high carbohydrate meal, and the most pronounced with no meal at all. Here, again, there was no parallelism between work (and work decrement) and the fatigue produced.

Among the visual mechanism functions, only critical flicker frequency showed any deterioration. These were greatest with no meal, and least after the standard meal. The fact that no changes in recognition time appeared was attributed in part to the choice of the illuminant (Verd-A-Ray lamp).

The ophthalmological tests (involving extrinsic eye muscles) consistently showed that the most deterioration occurred after the high carbohydrate meal, while accommodation improved. Whereas missing the meal produced the most discomfort (fatigue), two ophthalmological functions—adduction power and near-point accommodation—deteriorated the least.

In general, then, there was no superiority shown for the high carbohydrate meals as reported for other types of work by Haggard and Greenberg (1935). In fact, the high carbohydrate meal seems to be inferior. This is not surprising in light of the findings of Thorn, et al. (1943). The authors suggest that results might have been different for a type of work involving great energy expenditure.

GENERAL DISCUSSIONS AND REVIEWS

In addition to reports on single investigators, there is other literature that is useful to anyone interested in visual fatigue. Examples of these include the following: Bartley (1942, 1943, 1947, 1951, 1952, 1954, 1965), Bartley and Chute (1947), Bitterman (1948), Brozek (1948, 1949), Carmichael and Dearborn (1947), Demilia (1968), Florek (1967), Luckiesh (1944, 1948), Luckiesh and Moss (1938), Ryan (1947), Schmitke (1965), Simonson and Brozek (1951), Tinker (1946, 1948), Simmerman (1950), and Weber (1950).

GENERAL CONCLUSIONS

There is a great variety of ways of studying human activity. This activity can be divided into categories: 1. general metabolic processes; 2. vital processes in specific visceral and other organs, 3. specific sensory nonvisual processes, 4. processes in the visual mechanism, 5. overt motor processes (these have critical aspects of either energy expenditure or skill), and 6. experiential (sensory) processes having to do with perceiving the environment or evaluating the subject's own condition with reference to task performance. Summarizing, these forms of activity have to do with body maintenance, task performance and self-evaluation. The study of visual fatigue has some connection with all of these. Such study relates to these whether fatigue is defined as it originally was (a form of self-evaluation in connection with overt task performance) or whether the term fatigue loosely refers to work decrement, deterioration in body process as well.

The foregoing references to visual fatigue studies are by no means exhaustive, but to be that would require vast amounts of space. It is evident, however, that workers in fatigue have for some reason not seen the need strongly enough to come to general agreement on a consistent set of connotations for terms such as fatigue, tiredness, exhaustion, impairment, boredom and the like. As a consequence, no distinction has been generally accepted regarding a difference between the total organism as a person being the limiting condition for performance, and the change or breakdown in a limited process being the limiting condition. Historically, fatigue referred to the former, and impairment and related terms would seem to be appropriate for the latter. I refer to this here for it would seem that the establishment of some rational conventions in this case would immensely aid in the progress of research and understanding.

BIBLIOGRAPHY

Allphin, W.: The cost of seeing in a critical industrial task. *Illum Engn, 46*:530, 1951.
American Recommended Practice of Industrial Lighting: New York, Illum. Engn Soc, 1942.
American Standard Code of Lighting: New York, Illum Engn Soc, 1922.
American Standard Practice for School Lighting: New York, Illum Engn Soc, 1948.
Atkins, E. W.: The efficiency of the eye under different intensities of illumination. *J Comp Psychol, 7*:1, 1927.
Bartley, S. H.: The comparative distribution of light in the stimulus and on the retina. *J Comp Psychol, 19*:149, 1935.
Bartley, S. H.: A factor in visual fatigue. *Psychosom Med, 4*:369, 1942.
Bartley, S. H.: Conflict, frustration and fatigue. *Psychosom Med, 5*:160, 1943.
Bartley, S. H.: The basis of visual fatigue. *Am J Optom, 24*:372, 1947.
Bartley, S. H.: Fatigue and efficiency. In Helson, H. (Ed.): *Theoretical Foundations of Psychology*. New York, Van Nostrand, 1951.
Bartley, S. H.: What optometrists should know about fatigue. *Mich Optom, 31*:10, 1952.
Bartley, S. H.: Understanding visual fatigue. *Am J Optom 31*:29, 1954.
Bartley, S. H.: *The Mechanism and Management of Fatigue*. Springfield, Thomas, 1965.
Bartley, S. H., and E. Chute: *Fatigue and Impairment in Man*. New York, McGraw-Hill, 1947; reprinted—Johnson Reprint Corp., 1969.
Bartley, S. H., and G. A. Fry: An indirect method of measuring stray light within the human eye. *J Opt Soc Am, 24*:342, 1934.
Berens, C., and S. B. Sells: Experimental studies of fatigue of accommodation. II. *Am J Ophthalmol, 33*:47, 1950.
Berens, C., and E. K. Stark: Fatigue of accommodation. *Am J Ophthalmol, 15*:527, 1932.
Bitterman, M. E.: Heart rate and frequency of blinking as indices of visual efficiency. *J Exp Psychol, 35*:279, 1945.
Bitterman, M. E.: Transfer of decrement on ocular tasks. *Am J Psychol, 59*:422, 1946.
Bitterman, M. E.: Frequency of blinking in visual work: A reply to Dr. Luckiesh. *J Exp Psychol, 37*:260, 1947.
Bitterman, M. E.: Lighting and visual efficiency: The present status of research. *Illum Engn, 43*:906, 1948.
Bitterman, M. E., T. A. Ryan, and C. L. Cottrell: Muscular tension as an index of visual efficiency: A progress report. *Illum Engn, 43*:1074, 1948.
Bitterman, M. E., and E. Solway: Frequency of blinking as a measure of visual efficiency: Some methodological considerations. *Am J Psychol, 59*:676, 1946.
Blatt, N.: Weakness of accommodation. *Arch Ophthalmol, 5*:362, 1931.

Blount, W. P.: Studies of the movements of the eyelids of animals: blinking. *Quart J Exp Physiol, 18:*111, 1928.

Brozek, J.: Visual fatigue: A critical comment. *Am J Psychol, 61:*420, 1948.

Brozek, J.: Quantitative criteria of oculomotor performance and fatigue. *J Appl Physiol, 2:*247, 1949.

Brozek, J., and A. Keys: Flicker fusion frequency as a test of fatigue. *J Indust Hyg Toxicol, 26:*169, 1944.

Brozek, J., and E. Simonson: Visual performance and fatigue under conditions of varied illumination. *Am J Ophthalmol, 35:*33, 1952.

Brozek, J., E. Simonson, and J. C. Franklin: A note on methodological evaluation of selected visual tests. *Am J Ophthalmol, 31:*979, 1948.

Brozey, J., E. Simonson, and A. Keys: A work test for quantitative study of visual performance and fatigue. *J Appl Psychol, 31:*519, 1947.

Brozek, J., E. Simonson, and A. Keys: Changes in performance and in ocular functions resulting from strenuous visual inspection. *Am J Psychol, 63:*51, 1950.

Busch, G., K. Wachholder: Der Einfluss ermüdender geistiger Beanspruchung auf die Flimmerverschmelzungfrequenz. *Arbeitsphysiologie, 15:*149, 1953.

Carmichael, L., and W. F. Dearborn: *Reading and Visual Fatigue.* New York, Houghton Mifflin, 1947.

Chernilovskaya, F. M.: Izmenenie intensiõnosti oveschcheniga ak faktor povysheniya rabotosposobnosti cheloveka. (Change of intensity of illumination as a factor in raising working efficiency in man.) *Fiziologicheskii Zhurnal SSSR, 52:*1332, 1966.

Cogan, D. G., and F. C. Cogan: Color fatigue in the peripheral field. *Ophthalmologica, 96:*137, 1938.

Cogan, D. G., and F. C. Cogan: Recovery time from color fatigue in peripheral vision. *Ophthalmologica, 96:*267, 1939.

Collins, J. B., and B. Pruen: Perception time and visual fatigue. *Ergonomics, 5:*533, 1962.

Demilia, L. A.: Visual fatigue and reading. *J Educ, 151:*4, 1968.

Dodge, R.: The laws of relative fatigue. *Psychol Rev, 24:*89, 1917.

Fatigue of Workers: New York, Reinhold, 1941.

Ferree, C. E., and G. Rand: Intensity of light and speed of vision studied with special reference to industrial situations. *Trans Illum Engn Soc, 22:*79, 1927.

Ferree, C. E., and G. Rand: Visibility of objects as affected by color and composition of light. *Person J, 9:*475, 1931.

Ferree, C. E., and G. Rand: The effect of increase of intensity of light on the visual acuity of presbyopic and non-presbyopic eyes. *Trans Illum Engn Soc, 19:*296, 1934.

Ferree, C. E., and G. Rand: Intensity of light in relation to the near point and apparent range of accommodation. *Am J Ophthalmol, 18:*307, 1935.

Ferree, C. E., and G. Rand: Good working conditions for eyes. *Person J, 15:*333, 1937.

Ferree, C. E., and G. Rand: Work and its illumination. *Person J, 19:*93 (Pt. 1), 1940.

Florek, H.: Zmeny hranic binokularneho zrakoveho pola ako mozny ukazovatel unavy zrakoveho analyzatora. (Changes of binocular visual field range as possible fatigue indicator of the visual field analyser.) *Studia Psychologia, 7:*271, 1965.

Florek, H.: Some aspects of the determination of visual fatigue. *Studia Psychologia, 9:*46, 1967.

Florek, H.: Intermittentny svetelny podnet a zrakova anava. (Intermittent light stimuli and visual fatigue.) *Studia Psychologia, 11:*56, 1969.

Friedman, S., G. C. Carpenter, and A. N. Nagy: Decrement and recovery of response to visual stimuli in the newborn human. *Proc Annual Conv Am Psychol Assoc, 5:*273 (Pt. 1), 1970.

Fry, G. A., and S. H. Bartley: The relation of stray light in the eye to the retinal action potential. *Am J Physiol, 111:*335, 1935.

Geldard, F. A.: The measurement of retinal fatigue to achromatic stimulation. I and II. *J Gen Psychol, 1:*123, 578, 1928.

Haggard, H. W., and L. A. Greenberg: *Diet and Physical Efficiency.* New Haven, Yale U Press, 1935.

Halstead, W. C.: A note on the Bartley effect in the estimation of equivalent brightness. *J Exp Psychol, 28:*524, 1941.

Hartridge, H.: Some fatigue effects on the human retina produced by using coloured lights. *Nature, London, 160:*538, 1947.

Hofstetter, H. W.: An ergographic analysis of fatigue of accommodation. *Am J Optom, 20:*115, 1943.

Howe, L.: The fatigue of accommodation. *JAMA, 67:*100, 1916a.

Howe, L.: The fatigue of accommodation as registered by the ergograph. *Trans Sect Ophthalmol, JAMA, 67:*130, 1916b.

Howe, L.: Registration of fatigue of accommodation. *Trans Am Ophthalmol Soc, 15:*145, 1917.

Ives, J. E.: Study of the effect of degree of illumination on working speed of letter separators in a post office. Washington, Public Health Reports, Reprint #973, 1925.

Krivohlavy, J., V. Kodat, and P. Cizek: Visual efficiency and fatigue during the afternoon shift. *Ergonomics, 12:*735, 1969.

Kurtz, J. I.: The general and ocular fatigue problem. *Am J Optom, 14:*273, 308, 1937.

Lancaster, W. B., and E. R. Williams: New light on the theory of accommodation, with practical applications. *Trans Am Acad Ophthalmol,* p. 170, 1914.

Lighting for School Buildings. New York, Illum Engn Soc, 1917.

Lion, K. S.: Oculometric muscle forces and fatigue. *Illum Engn, 47:*388, 1952.

Lowenstein, O., and I. Givener: Pupillary reflex to darkness. *Arch Ophthalmol, 30:*603, 1943.

Luckiesh, M.: *Light, Vision and Seeing.* New York, Van Nostrand, 1944.

Luckiesh, M.: Reading and the rate of blinking. *J Exp Psychol, 37:*266, 1947.

Luckiesh, M.: Recommended footcandle levels for prolonged critical seeing. *J Opt Soc Am, 38:*712, 1948.

Luckiesh, M., and F. K. Moss: Fatigue of convergence induced by reading as a function of illumination intensity. *Am J Ophthalmol, 18:*319, 1935.

Luckiesh, M., and F. K. Moss: *The Science of Seeing.* New York, Van Nostrand, 1938.

Luckiesh, M., A. H. Taylor, and R. H. Sinden: Bearing of illumination intensity upon efficiency of visual operations. *Elec World, 78:*668, 1921.

Lybrand, W. A., T. G. Andrews, and S. Ross: Systemic fatigue and perceptual organization. *Am J Psychol, 67:*704, 1954.

McFarland, R. A.: Psycho-physiological studies at high altitudes in The Andes. II. Sensory and motor responses during acclimatization. *J Comp Psychol, 27:*227, 1937.

McFarland, R. A., A. H. Holway, and L. M. Hurvich: Studies of visual fatigue. Boston: Harvard U. Grad. School of Bus. Admin, 1942.

McFarland, R. A., C. A. Knehr, and C. Berens: Metabolism and pulse rate as related to reading under high and low levels of illumination. *J Exp Psychol, 25:*65, 1939.

Narasaki, S., J. Fukuda, and K., M., and T. Nobuko: On the fatigue of civil air transportation crews observed from their visual functions: II. *Japan J Aerospace Med Psychol, 6*:35, 1969.

National Research Council: Conference on Visual Fatigue. Washington, May 20-21, 1939.

Ponder, E., and W. P. Kennedy: On the act of blinking. *Q J Exp Physiol, 18*:89, 1927-28.

Rudolph, G.: Sur une variation de seuil differential de l'oeil sous l'influence de stimuli lumineux de courte duree: un phenomene de fatigue centrale. *Comp rend Soc Biol Paris, 145*:310, 1951.

Ryan, T. A.: *Work and Effort: The Psychology of Efficiency.* New York, Ronald, 1947.

Ryan, T. A., C. L. Cottrell, and M. E. Bitterman: Muscular tension as an index of effort: The effect of glare and other disturbances in visual work. *Am J Psychol, 43*:317, 1950.

Schmidtke, H.: Ueber die Messung der psychischen Ermüdung mit Hilfe des Flimmertests. *Psychol Forschung, 23*:409, 1951.

Schmidtke, H.: *Die Ermüdüng: Symptome, Theorie, Messversuche.* Stuttgart, Hans Huber, 1965.

Simmerman, H.: Visual fatigue. *Am J Optom, 27*:554, 1950.

Simonson, E., and J. Brozek: Effects of illumination level on visual performance and fatigue. *J Opt Soc Am, 38*:384, 1948a.

Simonson, E., and J. Brozek: Effect of spectral quality of light on visual performance and fatigue. *J Opt Soc Am, 38*:830, 1948b.

Simonson, E., and J. Brozek: Work, vision and illumination. Nat'l Tech Conf Illum Engn Soc, Washington, Preprint 35, 1951.

Simonson, E., J. Brozek, and A. Keys: Effect of meals on visual performance and fatigue. *J Appl Physiol, 1*:270, 1948.

Simonson, E., and N. Enzer: Measurement of fusion frequency of flicker as test for fatigue of central nervous system; observations on laboratory technicians and office workers. *J Indust Hyg Toxicol, 23*:83, 1941.

Shek, M. P.: Poteri informateii v zritel'norm andizatore v zavisinosti ot khoraktara utomleniha. (Loss of information in the visual analyzer as a function of fatigue.) *Voprosy Psikhologii, 9*:111, 1963.

Thorn, G. S., J. T. Quimby, and M. Clinton: A comparison of the metabolic effects of isolcaloric meals of varying composition, with special reference to postprandial hypoglycemic symptoms. *Ann Intern, 18*:915, 1943.

Tinger, M. A.: Illumination standards for effective and comfortable vision. *J Consult Psychol, 3*:11, 1939.

Tinker, M. A.: The effect of visual adaptation upon intensity of light preferred for reading. *Psychol Bull, 37*:575, 1940.

Tinker, M. A.: The effect of adaptation upon visual efficiency in illumination studies. *Am J Optom, 19*:143, 1942.

Tinker, M. A.: Illumination intensities for reading newspaper type. *J Edu Psychol, 34*:247, 1943.

Tinker, M. A.: Illumination standards. *Am J Public Health, 36*:963, 1946.

Tinker, M. A.: Trends in illumination standards. *Illum Engn, 43*:866, 1948.

Tinker, M. A., and D. G. Paterson: Influence of type form on speed of reading. *J Appl Psychol, 12*:359, 1928.

Tinker, M. A., and D. G. Paterson: Influence of type form on eye movements. *J Exp Psychol, 25*:528, 1939.

Travis, R. C., J. L. Kennedy, L. C. Mead, and W. Allphin: Muscle action potentials as a measure of visual performance cost. *Illum Engn, 46*:182, 1951.

Troland, L. T.: An analysis of the literature concerning the dependency of visual functions upon the illumination intensity. *Trans Illum Engn Soc, 26*:107, 1931.

Weber, R. A.: Ocular fatigue. *Arch Ophthalmol, 43*:257, 1950.

Weston, H. C.: Visual fatigue. *Optician, 124*:602, 1952.

Weston, H. C.: Visual fatigue, with special reference to lighting. In Floyd, W. F. and Welford, A. T. (Eds.): *Symposium on Fatigue.* London, Lewis, 1953a.

Weston, H. C.: Visual fatigue with special reference to lighting. *Trans Illum Engn Soc,* London, *18*:39, 1953b.

White, L. R., R. H. Britten, J. H. Ives, and L. R. Thompson: Studies in illumination. II. Relationship of illumination to ocular efficiency and ocular fatigue among the letter separators in the Chicago post office. Washington, Public Health Bull. No. 181, 1929.

Chapter 7

Use of Visual Methods for Measurement of General Fatigue

S. HOWARD BARTLEY and ERNST SIMONSON

SEVERAL ATTEMPTS TO STUDY the more general effect of visual work on nonvisual physiological functions, such as V_{O_2}, heart rate or muscle tension, have been discussed in Chapter 6, "Visual Fatigue." Visual tests have also been used as an index of general, mainly CNS fatigue in work without appreciable visual effort. Thus, visual receptors and other physiological functions appear to be linked by a mutual feedback in the response to work and fatigue.

CRITICAL (CFF) OR FUSION FREQUENCY (FFF) OF FLICKER

The CFF has been used more frequently than any other visual test as an index of general (CNS) fatigue.

It was proposed by Simonson and Enzer (1941) as a test reflecting subjective fatigue. Lapique (chronaxie, 1938), Bourguignon (1922), Wedensky (1886) and Ukhtomsky (1934) demonstrated the importance of the time parameter of excitability for the functional state of motor and sensory pathways. Since the CFF[1] is related to the time parameter of excitability of the visual pathways, its use as a fatigue test appeared to be logical. Simonson and Enzer found a significant drop of the CFF (−5.4 and −4.6 cps) in clerical workers and laboratory technicians, and a somewhat smaller, but still significant, drop in laundry workers, paralleling the sensation of subjective fatigue. Amphetamine (Simonson, Enzer and Blankstein, 1941) and Pervitin (Simonson and Enzer, 1942) prevented the drop, together with relief of subjective fatigue. It was suggested, therefore, that the drop of CFF (FFF) reflects subjective fatigue. However, in a subsequent investigation, the drop of CFF after alcohol ingestion was related to the alcohol content of blood rather than to sensation (Enzer, Simonson and Ballard, 1944), and it was concluded that the CFF is an index of the general state of excitability of visual pathways, primarily of the cortical visual centers,[2]

---

1. The CFF has been used extensively in the exploration of fundamental properties of the visual centers for the past 6 decades (reviewed by Simonson and Brozek, 1952), but not for fatigue research prior to Simonson and Enzer.
2. The localization of the CFF within the visual pathways has been controversial. Reviewing the extensive literature, Simonson and Brozek concluded that the experimental evidence speaks overwhelmingly for a central localization in the absence of ocular pathology.

and probably also of the general excitability of the CNS. This does not invalidate the CFF as a fatigue test. The "Introduction" in E. Simonson "Physiology of Work Capacity and Fatigue" (1971) includes a general discussion of this problem.

Obviously changes of the CFF are not specifically related to fatigue. They compete with effects of numerous other factors, synergistically or antagonistically, as will be discussed in the following:

In an attempt at clarification of the controversial literature, we will discuss the changes of the CFF in three main categories of work: 1. sedentary or light physical occupational work; 2. mental work; and 3. muscular work. As mentioned before, none of these categories of work involved appreciable visual effort. Application of the CFF to work involving visual strain such as discrimination of fine details was discussed previously in Chapter 6, "Visual Fatigue."

Sedentary or Light Physical Occupational Work[3]

As a rule, the FFF (CFF) was measured at the beginning and end of the work shift, and in some studies also before and after the lunch pause. The length of the working periods varied from 4 to 10 hours. It is in this work category that the results of the various studies are most controversial. Obviously, the working conditions are far less standardized and controlled than in laboratory work tests.

The significant decrease of the CFF in sedentary occupational work in Simonson and Enzer's study was confirmed by Schmidtke (1951) but not by Brozek and Keys (1944). Lee (1941) found a significant depression of the CFF in 528 truck drivers after 10 hours of driving; this is the largest and most comprehensive study performed. Of the numerous tests performed, only the CFF showed a significant change. On the other hand, there was no significant change of the CFF in pilot instructors after 8 hours work (Graybiel, et al., 1943). Wang Shu Mao (1965) measured the CFF in three groups of railway workers (5 key operators, 9 calculators and 36 dispatchers). There was a significant drop of the CFF in the key operators and calculators during work; the CFF increased slightly after short pauses at intervals of two hours, but never reached the initial values; and the lows and highs were consistently lower for the successive work interruptions (see Fig. 7-1). Without work interruptions, the CFF decreased continuously. There was no significant change of the CFF in dispatchers in the day shift, while there was a marked decrease after the night shift. It was concluded that the CFF may be used as a CNS fatigue test in railroad workers.

Steinhaus and Kelso (1943) found a significant decrease of the CFF

---
3. Under 50% of max. V_{O_2}.

178 Psychological Aspects of Work and Fatigue

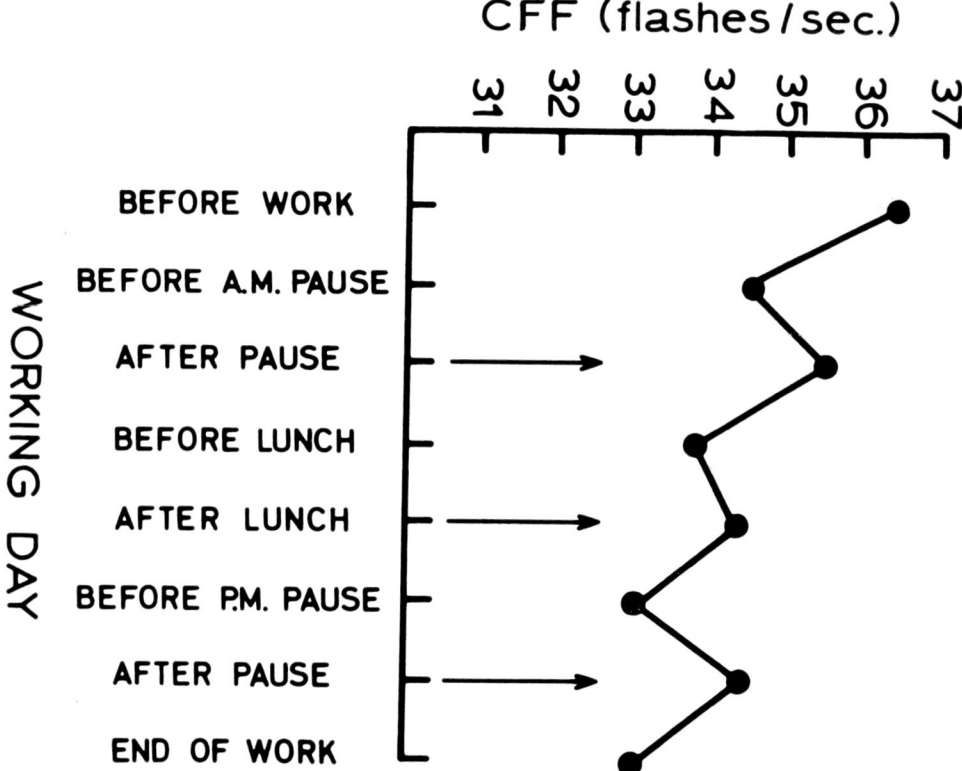

Figure 7-1. Decrease of CFF (ordinate: cps) during work day (8 hrs) in railroad workers. The decrease is partially reversed by pauses (Reproduced from Shu-Mao Wang, *Acta Psychol Sinica,* 4:307, 1965).

from morning to noon in 47 students and clerical workers. One of the most informative studies was performed by Busch and Wachholder (1953). While in the majority (10 of 17) of the subjects (students) the CFF dropped significantly during the working day, the results were variable, and in a few subjects an increase was observed at the end of work. The main series of their experiments was concerned with mental work and will be discussed later in this section. In view of the controversial results of the various authors, it is not surprising that they arrive at different conclusions regarding the usefulness of CFF as a test of CNS fatigue in occupational work. Some possible reasons for the discrepancies will be discussed at the end of this chapter, in context with the effects of other factors on the CFF.

There is agreement, however, that reading does not produce a significant depression of the CFF (Bitterman and Ryan, 1950; Schmidtke, 1951). It may be expected that the change of CFF in reading with adequate illumination and letter size depends largely on the subject matter. Reading of popular magazines for one hour was used as relaxation in an investigation of repeat variation of the ECG, blood pressure and plasma cholesterol (Simonson and Keys, 1970).

Oshima, et al. (1953) found a significant correlation between the decrease of the CFF during the day and the decrease during the week, indicating accumulation of fatigue. The decline in three days of night shift exceeded that in three days of day shift; it was most pronounced in steam boiler workers. None of the twenty occupations investigated involved any appreciable visual effort.

Trense (1962) applied the CFF in occupational work in noisy surroundings; 12,360 CFF measurements were made in 309 workers, probably the largest series yet performed. The investigations were performed in six industrial plants (metal, glass, chocolate, cement) with noise level up to 120 decibels. The work was either sedentary or physically light. The CFF was measured in 30 min. intervals over 4 hours. At noise levels exceeding 50 decibels, there was a progressive, marked decrease of the CFF, dependent on the noise level, most pronounced at 120 decibels (-7 cps). There was some recovery during intermittent 15 min. pauses (about $+3$ cps), but the initial level was not reached 30 min. after work. Protective devices reduced and retarded the drop of the CFF. Trense concluded that in noisy occupational work the CFF is a sensitive index of a CNS effect. Even more interesting from the point of control feedback mechanisms in fatigue is Trense's consecutive study (1963): sympathicomimetic drugs reduced or prevented the decrease of the CFF in noisy surroundings; in fact, sympathicomimetic drugs were about as effective as mechanical noise protective devices.

Mental Work (Laboratory Tests)

Arithmetic problems (additions, subtraction, multiplications) were used by all authors for the study of changes of CFF in mental fatigue in controlled laboratory conditions. The visual (reading) task was minimum and in some studies absent (blindfolded). Schmidtke (1951) found a continuous decrease of the CFF with duration of work (up to 180 min.) in general, parallel to the decrement of performance. Intermittent pauses and caffeine reduced and delayed the decrease of CFF. Davis (1955) found a small, but significant drop of the CFF in two hours of multiplications of two-digit numbers. The task was different from that in Schmidtke's experiment (Düker test, level D); whether the difference in the magnitude of the change is due to different task severity is conjectural. More precise information about the effect of task severity was provided by Bredenkamp (1966). He used for a light task the Düker test level A (example: $7 - 4 + 8$ ($= 11$) and for a severe task Düker's level F (example $5 - 3 + 6, 7 - 5 + 2, 6 + 5 -$

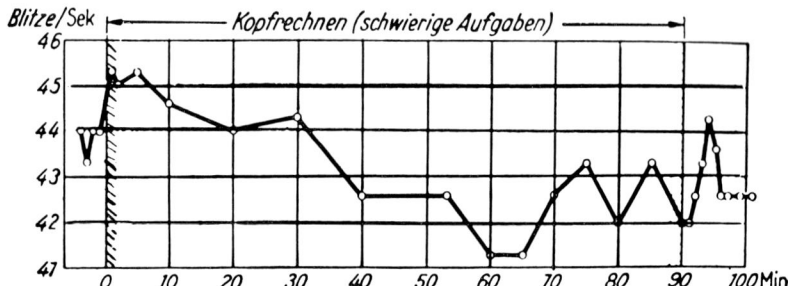

Figure 7-2. Flicker fusion frequency before, during and after ninety minutes of difficult mental work. The work period is marked by arrows (Reproduced from Busch and Wachholder, *Arbeitsphysiol, 15*:149, 1953, Fig. 3).

9 (= 2); the subtotals have to be memorized and only the final result is written down). Furthermore, in series 1, the subjects were advised to take their time while in series 2, they were instructed to calculate as fast as possible. Under conditions of high stress (series 2, level F), the FFF decreased linearly with time and with frequent intermittent short pauses varied around a linearly decreasing slope. At low level of effort, the CFF changes were not consistent. The reliability of the CFF after one hour of the simple task was low, but increases with duration of work. The author makes the interesting suggestion that the variations of the CFF may be more meaningful as fatigue index than its decline during work. Mücher (1960) found also a decrease of the CFF in mental work.

Busch and Wachholder (1953) investigated the changes during mental calculations at two different levels of severity. The CFF was measured in 5 and 10 min. intervals during the 90 min. work task. After an initial increase, the CFF dropped slightly in the light task with rather immediate recovery. During the difficult mental task, the drop of the CFF was more pronounced, followed by pronounced fluctuations during the last 30 min., which continued in the 10 min. recovery period (Fig. 7-2). The initial increase was interpreted as stimulation (arousal) phenomenon, and the terminal variations as imbalance of autonomic regulations. There is reason to believe that this is a spontaneous Orbeli[4] phenomenon, indicating transient reversal of fatigue changes as central feedback mechanism, to be discussed in somewhat greater detail later (Pupillography).

P. Rey's task (1971) of 30 min. duration was a combination of mental effort (requiring attention, concentration and choice reaction) and appreciable visual effort (Bourdon test: marking specified letters in intervals

---

4. The Orbeli phenomenon, a reversal of fatigue by sympathetic stimulation, is discussed in the volume "Physiology of Work Capacity and Fatigue," p. 198.

from several designated letters moving on a kymograph). Compared to Simonson and Brozek's somewhat similar task, the mental component is more pronounced, but the visual component is less strenuous. At a forced fast speed there was a highly significant decrease of the CFF. The decrease was smaller, but still highly significant, when the task was performed at a chosen convenient speed which was much slower. Marking the passage of small holes on a moving band decreased the CFF very slightly ($p = 0.05$). An auditory perception task (30 min.) did not change the CFF and also a verbal memory task was not effective. Rey concluded that decrease of the CFF is produced mainly by tasks involving visual perception at high repetitive frequency. There is not necessarily a discrepancy of Rey's results and those of Schmidtke (1951), Bredenkamp (1966), Busch and Wachholder (1953), since the mental component was different and more strenuous in the investigations of the German authors, while the visual component was more pronounced in Rey's studies. When the same test (Bourdon) was performed with room illumination flickering at a rate of 50 cps, the drop of the CFF and the increase of motor reaction time was more pronounced than with steady room illumination (Rey and Rey, 1964a). These results show indirectly the importance of the visual component. It appears then that primarily visual as well as primarily mental work depresses significantly the CFF, and that the changes of CFF are not specific for either component.

Wotzka and Grandjean (1968) investigated the CFF and tapping rate in sixty-eight traffic controllers at the Zürich airport (Switzerland). The work task is complex, involving visual attention (tracking radar screens and other types of visual information, 3½ hours per work day), 600 to 800 radio communications with pilots a day, amounting to a considerable mental strain in this highly responsible job. CFF as well as the tapping test showed a highly significant drop during 10 hours of work, more steeply during the last hours. There was a parallel trend in the self-rating score "refreshed-tired." The depression of the CFF (Enzer, Simonson and Blankstein, 1942) and of the tapping rate in circulatory insufficiency (Simonson and Enzer, 1941) and in hypothyroidism (Enzer, Simonson and Blankstein, 1941) is an interesting parallelism, indicating that both CFF and tapping rate reflect the functional state of the CNS. The strongest support for the suggestion made earlier that the CFF reflects the general state of excitability of the CNS, was provided by Hashimoto (1969). In a tracking task there was a highly significant negative correlation between the drop of the CFF and the alpha/beta ratio in the EEG, i.e. with fatigue, the frequency of the slower alpha waves increases and that of the faster beta waves decreases.

Physical Work

Strenuous, largely anaerobic, physical work (running to exhaustion) produced a marked depression of the CFF (Simonson, Enzer and Benton, 1943). This is consistent with Ishizuka's (1952) investigation who studied critical flicker frequency in relation to a motor performance (number of body inclinations per hour) and found that when more than 1000 inclinations were made, some relation between critical flicker frequency and inclinations appeared. It may be logical to assume that the depression of CFF in strenuous physical work is related to oxygen deficit, i.e. to the large O_2 debt. In Lambertsen's, et al. (1959) investigation of moderately heavy work (about 66% of max V_{O_2}) there was no evidence of cerebral ischemia, but this does not exclude cerebral ischemia in severe work close to or exceeding maximum V_{O_2}. Observations of amnesia after strenuous athletic performance are strongly suggestive of cerebral ischemia. There is a striking parallelism in the decrease of cerebral blood flow and the decrease of CFF with age (Simonson, 1958). Even a slight degree of hypoxia (arterial O_2 saturation 90%) (simulated high altitude) decreases significantly the CFF (Winchell and Simonson, 1951). It appears probable that the decrease of CFF in strenuous work is due to cerebral ischemia.

There was no consistent change of the CFF in moderate physical work in Simonson's, et al. investigations (1943). Brozek, Simonson and Keys (1950) reported no significant change of the CFF in hard work, but since it was continued over several hours, it must have been at or below 50 percent max V_{O_2}, i.e. essentially aerobic. Therefore, there is no contradiction to the decrease of CFF in strenuous short exercise exceeding this level of severity, so that it can be maintained only for several minutes. It increases in static work (Simonson, Enzer and Benton, 1943) probably due to central sympathetic stimulation, as shown by the pronounced increase of arterial blood pressure.[5]

Flicker (Phosphenes) Produced by Electrical Stimulation of the Eye

Suzuki (1950) attempted to obtain a measure of fatigue by using rectangular electric pulses delivered to the eye (Motokawa and Iwama's method, 1949). The concept of fatigue in his investigation covered the feeling of tiredness.

The performances included in the investigation were transmitting and

---

5. The CFF does not respond to acute starvation, but there was a small but statistically highly significant decrease after six months of caloric semi-starvation (about one half of the caloric requirement). There was no significant change of the CFF in acute thiamine deficiency and sleep deprivation (Brozek, Simonson and Keys, 1950). The effect of these various stresses is not relevant for fatigue.

receiving telegrams, telephone operators on duty, booking clerks at work, locomotive engineers and assistant engineers at work, stokers and coalies at work.

The experimental stimulus was applied at 20 cycles per second. The difference in the voltage of the electrical stimulus needed just to produce flicker and then the voltage at which flicker just disappeared as voltage was reduced was taken as the reference. The value of this difference during work and after recovery, minus the reference value was taken as a measure of fatigue (fatigue indicator).

The subject's activity was put into three degrees of severity: ordinary, a "little severe," and "very severe." It was found that the indicator voltage values varied in accord with the degree of severity and amount of the work, and corresponded well with the feeling of fatigue in many cases.

The author pointed out that the present technique of electrical stimulation of the eye proved to be an effective indicator of fatigue. It should be noted that all types of work investigated were sedentary or physically light to moderate, probably well under 50 percent of max V_{O_2}, so that V_{O_2} is not a reliable indicator of fatigue.

Motokawa and Iwama (1949) claim that intermittent electrical stimulation of the eye to produce the experience of flicker is a very sensitive measure of oxygen deficiency in the human subject. In fact, they found it to be more sensitive than using photic intermittent stimulation for the same purpose, which is somewhat at variance with Simonson and Winchell's (1951) results as mentioned above. Furthermore, intermittent electrical stimulation has additional advantages: 1. it can be used in a lighted room; 2. there is no need to wait for dark adaptation; 3. it takes only a few seconds to make a measurement and can be repeated without any extended interval between trials; 4. measurements can be taken when subjects are remotely situated from the investigator; 5. the rapidity of taking this electrical threshold provides for following rapid changes in oxygen deficiency as equivalent altitudes are increased.

Bujas, Petz and Karkovic (1952) used a series of electrical pulses to the eye and were unable to show that critical flicker frequency was related to fatigue. Here it was not visual fatigue itself that was at issue but something entirely nonvisual. "Exhaustion" was produced in a step test, and "mental fatigue" produced by 90 minutes of adding two-digit numbers. Electrical critical flicker frequency was not affected by these tests which presumably produced fatigue. Twenty-four hours of sleep deprivation did not affect the electrical critical flicker frequency either.

It appears that the effect of fatigue on the fusion frequency of intermittent electrical stimulation is controversial. However, the type of work in Bujas and Suzuki's investigations was quite different. Compared to the large material on the optical CFF, the number of investigations with the electrical CFF is still very small. The results of the Japanese authors are encouraging for further research.

Possible Reasons for Controversial Results of CFF Fatigue Studies

The results in laboratory experiments are fairly uniform; in most studies with strenuous visual work, strenuous mental work, and strenuous physical exercise there was a significant drop of the CFF.

In contrast, discrepancies were observed in occupational work performed for 4 to 10 hours with infrequent measurements of the CFF (as a rule at the beginning and end of work). As already mentioned, the less perfect control of the conditions in occupational work is probably one of the major factors which explain in part the discrepancies of results in the various studies. Another factor is the lack of standardization of the technique of CFF determination. The CFF depends on the size, brightness and color of test patch, surrounding illumination, state of adaptation, light:dark ratio and other variables (reviewed by Simonson and Brozek, 1952). While in most investigations the range of CFF was similar, i.e. between 30 and 45 cps, it is not certain that the changes of the CFF at different testing arrangements will be identical even at a similar range of CFF. The effect of different technique of CFF determination during a visual-mental task (Bourdon test) was investigated by P. and J. P. Rey (1964b). The CFF was determined 1. with continuous ascending, 2. continuous descending flicker rate and 3. successive stepwise approximation of CFF with variation of flicker rates below and above CFF. Method 3 was superior both in regard to repeat variation at rest as well as to magnitude and significance of the decrease of the CFF during work. This study is encouraging for investigation of the effect of other variables on the change of CFF during work.

Busch and Wachholder (1953) suggested that diurnal variations of the CFF may interfere with fatigue trends.

The most powerful factor to account for the discrepancies of results is probably the effect of central sympathetic stimulation. We mentioned that the CFF is related to the excitability of the visual pathways and CNS in general, rather than specifically to fatigue. Thus, depression in fatigue may be reversed by sympathetic stimulation.

Already in the early investigations, Simonson, et al. (1941, 1942) found that central sympathicomimetic drugs (amphetamine, Pervitin®) reduced or eliminated the decrease of CFF at the end of the working day. Schmidtke (1951) obtained similar results with caffeine, and a sympathicomimetic drug reduced also the decrease of CFF in noisy occupational work (Trense, 1963). A cold hip bath (Steinhaus and Kelso, 1943) and immersion of one arm in ice water (Simonson, 1958) increased significantly the CFF, due to sympathetic stimulation evidenced by the highly significant increase of blood pressure. The same is true also for the stimulating effect of static work (Simonson, Enzer and Benton, 1943).

Stimulation from other sensory receptors (sound, smell and taste) also increases the CFF (Krakov, quoted from Landis, 1954). Busch and Wachholder (1953) found an increase of the CFF in tasks requiring concentration, and they explained the initial increase of the CFF in difficult mental work as a stimulating effect of the challenging task situation. In Hashimoto's (1969) study the CFF decreases continuously in a tracking task. When a chime was rung at 7 minute intervals (which the subject had to turn off after 1 minute) the CFF was maintained at a higher level. In our experience (unpublished) such stimuli as slamming the door or a person entering the room produced frequently a transient increase of the CFF. In a newspaper company, articles were transmitted by telephone to branch offices. The CFF did not change significantly from 10 A.M. to 6 P.M. When the work was mechanized by a teletype system and thus became more monotonous, the CFF decreased significantly together with more frequent complaints about subjective fatigue (Hashimoto, 1969). It is reasonable to assume that the effects of the various stimuli are due to central sympathetic stimulation. This concept agrees well with Grandjean's hypothesis of CNS fatigue, i.e. stimulation of cortical centers from the activating system in the reticular formation of the midbrain (Moruzzi and Magoun, 1949; Bremer and Terzuolo, 1954) counteracting the depression produced by fatigue. The effect of sympathetic stimulation has been explored more systematically by Lowenstein and Loewenfeld with the pupil reflex (reviewed in "Physiology of Work Capacity and Fatigue" p. 200-207), which is a superior method because there is a large body of information about the central and peripheral sympathetic and parasympathetic pathways of the pupil reflex (see following part). However, the similarity of responses of the CFF and pupil reflex to sympathetic stimulation is striking. The increased variability at the end of the difficult mental task in Busch and Wachholder's (1953) investigation may be explained as a spontaneous Orbeli phenomenon, i.e. as a feedback mechanism triggered by decrease of the excitability to a certain and probably individually variable threshold level, following Lowenstein and Loewenfeld's (1952) suggestion for the pupil reflex.

Thus we agree with Bredenkamp's suggestion of the significance of CFF variability as index of fatigue even in the absence of a decrease.

It appears then that the inconsistency of results of CFF in occupational work is most likely due to the effect of various uncontrolled extraneous stimuli, and probably different individual sensitivity to such stimuli. Since intervening stimuli are hard to control in occupational work, the application of the CFF as a fatigue test is somewhat questionable, particularly in stimulating work tasks. The results are more consistent in monotonous work situations (Grandjean, 1970) and in laboratory experiments. Hashimoto, Kogi, et al. (1967) found that the level of the CFF in bus drivers during 3.5 hours of driving on an expressway was higher at a speed limit of 100 km/hr than at 80 km/hr, and explained this with a stimulating effect of the higher speed. It should be noted, however, that in the majority of studies the CFF declined during prolonged occupational work. Rey (1971) concludes after a critical discussion of the significance of CFF changes, "if all precautions are taken to eliminate the influence of any other factor, a decline in CFF following a tiring mental task can reasonably be attributed to mental fatigue." Grandjean concurs with this conclusion and considers the CFF as "a useful indicator of the cortical activity of the brain."

PUPILLOGRAPHY

The effects of intermittent photic stimulation on pupillary movements were discussed from the aspect of conflicts (Chapter 6, "Visual Fatigue"). The frequency was too fast for the total duration of about 1 sec. for the pupillary contraction and about 2 sec. for the redilation phase.

Lowenstein (1937) investigated the fatigue of the pupillary reflex in successive light flashes at 3 sec. intervals until fatigue which occurred in healthy subjects after 70 to 100 consecutive light stimuli. In the experiment shown in Figure 47 (Physiology of Work Capacity and Fatigue) the reaction was practically absent after 100 stimuli, but was immediately restored by an acoustic shock. Other sensory stimuli (tactile pain stimulus or fear suggestion) also restored the pupillary reflex ("psychic restitution effect"). This is in effect a reproduction of the Orbeli phenomenon observed in muscular fatigue. The pupil reflex is ideal for fatigue studies, since the sympathetic (dilatation) and parasympathetic (contraction) peripheral and central pathways are anatomically well defined; moreover, Lowenstein and Loewenfeld have localized their involvement in the four phases of the pupil reflex (fast and slow contraction phase, fast and slow redilation phase). They demonstrated disintegration of autonomic regulation in fatigue by this method.

There is a close relationship between fatigue produced by prolonged mental work and changes in the pupil reflex. In a state of general fatigue, the fatigue of the pupil reflex was accelerated. The authors also demonstrated that the fatigue of the pupil reflex is central, which explains the summation effect with general fatigue. Together with faster fatigue, the variability of the pupillary reflex movement was greatly increased after 8 hours of uninterrupted mental work (Fig. 7-3). There is some similarity to

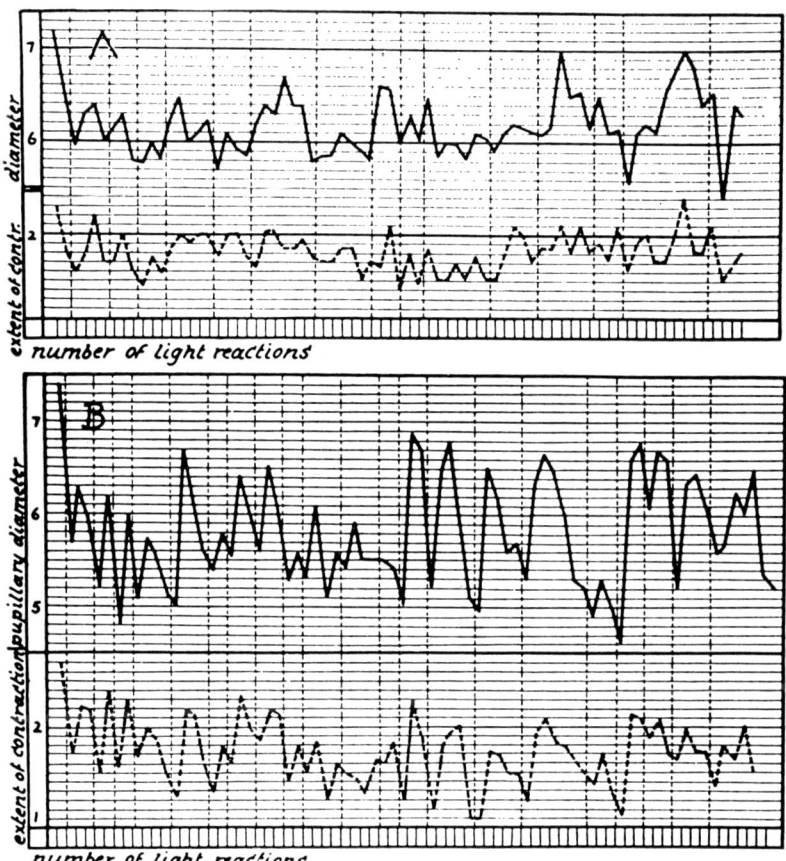

Figure 7-3. Effect of generally fatiguing work on the natural rhythm in the deterioration of the reflex to light. The spontaneous rhythm in a normal man twenty-four years of age before (A) and after (B) an eight-hour day of uninterrupted work. The solid line represents pupillary diameter at the beginning of each reaction to light, and the broken line represents extent of contraction in each reflex. The abscissa represents the number of reactions and the ordinate, millimeters. (From Lowenstein and Loewenfeld, *J Nerv Ment Dis, 115 (2)*:121, 1952, Fig. 6).

the increased variability of the CFF as discussed earlier, indicating imbalance of autonomic regulation. The transient peaks were interpreted by Lowenstein and Loewenfeld as spontaneous brief "restitution phenomenon," on the basis of central feedbacks from various sensory and emotional stimuli (fear, joy, apprehension, spontaneous thoughts, etc.). Thus, mental fatigue, according to these observations, is a discontinuous process (the pupillographic studies of Lowenstein and Loewenfeld are discussed in somewhat greater detail, pp. 200-207, E. Simonson, "Physiology of Work Capacity and Fatigue").

DARK ADAPTATION

Bodansky and Hendley (1946) found that quite strenuous bicycle ergometer exercise (20,000-35,000 foot pounds over a period from 3 to 5 minutes) produced a rise in the rod thresholds after 5 to 10 min. both in normal and methemoglobinemic individuals. Wendland (1948) investigated the effect of moderate (bicycle ergometer, 10 and 35 min.; genuflections, 3 min.), and severe exercise (running "all out") on visual thresholds after dark adaptation in 35 healthy college students from 17 to 29 years. In all subjects there was an increase of the threshold, more so after the strenuous exercise, beginning 1 to 5.75 min. after exercise and lasting from 1 to 16 min., with considerable individual variation (from 0.08 to 0.56 log units), with a mean increase of 0.26 log units. The maximum increase of the threshold of 0.56 log units represents almost a fourfold change of sensitivity.

Pilocarpine fixation or use of an artificial pupil did not influence the results. There was no difference in the response between physically trained and untrained subjects, and between men and women. The maximum increase of the final rod threshold by heavy exercise was equivalent to the effect of an altitude of 15,000 feet. There is some parallelism to the effect of strenuous exercise on the CFF, and to the effect of respiratory acidosis produced by breathing air with 5% CO_2 on the CFF (Simonson and Winchell, 1951) on the final rod threshold (Wald, et al., 1942). Thus, oxygen debt and increased CO_2 production may be involved in the increase of visual thresholds and decrease of CFF in severe exercise at or exceeding the max V_{O_2}.

BIBLIOGRAPHY

Bitterman, M. D., and A. T. Ryan: Changes in C.F.F. resulting from prolonged visual work under high and low illumination. Eastern Psychol Assoc Meeting, 1950.

Bodansky, O., and C. D. Hendley: Effect of methemoglobinemia on the visual threshold at sea level and high altitudes and after exercise. *J Clin Invest, 25:*717, 1946.

Bourguignon, G.: *La Chronaxie Chez L'homme.* Paris (Masson et Cie), 1922.

Bredenkamp, J.: Eine Analyse der Flimmerverschmelzungsfrequenz als Ermüdungsindikator. Zeitschrift exp. u. angew. *Psychologie, 3:*200, 1966.

Bremer, F., and C. Terzuolo: Contribution a l'étude des mecanismes physiologiques due mainien de l'activité vigile. *Arch Int Physiol, 62:*157, 1954.

Brozek, J., and A. Keys: Flicker fusion frequency as a test of fatigue. *J Indust Hyg Toxicol 26:*169, 1944.

Brozek, J., E. Simonson, and A. Keys: Changes in performance and in ocular functions resulting from strenuous visual inspection. *Am J Psychol, 3:*51-66, 1950.

Bujus, Z., B. Pets, and A. Karkovic: Can the critical frequency of interrupted electrical stimulation of the eye serve as a test of fatigue? *Archiv Hig Rada, 3:*428, 1952.

Busch, G., and K. Wachholder: Der Einfluss ermüdender geistiger Beanspruchung auf die Flimmerverschmelzungfrequenz. *Arbeitsphysiologie, 15:*149, 1953.

Davis, S. W.: Auditory and visual flicker fusion as measure of fatigue. *Am J Psychol, 68*:654, 1955.
Düker, H.: Verfahren zur Untersuchung der psychischen Leistungsfähigkeit. *Psychol Forsch, 23*:10, 1949.
Enzer, N., E. Simonson, and G. Ballard: Effect of small doses of alcohol on the central nervous system. *Am J Clin Pathol, 14*:333, 1944.
Enzer, N., E. Simonson, and S. S. Blankstein: The state of sensory and motor centers in patients with hypothyroidism. *Ann Intern Med, 15*(4):659, 1941.
Enzer, N., E. Simonson, and S. S. Blankstein: Fatigue of patients with circulatory insufficiency investigated by means of the fusion frequency of flicker. *Ann Intern Med, 16*:701, 1942.
Grandjean, E. P.: Fatigue. *Amer Industr Hyg Ass J, 31*:1, 1970.
Hashimoto, K.: *Physiological Features of "Monotony" Manifested under High Speed Driving Situations.* Railway Labour Science Institute, Japan National Railways, 1969.
Hashimoto, K., K. Kogi, et al.: Physiological strain of high speed bus driving on the Mei-Shin Expressway and the effects of moderation of speed restrictions. *J Railway Lab Sci, 20*:1, 1967.
Ishizuka, T.: Studies on flicker phenomena. *Osaka Daigaku Igaku Zassi (Osaka), 4*:33, Issues 5 & 6, 1952.
Lambertsen, C. J., S. G. Owen, H. Wendel, M. W. Stroud, A. A. Lurie, W. Lochner, and G. F. Clark: Respiratory and cerebral circulatory control during exercise at .21 and 2.0 atmospheres inspired po_2. *J Appl Physiol, 14*:966, 1959.
Landis, C.: Determinants of the critical flicker-fusion threshold. *Physiol Rev, 34*:259, 1954.
Lapique, L.: *La Chrononaxie et ses Applications Physiologiques.* Hermann and Cie (Eds.), 6, Rue de la Sorbonne, 6, Paris, 1938.
Lee, R. H.: Fatigue and hours of service of interstate truck drivers. Critical fusion frequency of flicker. *Public Health Bull No. 265*:195, 1941.
Lowenstein, O.: Der psychische Restitutionseffekt. Das Prinzip der psychischen Wiederherstellung der Ermüdeten, der Erschöpften und der Erkrankten Funktion, Basel, Benno Schwabe and Co., 1937.
Lowenstein, O., and I. E. Lowenfeld: Disintegration of central autonomic regulation during fatigue and its reintegration by psychosensory controlling mechanisms; disintegration, reintegration; pupillographic studies. *J Nerv Ment Dis, 115*:121, 1952.
Moruzzi, G., and H. W. Magoun: Brain stem reticular formation and activation of the EEG. *Electroenceph Clin Neurophysiol, 1*:455, 1949.
Motokawa, K., and K. Iwama: The electrical excitability of the human eye as sensitive indicator of oxygen deficiency. *Tohoku J Exp Med, 50*:319, 1949.
Mücher, H.: Über die Abhängigkest der Visuellen verschmelzungsfrequenz von leichter geistiger. *Arbeit Psychol Beitr, 4*:530, 1960.
Oshima, M., K. Endo, H. Yamanaka, and T. Shibuya: Flicker value in relation to fatigue and working conditions. *Reports Inst Science of Labor,* Tokyo *47*:1, 1953.
Rey, P.: The interpretation of changes in critical fusion frequency. In Singleton, W. T., Fox, J. G., and Whitefield, D., (Eds.): *Measurement of Men at Work.* London, Taylor and Francis, 1971, p. 115.
Rey, P., and J. P. Rey: La frequence de fusion optique subjective: comparison de trois methodes de mesure avant et apres le travail. *Le Travail Humain 26*:135, 1964a.
Rey, P., and J. P. Rey: Pourqoi certain taches visuelles abaissent-elles la frequence de fusion optique subjective? *Le Travail Humain, 26*:293, 1964b.

Schmidtke, H.: Üeber die Messung der psychischen Ermüdung mit Hilfe des Flimmertests. *Psychol Forschung, 23:*409, 1951.
Simonson, E.: Functional capacities of older individuals. Clinical medicine symposium. *J. Gerontol, 13* (Suppl 2) (3):18, 1958.
Simonson, E.: Effect of local cold application on the fusion frequency of flicker. *J. Appl Physiol, 13*(3):445, 1958.
Simonson, E.: Performance as a function of age and cardiovascular disease. In Welford, A. T., and Birren, J. E. (Eds.): *Behavior, Aging and the Nervous System.* Springfield, Thomas, 1965, pp. 401-434.
Simonson, E.: Introduction in Simonson, E. (Ed.): *Physiology of Work Capacity and Fatigue.* Springfield, Thomas, 1971.
Simonson, E., and J. Brozek: Flicker fusion frequency: Background and applications. *Physiol Rev, 32:*349, 1952.
Simonson, E., and N. Enzer: The state of motor centers in circulatory insufficiency. *Arch Intern Med, 68:*498, 1941.
Simonson, E., and N. Enzer: Measurement of fusion frequency of flicker as test for fatigue of central nervous system; observations on laboratory technicians and office workers. *J Indust Hyg Toxicol, 23:*83, 1941.
Simonson, E., and N. Enzer: Effect of pervitin (desoxyephedrine) on fatigue of the central nervous system. *J Industr Hyg Toxicol, 35*(7):205, 1942.
Simonson, E., N. Enzer, and R. W. Benton: The influence of muscular work and fatigue on the state of the central nervous system. *J Lab Clin Med, 28:*1555, 1942.
Simonson, E., N. Enzer, and S. S. Blankenstein: The effect of amphetamine on fatigue of the central nervous system. *War Med, 1:*690, 1941.
Simonson E., and A. Keys: Repeat variations of electrocardiogram, blood pressure, and blood cholesterol within one hour and six months. *Br Heart J, 22:*660, 1970.
Simonson, E., and P. Winchell: The effect of high carbondioxide and of low oxygen concentration on the fusion frequency of flicker. *J Appl Physiol, 3:*637, 1951.
Steinhaus, A. H., and A. Kelso: Improvement of visual and other functions by cold hip baths. *War Med, 4:*610, 1943.
Suzuki, K.: Professional differences of fatigue as revealed by the method of electric flicker. *Tohoku J of Exp Med, 52:*1, 1950.
Trense, E.: Erfahrungen mit dem Flimmertest bei Lärmarbeitern. *Int Arch f Gewerbepath u Gewerbehyg, 19:*226, 1962.
Trense, E.: Zur Bekämpfung von Lärmschaden durch ein Sympathicomimeticum. *Zeitschr f Arztl Fortbildung, 52:*(8), 1963.
Ukhtomsky, A. A.: Excitation, fatigue, inhibition. *Fiziol Zh SSSR Sechenov, 17:*1114, 1934 (Russ).
Wald, G., L. Brouha, and R. E. Johnson: Experimental human vitamin A deficiency and ability to perform muscular exercise. *Am J Physiol, 137:*551, 1942.
Wang, Shu-Mao: Critical flicker frequency as an indicator of fatigue in railroad workers. *Acta Psychol Sinica, 4:*307, 1965.
Wedensky, N. E.: O sootnoshenii mezhdr razrashenium i vozbuzhdeniem pri tetanuse (On relation between stimulation and excitation during tetanus). *Zap Akad Nauk* (Addition 3), SPB, 1886 (Russ).
Wendland, J. P.: Effect of muscular exercise on dark adaptation. *Am J Ophthalmol, 31:*1429, 1948.
Wotzka, F., and E. Grandjean: Physiologische med pathologische Ermudüngsmessungen bei Flugverkehrsleitern. *Z Preventiv med, 13:*204, 1968.

SECTION FOUR
ASPECTS OF CENTRAL PROCESSING

Chapter 8

Vigilance

HEINZ SCHMIDTKE[1]

INDUSTRY'S TECHNICAL DEVELOPMENT toward increasing automation has resulted in occupations that mainly involve supervision and control functions. Here, alertness and readiness for action are more important than the perception of environmental stimuli and their subsequent mental processing and transfer to motor reaction. The work of the control panel operator in a modern chemical plant may serve as an example. The delivery of raw material, intermediate and semifinished products to the various production units, and transport of finished products is accomplished by means of control and regulation panels. The operator receives information about the state of the actual production process at any given time by means of meters, monitors, TV and microphones, but action is only expected in case of technical defects in any of the control systems. Thus, the operator essentially has the function of a "monitor of a superior order" which contributes to the redundancy of the whole system.

This type of activity may approach the dreams of some political philosophers of the last century. However, experience has shown that the forced sedentary job activity results in many problems, since a satisfactory level of vigilance for the whole working period is not always possible. To explain deficiencies in human performance at such working places, low working morale has been frequently suggested. One of the purposes of this chapter, based on the results of vigilance research, attempts to find a more realistic appraisal of human performance under conditions of deprivation of stimuli and activity (monotony). Also, an attempt will be made to discriminate between a decrement of performance produced by mental overexertion from a decrease due to underexertion.

According to Head (1926), vigilance can be understood as a definite state of the central nervous system whose level of excitation can vary. N. H. Mackworth (1957) characterizes vigilance as "state of readiness to detect and respond to certain specified small changes occurring at random time intervals in the environment." On the basis of the present state of knowledge, the "readiness to detect and respond" must be interpreted as a function of the activation and arousal level of external stimulation and motivational factors.

One of the first thorough analyses of performance in an environment

---
1. Translated by Ernst Simonson and Philip Weiser, Editors.

having stimuli deprivation was done during World War II by the British Air Force, who investigated the relationship between frequency of submarine localization by means of radar and watch time of the radar observers (Anonymous, 1944). Statistical evaluation of the logbooks (start of duty of observer and time of contact reports) over the 24 hour period showed that 50.5 percent of all reported contacts were made in the first 30 minutes of a watch. The remaining 49.5 percent were distributed (Fig. 8-1) throughout the following 90 minutes. This striking result prompted N. H. Mackworth's (1950) classical study which started psychological vigilance research.

N. H. Mackworth (1950) simulated a pronounced monotonous (low stimulation level) activity in the laboratory, comparable to that of the radar observers. The task consisted of observing an electrical clock (clock test) with the pointer progressing in 100 steps per revolution (1/100 min. dial). Each of these normal time steps was a neutral, i.e. noncritical signal. Occasionally, the pointer made a double step jumping to the second next mark without interruption. This was the critical signal requiring a response. There were 12 critical signals per each 30 min. during the 2 hour task, in intervals from 45 sec. to 10 min. Sailors and cadets of the British

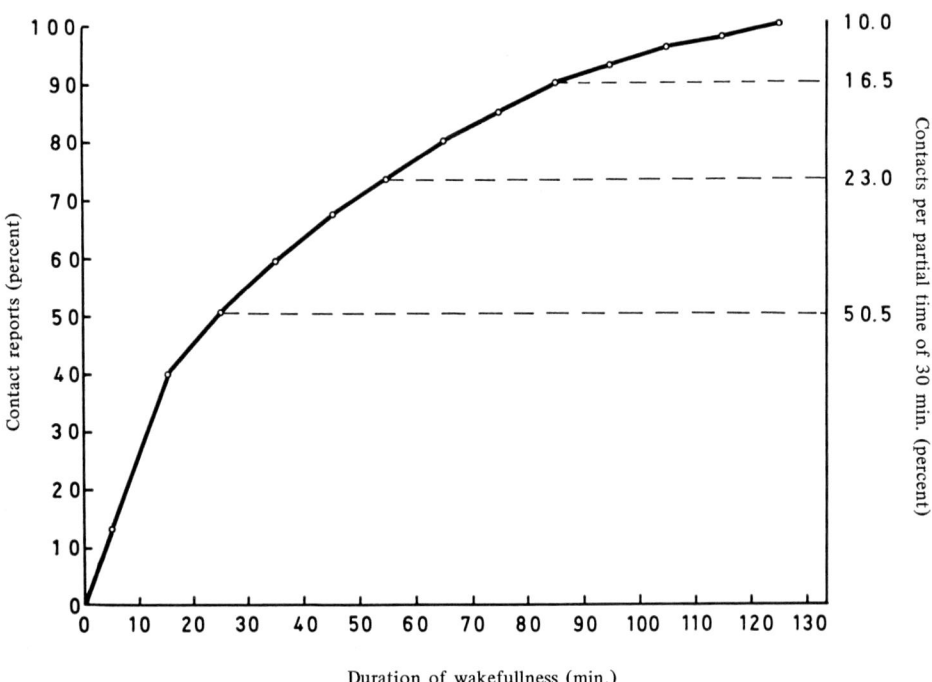

Figure 8-1. Relationship between watch time of radar observers and contact reports (according to Baker's data).

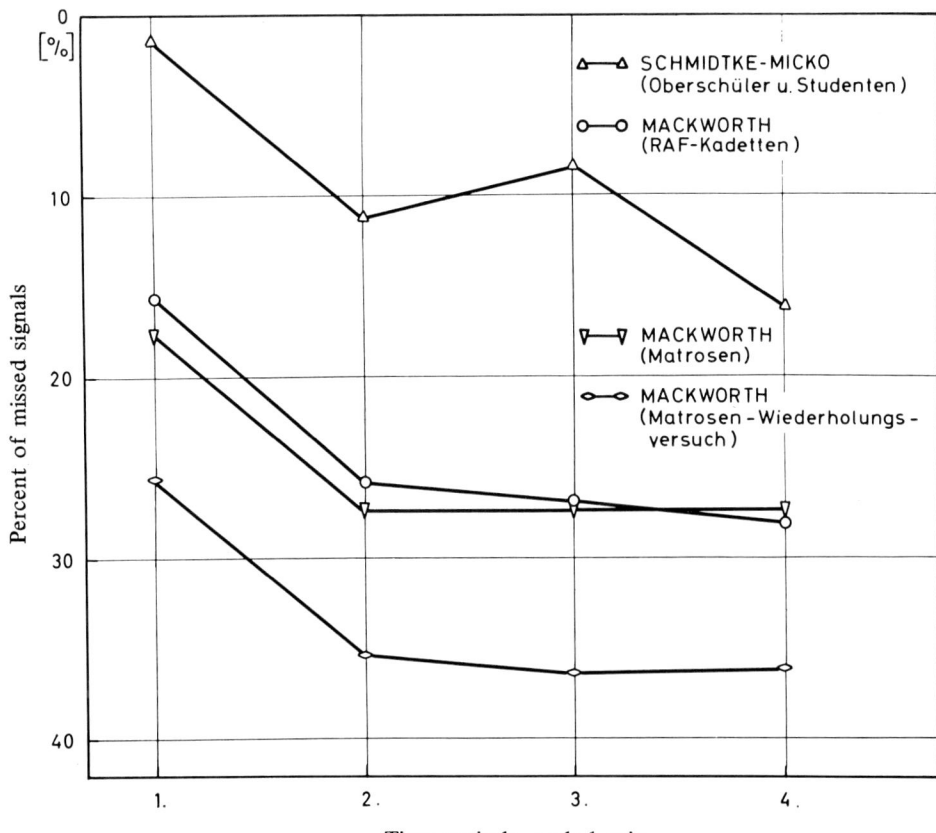

Figure 8-2. Time course of performance during two hours observation with the clock test (according to N. H. Mackworth, and Schmidtke & Micko).
  SCHMIDTKE-MICKO (High school and university students)
  MACKWORTH (RAF cadets)
  MACKWORTH (Sailors)
  MACKWORTH (Sailors—repeat experiment)

navy served as subjects. The performance showed the same decrement of vigilance as in the submarine localization of radar observers during the war i.e. a pronounced drop in the first time periods of the vigilance task. However, there were some differences between the experimental groups: the group of conscripted soldiers made more observational errors than the group of cadets. A repetition of this seemingly uninteresting test with the same subjects revealed an even more significant performance decrement. In a repeat study by Schmidtke and Micko (1964), the performance of students who were interested in the results, was even better. It may be concluded that performance motivation may be an important factor for observer activity in an environment with low level of stimulation (Fig. 8-2).

Based on N. H. Mackworth's investigations, numerous experiments were performed with the purpose of classifying the dependence of vigilance on the type and number of signals (for ref. see Singer, 1969 and J. F. Mackworth, 1969). At the present time, we are still far from a comprehensive vigilance theory with satisfactory explanation of all results. Nevertheless, the effect of some variables has been more or less clarified including (among other factors) the signals impinging on the observer which can be differentiated as

A. critical signals, requiring a response of the observer;
B. neutral signals which are nonspecific for the task and can be characterized as background noise;
C. noncritical signals, which are nonspecific for the observation task, but are markedly different from the spectrum of neutral signals;
D. noncritical additional signals, which are artificially inserted into the field of observation but do not require a response of the observer, and are different from the critical and neutral signals (for instance, having entirely different physical parameters);
E. critical additional signals, corresponding to category of "D" but requiring a response of the observer.

In addition to the type and number of signals, the effects of location in space, intensity, duration and regularity of timing of signals (i.e. variation of intervals) have been investigated. Other variables were the uninterrupted duration of the observation task, length and frequency of pauses, type and extent of success or failure reports, degree of preceding load or sleep deprivation, effect of drugs and additional environmental stress (noise, temperature, etc.). Some of the results of these complex investigations will be briefly outlined in the following sections.

TYPE AND FREQUENCY OF SIGNALS

One of the most frequently analyzed variables in vigilance experimentation is the frequency of signals. Here the results of N. H. Mackworth (1950), Deese and Ormond (1953), Jenkins (1958), Wiener (1963), Schmidtke and Micko (1964) and other investigators are quite consistent: the observational performance is the better, the higher the frequency of critical signals which require a response. This is true up to an optimum signal frequency, which Micko (1963) found to be 120 and Schmidtke (1966) about 300 critical signals per hr. If this frequency is exceeded significantly, a stress situation developed resulting in increasingly missed signals. Therefore, we can start from the fact that there is an approximately inverse U-shaped relationship between the frequency (per unit of time) of critical signals and observer performance (Fig. 8-3).

Whether the improvement of performance with increasing signal fre-

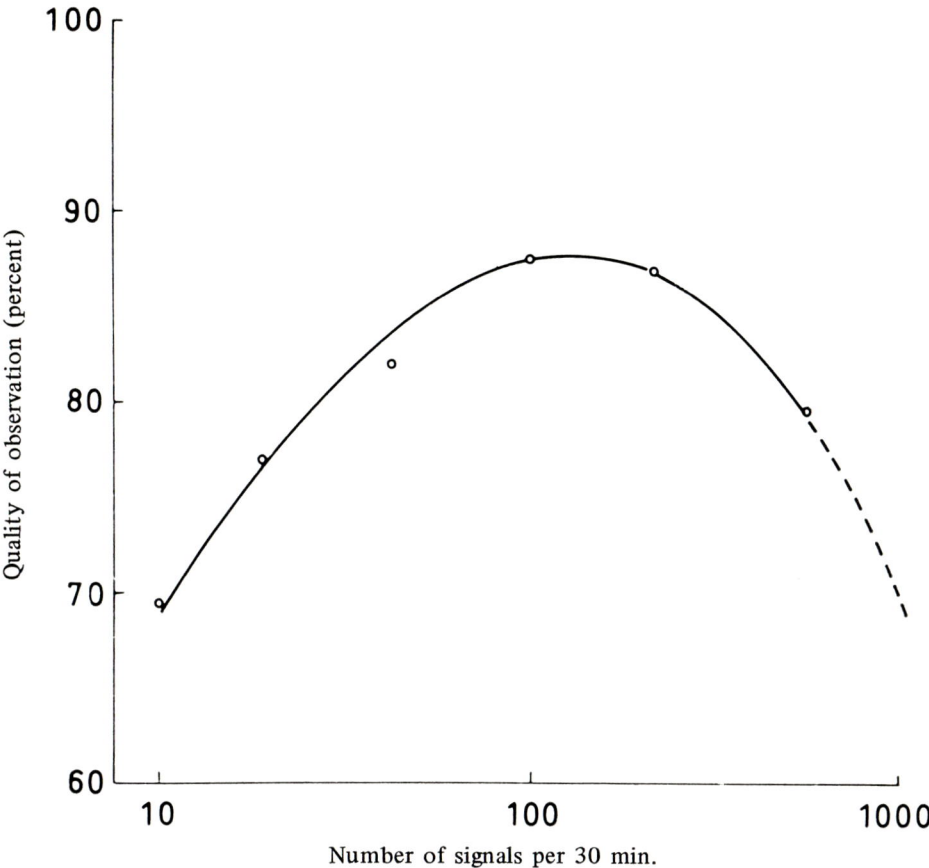

Figure 8-3. Relationship between signal frequency and quality of observer performance (according to Schmidtke).

quency (ascending limb of the U curve) is due to the increased stimulation level of activity, is doubtful (Colquhoun, 1961). According to this author, it must be noted that with a change of the frequency of critical signals (relative to neutral or noncritical signals), there is a change of the probability that a given signal will be a critical signal. Therefore, the better performance with greater frequency of critical signals may be due to the greater probability that a critical signal will occur, provided that there are also neutral and noncritical signals along with the critical signals.

The significance of neutral and noncritical signals for the observer performance has been investigated by numerous authors in vigilance research, starting from the question of whether the improvement of performance with higher frequency or probability of critical signals could also be achieved by means of artificially added stimuli. Unfortunately, the results still are not consistent. However, there appears to be the following tendency: improvement of performance can always be expected when the observer situation is characterized by paucity of stimuli, when the additional stimuli have a certain regularity, when the additional signals are distinctly different from the critical and neutral signals, and when the observer received information whether he has or has not correctly responded to the additional stimulus.

In the absence of these conditions, additional stimuli have no positive effect. On the contrary, some findings suggest that the decision times lengthen, because the observer has to examine in each case whether the signal is critical or additional. It should also be noted that the necessity to respond to noncritical additional signals may be interpreted as "Occupational therapy" with all consequent negative effects on the performance motivation of man.

The present experimental results concerning the variables mentioned above have been summarized by Schmidtke and Micko (1964) as shown in Figure 8-4: Variable I: In case of infrequent critical signals, the observer performance improves with increasing frequency of critical signals per unit of time; however, if the frequency of critical signals exceeds that of neutral signals, a reversal in performance occurs. In this condition, the reaction to critical signals becomes the same as that of neutral signals which elicit an automatic response, while for the few neutral signals, now acting

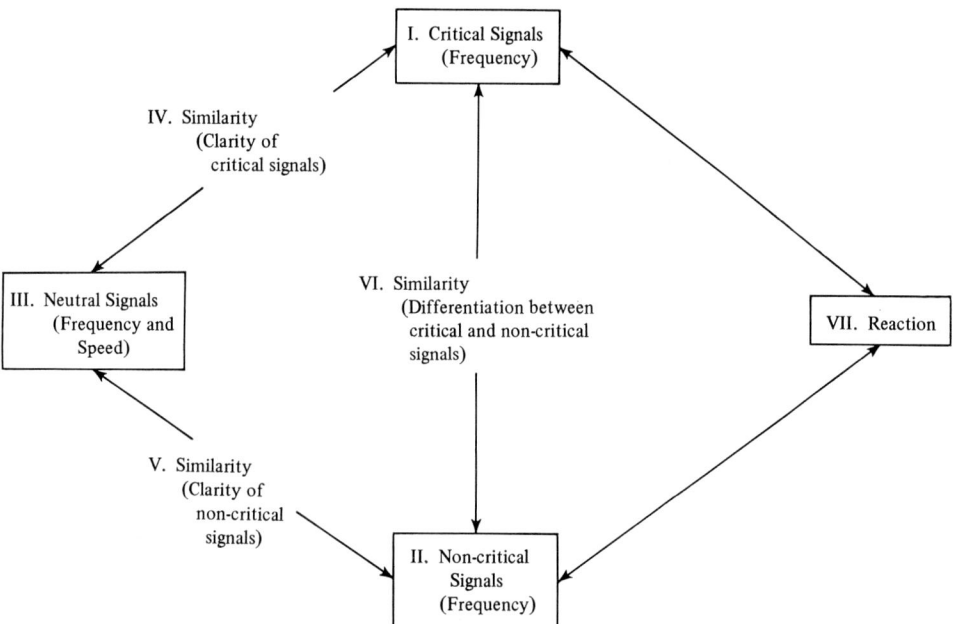

Figure 8-4. Schematic sketch of variables affecting quality of observation (according to Schmidtke & Micko).

like critical signals, the response should be suppressed. The effect of variable I probably depends on variables II and III. Variable II: It appears that the frequency of noncritical signals affects the observer performance; however, the results are not consistent. The effect of variable II certainly depends to a large degree on nearly all other variables. Variable III: The frequency of neutral signals, i.e. the speed of their sequence, is probably another significant variable. Possibly, there is some interaction between variables I and III. Variable IV: The similarity of critical and neutral signals, or in other words, the clarity of critical signals, determines performance. It could be shown that distinct signals can be more easily detected resulting in a slower drop of performance. It is not yet entirely certain whether the clarity of critical signals depends not only on the relationship: intensity of critical signals/intensity of neutral signals, but also on the absolute value of these two intensities. The variables I and IV are apparently mutually independent, aside from the existence of a plateau effect. If the critical signals are made so distinct that all are detected, the frequency ceases to play a role. Variable V: There are not yet reliable investigations on the clarity of noncritical signals. In any case they are differentiated from the true (critical) signals only because they are distinctly different from the neutral signals. If they are supposed to be "arousing stimuli," their effect probably increases with their strength (intensity), provided that they have no aversive effect. Variable VI: With these variables one has to decide whether the noncritical signals look exactly like the critical ones or whether they are more or less similar. If they look alike, the noncritical signals will appear to the observer as critical signals, and their presentation has the same effect as an increased frequency of the critical signals. If critical and noncritical signals are distinctly different, their effect can be quite variable. This variable depends also on whether and how the observer has to respond. Variable VII: This is concerned with the question of whether critical and noncritical signals require the same or different reaction, or no reaction at all. So far there is not a sufficiently reliable investigation available to demonstrate that under otherwise identical conditions, the same response to critical and noncritical signals is more advantageous. However, there is some indication that it will make no difference whether noncritical signals should require a different reaction or no response at all.

INTERACTIONS

I and II: From Colquhoun's (1961) findings it can be concluded that the observer performance does not depend on the frequency of the critical or noncritical signals, but on the relationship: frequency of critical signals/frequency of noncritical signals. Still not resolved is whether this is a general rule or whether this relationship depends on variables III, IV, V,

VII and particularly VI. In Colquhoun's experiments critical and noncritical signals were very similar, and both were distinctly different from neutral signals. No response to noncritical signals was required.

I and III: Colquhoun apparently concludes that the mutual dependence between the effect on the vigilance of variables I and III is the same as between variables I and II. This would mean that the detection performance does not really depend on the frequency of the critical and neutral signals, but on the relationship: frequency of critical signals/frequency of neutral signals. The results showed that more critical signals were detected, if this ratio is changed, either by increased frequency of critical signals (see I), or decrease of frequency of neutral signals (III). It is still open whether the observer performance remains the same with change of the number of critical and neutral signals provided that the ratio is constant.

VI and VII: In case that critical and noncritical signals require a different response, the performance is better if they are as dissimilar as possible (Baker, 1961); Schmidtke and Micko, 1964). If they require the same response, the similarity does not seem to be important (Garvey, et al., 1959).

The mutual dependence of clarity or similarity of critical and noncritical signals, i.e. the interaction of variables IV, V and VI, has not been sufficiently explored. Therefore, there is little general information as to whether any, few or the absence of noncritical signals are more favorable. The differing results obtained by Colquhoun and by Weiner and Ross (1962) are not necessarily a consequence of the different criterion of vigilance— probability of signal detection (Colquhoun) and frequency of observer responses (Weiner and Ross)—but may be due to differences in variables IV, V and particularly VI.

SIGNAL INTENSITY

If the intensity of a signal impinging on a defined receptor system falls below a critical value (absolute or differential threshold), it cannot be perceived and processed. The occasionally reported story of a subconscious influence on opinions, for instance by the presentation of optical information in a film or on TV for a few msec, lacks any solid basis. For the threshold, i.e. absolute or relative visual threshold, the Bunse-Roscoe equation $I \times t^p = K$ applies, i.e. the biological effect of an electro-magnetic radiation is determined by the product intensity $\times$ time, where time has an exponent (Schwarzschild's exponent). Suprathreshold stimuli are, in general, recognized faster and more reliably, the higher their intensity.[2]

---

2. Footnote of editor: This corresponds to Lapique's chronaxie, originally developed for muscle and nerve, but later also applied to visual and other sensory stimuli (Bourguignon, 1922).

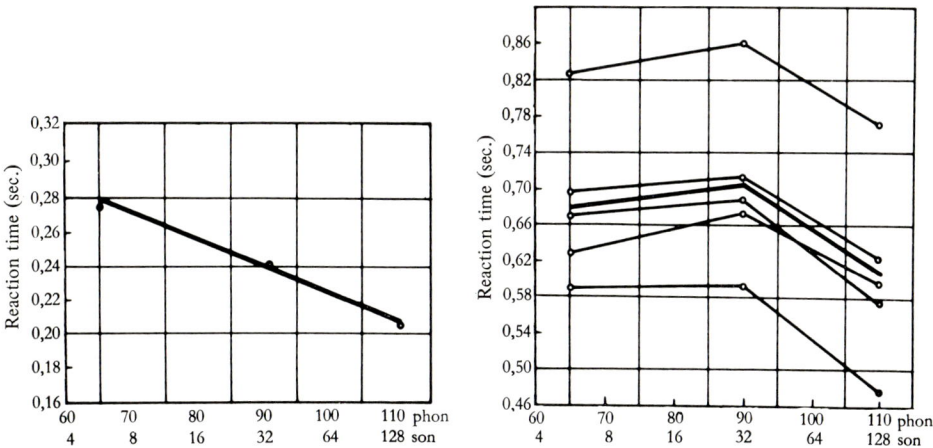

Figure 8-5. Effect of loudness of an acoustic stimulus on the reaction time; left: simple stimulus; right: choice reaction situation (according to Schmidtke).

This may be illustrated by two examples. In a former study of reaction time by the author (Schmidtke, 1961a), it could be shown that the simple reaction time (R_t) to acoustic stimuli decreases approximately with increasing loudness (phones) ($Rt = 0.38 - 1.53 \times 10^{-3}$; x = phon value; range of validity 65 x to 110 phon, Fig. 8-5). During discrimination of successive consecutive stimuli having different loudness, this proportionality is lost because additional choice reactions are necessary (for instance, stimulus 2 is louder than stimulus 1, but lower than stimulus 3). However, the right part of Figure 8-5 shows that also under condition of a choice reaction, a signal of 110 phon elicits a significantly faster response than a stimulus of 65 phon.

From these results it can be concluded that for signal detection a stimulus intensity as high as possible—or a high difference between intensity of critical and neutral signals, is desirable. Extreme intensities, however, should be avoided because they may produce an aversive reaction. The demand for high stimulus intensity is particularly justified when in prolonged observer performance a decrease of vigilance level is expected. Hartman (1963) showed in experiments on the illumination level necessary for recognition of a test figure during automobile driving on a highway at night, that during the first 90 minutes an average illumination of 2 Lux was necessary, which had to be increased to 5 Lux between the 210th and 300th minute of driving in order to produce response of the driver (Fig. 8-6). This shows the close relationship between necessary signal intensity and preceding work load (see Chapter on Information Acquisition).

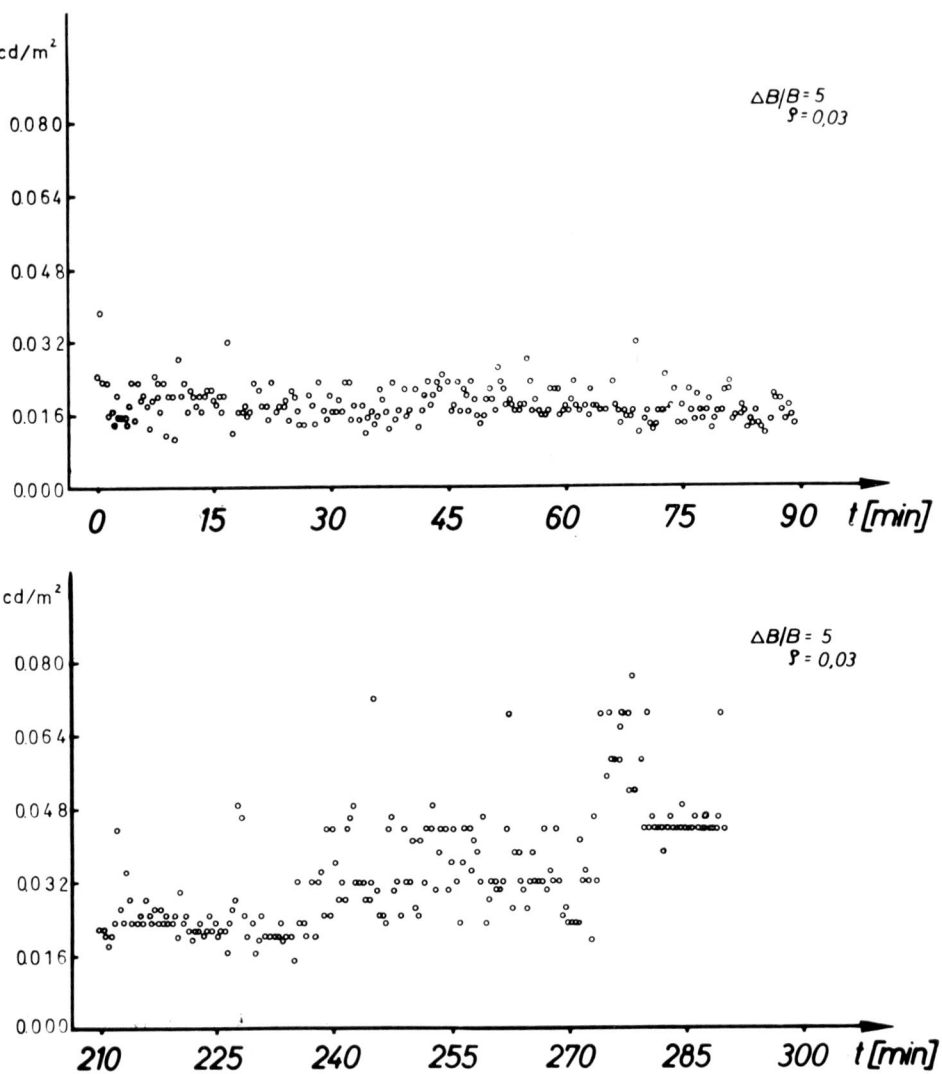

Figure 8-6. Effect of uninterrupted time of driving on a highway at night on the illumination necessary for recognition of a test figure (according to Hartmann).

DEGREE OF PRECEDING WORK LOAD

Among the variables affecting performance during prolonged observational tasks, the degree of preceding work load plays an important role. The greater the fatigue, the more is the decrement in the ability to concentrate on the content of certain information. Effects of sleep deprivation on signal detection have been studied quite thoroughly. Baker, Ware and Sipowicz (1962), for example, instructed subjects to record brief interruptions of an otherwise continuously lighted signal lamp. Figure 8-7 shows the results: from an average detection performance of about 90 percent in the first hour the detection rate drops to minimum values of about 30 percent after 20 hours of observation time. It is remarkable that there was a certain stabilization of performance in the last third of this experiment with the subjects remaining awake for the total time (24 hours) of the experiment. The subjects who were less resistant to the monotonous situation slept for short intervals from time to time; their performance declined continuously until a few hours before the termination of the experiment. The implication for extremely long work shifts under monotonous conditions is obvious.

In work begun after a period of sleep deprivation, the decline of observer performance was even more pronounced than in Baker's, et al. experiments with extremely long uninterrupted work periods. As an example, we refer to Wilkinson's (1960) study, whose subjects had to react to a spot of light which could appear in eight different locations. The sleep-deprived group missed 25 percent of the signals, although they observed the display, further 12 percent by looking away from the display and another 12 percent during brief sleep periods. The error rate of 49 percent compares with that of 26 percent of the rested control group.

In general, one can conclude from the broad spectrum of sleep deprivation experiments that in an environment with low level of stimulation the

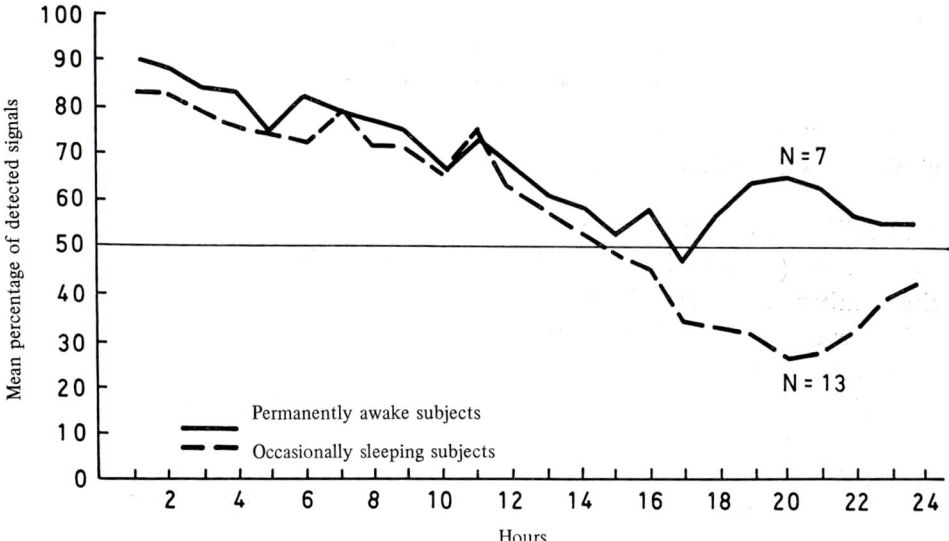

Figure 8-7. Dependence of signal detection on type of activity of observer (according to Baker, Ware, and Sipowicz).

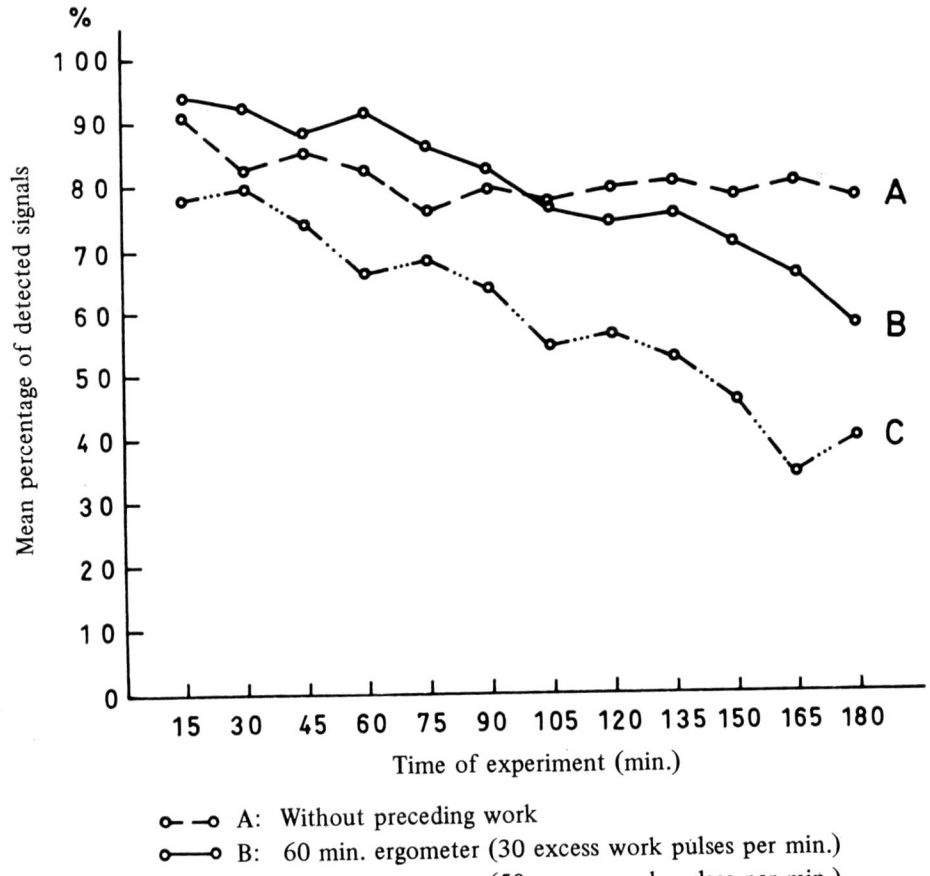

○——○ A: Without preceding work
○———○ B: 60 min. ergometer (30 excess work pulses per min.)
○----○ C: 60 min. ergometer (50 excess work pulses per min.)

Figure 8-8. Signal detection performance in a 3 hour experimental period after strenuous physical work (after Schmidtke).

probability of sleeping increases together with the number of true observation errors (overlooking of critical signals requiring a response) and with the number of false reactions (reactions without signals).

However, not only sleep deprivation results in a decline of vigilance. My own observations have showed that preceding heavy muscular work also had a considerable effect on performance in the clock test (Schmidtke, 1973). Each subject had to go through three experimental conditions in random order: A—without preceding work;[3] B—after preceding bicycle ergometer work close to the individual limit for prolonged work;[4] C—after bicycle ergometer work with a higher load. The load was so regulated by changing

---

3. Probably closer to 50% max $\dot{V}_{O_2}$.
4. Probably about 70-80% max $\dot{V}_{O_2}$.

of the brake resistance that the heart rate of the subject increased by 30 beats/min. (B) or by 50 beats/min. over the resting heart rate (C). Figure 8-8 gives a summary of the results. Curve A is not essentially different from the start of the curve in Figure 8-7. Curve B shows that preceding metabolic load close to the individual limit for prolonged performance exerts a rather positive effect during the first minutes of the experiment. With progressing time the positive stimulation effect is increasingly obscured, and finally the performance is significantly poorer as compared to A. A preceding workload significantly higher than the individual limit for prolonged performance (condition C), produces a massive deterioration of vigilance.

EXTERNAL STRESS FACTORS

It is known from industrial work physiology and from N. H. Mackworth's early investigations that external environmental stress factors (temperature, noise, etc.) affect not only physical work capacity (Simonson, 1971 PWCF, Chaps. 7, 13 and 14) but also mental work performance. Within the scope of this chapter we limit ourselves to a small selection of reports from a very large number of investigations. Mackworth (1950) made an interesting contribution to this problem. Trained Navy telegraph operators were tested for three hours under different climatic conditions. In addition to the expected time effect, two other variables could be isolated: the climate (T°) in the laboratory room and the individual performance level. These variables were not mutually independent. The lower the individual performance level, the more pronounced is the decline of performance with time and with increasing climatic stress (Fig. 8-9). Since extreme climatic stress produces a considerable cardiovascular load (see Chaps. 7 and 11, Simonson, 1971), it is not surprising that this effect on human performance is similar to the decrements seen after strenuous physical activity.

Figure 8-10 shows N. H. Mackworth's observations (1950), as well as the results of Viteles and Smith (1946) on nearly nude men, who were engaged in mainly mental activities over several hours in the heat. We refer here to performance in a neutral climate as 100 percent. One may conclude from the results that above an effective temperature of about 27° C, performance drops markedly. However, the extent of performance decrement depends on many other important environmental factors in addition to the thermal stress. For instance, the type of mental work, subject motivation, and the presence of other environmental stresses all pay an important role (Wenzel, 1974).

Wilkinson and Associates (1964) pointed out another aspect. The subject had to accomplish two tests in four successive experimental periods. In addition to a control experiment the subjects were exposed to three different body temperatures (37.3° C, 37.9° C and 38.5° C). Aside from a general positive practice effect, performance in an addition test depended on the body temperature: the performance was at the lowest level and errors were most frequent at the highest body temperature. The situation was reversed with a signal detection test. A repetition of the experiments resulted not only in

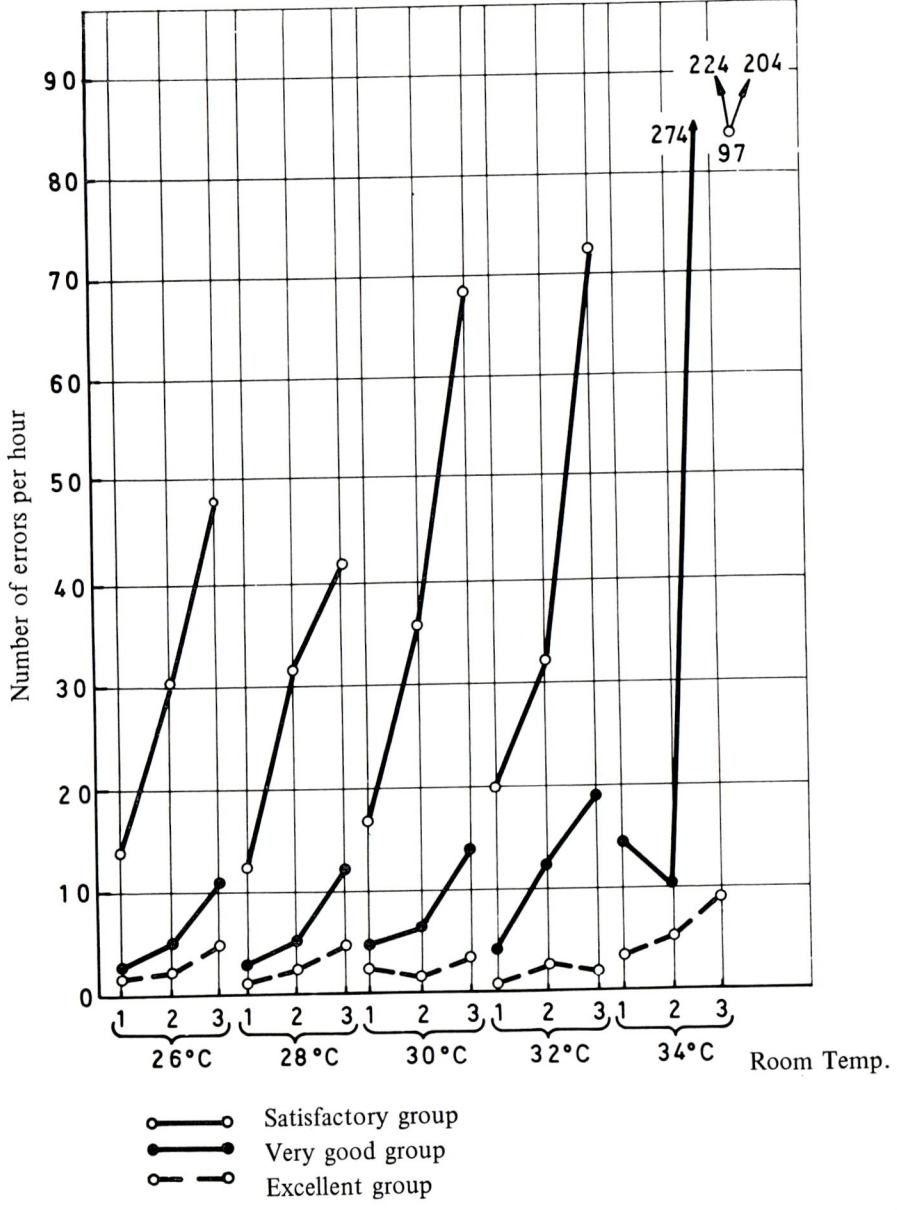

Figure 8-9. Effect of climatic stress (heat) on performance of telegraph operators with different performance levels (after N. H. Mackworth).

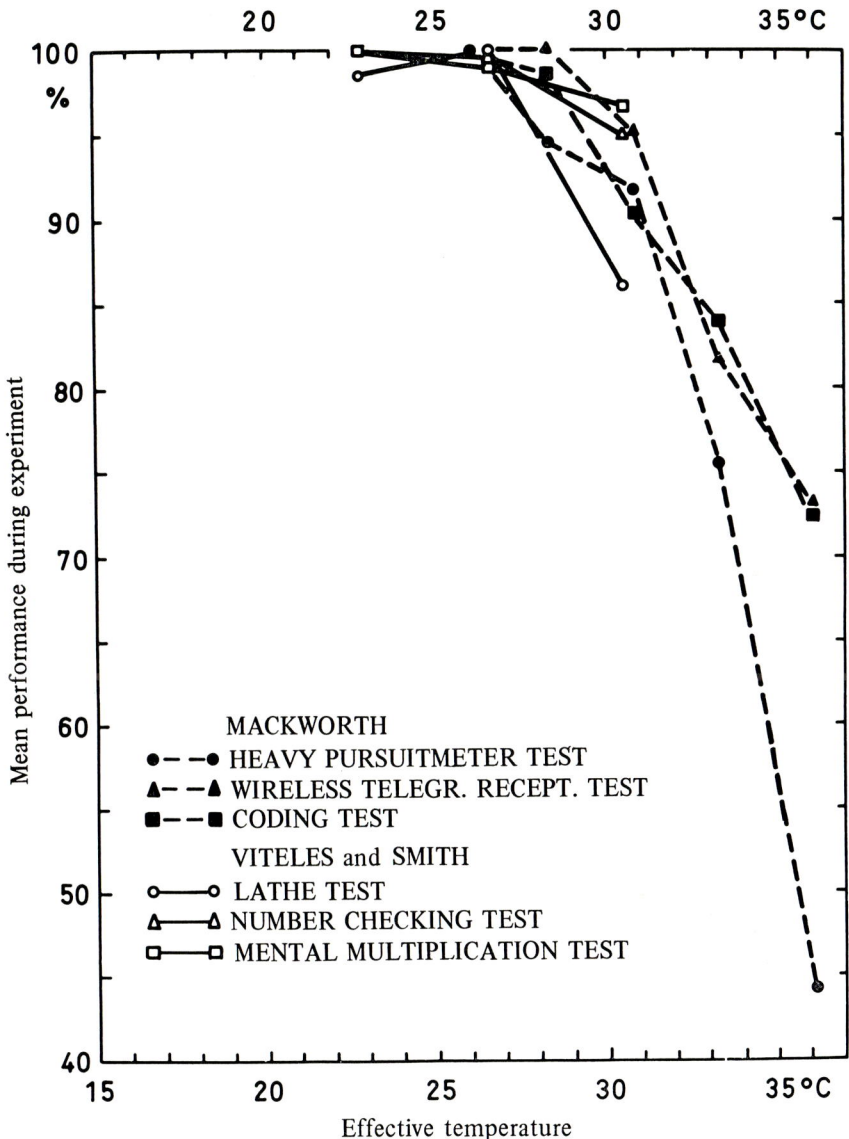

Figure 8-10. Performance of nearly nude men in various types of prolonged (several hours) psychological and psychophysiological performance at different effective temperatures (according to N. H. Mackworth and Viteles & Smith).

a negative practice effect, but the results were reversed: all signals were detected in shorter time periods at higher body temperature. Obviously, the environmental thermal stress produces a higher degree of activation in the already quite stimulating addition test leading to a hyperactivation with characteristic feedback effect on mental performance, while the lower level of activation in a monotonous vigilance test is increased by the external stresses as secondary favorable effect on performance.

Very similar results have been found regarding the effect of noise on the vigilance level. Kirk and Hecht (1963) have shown that vigilance performance under the effect of variable noise is significantly better than under the effect of constant noise or under quiet conditions. McBain (1961) found that under the effect of random noise, the number of errors was diminished in monotonous tasks. These results agree with those of Broadbent and Gregory (1963, 1965) who suggested on the basis of their experiments that noise sensitizes the subject's ability to detect signals. This situation probably applies to the observation that sensory deprivation has no negative effect on the reaction performance during perceptual isolation (Smith, et al., 1967). In contrast, the performance of detection tasks decreases in more prolonged isolation periods as shown by Zubek, et al., 1961, 1966. However, this may be due to central nervous hyperactivation which occurs when a subject is exposed to a normal environmental stimulus level after a long period of stimulus deprivation.

Finally, we come to the discussion of another external stress factor: hypoxia. It is known for a long time that oxygen deficiency has a pronounced effect on human behavior in addition to the physiological effects. Lottig (1936), Goralewski (1936), and Diringshofen (1942) and other investigators found impairment of motor performance and McFarland (1937) found considerably prolonged choice reaction time, as well as particularly more important disturbances in attention and learning, and Gerathewohl (1954) found a disturbance in the processing and transformation of information. In the experiments of Gerathewohl it can be seen that at an altitude over 5000 meters the number of errors increases slowly but markedly above altitudes of over 7000 meters. Even more distinct is the effect of oxygen deficiency on the consistency of performance. As shown in Figure 8-11, if the critical threshold of oxygen deficiency corresponding to an altitude of about 6000 meters is exceeded, the variability of performances increases markedly. One of the symptoms the subject experiences at this altitude, is the sensation of sleepiness, which interferes with appraisal of reality and marked disturbance of vigilance.

From the examples as described above, it can be seen that external stresses do not necessarily interfere with vigilance. In somewhat simpler terms it can be said a mild stress situation may have a stimulating effect while a strong stress produces a greater strain of the organism and depresses the level of vigilance. However, this is only a general rule. It has always been demonstrated that the ability for maintenance of a certain level of vigilance varies from one individual to another. However, it has

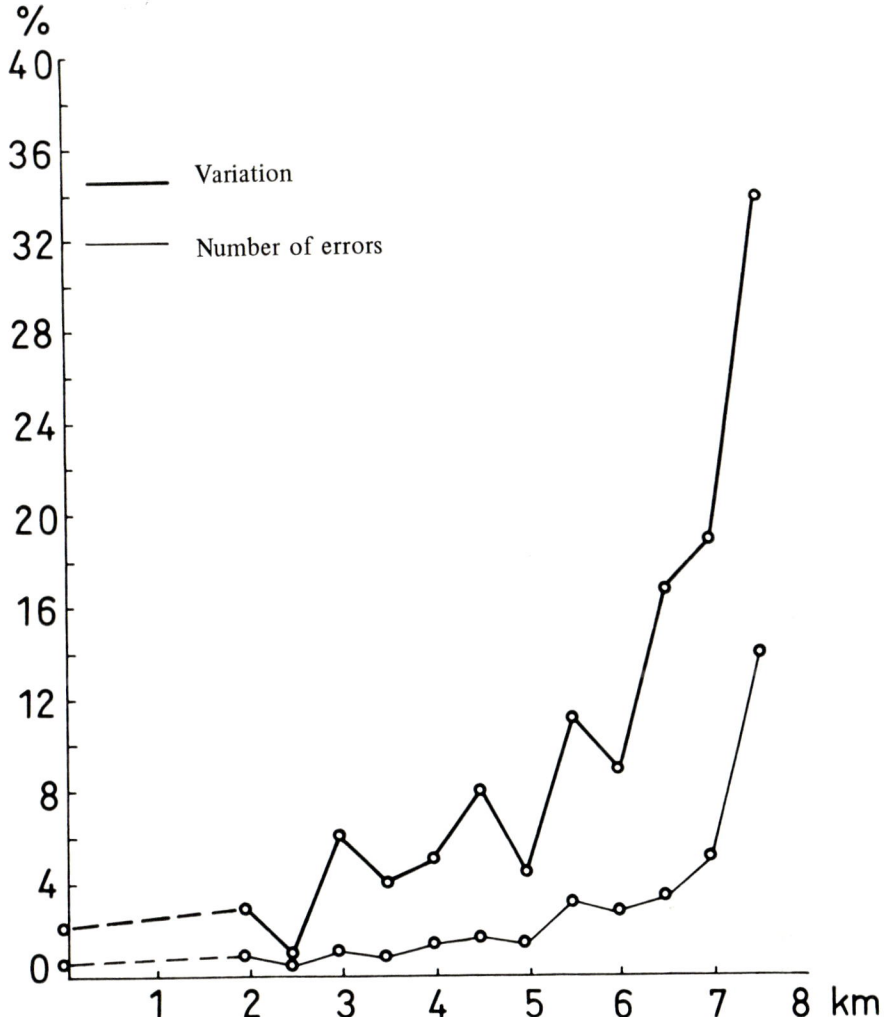

Figure 8-11. Increase in number of errors during a prolonged reaction experiment with increasing intensity (according to Gerathewohl).

not been possible, so far, to find with any satisfactory way, some personal characteristic which would be covariant with the vigilance performance which would permit a prognosis of ability. This may be in part due to the fact that the reliability of vigilance criteria is not particularly encouraging.

EFFECT OF DRUGS

It is not possible within the scope of this chapter to give even an approximately complete review of the effect of drugs on vigilance. Therefore, we give only a few examples of some results. There is agreement of various authors (N. H. Mackworth, 1950; J. F. Mackworth, 1970; Eysenck, et al., 1957; Jerison, et al., 1965; Loeb, et al., 1965; Düker, H. and E. Düker, 1953; Düker, H. and H. Wieding, 1960; Neal and Pearson, 1966; Seashore and Ivy, 1953; Simonson and Enzer, 1941) that stimulants like amphetamine have a positive effect on performance types which are related to vigilance (i.e. signal detecting, proof reading, operating motors, etc.). The EEG shows an increased activation desynchronization suggesting that amphetamine acts upon the reticular formation (French, 1960). Therefore, amphetamine has been occasionally applied in military situations to compensate for effects of sleep deprivation or insufficient sleep.

Tranquilizers and depressants like chlorpromazine, benadryl, meprobamate, or barbituates have the opposite effect, producing a cortical deactivation and inhibition of reticular activity. This has been shown, for example, by a significant depression of the flicker fusion frequency (Schmidtke, 1951) and a decrease of performance in an auditory vigilance task (Loeb, et al., 1965; Bakan, 1961) and an increase in reaction time without stimulus, i.e. in false alarms or false responses (Neal and Pearson, 1966; Kornetsky and Bain, 1965). Alcohol also produces a definite decrement in vigilance. As H. Düker (1963) clearly has shown, small doses of alcohol increased per-

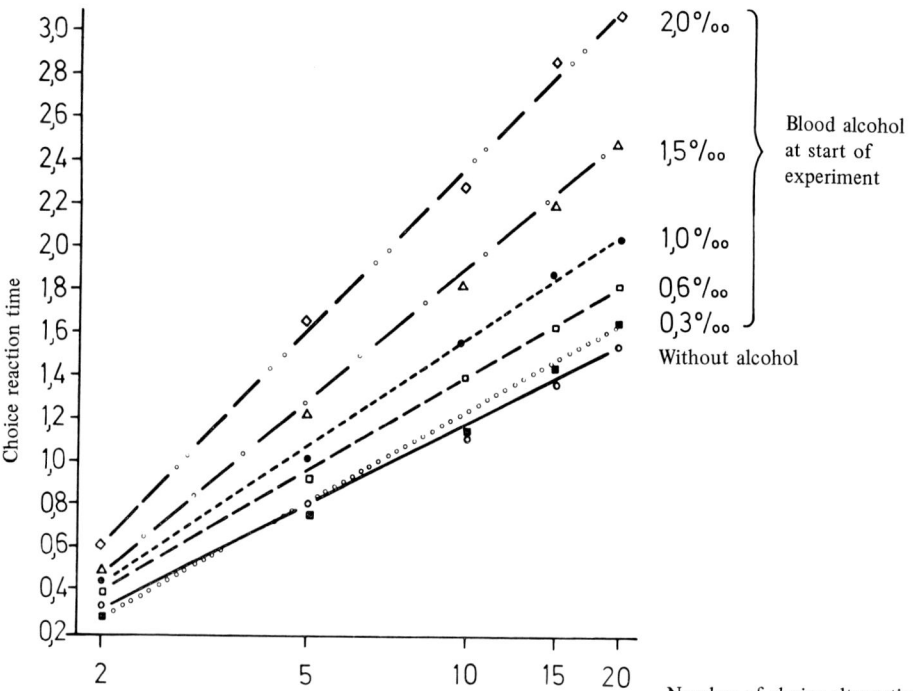

Figure 8-12. Effect of number of choice alternatives on choice reaction time as a function of blood alcohol concentration (according to Schmidtke).

formance, which may be due to disinhibition or as suggested by Düker to an increased concentration after realizing that alcohol had been consumed which may have resulted in a reactive increase of performance. Larger doses of alcohol, however, exert a massive depression in activity, narrowing of the visual field, prolongation of the choice reaction time, and even a more pronounced disturbance of vigilance performance (e.g. see Graf, 1932; Abele, 1958; Drew, et al., 1958; Elbel, 1961; Harper and Albers, 1964; Grechow, 1968; Liske, 1971). Figure 8-12 summarizes the results of an unpublished study of the effect of alcohol on the performance in a choice reaction test. Twenty six untrained subjects participated in this experiment. The subjects had to observe the illumination of a number on a display board, press the corresponding number on a key board which contained 2, 5, 10, 15 or 20 alternatives. The blood alcohol concentration was determined immediately before the start of the experiment (maximum deviation from designated group value was 10 mg %). As shown in Figure 8-12, small doses of alcohol shortens slightly the reaction time (slightly but not significantly) in the presence of only a few alternatives, but large doses produce massive prolongation in reaction time.

VIGILANCE THEORIES

The results of vigilance research as briefly discussed above have resulted in several attempts of theoretical organization. However, at present there is no comprehensive theory which can explain all observations. To summarize the various theoretical approaches, the following principles of organization can be differentiated (also see Schmidtke and Hoffman, 1964): theories explaining the decline of vigilance primarily or secondarily by fatigue, and theories with the model of an adaptation process in the broad sense.

Theory of Vigilance Decrease as Result of Fatigue

Decline of vigilance in mental fatigue has, as a rule, not only different causes (in one case, understimulation; in another case, excessive load), but also could lead to different behavior with change of the load level. The disturbance of vigilance usually disappears rapidly with change of working condition while symptoms of fatigue are much less affected. The only theoretical attempt which permits an interpretation of vigilance decrement as a result of fatigue goes back to Bills (1931).

According to the blocking theory, arrived from experiments on prolonged tasks involving attention in monotonous mental activity with primarily visual stress, the orientation toward the task objective is interrupted for short intervals with increasing frequency. These phases of blockade produce not only significant prolongation of the reaction time but also the missing of critical signals of short duration. There is some indication that such blocks are due to functional disturbances of the CNS as consequence of fatigue (See Chap. 10). However, the block theory does not give any reliable prognosis as to when and under what condition such absences occur in the course of prolonged observer activity.

Theory of Vigilance Decline as Result of Adaptation

We can define adaptation as an adjustment of the organism to a specific environmental condition. Adaptation is possible not only to a low level of illumination or to certain background noise but also to stimuli which are repeated in a regular or similar sequence and therefore, have a decreasing novelty value. The activation theory starts from the point that the critical arousal level and consequently, vigilance, is affected to a significant degree by sensory stimuli conducted over several pathways to the CNS. Moruzzi and Magoun (1949) discovered that the nervous impulses from the periphery of the body are conducted to the cerebral cortex not only directly but also through collaterals of afferent neurons that stimulated the reticular formation of the medulla and the mid brain. From stimulation of the reticular formation, impulses are conducted through ascending nonspecific conduction pathways to the cortex serving as an important determinant for cortical excitation. In the absence of reticular formation stimulation, either in monotonous work situations with absent external stimuli or due to adaptation to an existing level of stimulation, the arousal level declines. As a result, vigilance level declines. However, it is possible that mental processes, even with insufficient sensory stimulation arising from the cortex, may stimulate the reticular formation through an internal feedback circuit and produce transient stimulation of the reticular formation. However, the internal stimulation cannot compensate for the lack of external sensory stimuli in the long run.

There is no doubt that the results of a large number of vigilance experiments can be explained on the basis of this activation theory. This is not surprising because the ascending reticular activation system (ARAS) has profound biological functions. At the same time, this is also the weakness of the theory. The biological basis is so broad that this theory may obscure contradictory results and also makes the formulation of more precise hypotheses difficult.

The theory of self-stimulation proposed by Bakan (1957) has a close connection to the activation theory. This theory starts from the observation that at a very low external level of stimulation, slowly develops a phase of sleep-like condition. However, factors arriving from the working situation, such as responsibility for production, social expectations and so on, counteract sleepiness, producing so to speak, as a defense reaction, day dreams, motor activities and side-occupations. This certain level of vigilance can be maintained, however, only at the expense of the task. The more the subject has to occupy himself in order to keep awake, the more his attention is diverted from the stimuli relevant for the task. Taken alone, the value of the theory of self-stimulation is not high. However, in connection with the activation theory, a synthesis of both aspects, that is activation and diversion may explain the finding that in prolonged observation activity, performance decreases and motor activity increases (Singer, 1969).

Broadbent (1958) has proposed a filter theory starting from an entirely different conceptual model. He begins from the assumption that the CNS can only process a very limited part of the multitude of environmental stimuli. In other words, it acts like a channel of communication with an electrical filter at the entry passing only signals of defined characteristics. The probability of conduction of the signal depends on its intensity, its biological significance and novelty. The filter is adapted specifically to the task, but the critical signals have a high priority within the probability of being processed. With continuing time of activation, however, more and more noncritical signals pass through the filter, either because of their higher intensity or because of a higher novelty value. By processing noncritical stimuli, however, relevant critical signals are missed due to the limited capacity for processing. In addition, the threshold of critical signals increases with increasing repetition. Therefore, the filter theory explains the actual vigilance as a function of novelty of critical signals and the decline of vigilance as adaptation to these signals.

N. H. Mackworth's (1957) inhibition theory has more historical interest. Essentially, it goes back to Pavlov and can be easily reconciled with a more general concept of reinforcement theory. The starting point of this theory is the assumption that reactions to critical signals are voluntary reactions which can be conditioned by practice and instruction. However, in observer activity there is in general no information available whether the reaction is correct or wrong. Therefore, the inhibition of reaction occurring with each repetition of the signal cannot be compensated by the reinforcement effect of success or failure. Thus, absent reinforcement ultimately leads to unlearning the conditioned reaction and to a decline of performance. According to these theories, vigilance is a function of the frequency of successes associated with correct reactions. If such reinforcement affects are absent due to low frequency of stimuli or reports of success, the vigilance level decreases.

The expectation theory of Deese (1955) and Baker (1959) is a modification of the reinforcement theory. Already, Mackworth suspected that man formulates on the basis of experience in an observer situation a certain expectation as to when the next critical signal may be expected. If signal expectation and signal occurrence coincide, the vigilance level is reinforced.

On the other hand, if signals are given at times when they are not expected, they meet a reduced vigilance with the result that the probability of detection is small. Thus something like time discrimination learning enters the expectation theory. According to the expectation theory, vigilance depends on the probability that a critical signal occurs in the next moment. However, critical signals are often rare. Then the subjects learn quite rapidly to evaluate the chance of signal occurrence to be small and the vigilance level drops.

Considering all vigilance theories together, the question that deserves foremost attention is, under which conditions the performance of long observation tasks is best. The quality of performance may be regarded as the psychophysiological variable of the vigilance level. However, whether the so-called vigilance is really a uniform variable still has to be examined. In comparing different vigilance criteria, for example, the number of detected signals, of false responses, the latent period, the reliability of response, the perception threshold for signals, and the frequency of observer reactions, it appears that these criteria do not measure the same variable. Already, Broadbent (1960) noticed that their correlation is lower than expected. It may be concluded, therefore, that in vigilance tasks, different types of activity and performance must be discriminated because they depend on these different vigilance criteria in a different manner.

One cannot rule out that the detection and the identification of a signal must be differentiated exactly like the performance rate of the observer (termed by Holland [1958] "detection frequency") and the speed of recognition. It is difficult to prove whether an observer has noticed a signal. However, a signal can be identified in case of a specific reaction. Between noticing and identification of a signal there is a certain time interval whose duration may depend on other factors than the latent period of detection. Increase of noncritical signals increases the frequency of observation (Elliot, 1960); however, as a consequence of the increasing number of alternatives, the time for identification and response also increases (Merkel, 1885; Hick, 1952; Crossman, 1953; Hyman, 1953; Welford, 1960; Schmidtke, 1961b). Since the type of the most frequently used noncritical signals does not allow a discrimination between detection and identification, this difference has not been considered in the vigilance theories as discussed above.

In contrast to all other theories, the blocking theory is not concerned with the underlying cause for the variations of vigilance, but it describes what happens in a vigilance experiment. It is surprising that Bills did not discuss the problems inherent in the definition of "blocks."

The expectation theory is the only theory which provides an explanation why the performance according to quality and regularity is about the same when the intervals between the signals are approximately identical. Neither the activation theory nor the filter theory permit any definite prediction of the vigilance performance. The reinforcement theory is based on the assumption that in addition to the process of unlearning there must be a process of learning time discrimination. However, not all aspects of the vigilance problem can be explained by learning of time discrimination. If the learning of time discrimination is made more difficult by waking stimuli, distractions, and pauses, performance is by no means always disturbed. Dardano (1962) showed that an essential prerequisite of the expectation theory, i.e. the improvement of vigilance with lengthening of the time interval from the last signal, loses its meaning in case of irregular sequel of signals.

The decline of performance in vigilance tests that exclude the learning of time discriminations, can be explained by the activation theory as well as the inhibition theory. Both theories have the common assumption that the drop of vigilance is due to the decrease in attention for the appearance of rare critical signals. It is the result of the rarity of signals with a lack of success or lack of information that the detection of critical signals is not reinforced. As a consequence, noncritical or neutral signals can evoke a response.

Distraction is the central point of the filter theory as well as the reinforcement theory. If the intensity of the signal or the reaction potential of the required observation activity decrease, other reactions, activities or stimuli whose reaction potentials are not disturbed come into the foreground. The inhibition theory or the theories of unlearning say only that the reaction to critical stimuli is more disturbed than the reaction to noncritical stimuli.

In contrast, the activation theory predicts an uniform decline of any type of mental activity if sensory stimulation decreases. It is relatively unimportant whether the decrease of stimulation involves critical or task-specific stimuli. All findings which show a dependence of the vigilance level on the extent of irrelevant stimulation, support the activation theory.

With prolonged observation tasks other sectors in the observation field are more preferred than they were at the start of the task (Broadbent, 1950 and 1951) together with increasing motor unrest (Bakan, 1957, Baker, 1958). There is not only a change of the activation level in direction of deactivation, but at the same time, a change of the whole activity and its distribution. Therefore, an argument can be made that one cannot ignore entirely the theory of unlearning.

From this brief discussion it may be concluded that nearly all theories permit a prediction of some experimental results. However, no theory is sufficiently comprehensive to explain all results of vigilance research. This may be due to the absence of a theory of a superior order. The suggestion that human vigilance is not a single, uniform variable, as generally assumed, has about the same probability. If this is the case—and there are several indications in this direction—the differences in the attempts of theoretical interpretations may be easily clarified.

BIBLIOGRAPHY

Abele, G.: Die Lenkbewegungen des Kraftfahrers unter Alkoholeinfluß. *Dtsch Z ges gerichtl Med, 48*:58, 1958.

Anonymous: Changes in efficiency during ASV watches. RAF/ORS/CC Report No. 285, 1944.

Bakan, P.: Discussion III. Symposium on vigilance. *Adv Sci,* 410, 1957.

Bakan, P.: Effect of meprobamate on auditory vigilance. *Percept Mot Skills, 12*:26, 1961.

Baker, C. H.: Attention to visual displays during a vigilance task. Med Res Council, APU-Report 294, 1958.

Baker, C. H.: Towards a theory of vigilance. *Can J Psychol, 13*:35, 1959.

Baker, C. H.: Maintaining the level of vigilance by means of knowledge of results about a secondary vigilance task. *Ergonomics, 4*:311, 1961.

Baker, R. A., J. R. Ware, and R. R. Sipowicz: Signal detection by multiple monitors. *Psychol Record, 12*:133, 1962.

Bills, A. G.: Blocking: a new principle of mental fatigue. *Am J Psychol, 43*:230, 1931.

Bourguignon, G.: *La Chronaxie Des L'homme.* Paris, Masson et Cie, 1922.

Broadbent, D. E.: The twenty dials test under quiet conditions. Med Res Council, APU-Report 130, 1950.

Broadbent, D. E.: The twenty dials and the twenty lights test under noise conditions. *Med Res Council,* APU-Report 160, 1951.

Broadbent, D. E.: *Perception and Communication.* London, Macmillan, 1958.

Broadbent, D. E.: The effect of signal frequency in a checking task. *Ergonomics, 3*:277, 1960.

Broadbent, D. E., and M. Gregory: Vigilance considered as a statistical decision. *Br J Psychol, 54*:309, 1963.

Broadbent, D. E., and M. Gregory: Effects of noise and of signal rate upon vigilance analysed by means of decision theory. *Hum Factors, 7*:155, 1965.

Colquhoun, W. P.: The effect of unwanted signals in a vigilance task. *Ergonomics, 4*:41, 1961.

Crossman, E. R. F. W.: Entropy and choice time: the effect of frequency unbalance on choice-response. *Q J Exp Psychol, 5*:41, 1953.

Dardano, J. F.: Relationship of intermittent noise, intersignal interval and skin conductance to vigilance. *J Appl Psychol, 46*:106, 1962.

Deese, J.: Some problems in the theory of vigilance. *Psychol Rev, 62*:359, 1955.

Deese, J., and E. Ormond: Studies of detectability during continuous visual search. Wright Air Dev. Center, Techn. Report No. 53-8, 1953, Wright Patterson Air Force Base, Ohio.

Diringshofen, H. von: Vorschläge zur Bezeichnung der Wirkungsschwellen und Phasen bei Sauerstoffmangel im Höhenversuch. *Luftfahrtmedizin, 6*:149, 1942.

Drew, G. C., W. P. Colquhoun, and H. A. Long: Effect of small doses of alcohol on a skill resembling driving. *Br Med J 2*:993, 1958.

Düker, H.: Über reaktive Anspannungssteigerung. *Z exp angew Psychol, 10*:46, 1963.

Düker, H., and E. Düker: Über die Wirkung von Pervitin auf die psychische Leistungsfähigkeit. *Z exp angew Psychol, 1*:32, 1958.

Düker, H., and H. Wieding: Über die Dauer der leistungssteigernden Wirkung des Pervitins bei geistiger Tätigkeit. *Psychol Beitr, 5*:23, 1960.

Elbel, H.: Neue Ergebnisse der Blutalkoholforschung. *Hefte Unfallheilkunde, 66*:74, 1961.

Elliot, E.: Perception and alertness. *Ergonomics, 3*:357, 1960.

Eysenck, H. J., S. Casey, and D. S. Trouton: Drugs and personality, II. The effect of stimulant and depressant drugs on continuous work. *J Ment Sci, 103*:645, 1957.

French, J. D.: The reticular formation. In *Handbook of Physiology*. Washington, American Physiological Society, 1960, Chap. 52, pp. 1281-1305.

Garvey, W. D., F. V. Taylor, and E. P. Newlin: The use of artificial signals to enhance monitoring performance. US-Naval Res Lab Report 1959.

Gerathewohl, S. J.: Die Psychologie des Menschen im Flugzeug. München, 1954.

Goralewski, G.: Die experimentelle Erzeugung zentralnervöser Ausfallerscheinungen durch Sauerstoffmangel bei normalem Atmosphärendruck. *Luftfahrtmed Abhandl 1,* 189, 1936.

Graf, O.: Über den Zusammenhang von Alkohol-Blutkonzentration und psychischer Alkoholwirkung. *Z Arbeitsphysiol, 6*:137, 1932.

Grechow, J.: Alkohol und Verkehrstüchtigkeit. In Wagner, K., and Wagner, H. J. (Eds.): *Handbuch der Verkehrsmedizin*. Berlin, Heidelberg, New York, 1968.

Harper, C. R., and W. R. Albers: Alcohol and general aviation accidents. *Aerospace Med, 35*:462, 1964.

Hartmann, E.: Disability glare and discomfort glare. In Ingelstam, E. (Ed.): *Lighting Problems in Highway Traffic,* Oxford, London, New York, Paris, 1963, Vol. II.

Head, H.: *Aphasia*. Cambridge, 1926.

Hick, W. E.: On the rate of gain of information. *Q J Exp Psychol, 4*:11, 1952.

Holland, J. G.: Human vigilance. *Science 128*:61, 1958.

Hyman, R.: Stimulus information as a determinant of reaction time. *J Exp Psychol, 45*:188, 1953.

Jenkins, H. M.: The effect of signal rate on performance in visual monitoring. *Am J Psychol, 71*:647, 1958.

Jerison, H. J., R. M. Pickett, and H. H. Stenson: The elicited observing rate and decision processes in vigilance. *Human Factors, 7*:107, 1965.

Kirk, R. E., and E. Hecht: Maintenance of vigilance by programmed noise. *Percept Mot Skills, 16*:553, 1963.

Kornetsky, G., and G. Bain: The effects of chlorpromazine and phenobarbital on sustained attention in the rat. *Psychopharm, 8*:277, 1965.

Liske, E.: Clinical aspects of aerospace neurology. In Randel, H. W. (Ed.): *Aerospace Medicine,* 2nd ed., Baltimore, Williams & Wilkins, 1971.

Loeb, M., G. R. Hawkes, O. W. Evans, and E. A. Alluisi: The influence of d-amphetamine, benactycine, and chlorpromazine on performance in an auditory vigilance task. *Psychol Sci, 3*:29, 1965.

Lottig, H.: Über den diagnostischen Wert der Höhentauglichkeitsprüfung. *Luftfahrtmed Abhandl 1*:65, 1936.

Mackworth, J. F.: *Vigilance and Habituation*. Middlesex, Harmondsworth, 1969.

Mackworth, J. F.: *Vigilance and Attention: A Signal Detection Approach*. Middlesex, Harmondsworth, 1970.

Mackworth, N. H.: Researches on the measurement of human performance. London, 1950. Med. Res. Council Spec. Report Series No. 268 (H. M. Stationary Office), 1950.

Mackworth, N. H.: Some factors affecting vigilance. Symposium on vigilance. *Advancement of Science, 53*:389, 1957.
McBain, W. N.: Noise, the "arousal hypothesis" and monotonous work. *J Appl Psychol, 45*:309, 1961.
McFarland, R. A.: Psychophysiological studies at high altitudes in the Andes, I. and II. *J Comp Psychol, 23*:191 and 227, 1937.
Merkel, J.: Die zeitlichen Verhältnisse der Willenstätigkeit. *Philos Studien, 2*:73, 1885.
Micko, H. Ch.: Über den Einsatz zweier Beobachter bei Dauerbeobachtungstätigkeiten. *Z exp angew Psychol, 10*:35, 1963.
Moruzzi, G., and H. W. Magoun: Brain stem reticular formation and activation of the EEG. *EEG Clin Neurophysiol, 1*:455, 1949.
Neal, G. L., and R. G. Pearson: Comparative effects of age, sex, and drugs upon two tasks of auditory vigilance. *Percept Mot Skills, 23*:967, 1966.
Schmidtke, H.: Über die Messung der psychischen Ermüdung mit Hilfe des Flimmertests. *Psychol Forschung, 23*:409, 1951.
Schmidtke, H.: Der Einfluß der Reizintensität auf die Reaktionszeit. *Psychol Beitr, 2*: 277, 1961a.
Schmidtke, H.: Zur Frage der informationstheoretischen Analyse von Wahlreaktionsexperimenten. *Psychol Forschung, 26*:157, 1961b.
Schmidtke, H.: Leistungsbeeinflussende Faktoren im Radar-Beobachtungsdienst. Köln/Opladen, 1966.
Schmidtke, H.: Wachsamkeitsprobleme. In Schmidtke, H. (Ed.): *Ergonomie 1*. München, 1973.
Schmidtke, H., and H. Hoffmann: Untersuchungen über die Dauerbeanspruchung der Aufmerksamkeit bei Überwachungstätigkeiten. Köln/Opladen, 1964.
Schmidtke, H., and H. Ch. Micko: Untersuchungen über die Reaktionszeit bei Dauerbeobachtung. Köln/Opladen, 1964.
Seashore, R. H., and A. C. Ivy: Effects of analeptic drugs in relieving fatigue. *Psychol Monog, 67*:no. 15, 1, 1953.
Simsonson, E., and N. Enzer: The effect of amphetamine (benzedrine) sulfate on the state of motor centers. *J Exp Psychol, 29*:517, 1941.
Singer, R.: Der Einfluß von zusätzlichen Signalen auf die Entdeckungsleistung bei einer akustischen Vigilanz-Aufgabe. Dissertation, Regensburg, 1969.
Smith, S., T. I. Myers, and D. B. Murphy: Vigilance during sensory deprivation. *Percept Mot Skills, 24*:971, 1967.
Viteles, M. S., and K. R. Smith: An experimental investigation of the effect of change in atmospheric conditions and noise upon performance. *Heat Pip Air Condit, 18*:107, 1946.
Weiner, H., and S. Ross: The effect of "unwanted" signals and D-amphetamine sulfate on observer responses. *J Appl Psychol, 46*:135, 1962.
Welford, A. T.: The measurement of sensory-motor-performance: a survey reappraisal of twelve years progress. *Ergonomics, 3*:189, 1960.
Wenzel, H. G.: Klima. In Schmidtke, H. (Ed.): *Ergonomie 2*. München, 1974.
Wiener, E. L.: Knowledge of results and signal rate in monitoring: A transfer of training approach. *J Appl Psychol, 47*:214, 1963.
Wilkinson, R. T.: The effect of lack of sleep on visual watch-keeping. *Q J Exp Psychol, 7*:36, 1960.

Wilkinson, R. T., R. H. Fox, R. Goldsmith, I. F. G. Hampton, and H. E. Lewis: Psychological and physiological responses to raised body temperatures. *J Appl Physiol, 19*:287, 1964.

Zubek, J. P., D. Pushkar, W. Sansom, and J. Gowing: Perceptual changes after prolonged sensory isolation (darkness and silence). *Can J Psychol, 15*:83, 1961.

Zubek, J. P., and M. MacNeill: Effects of immobilization: behavioral and EEG-changes. *Can J Psychol, 20*:316, 1966.

Chapter 9

Disturbance of Acquisition of Information

HEINZ SCHMIDTKE[1]

A SUITABLE ORIENTATION to one's environment and an efficient performance of work tasks are only possible if the impulses impingent from the environment are correctly received by various receptor systems. The correct reception of environmental stimuli depends on several conditions. First of all, the modality of the physical stimuli impingent on the receptor systems must be in agreement with the encoding parameters of the sensory organs. A further condition is the degree to which the receptor systems are functional. Finally, the function of many receptors must be considered as time dependent, and moreover, the whole process of information acquisition may be disturbed by mental stresses. In the following, we will examine how far disturbances of receptor and perception mechanisms can be regarded as evidence of disturbance of mental functions.

The research in the field of the problem of mental fatigue has resulted in such extensive literature about the alterations in receptor functions during stressing of sensory organs or during general mental stress that an encyclopedic discussion would far exceed the scope of this volume. The major part of the investigations were concerned with visual and auditory perception, and it is certainly not a coincidence that an increasing proportion of these studies has been performed in the military research laboratories. For a review of these extremely widely scattered and, so far as methods are concerned, very heterogenous material, we will first review the studies concerned with disturbance of reception by the most essential sensory functions, and then we attempt to relate perceptual disturbances to the preceding mental stress.

PERCEPTUAL PROCESSES DURING WORK AND FATIGUE
Vision

The process of seeing is of primary importance for orientation of man in his environment and for his performance at his working place. The increasing demand of precision work and progressive miniaturization of many products often results in visual stress at or above the functional performance limit of the visual apparatus. Therefore, it is not surprising that reports of visual fatigue and its symptoms are accumulating in the professional literature.

---

1. Translated by Editors.

We will operationally define fatigue as a loss of sensitivity resulting from prolonged stimulation, with the visual photochemical processes playing a secondary role. However, in many reports the phenomena of adaptation and fatigue are not sufficiently differentiated. In the process of adaptation, i.e. adaptation of the eye to a given level of surrounding illumination, photochemical and nervous regulatory mechanisms are involved.

Specifically, the differentiation between adaptation and fatigue in the older investigations of Helmholtz (1911), Grindley (1926), Fröhlich (1929), in the review of Durig (1927) and of Carmichael and Dearborn (1947) was not sufficiently rigorous. Therefore, the fatigue phenomena described by these authors can be interpreted only with reservation. This is supported by investigations of Schober (1964), Granit (1947), Weber (1950) and others, who emphasize that with exception of extremely strenuous visual conditions the fatigue of the retinal receptors is minimal and of little consequence for the function of the eye. Based on the present state of research into sensory perception, the visual fatigue must be primarily due to muscular (Gerathewol, 1952 and Weston, 1952) or central nervous components (Chaps. 6 and 7).

Visual Receptors

There are some indications of receptor system fatigue such as the time dependent variations of visual acuity. White, Britten, Ives and Thompson (1929) and Solowjewa (1960) found changes of visual acuity during the working day; however, the illumination level was not constant (varying in the White, et al., investigation between 2, 4, and 10 foot-candles). Since visual acuity depends on the illumination level (density of reflected brightness) (Luckiesh and Moss, 1938 and Schober, 1964, to name but a few), the changes of visual acuity in the experiments of White, et al., and Solowjewa may be due to changes of the illumination level rather than to fatigue. In fact, the results of Simonson and Brozek (1948, 1952), Weber (1950), Saldanha (1955, 1957) and Simmerman (1950), and Kroebel (1958A, 1958B) are at variance with the view that a decrease of visual acuity is associated with fatigue. Kroebel, who investigated the effect of contrast on visual performance, demonstrated that with a decrease of illumination and contrast, there is a deterioration of visual acuity as well as brightness discrimination. There is a wealth of information about the relationship between surrounding and target illumination contrast, target size, etc. (see Luckiesh and Moss, 1938).

Another change related to ocular perceptual performance has been reported by Graefe, Mazzi, Kyreileis and Siegert (from Schober, 1964) as a progressive narrowing of the visual field resulting from prolonged observation and inspection tasks. This phenomenon, observed frequently in patients with brain damage (Forster's "Verschiebungstyp"), was considered by these authors as an index of fatigue. Baur (1910) reported a similar phenomenon also in healthy subjects. However, reliable quantitative information is not yet available.

Probably, the occasionally observed uncertainty of color recognition and the phenomenon of color-asthenopie has also a low diagnostic validity as fatigue index. Although both phenomena have been occasionally related to fatigue, the underlying photochemical processes are largely unknown (Hartridge, 1947).

To summarize the investigations of visual receptor performance which so far have been related to fatigue, it can be said that neither the variations of visual acuity and of the visual field, or the reliability of color recognition after prolonged visual stress are unquestionably due to fatigue.

In this connection, we also refer the readers to the numerous investigations of the fusion frequency of flicker (FFF). In contrast to visual acuity, visual field, color and brightness discrimination, the FFF is not directly involved in visual performance. Rather, it is an expression of CNS fatigue with some similarity to pupillary reflex fatigue. Therefore, the discussion of this large and somewhat controversial literature on the changes of the FFF in fatigue is to be found in Chapter 7.

Ocular Muscle Function

For visual perception, ocular muscle functions are of fundamental importance for sensory reception, particularly in accommodation, pupillary movements, binocular fusion, and blinking. Observations of accommodation fatigue have been reported by Bitterman (1946), Hirsch (1958), Weber (1950), Berens (1950), and Hofstetter (1943). These authors agree that visual work with continued forced changes of accommodation produces a significant decrease of the range of accommodation. However, Hofstetter points out that the reproducibility of these results is poor and that the fatigue effect is of short duration; it disappears even with the increase of subjective effort. On the basis of these results, Hofstetter suggests that disturbances of accommodation are centrally located rather than peripherally in the muscles. This hypothesis is supported by the fact that work involving accommodation changes for 15 minutes reduces the range of accommodation from 10 to 3.5 diopters, but it is completely restored after a pause of a few seconds with closed eyelids (see Fig 9-1). It is questionable whether this would be possible in true muscular fatigue.

In addition to investigations of the change in the range of accommodation that is dependent on the duration of visual work, there are several, though controversial, studies of the time course of accommodation. Reit-

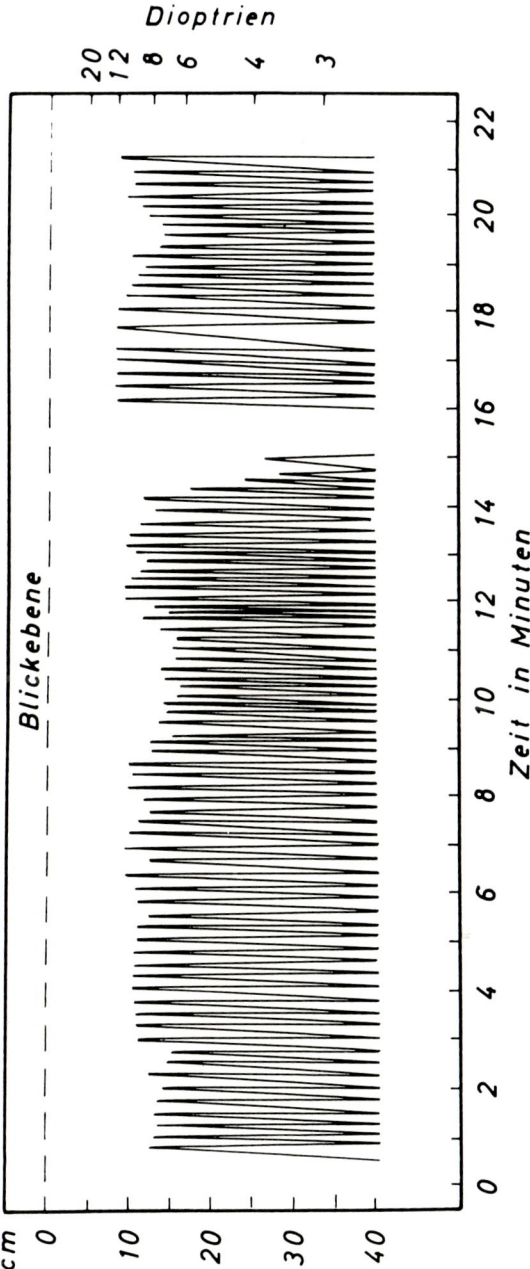

Figure 9-1. Diagram of variation of accommodation range in experiments with continuous change of reading distance. Abscissa time in minutes. Ordinate diopters. o = level of target (From H. W. Hofstetter, "An Ergographic Analysis of Fatigue of Accommodation," *American Journal of Optometry and Archives of American Academy of Optometry, 20*:115, 1943).

nauer (1957) found that visual strain by reading for a whole day did not produce fatigue of accommodation, so far as its time course is concerned.[2]

Changes in accommodation speed which can be interpreted as fatigue, occurs only after pronounced stress of the skeletal muscles. Reitnauer's results are at variance with those of Ferree and Rand (1936), Strughold (1951), Collins (1959), and Collins and Pruen (1962). The latter authors emphasize that inspection work over two hours with high level of precision (fine adjustment of a mark on a measuring scale) produced significant prolongations of the time for accommodation from distant to near vision, which could be interpreted as result of fatigue.

In connection with these results, it may be mentioned that after four hours of strenuous visual work involving the recognition of fine details moving at a constant distance in dim illumination, there was no change in the accommodation near-point, routine ophthalmological tests of abduction, and positive vertical divergence (Brozek, Simonson and Keys, 1950). In contrast, there was a highly significant deterioration of the convergence near-point.

Also, we refer here to the extensive work of Lowenstein and Loewenfeld on the fatigue of the pupillary reflex, discussed in detail in *Physiology of Work Capacity and Fatigue*. Briefly, fatigue of the pupil reflex elicited by a series of light stimuli, occurs after a variable number of stimuli dependent on the condition of the subject. Together with the gradual decline of the amplitude of pupillary movements there are changes of the contour from which localization of its components is possible (sympathetic and parasympathetic, peripheral and central). After complete or partial fatigue, the pupil reflex can be restored by strong sensory stimuli (psychological restitution phenomenon). Significant changes in the fatiguability of the pupil reflex have been observed after prolonged mental work. Fatigue of the pupil reflex may conceivably occur in conditions of rapidly changing illumination, but such conditions are extremely unusual. The fatigue of the pupil reflex is used as an experimental clinical procedure (See *Physiology of Work Capacity and Fatigue,* Chap. 9).

Pronounced mental fatigue may also produce strabismus divergens. It occurs after prolonged stress of the ocular muscles or cortical centers when the fusion impulses to the eye muscles become insufficient for normal eye muscle coordination. O. and L. Prokop (1955) regard the double images due to strabismus divergens as early symptom of mental fatigue, and point out that this is associated with subjectively annoying weakness of convergence and sensation of foreign bodies in the eye. The development of

---

[2]. It should be noted that the stress of reading depends on letter size (visual angle), illumination level, and contrast. Reading of ordinary letter size with adequate illumination, even continued for many hours, cannot be considered as visual strain. (ref)

strabismus divergens is facilitated in persons with heterophoria, necessitating greater effort of the external eye muscle for normal seeing. In the absence of a careful correction of heterophoria, a much earlier occurrence of strabismus divergens must be expected than in persons with normal vision. According to Borges Dias (1940) evidence is available that prolonged flight duration produces pronounced heterophoria in pilots as a fatigue phenomenon.

Quite similarly, Hafemann and Holfeld (1956), Siemes (1957), Hafemann (1957), Wieland (1957), Demmel (1957) and Rohrer (1958) reported that prolonged work produced a significant decrease of the range of fusion (sum of maximum divergence and convergence in terms of diopters for each eye) in school children and workers engaged primarily in muscular exertion. However, this was not confirmed in control experiments by Schmidtke (1959). It was suggested that the discrepancy of results is, in a small part, due to a low sensitivity of the variation of the range of fusion as fatigue index than to inadequacy of the method in view of the liability of this visual function. The phoria studies of Bartlett, Beinert and Graham (1953) also do not show any significant change of the range of fusion after a radar observation over several hours.

The rate of voluntary horizontal eye movements between two targets decreased significantly after two hours of strenuous visual work that involved recognition of fine details under inadequate illumination of 2 ft-c (Brozek, Simonson, and Keys, 1950). Of the various criteria of precision of eye movements used in this study, the prolongation of the fixation phase of lateral eye movements was the most sensitive one to the visual strain.

Finally, in connection with the complex of functional disturbance of eye muscles, investigations of the changes of the blinking rate should be mentioned as a possible symptom of mental fatigue. According to Luckiesh and Moss (1938) the blinking rate increases under inadequate illumination and with the duration of work. Results of Tinker (1937), McFarland, et al. (1942), Bitterman (1945) and Simonson and Brozek (1948) disprove the claim of Luckiesh and Moss that the increase of the blinking rate is a valid index of fatigue. Thus, there is a lack of consistency in the changes of the blinking rate. Poulton (1958) in his interpretation of the results of Carmichael and Dearborn (1947) points out that their conclusion of no significant change of the blinking rate even after long working periods, contrasted to their published curves. In fact, Poulton suggested that the results of Carmichael and Dearborn support the view of Luckiesh and Moss. In view of the controversial results it is difficult to arrive at a final conclusion about the significance of the blinking rate as an index for mental fatigue. However, the best evidence speaks against it. In the most strenuous visual work task yet performed over four hours, there was no

TABLE 9-I

INITIAL PERFORMANCE AND PERFORMANCE DECREMENT AT DIFFERENT LEVELS OF ILLUMINATION, IN TERMS OF NUMBER OF CORRECTLY IDENTIFIED LETTERS OUT OF 200

Foot Candle Level	Score Initial	Decrement
2	162.0	26.0
5	176.6	14.1
15	187.8	9.8
50	193.6	9.9
100	192.9	6.8
300	193.7	10.0

significant change of the blinking rate (Brozek, Simonson and Keys, 1950).

In the comprehensive study of Simonson and Brozek (1948, 1950, 1952), the performance drop in strenuous visual work involving recognition of small letters with limited exposure time is the most pertinent index of fatigue in well motivated subjects. Table 9-I shows a condensation of the results. The initial performance increases with the illumination up to 50 foot candles, reaching a plateau. The performance decrement is largest at the lowest illumination level as may be expected, reaches an optimum at 100 ft-c, and increases again at 300 ft-c. Together with the decrement, there is an increased variability of performance at the end of the work period of two hours.

Audition

Several authors have attempted to use variations in auditory reception as indexes of mental fatigue. However, these efforts have been even less successful than the visual investigations. Herwig (1955) for instance, measured the upper audible frequency limit with conventional audiometric methods for testing of hearing. These threshold measurements were performed in occupational work, with consideration of duration and intensity of effort. However, control experiments of Graf (1955) suggest that the decrease or recovery of the upper frequency threshold is more closely correlated to variations of auditory adaptation than to changes in mental work capacity.

In a manner similar to the visual FFF, Davis (1955) developed a method for determination of the auditory fusion frequency, following investigations of Miller and Taylor (1948). Davis found that the response of the auditory fusion frequency to mental work (arithmetic problems) exceeds that of the simultaneously measured optical FFF. Control experiments have not yet been reported. An appraisal of Davis' results is difficult in view of the inadequate information about the method. Simonson (unpublished) also attempted to measure the auditory fusion frequency, but due to the much greater mechanical inertia of the microphone or to multiple sources of sound production, the measurement of the auditory fusion point was far less accurate than that of the FFF, and the attempt was abandoned.

The literature about the relationship between noise and work capacity is extremely voluminous. The review of Kryter (1950) does not indicate any impairment of the inner ear receptors with mental fatigue. It is much more probable that the variations of auditory reception is related to adaptation or temporary deafening effects. However, the term "auditory fatigue" has been commonly used in recent investigations of damage of the ear by noise so that misconceptions are widespread. It is unfortunate that in this field the term "fatigue" is synonymously used with adaptation and deafening. Bartley (1957) already has criticized this lack of clarification which shows up in the investigations of Harris (1954), Carterette (1955), Greisen (1951), Egan (1955), Dix, et al. (1949), Gardner (1947), Hirsh and Ward (1952), Huizing (1948), Meyer (1954), Wilson (1950) and others. Although these and other authors explain the decrease of auditory performance by noise as due to fatigue, nobody has shown that these variations have anything to do with fatigue. However, according to results of Laird (1933) and Jansen (1959) there is no doubt that intense noise produces vegetative reactions which may exert an indirect effect on the development of fatigue.

As a consequence of the investigations on disturbances of reception discussed above, we conclude that true fatigue processes of sensory organs have hardly been observed so far in the degree of effort usual in occupational work. If the term fatigue has been used, there was, as a rule, some kind of adaptation phenomenon involved, with the exception of investigations concerned with eye muscles, where functional changes were indeed observed which could be considered as fatigue in a more rigid definition. Finally, investigations of the FFF have shown that some phenomena labelled as "visual fatigue" are of central genesis, i.e. related to changes within the CNS. Even such tests of retinal functions as brightness and color discrimination, visual acuity, etc., involve the whole visual pathway.

This is probably valid, cum grano salis, for the whole complex of disturbance of perception, extending from minor distortions of environmental information to psychopathologic disturbances of sensations. Although elements of information processing are included in the processes of perception, for instance association of excitation patterns corresponding to physical stimuli with stored memory patterns of comprehension and content, the center of gravity for these processes must be regarded as being located at the acquisition (place of entry) of information. Therefore, it appears to be legitimate to discuss disturbances of perception in this part. Also see Chapter 14 for a discussion on the role of internal information acquisition during physical work.

PERCEPTUAL DISTURBANCE
Optical Illusions

In the past it was occasionally attempted to relate changes in the degree of geometric optical deception to disturbances of perception as a result of fatigue. However, an introductory remark regarding these experiments should be made. A priori, geometric-optical deceptions have nothing to do with disturbances of perception. The appearance of such deceptions only proves that the Euclidian laws of geometry are not valid for the sphere of subjective perception. For instance, the parallels in the well known Hering's illusion pattern intercept an already finite and not in an infinite space. Starting from the reference system of the geometrically defined visual field, an illusion exists in the direct sense of common usage of language, i.e. a deception which is rejected at repeated confrontation. In the subjective space of seeing a man, however, the lack of parallelism of straight lines in Hering's pattern is preserved, independent of his knowledge of the parallelism of the straight lines in the geometrically defined visual field. From this aspect the use of deception patterns is questionable, because of abstraction of the subjective space of perception from the "Eigenstandigkeit" (self-sufficiency) of geometry. On the contrary, the discrepancy between the physical object of presentation and the perception of the object points to incompatibility between subjective and objective space of seeing. Therefore, a "deception" is not actually involved here nor (for comparison) in the phenomenon of dimensional or color consistency (see Gunther, 1955; von Holst, 1957; Tausch, 1954; and others).

From the history of psychology it is well known that the adherents of "Gestaltpsychologie" (for example Ehrenstein, 1943, 1947; Riemann, 1933; and others) consider that optical illusions are an index for the whole entity of man's conscience structure. The degree of perceptual entity is greater in early developmental phases (for instance, in children) than in healthy adult subjects whose perception is to a greater degree characterized by analytical perception of objects (except in some exceptional situations: disease, alcoholic intoxication). Investigations of alcohol intoxication on human perception have revealed that in this condition, the characteristics of perception change from a mainly analytical to a synthetic-entity type of information acquisition. Therefore, the hypothesis was plausible that such a change may be due to fatigue. This hypothesis was verified by Bier (quoted from Ehrenstein) by a series of experiments on workers in industry. At the start and the end of the work, these workers engaged in inspection and assembly work, were given models with optical illusion figures after Oppel, Ehrenstein, Muller-Lyer and Poggendorf which they had to adjust for subjective compensation of the original illusion. Thus, the experimenter could read on metric scales the actual degree of illusion without knowledge of the subjects. The results showed that during the working day the degree of illusion increased on the average between 33 and 69 percent, dependent on the particular illusion pattern used. This increase suggests that mental load interferes with the analytical perception of objects after eight hours of work and could be due to fatigue of those brain centers which regulate the spontaneous activity of human visual perception. Similar observations have been reported by Tussing (1941), Lybrand, Andrews and Ross (1954), while Nack (1947) was not able to confirm these results.

Degree of Wakefulness

The more the critical-analytical approach of man in his environmental orientation declines, the greater he becomes exposed to the risk of incomplete or false interpretation of defined contents of perception. Not rarely, this leads to violations of social behavior. The analysis of causes of automobile accidents and testimony of persons involved in accidents in the traffic courts frequently show that traffic signs were overlooked, not correctly seen, or misinterpreted, although, as a rule, little weight is given to such testimony. It cannot be ruled out that after mental stress drivers may suffer from disturbances of perception resulting in or contributing to accidents. However, it should be emphasized that no systematic investigations on the relationship between disturbances of perception caused by fatigue and automobile accidents have yet been reported.

However, the possibility of such relationship is supported by a study of Hartmann (1963). Hartmann investigated the changes of the perception threshold of an illuminated test figure in relationship to the duration of uninterrupted automobile driving. The investigations were performed during night on German highways (Autobahn). A rather large test figure (Landolt-ring) was mounted on the back of an automobile, which was illuminated in irregular time intervals. The passenger of an automobile following at a constantly maintained distance served as subject. He had to report the perception of the test figure by radio communication to the preceding automobile. In case this communication was not received within a given time, the illumination level of the test figure was stepwise increased until recognition by the subject. The results of Hartmann are summarized in Figure 9-2. It can be seen that within the first 90 minutes the perception threshold of the test figure varies within relatively narrow limits of 0.02 cd/m^2, but after 210 to 290 minutes the threshold significantly increased in the direction of higher intensities of illumination. Starting from the hy-

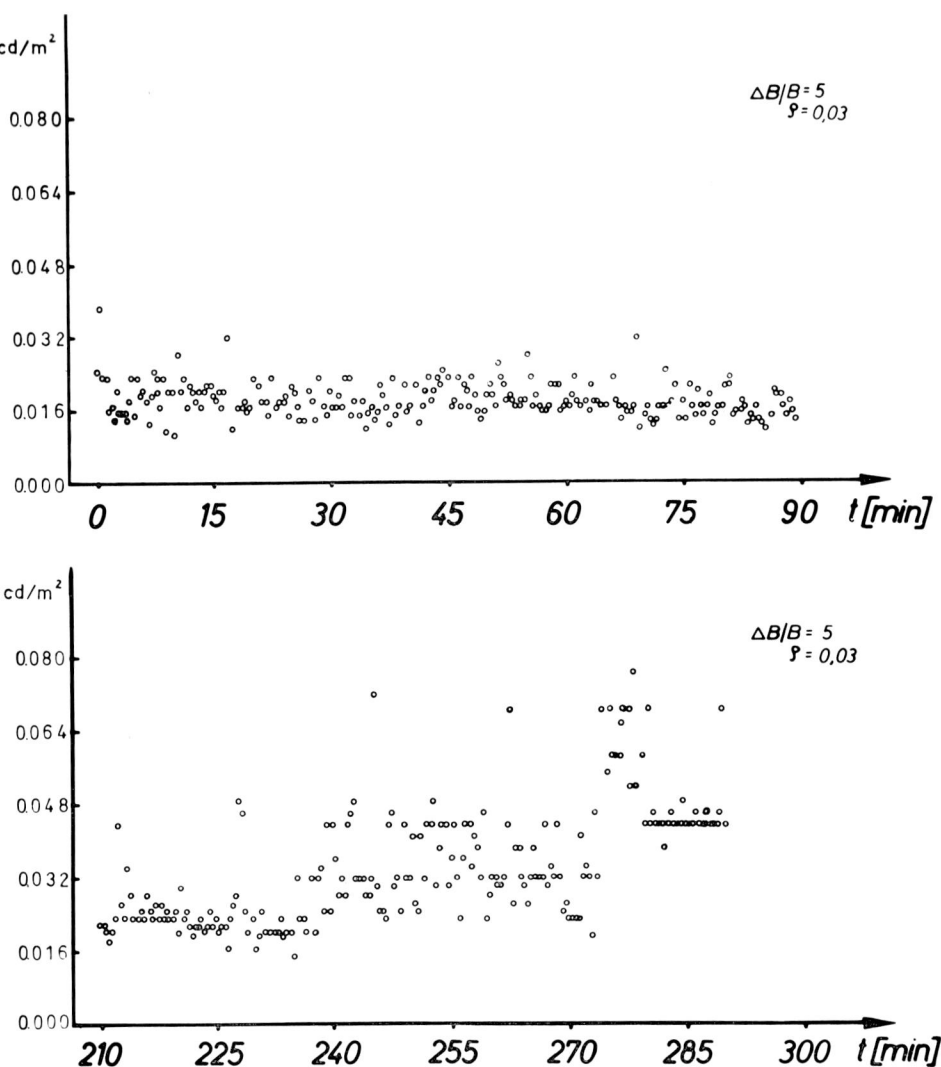

Figure 9-2. Recognition threshold of a test target (Landolt ring, mounted on the back side of an automobile) during the first 90 minutes (upper part) and from 210 to 300 minutes (lower part) of night driving. The subject was a passenger in an automobile following the one on which the target was mounted (From E. Hartmann, "Disability Glare and Discomfort Glare," in E. Ingelstam, ed., *Lighting Problems in Highway Traffic* [Oxford, 1963] p. 95).

pothesis that the parameter of regression indicates the degree of fatigue and that the parameter of variability of the measurements indicates the level of attention (wakefulness), Hartmann concluded that in the first 90 minutes there was little fatigue and the level of wakefulness was high while later a progressive increment of fatigue was associated with a decrease of wakefulness must be assumed. Independent of the question of the justification of such far reaching interpretation of the results, the fact remains that the driver after several hours of uninterrupted driving needs a higher illumination level for perception of critical environmental signals than in fresh condition.

Another approach in this direction comes from investigations regarding the signal detection theory (Schmidtke, 1968, in part yet unpublished). The starting point here is the hypothesis that the probability of detecting a signal in the visual field depends on the space-time course of ocular search movements as well as the difference between target illumination and surrounding illumination. The larger the spatial distance between the signal and the fixation point (F_x) of the eye, the lower is the expected probability of detection of the signal at the time (t_x). An experimental verification of this hypothesis would lead to the formulation of a theory of signal detection on the basis of the search movements of the eye. The critical value for probable detection of the signal would be expressed by the equation: the distance $|F_{n-1} - F_n|$ (in arc) = a. The critical visual angle a would be a function of the illumination difference between target and surrounding illumination and, among other variables, of the mental load.

For examination of this hypothesis, the subject was seated 2 m before a transparent square test area (horizontal and vertical visual angle 28°, diagonal 39°) and had to look at this field (illuminated with 7.6 Apostilb) for a signal (circle of 2 cm diameter, corresponding to a visual angle of 33.6 arc minutes, with an illumination of 8.4 Apostilb). The position of the signal was systematically varied according to the experimental schedule. For determination of the ocular search movements, a narrow beam from an infrared lamp, pupillo-motorically inert, was projected on the cornea, and its reflection was photographed. The fixation of the head was rigidly maintained. Before the start of each ocular search the light of a small red test mark in the center of the visual field was switched on as a fixation point of the observer (F_1). Simultaneously, with switching off the light of this test mark, the signal was projected into the search field. Thus, for each measurement comparable starting conditions were provided. Twenty measurements (signal presentations) were performed per experiment.

After conclusion of this series of measurements (in fresh condition), the subject had to work for a period of two hours on a binary choice reaction consisting in the presentation of high (1200 Hz) and low frequency (700 Hz) sounds in arbitrary sequence. The subject had to respond by pressing one of several levers corresponding to high or low tones, dependent on the sound presented. Eighty-four auditory stimuli were presented per minute. After the two hours' mental work, another series of signal detection followed each 20 signal presentations. The change of both measurement indices 1. "number of changes of fixation until signal detection" and 2. the "critical radial distance $|F_{n-1} - F_n|$" was then analyzed. The following results were obtained: after a mental load without stress of the visual apparatus the mean number of fixation changes necessary for signal detection increase from 7.37 ± 3.12 to 9.84 ± 3.71, together with an increase of the mean distance between two consecutive fixations from $6° 12' \pm 1° 56'$ to $7° 53' \pm 2° 09'$. Closely associated with the change in the number of fixation changes was the change in critical radial distance $|F_{n-1} - F_n|$ which dropped from a mean of $4° 08' \pm 1° 22'$ to a mean of $3° 12' \pm 1° 17'$ after the mental work period. The simultaneous changes of the number of fixation changes and distance is not surprising, because both indices are related.

As a possible interpretation of these results, a hypothesis that intense mental load changes the stimulation threshold is proposed. This hypothesis predicts changes that are similar to Hartman's results. Since the stimulus intensity in these experiments was kept constant, the effect of fatigue showed up in a lengthening of the search period due to the smaller critical radial distance $|F_{n-1} - F_n|$.

Thus, the increase of the degree of illusion in the geometric-optical illusion experiments, the misinterpretation of perception, and the increase of the threshold for perception for visual stimuli all suggest a cerebral location of these disturbances. They were interpreted by von Bracken (1952) as a symptom of loosening the functional integrity of personality in ontogenetically and/or phylogenetically regressive direction of lower, earlier levels of organization. Haider's (1957) experiments of the effect of mental work on the time course of negative after-images support the thesis proposed by "Gestalt"-psychologists and by von Bracken. After a Kraepelin test (additions) of 90 minutes the red-green after-image was prolonged, the average, by 8 percent and the black-white after-image by 25 percent in well motivated subjects. In this connection we refer also to similar results of Weil (1929) and McFarland (1937).

Blocking

Under conditions of extreme mental work, a true blocking within the processes of information acquisition cannot be ruled out. However, there is hardly any experimental documentation for this assumption if one disregards sleep deprivation experiments or pharmacological studies. Nevertheless, such phenomena have occurred in self-observations. Thus, after driving for several hours immediately after a prolonged conference several years ago, the author (H. S.) observed an apparently private automobile going in the same direction. On closing the distance the automobile proved to be a furniture truck with the name and location of the company readable on the back. However, the most critical decision for traffic safety, the overtaking maneuver, was not started. Only due to the shock reaction of the passenger were the brakes applied so that the accident damage was light. In this example the transmission of afferent stimulus was functioning, but the transformation of the information into the corresponding motor action pattern was entirely blocked. Blocking will be discussed in greater detail in the following chapter on information processing.

Illusions and Hallucinations

Finally, the observations associated with the concept of illusion and hallucination fall into the field of disturbances of perception. Korbsch (quoted from von Bracken, 1952) and McCandless (1958), among others, have reported misinterpretations of perception contents which approach the definition of illusion. Korbsch reported a common observation from military physicians in the First World War that units who were in combat for a prolonged time, often considered other friendly units as enemies which resulted in bitter fighting with high losses, in spite of signals which should have identified the units. A particularly clear example for fatigue illusions has been presented by McCandless. He describes a unit of the American Navy operating in the Second World War in the Aleutians. There was information about possible contacts with Japanese ships. Some of the American ships detected with the aid of radar six objects in a distance of 15 nautical miles, moving in a certain course with a speed of 15 nautical m.p.h. On the basis of this exact localization three cruisers and two battleships opened heavy fire which was maintained for 30 minutes in "the battle of the pips." This "sea-battle" has been recorded in the history as a "naval engagement that lacked only one thing to be a great victory—the enemy." According to McCandless, other ships in the same American unit did not participate in the fight because their radar operators were not able to detect any targets. It is quite obvious that the radar operators of the ships involved in this sea-battle suffered from disturbances of perception, on the borderline between illusions and hallucinations, due to anticipation of the enemy after the psychophysical stress of a long cruise under alarm conditions.

The disturbances of perception observed by Kleitman (1939) resulted from prolonged sleep deprivation and other conditions and described as light hallucinations fall also into this category. These hallucinations consisted in seeing certain objects in the working space, which actually did not exist, or in reporting actions as finished, although they were not performed by the subjects. A similar example was given by Eagles, Halliday and Redfearn (1953): an experimental subject had a quarrel with the experimenter, after prolonged sleep deprivation, the subject maintained that he had given the experimenter packs of sorted cards, although the cards were laying unsorted before the subject. A perception of nonexistent events (as in McCandless' example), or the misinterpretation of perception (as in Eagles, et al., observations) must be regarded, besides its psychopathological significance, as symptoms of mental fatigue.

The visual hallucinations of automobile drivers in connection with prolonged driving time, reported by Moseley (1953) fall also into the field of perceptual disturbances resulting from fatigue. A common feature of these hypnagogic hallucinations is the recognition of objects which do not exist. According to Moseley, automobile drivers have said that they had seen objects or animals on the road and consequently made steering movements for evasion, or stopped the vehicle, and then recognized that there was no reality in their observations. This symptom occurred particularly frequently after driving at night or over long distances, at diminished tension of attention and pronounced sensation of fatigue. Just how important this insight can explain such disturbances of perception is shown by noting the relatively small sample of subjects investigated by Moseley: two traffic accidents occurred for which hallucinations must have been responsible. Almost all forms of perception disturbances due to load (mental or severe physical work) are distinguished by "primitivisation" of perception processes. As a consequence of primitivisation, there is a fixation of the partial contents of an observation at the expense of selectivity and accentuation, leading to incomplete or false interpretation of the content of the observation. Besides the fixation of partial contents of the observation, the primitivisation of the processes of perception is also noticeable in premature hypotheses to which the subject adheres rigidly (see McCandless' example). For this interpretation, Voigt (1956) has provided elegant support. After a pronounced mental load, Voigt presented photographic pictures to his subjects. For each picture there was a series of photos with different sharpness. Every series started with an entirely unclear photo without the possibility of picture recognition and ended with a clear picture, sharply focussed. In fatigued condition, the subjects gave descriptions of the content at a much greater degree of unclarity than in fresh condition. The premature formation of opinion of the content of perception and the uncritical adhering to such opinion may be considered as essential symptoms of disturbance of acquisition of information due to fatigue.

BIBLIOGRAPHY

Bartlett, C. S., R. L. Beinert, and J. R. Graham: Study of visual fatigue and efficiency in radar observation. Final Rep. Hobart College, Geneva, RADC-TR 55-100, 1953.
Bartley, S. H.: Fatigue and inadequacy. *Physiol Rev, 37*:301, 1957.
Baur, A.: Die Ermüdung im Spiegel des Auges. Langensalza, 1910.
Berens, C.: Experimental studies of fatigue of accommodation II. *Am J Ophthalmol, 33*:47, 1950.

Bitterman, M. E.: Heart rate and frequency of blinking as indices of visual efficiency. *J Exp Psychol*, 35:279, 1945.
Bitterman, M. E.: Transfer of decrement in ocular task. *Am J Psychol*, 59:422, 1946.
Borges Dias, A.: Heterophoria due to fatigue from flying. *Ophthalmos* (Rio de J.), 1:553, 1940.
Bracken, H. von: Zur Psychopathologie der Ermüdung. In Bornemann, E.: *Ermüdung*. Lüneburg, 1952.
Brozek, J., E. Simonson, and A. Keys: Changes in performance and in ocular functions resulting from strenuous visual inspection. *Am J Psychol*, 63:51, 1950.
Carmichael, L., and W. Dearborn: *Reading and Visual Fatigue*. Boston, 1947.
Carterette, E. C.: Prestimulatory auditory fatigue for continuous and intermittent noise. *J Acoust Soc Am*, 27:103, 1955.
Collins, J. B.: Visual fatigue and its measurement. *Ann Occup Hyg*, 1:228, 1959.
Collins, J. B., and B. Pruen: Perception time and visual fatigue. *Ergonomics*, 5:533, 1962.
Davis, R. C.: Auditory and visual flicker-fusion as measurement of fatigue. *Am J Psychol*, 68:654, 1955.
Demmel, W.: Die Beziehungen der Fusionsfähigkeit zur Leistungsbereitschaft. Bonn, Diss, 1957.
Dix, M. R., et al.: Auditory adaptation in the human subject. *Nature* (London), 164:59, 1949.
Durig, A.: Theorie der Ermüdung. In Atzler, E.: *Körper und Arbeit*. Leipzig, 1927.
Eagles, J. B., A. M. Halliday, and J. W. T. Redfearn: The effects of fatigue on tremor. In Floyd, W. F., and A. T. Welford (Eds.): *Symposium on Fatigue*. London, 1953.
Egan, J. P.: Prestimulatory fatigue as measured by heterophonic loudness balance. *J Acoust Soc Am*, 27:110, 1955.
Ehrenstein, W.: Die optischen Täuschungen als Kriterium der Ermüdung. *Industr Psychotechnik*, 20:18, 1943.
Ehrenstein, W.: Probleme der ganzheitspsychologischen Wahrnehmungslehre. 2. Aufl. Leipzig, 1947.
Ferree, C. H., and G. Rand: An instrument measuring dynamic speed of vision, of accommodation and ocular fatigue. *Arch Ophthalmol*, 15:1072, 1936.
Fröhlich, F. W.: Die Empfindungszeit. Jena, 1928.
Gardner, M. B.: Short duration auditory fatigue as a method of classifying hearing impairment. *J Acoust Soc Am*, 19:178, 1947.
Gerathewohl, S. J.: Eye movements during radar operations. *J Aviat Med*, 23:597, 1952.
Graf, O.: Erforschung der geistigen Ermüdung und nervösen Belastung. Köln-Opladen, 1955.
Granit, R.: Sensory mechanism of the retina. Oxford, Hafner, 1947.
Greisen, L.: Comparative investigations of different auditory fatigue test. *Acta otolaryngol*, 39:132, 1951.
Grindley, W.: Retinal fatigue in protracted subjective tests. *Optician*, 72:42, 1926.
Günther, N.: Die Struktur des Sehraumes. Stuttgart, 1955.
Hafemann, G.: Das Leistungsverhalten der Fusionsbreite als Maß der Leistungsbereitschaft im Schichtunterricht. *Münch med Wochenschr*, 99:43, 1957.
Hafemann, G., and L. Holfeld: Über Objektivierung und Beeinflussung von Ermüdungserscheinungen bei Schulkindern. *Der Öffentl Gesundheitsdienst*, 18:9, 1956.
Haider, M.: Experimenteller Beitrag zum Verhalten des negativen Nachbildes bei Ermüdung. *Z exp angew Psychol*, 4:94, 1957.

Harris, J. D.: Roles of sensation level and sound pressure in producing auditory fatigue. *Laryngoscope, 64*:89, 1954.

Hartmann, E.: Disability glare and discomfort glare. In Ingelstam, E. (Ed.): *Lighting Problems in Highway Traffic.* Oxford/London/New York/Paris, 1963, p. 95, Vol. 2.

Hartridge, H.: Some fatigue effects on the human retina produced by using coloured lights. *Nature* (London), *160*:538, 1947.

Helmholtz, H. v.: Handbuch der physiologischen Optik, 3. Aufl. Leipzig. 1911.

Herwig, B.: In *Arbeitsablauf und Arbeitsbelastung.* RKW-Berichtsreihe C 5. Berlin/Köln/Frankfurt, 1955.

Hirsch, J. A.: Accommodation fatigue in the aging radar observer. USAF Aero Medical Lab. Wright-Patterson AFB, Ohio, USA. WADC-TR-58-24, 1958.

Hirsh, I. J., and W. D. Ward: Recovery of the auditory threshold after strong acoustic stimulation. *J Acoust Soc Am, 24*:131, 1952.

Hofstetter, H. W.: An ergographic analysis of fatigue of accommodation. *Am J Optom, 20*:115, 1943.

Holst, E. von: Aktive Leistungen der menschlichen Gesichtswahrnehmung. *Studium Generale, 10*:231, 1957.

Huizing, H. C.: Relation between auditory fatigue and recruitment. *Acta oto-laryngol* Suppl., *78*:169, 1948.

Jansen, G.: Zur Entstehung vegetativer Funktionsstörungen durch Lärmeinwirkung. *Arch Gewerbepath und Gewerbehyg, 17*:238, 1959.

Kleitman, N.: *Sleep and Wakefulness.* Chicago, 1939.

Kroebel, W.: Das Sehvermögen des menschlichen Auges bei Schwarz-Weiss-Bildern. *Naturwiss, 45*:105, 1958A.

Kroebel, W.: Über die physikalischen Grundlagen der Gütebeurteilung photographischer Bilder. *Naturwiss, 45*:284, 1958B.

Kryter, K. D.: The effects of noise on man. *J Speech Hear Disord,* Monograph Supplement 1, 1950.

Laird, D.: The influence of noise on production and fatigue as related to pitch, sensation level, and steadiness of noise. *J Appl Psychol, 17*:320, 1933.

Luckiesh, M., and F. M. Moss: *The Science of Seeing.* New York, 1938.

Lybrand, W. A., T. G. Andrews, and S. Ross: Systematic fatigue and perceptual organization. *Am J Psychol, 67*:704, 1954.

McCandless, B.: The battle of the pips. US Naval Inst. Proceedings, *84*:49, 1958.

McFarland, R. A.: Psychophysiological studies at high altitude in the Andes. I. The effect of rapid ascents by aeroplane and train. *J Comp Physiol, 23*:191, 1937.

McFarland, R. A., A. H. Holway, and L. M. Hurvich: Studies of visual fatigue. Harvard School of Bus. Adm., 1942.

Meyer, M. F.: Auditory fatigue beyond and within the compass of the voice. *Am J Psychol, 67*:538, 1954.

Miller, G. A., and W. G. Taylor: The perception of repeated bursts of noise. *J Acoust Soc Am, 20*:171, 1948.

Moseley, A. L.: Hypnagogic hallucination in relation to accidents. *Am Psychol, 8*:407, 1953.

Nack, G.: Experimenteller Beitrag über geometrisch-optische Täuschungen als Kriterium der Ermüdung. Diss. Wien 1947.

Poulton, E. C.: On reading and visual fatigue. *Am J Psychol, 71*:609, 1958.

Prokop, O., und L. Prokop: Ermüdung und Einschlafen am Steuer. *Dtsch Z ger Med, 44*:343, 1955.

Reitnauer, P. G.: Zeitverhältnisse der Akkommodation des menschlichen Auges und ihre Veränderungen unter experimentellen Ermüdungsbedingungen. *Z f Psychol, 161*:107, 1957.

Riemann, H.: Über Messungen des Täuschungsbetrages bei geometrisch-optischen Täuschungen und deren Verwendbarkeit als Mittel der typologischen Diagnose. Diss. Danzig, 1933.

Rohrer, H.: Vergleichende Untersuchungen über Ermüdung, Leistungsabfall, Unfallhäufigkeit bei verschiedenen Arbeitsformen. Med. Diss. Bonn, 1958.

Saldanha, E. L.: An investigation into the effect of prolonged and exacting visual work. Med Res Council, APU Rep. 243, 1955.

Saldanha, E. L.: Alternating an exacting visual task with either rest or similar work. Med Res Council APU Rep. 289, 1957.

Schmidtke, H.: Über Ermüdungsmessung mit dem Synoptophor. *Int Z angew Physiol einschl Arbeitsphysiol, 17*:490, 1959.

Schmidtke, H.: Beitrag zur Theorie der Signalentdeckung. *Psychol Beiträge, 3*:464, 1968.

Schober, H.: Das Sehen, Band II. 3. Aufl. Leipzig, 1964.

Siemes, M.: Über den Einfluß von Traubenzuckergaben auf die Ermüdung, nachgewiesen mit einer sinnesphysiologischen Methode an Lehrlingen. *Zbl Arbeitsmed und Arbeitsschutz, 7*:15, 1957.

Simmerman, H.: Visual Fatigue. *Am J Optom, 27*:554, 1950.

Simonson, E., and J. Brozek: Effects of illumination level on visual fatigue. *J Opt Soc Am, 38*:384, 1948.

Simonson, E., and J. Brozek: Beleuchtung und Ermüdung des Sehens. *Zbl Arbeitswiss, 4*:49, 1952 und *5*:70, 1952.

Solowjewa, W. P.: Fisiologitscheskaja ozenka razionalisazii reschima truda pri naprjaschennoi umstwennoi rabotje (korrektorü tipografii). In Letaweta, A. A., and Kosilowa, S. A.: *Materialü k fisiologitscheskomu obosnowaniju trudowüch prozessow.* Moskau, 1960.

Strughold, H.: The human time factors in flight. Handbook of Human Engineering Data. 2. Aufl. US Naval Research Laboratory 1951.

Tausch, R.: Optische Täuschungen als artifizielle Effekte der Gestaltungsprozesse von Größen- und Formkonstanz in der natürlichen Raumwahrnehmung. *Psychol Forsch, 24*:229, 1954.

Tinker, M. A.: Validity of frequency of blinking as a criterion of readability. *J Exp Psychol, 36*:453, 1937.

Tussing, L.: Perceptual fluctuations of illusions as possible physical fatigue index. *J Exp Psychol, 29*:85, 1941.

Voigt, J.: Die Aktualgenese in der psychologischen Diagnostik. *Psychol Beiträge, 2*:586, 1956.

Weber, R. A.: Ocular fatigue. *Arch Ophthalmol*, Chicago *43*:257, 1950.

Weil, H.: Sinnespsychologische Kriterien menschlicher Typen. *Z Psychol, 110*:51, 1929.

Weston, H. C.: Visual fatigue. *Optician 124*:602, 1952.

White, L. R., R. H. Britten, J. H. Ives, and L. R. Thompson: Studies in illumination. II. Relationship of illumination to ocular fatigue among the letter separators in the Chicago post office. Public Health Bull. No. 181. Washington, 1929.

Wieland, H.: Ein Beitrag zur Leistungsmessung. *Zbl Arbeitsmed und Arbeitsschutz, 7*:11, 1957.

Wilson, W. H.: Determination of susceptibility to abnormal auditory fatigue. *Ann Otol, 59*:399, 1950.

Chapter 10

Disturbance of Processing of Information

HEINZ SCHMIDTKE[1]

MANY OF THE ENVIRONMENTAL stimuli perceived by the sensory systems have a meaningful content for the individual. Consequently, they have to be compared to the stored memory patterns in the process of identification. Disturbances in the processing of information, therefore, may result in insufficient or faulty association of stimuli-memory and behavioral patterns. This aspect of disturbances of information processing overlaps widely with the disturbances of perception, as discussed in the preceding part. Disturbances of information processing, however, may be entirely internal, so that under the influence of the predetermined tendencies for association, the process of idea formation or the reproduction of memory patterns is impaired.

The classical investigations of these types of disturbances date back essentially to Kraepelin. The extremely voluminous studies of Amberg (1896), Rivers and Kraepelin (1896), von Voss (1899), Hylan and Kraepelin (1904), Heumann (1904) and Graf (1922) have provided the basis for the recognition of regularities in the disturbances of mental processes that are dependent on the duration of work. These authors demonstrated in difficult experiments that with an intense mental load, the correlation of associations and memory patterns becomes disorderly-fluctuating. It is logical that Aschaffenburg (1899) in the course of his investigations on associations, related the disturbances of thinking in fatigue to the pathological symptom of "Ideenflucht" (flight of ideas).

Similar to this pathological condition, prolonged, monotonous mental work leads to increasing disorder in associational processes. This is primarily due to the fact that, along with an intended thought object or focal image (Zielvorstellung), there is an influx into conscious experience of task-unrelated associations, images or ideas, many times necessitating a new start of mental operations. Furthermore, a voluntary screening against foreign disturbing associations is necessary for a positive motivation which affects the performance. According to von Voss (1899), Pauli (1936), Düker (1931, 1934) and others, this situation shows up in increasing duration and variations of the time for additions in mental arithmetic work.

Schmidtke (1963) has reported an approach for quantitative analysis of disturbance of the mental processes in fatigue. Using Düker's concentra-

---

1. Translated by Editors.

tion-performance tests, an attempt was made to measure the recovery time needed for compensation of mental fatigue that was related to the duration of uninterrupted work and to the required level of performance (number of arithmetic problems per unit of time). Based on a work task lasting 4 hours, first the upper limit for prolonged performance was defined as the highest speed of arithmetic problems that could be done with a sum of errors and missed problems at or below 5 percent of all problems presented. This mental work (blindfolded) is of the type $\frac{6+3-7}{9-4+3}$. First the result of the first line is determined and memorized. After solving the problem of the second line, the difference between both results (8 − 2 = 6) is determined and pronounced or recorded.

After determination of the limit of prolonged performance, experiments were performed with forced speed of calculations above this limit, but of shorter duration without pauses (30, 20, 15, 10 or 5 minutes). After such a period of calculation, the length of a pause needed for full compensation of the fatigue produced by exceeding the limit of prolonged performance was determined for the designated speed, so that with intermittent work periods and pauses, a work duration of 4 hours could be

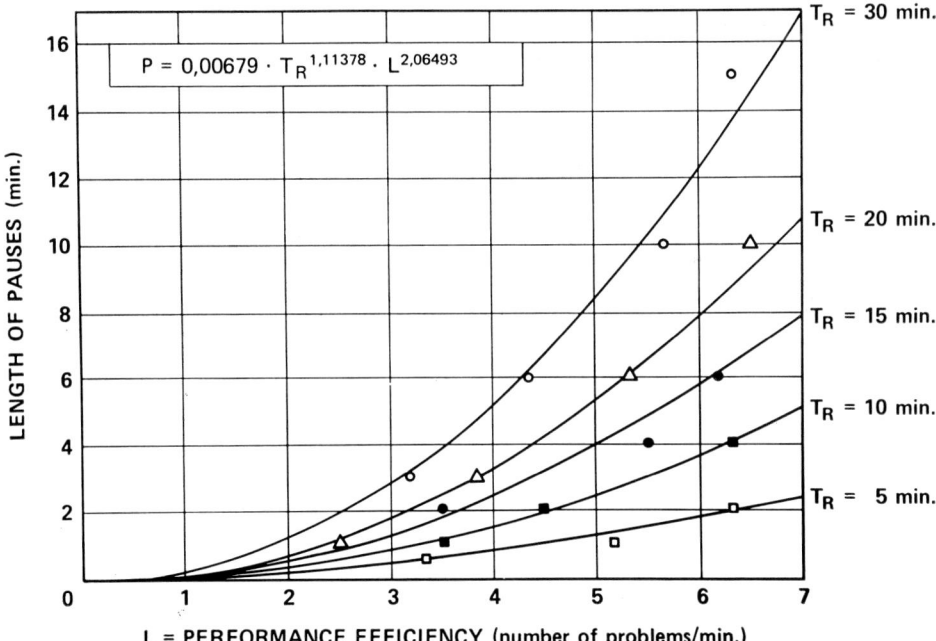

Figure 10-1. Relationship between performance (arithmetic problems per min.)—abscissa —in uninterrupted working time (right ordinate) and necessary length of pauses per min (left ordinate) (From H. Schmidtke, "Untersuchungen uber den Erholungszeitbedarf bei psychisch beanspruchender Tätigkeit," in *Arbeitsstudien heute und morgen* [Berlin/Koln/Frankfurt] 1963).

maintained. The results showed that the length of pauses needed for compensation of fatigue increases exponentially with the work duration and the speed of calculation and can be expressed by the equation $P = k \cdot T_R^a \cdot L^b$ where P = length of pauses (min.), T_R = duration of the single work periods (min.), L = effective performance limit for prolonged continued performance (problems/min.), K = constant (min./problems), a and b constants (dimensionless). Figure 10-1 indicates that the length of pauses necessary for prolonged performance versus performance as work duration is increased and can be expressed by the equation

$$P = 0.0068 \times T_R^{1.114} \times L^{2.065}$$

Starting from the hypothesis that the length of pauses determined in this manner is a suitable, though indirect, expression for the degree of interference with information processing, there appears to be a general similarity between mental and physical work.

TRANSIENT REACTIVITY FAILURE

Intense mental stress may quite often produce a phenomenon which can be described as transient reactivity failure. That is, this type of work is associated with a short loss of *rapport* to the task. Bills (1931) has thoroughly explored this situation. He proposed the hypothesis that the phases of reactivity failure regularly appearing in mental work are due to blocking of central nervous processes, so that even with high motivation, the subject is unable to process mental tasks during such blocks. Bills arrived at the following conclusions: a. Transient blocks may be considered as forced pauses facilitating recovery, preventing a fast performance decrement in mental work. (Thus, transient blocks are functionally similar to the pauses in dynamic work due to the alternating activity of flexors and extensors.) b. The rhythmic fluctuations of both the degree of and the direction of attention corresponding to fluctuations of mental performance cannot be ruled out. c. From observations of the cumulative prolongation of the refractory period of peripheral nerves at high stimulation frequencies, it was concluded that prolongation of transmission time is also possible within the CNS. d. Such phases of decreased mental capacity (provided that they occur), may significantly affect the number of errors so that it may be possible to propose a hypothesis for the causes of performance decrement.

Bills used relatively simple continuous tasks, i.e. arithmetic additions and subtractions, looking for inversion of cube patterns, naming of colors, naming of antonyms, or substitution of numbers by letters. The time interval from stimulus presentation to reaction was recorded. A reaction pause exceeding at least twice the average reaction time of a given subject was operationally defined as "mental block." Dependent on the individual rate, the delay of the reaction had to be two to four seconds for interpretation of the block. It appears surprising today that Bills did not discuss the underlying causes and the problems of definition for "mental block"; however, the results are stimulating and important enough for discussion in the context of this chapter.

Bills' experiments, as briefly described above, produced essentially the following results: in homogenous and continuous mental activities, block of reactivity occurs in a certain rhythm. The time of such blocks, dependent on the task, extend from two to six times the reaction time. Training reduces the frequency as well as direction of blocks. It is important to note that errors are recorded in connection with blocks because of the possibility of an alternative interpretation (see also the following discussion of the time course of awareness of errors in typing). With reference to Figures 10-2 and 10-3 it should be noted that during mental fatigue, the frequency as well as the length of the blocks increases with increasing duration of the work task. While guarding against overinterpretation of Bills' results, these observations suggest the hypothesis that the blocks may be considered as forced autonomic pauses of the organism with the purpose of maintenance of optimal neural activity over a prolonged time.

Since blocks appear only after a series of undisturbed reactions, as shown in Figures 10-2 and 10-3, they certainly cannot be explained by a simple prolongation of the refractory period. It may be assumed, with refer-

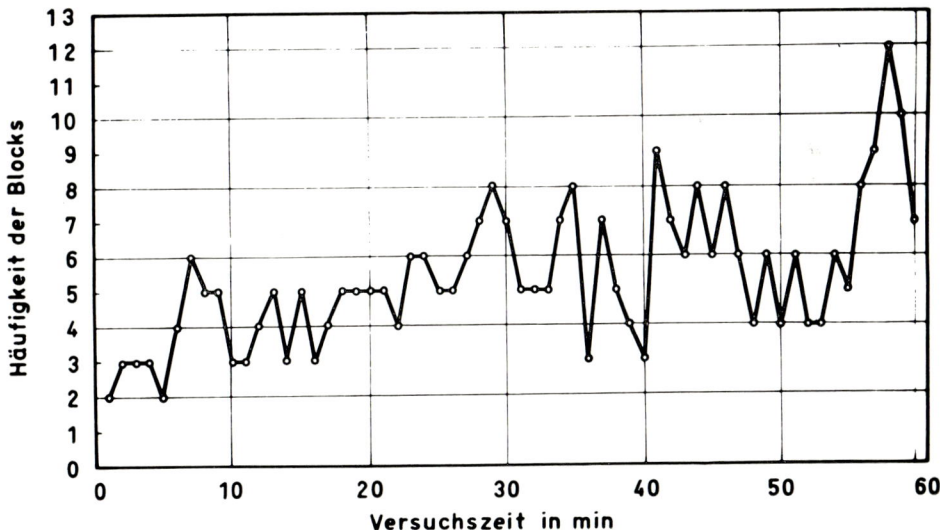

Figure 10-2. Relationship between duration of experiment (min.—abscissa—) and frequency of blocks (ordinate) (From A. G. Bills, "Blocking: A New Principle of Mental Fatigue," *American Journal of Psychology*, 43:230, 1931).

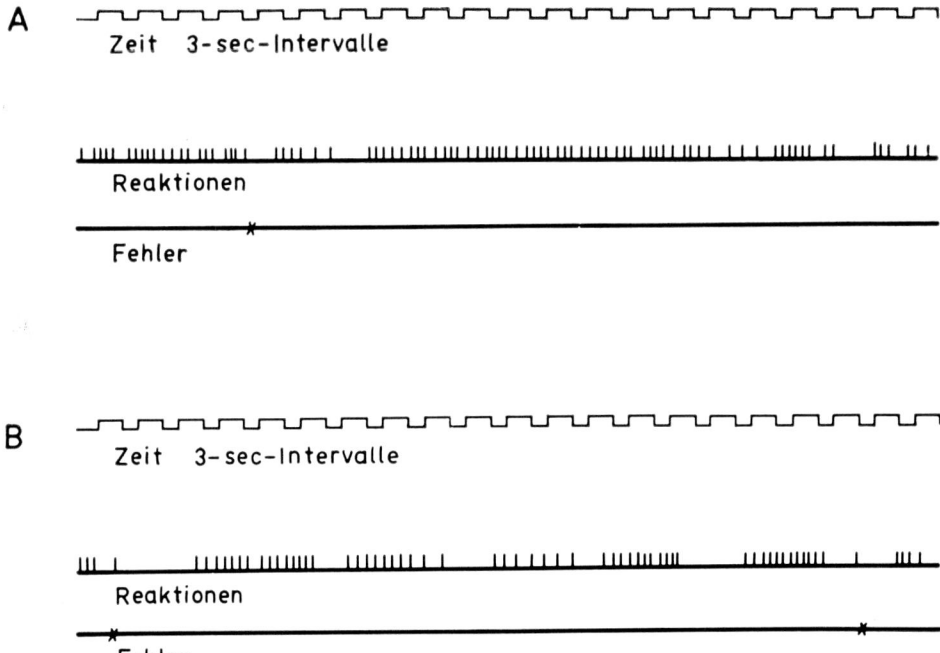

Figure 10-3. Records of blocking experiments. A—During the first 15 min. of experiment; B—During the last 15 min. of experiment; Both A and B—Upper tracing time (3 sec. intervals); Middle tracing—Reactions; Bottom tracing—Errors (From A. G. Bills, "Blocking: A New Principle of Mental Fatigue," *American Journal of Psychology, 43*:230, 1931).

ence to Lashley (1938) that the blocks are an expression for periodic failures of central integration mechanisms.

An Information Theory Explanation

A psychological analysis, on the basis of information theory, appears to be the most suitable approach for explaining these disturbances of integration (Bäumler, 1967). This explanation leads to the conclusion that blocks are disturbances in the information processing (related to a given task) that occur in various locations (acquisition, integration, reaction).

In a critical analysis of Bills' method, Bäumler showed that the criterion for blocks is not suitable for most experimental problems. Furthermore, all definitions of blocks that were based only on performance data are questionable, and they are meaningful only when they are observed doing certain mental tasks. When the criterion is typically used, it refers to the output characteristics in rapid sequences of reactions, and procedures for elimnination (or reduction) of the variability in the measurements by a suitable transformation of variables are needed. In the so-called "Partial Moment

Criterion," Bäumler related different segments of the distribution to one another. This method was more reliable and more sensitive for the detection of blocks than Bills' original method. The separation of mixed distributions (the populations of normal reactions and blocks) was also proposed, particularly for prolonged experiments with a large number of reactions.

The replication of some of Bills' experiments confirmed part of his results (for example, the increase of blocks with fatigue), while other results (effect of training) were disproved.

In further experiments Bäumler showed that blocks can also be elicited by orientation reactions that are similar to the well known effects of attention diversion. Essential factors for the appearance of blocks were those of motivation and expectation, such as relative novelty, habituation, disinhibition, saturation, apprehension of failure and of other anxieties regarding tangible expected results, external stimuli with extreme emotional content as well as spontaneous ideas and motives.

Bäumler suggested that any reduction of a theory of blocking to a special causal category such as refractoriness theory, saturation theory, special motivation theories, theory of orientation reactions, narcoleptic theory, and activation theory, is not possible. More promising is a general model based on the psychology of information or regulations. Thus, blocking would be a result of information overload (so-called catastrophe collapse) (Miller, 1960, 1961). This overload-inhibition is not necessarily a protective inhibition, it may well be, for instance in fatigue, a symptom of inadequate compensation for central nervous disturbance (Schmidtke, 1965).

An essential factor leading to blocking is the fact that the capacities for simultaneous processing of information are quite low in man. This limitation, also called one channel perception, is directly related to the principle of the limitation of consciousness (Pauli, 1924; Broadbent, 1957). This principle is also suggested by neurophysiological investigations (Hernandez-Peon, et al., 1956), and it appears to be identical with the principle of singularity of response, or the final common pathway, well known from the classical study of neural reflexes (Sherrington, 1905).

This principle indirectly implies the effectiveness in a hierarchy of motives and the conflict between different goals. According to Bäumler, blocking is an expression of the dynamics of motives and resulting interference of reaction tendencies. It is characterized by critical reversal values for these factors when the information capacity is exceeded by additional information, such as a new motive or a new task. The cause may be external as well as internal interference stimuli that affect motivation and produce an unexpected discrepancy in the performance goal. In the frame of regulatory processes used for the maintenance of homeostasis, elicited by the interference, blocking may be a negative (decrease of performance) as well as positive (protective) function.

Similarly to Bills and Bäumler, Broadbent (1950) also observed a short depression of the concentration level in choice reactions. Thus, the results confirmed the increment of time of performance and increased variability in mental work (additions) described in detail by Kraepelin and associates.

CHOICE REACTION SITUATIONS

The time dependence of information processing can be demonstrated particularly well in choice reaction experiments. It is not surprising that in the past an extremely large number of experiments of this type were performed. It is impossible to discuss them all within the scope of this volume. We limit ourselves to the description of several results which are little known in the English literature on this subject.

In an extensive study by Schmidtke (1960), the effect of training and fatigue on the reaction time in choice reaction situations was investigated. This study was different from the early experiments of Merkel (1885), Hick (1952) and Hyman (1953), regarding the number of choice alternatives which varied between 2 and 36. The experiments confirmed Merkel's findings that there is a relationship between the reaction time and the logarithm of the number of possible choice reactions. However, this relationship holds only as long as the subjects are not trained in choice reactions. After they have arrived at a training plateau so that there is no further progress in learning during successive experiments, the relationship is entirely different. With few choice alternatives (about 8), the difference of reaction time in untrained and trained conditions is small, but with increasing number of choice alternatives the difference between the start and end of training values increases. Intensive mental work (alternating 30 min. periods of Düker's concentration test and an inspection test similar to Bourdon's) over a period of four hours produces an effect corresponding to a pronounced loss of training (Fig. 10-4). However, the reaction times with a small (2-6) number of choice alternatives show, after four hours of mental work, only slight differences from those measured in the first phase of training without proceeding work. Therefore, it appears unlikely that the fatigue produced in mental work has any effect on the muscular contraction or neural conduction times, because in fatigue longer reaction times than in fresh condition should be expected also with a small number of choice alternatives. If, on the other hand, at a large number of choice alternatives the reaction times after mental work increase to an extent that they approach the times at the beginning of training, it must be concluded that the prolongation is located in the opto-motive information centers, i.e. in the centers of information processes, provided that possible receptor fa-

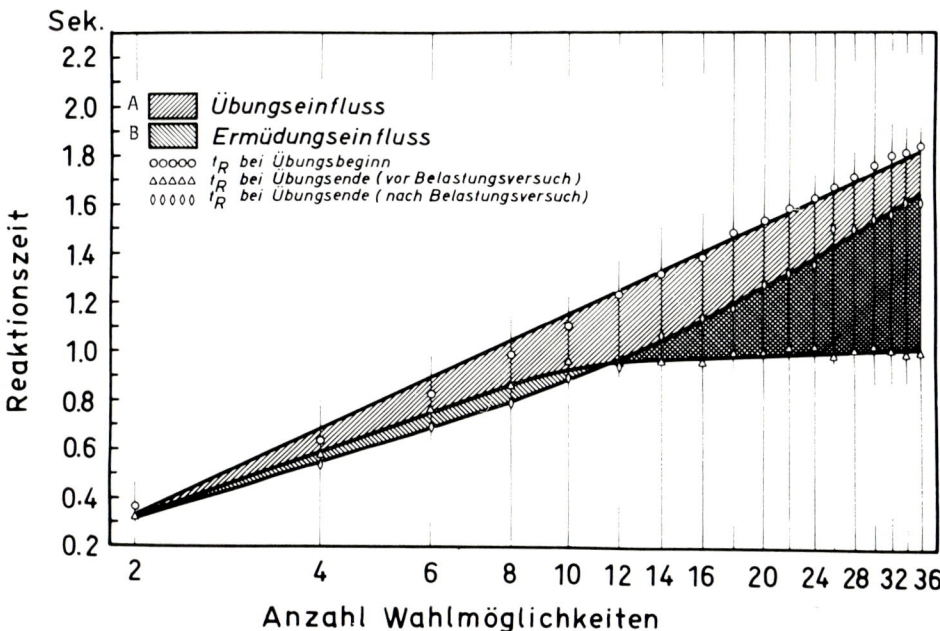

Figure 10-4. Effect of training and fatigue on choice reaction time. A—Effect of training; B—Effect of fatigue; ooooo—Start of training; ΔΔΔ—End of training before load; 000 —End of training after load; Abscissa—number of choices; Ordinate—Reaction time (sec.). From Schmidtke.

tigue can be ruled out. Therefore, the hypothesis was proposed that the effect of training, shortening of the reaction time, is lost more and more in central fatigue, i.e. mental fatigue is equivalent to a loss of training.

Babadschanjan, et al. (1960) arrived at similar conclusions from choice reaction time experiments with strenuous mental load in railroad employees. Their subjects had to select a critical color hue out of five different blue hues, moving behind a slit, and press a lever on its appearance before and after a work shift of 12 hours. With this experimental procedure, the speed of reaction, the reaction time, and the errors could be measured. A significant increase of errors (missing reactions or reactions to a false hue) was observed after the work, as well as a prolongation of the latent period and reaction time. Table 10-I shows a condensation of some of Babadschanjan's, et al., results. The pronounced prolongation of the choice reaction time speaks for massive disturbance of information processing and obviously a high degree of mental fatigue as a result of the prolonged work.

In his investigations on mental load problems Kalsbeek (1964, 1965, 1967) thoroughly investigated the effect of work duration on mental performance capacity. In binary choice reaction situations with motor re-

TABLE 10-I

PROLONGATION OF LATENT PERIOD AND REACTION TIME AFTER
12 HOURS WORK OF TRAIN ENGINEERS

Subjects	Latent Period Before Work	After Work	Reaction Time Before Work	After Work
S-n	0.188 sec	0.289 sec	0.311 sec	0.682 sec
K-ow	0.108 sec	0.350 sec	0.250 sec	0.648 sec
M-ing	0.134 sec	0.148 sec	0.362 sec	0.503 sec

Recalculated from M. G. Babadschanjan, et al., "Isutschenije pritschin utomljajemosti dispetscherow," in A. A. Letaweta, and S. A. Kosilowa, *Materialü k fisiologitscheskomy obosnowaniju trudowüch prozessow* (Moskau, Medgis, 1960) p. 154.

sponses of highly trained subjects to visual or auditory signals, there were differences in the performance dependent on the prolongation of the work time, with the use of a quality criterion (maximum of 3 errors per experiment). During a time of only 3 minutes, 76 ± 7.2 signals could be processed. However, with an experimental time of 4 hours the maximum rate of processing dropped to 20 signals/min. (Fig. 10-5), if the quality criterion was fulfilled over the total experimental time. Obviously, a quite uniform tendency in the results of all choice reaction time experiments can be noted:

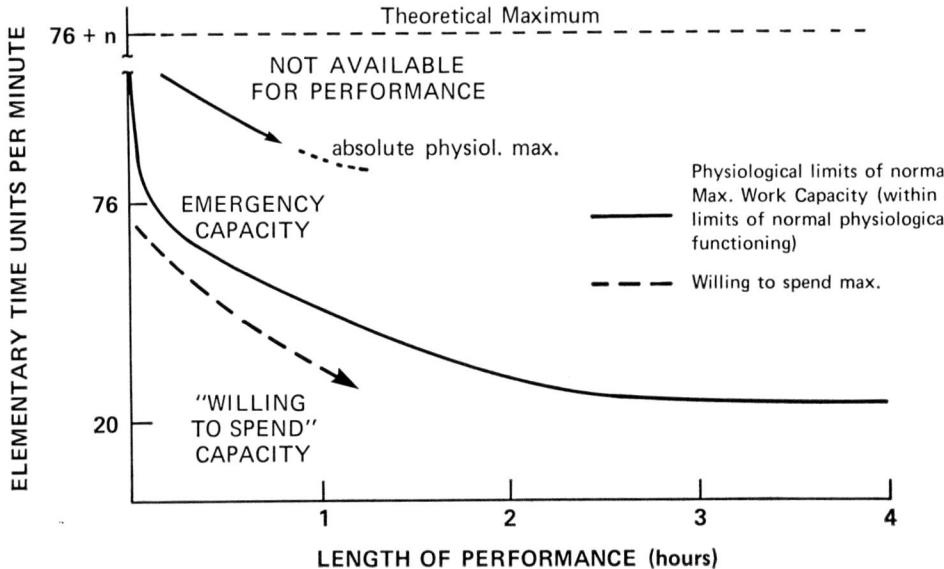

Figure 10-5. Diagram of maximal mental capacity, expressed in elementary time units/min. i.e. minimal lapse of time needed to organize an output in a binary choice task (From J. W. H. Kalsbeek, and J. H. Ettema; "Physiological and Psychological Evaluation of Distraction Stress," Proceedings of 2nd Int Congress on Ergonomics, Dortmund 1964, Supplement to *Ergonomics*, 443).

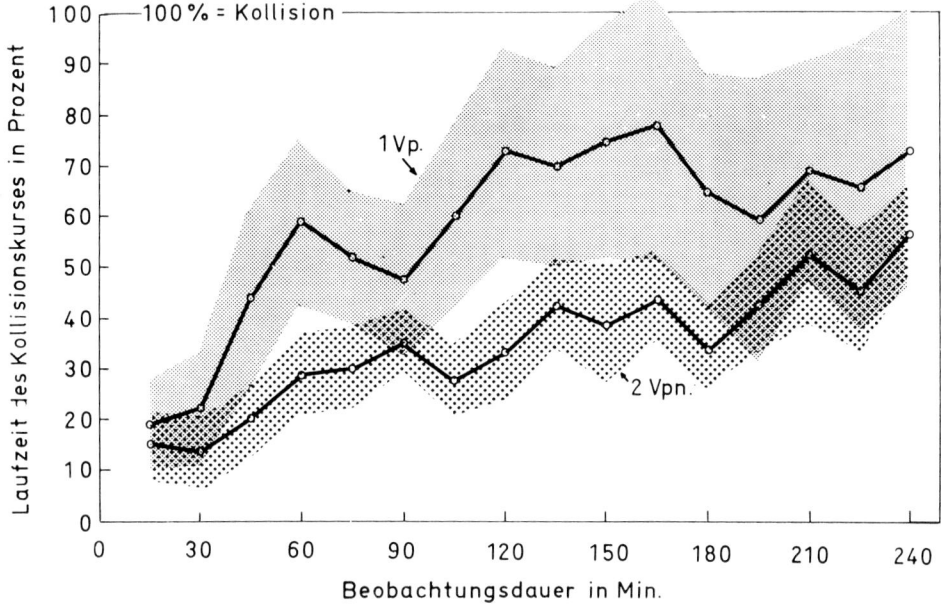

Figure 10-6. Effect of observation time (min.) (abscissa) on recognition of collision course (in percent) (ordinate) in single (upper tracing) and group experiments (lower tracing) (From Schmidtke).

with increases in work time and mental strain, there is a decrease in the number of information units that can be correctly processed.

Tasks with a high content of decision-making, for instance, are involved in radar control of air traffic or coastal navigation. In a traffic situation requiring observation by trained observers of about 25 objects on a radar screen for possible collision courses, a significant deterioration of performance had occurred after a relatively short time (Fig. 10-6). The recognition of collision courses involves a sequence of connected reactions: recognition of a possible danger situation, marking of echoes on the screen for time t_o, plotting for a somewhat later time t_1, determination of the course for both objects, measurement of the distances between t_o and t_1 for both objects, calculation of the respective speeds, and finally the decision based on the course and speeds of both objects, whether there is a risk of collision. Obviously, disturbance on any place in the sequence of actions may result in decision error or loss of precious time, thus interfering with performance. It is characteristic for these experimental results (Schmidtke, 1966), that with increasing duration of work the mean performance time slows down considerably along with increasing variability. Even after a work duration of several hours, however, there are always interspersed periods with relatively fast reactions. Nevertheless, there is an increasing frequency of entirely missed danger situations, or delayed reactions so that the effect of course correction would have been questionable. It is of interest that a work organization with two parallel tasks by two observers on two identical radar screens largely eliminates these fatigue effects.

Not only mental loads produce disturbance in the information processing. Physical loads also may play an interfering role. For instance, Behr (1970) showed that with increasing load in severe dynamic work (expressed in terms of kpm/sec. or excess pulse rate per min. over the resting level) the performance in a binary decision test drops progressively. According to Figure 10-7 the decline of performance increases with the number of decisions per minute. However, there are also numerous indications of a reversed U-form relationship between muscular exertion and mental performance (Courts, 1939; Shore, 1958; Eason and White, 1961; Eason, 1963; Eason and Branks, 1963; Burgess and Hokanson, 1964; Doerr and Hokanson, 1965;

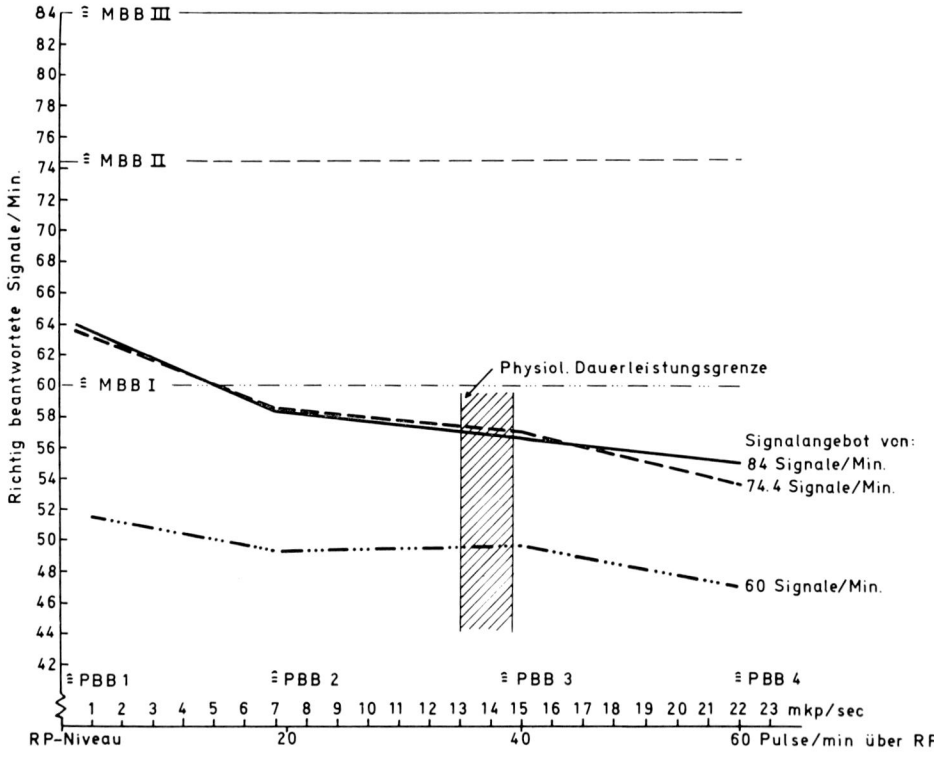

Figure 10-7. Effect of physical exertion on mental work (From E. Behr, *Beitrag zur Untersuchung der mentalen Leistungsfähigkeit bei definierter physischer Belastung.* München, Diss, 1970. Correct responses per min.; ordinate) at different rate of signals (84, 74.4, 60 signals per min.: MBB III, II, I) and at different circulatory load, MBB = degree of mental load, PBB = degree of physical load, RP = resting pulse rate (abscissa) Upper margin of straited column: Physiological limit for prolonged work.

Wood and Hokanson, 1965). Such relationship would speak for an increase of the activity level of the organism in light work, with a secondary favorable effect on the mental work capacity, whereas heavy work results, possibly through hyperactivation or inadequate cerebral oxygen supply, in disturbance of the decision processes. Possible cerebral ischemia in fatigue in heavy work is discussed in the section "Ischemic Fatigue" in *Physiology of Work Capacity and Fatigue*. There is no evidence of cerebral ischemia in moderately heavy work, but some indirect evidence is suggestive of cerebral ischemia in severe dynamic work such as running to exhaustion.

REGULATION OF SOCIAL BEHAVIOR

Closely related to, though not identical with the processing of information, are processes of regulation of social behavior. After intensive mental load not only a certain carelessness in regard to errors can be observed (Davis, 1946) but also disturbances of behavior in some ways similar to expansive hypomanic phenomena and to progressive disinhibition in alcohol intoxication. For example, the experiments with sleep deprivation of Eagles, Halliday and Redfearn (1953) and of Tyler (1955) as well as extensive military experiences have shown that after prolonged work, the slow development of general fatigue in man leads to unmotivated foolishness as well as to lack of discipline both in regard to their own safety and behavior to superiors. Even with children, frequent and unmotivated laughing, changing quickly to defiance reaction, may be interpreted as a symptom of fatigue. Observing children at play during the day, provided they have reached the respective play age and sufficient toys are available, it can be noticed that they cooperate intensively and harmoniously so that they are oblivious to the environment. With increasing fatigue in the late afternoon the picture changes radically. The previously smooth social contact deteriorates increasingly with appearance of egocentric tendencies in some, and of increasingly crude behavior in others. These social tendencies terminate in fights with dissolution of the play group.

However, the social contacts suffer also in adults in fatigue and external stress. Thus, one of the authors (Schmidtke, 1973) was able to demonstrate that in a group of 4 subjects working as a team in intense heat (mean effective room temperature 32°C), there was an increasing frequency of social offenses (Fig. 10-8) such as disturbances of behavior resulting in quarrels or cursing between two or more members of the team. Inadequate regulation of social behavior is probably related to inadequately functioning decision processes. In case of disturbance of information processing by fatigue, exaggerated affective or undisciplined behavioral reactions may appear in the field of social interactions interfering with the inter-individual communication. If this hypothesis is correct, a planned fatigue prophylaxis

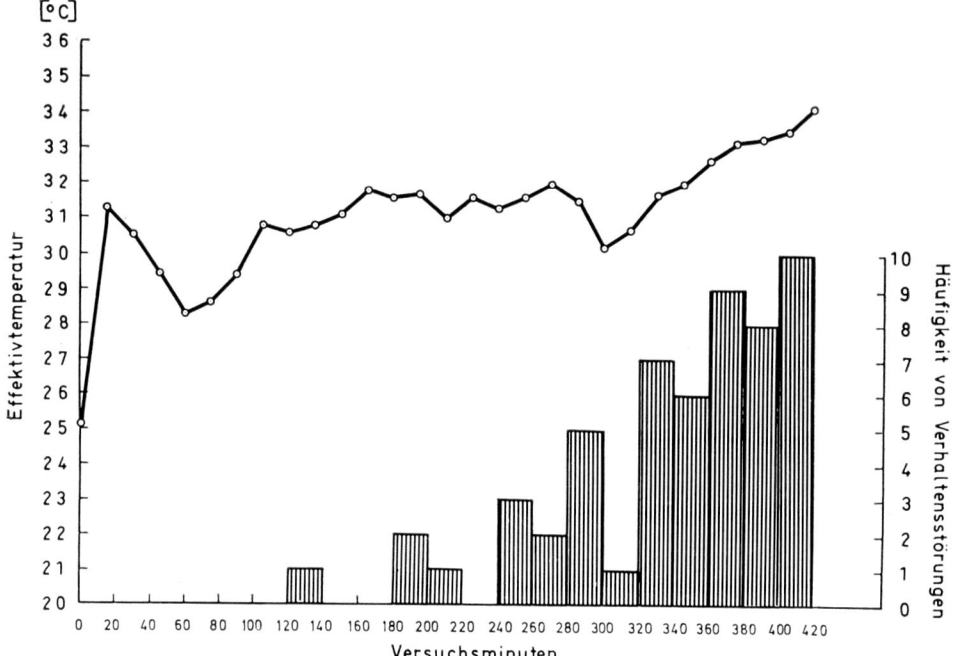

Figure 10-8. Effect of working time (abscissa) and climate stress, effective temperature (left ordinate) on frequency of disturbances of social behavior (right ordinate) (From H. Schmidtke, "Mentale Beanspruchung," in H. Schmidtke, *Ergonomie I*, München, 1973).

should not only result in improvement of the individual work capacity, but also should contribute to decrease the avoidable tensions and frustrations in the inter-individual relationship.

In a summarizing conclusion, it can be stated: it may not be justifiably certain that the disturbances of social behavior are related to disturbances in the processing of information. It is certain, however, that these two phenomena are not independent. Therefore, we feel that it is justified to discuss these types of disturbances within this part.

BIBLIOGRAPHY

Amberg, E.: Über den Einfluß von Arbeitspausen auf die geistige Leistungsfähigkeit. *Psychol Arbeiten*, 1:300, 1896.

Aschaffenburg, G.: Experimentelle Studien über Assoziationen II. *Psychol Arbeiten*, 2:1, 1899.

Babadschanjan, M. G., W. N. Sokolowa, J. I. Kostina, M. I. Mamazaschwili, and W. J. Tschirkow: Isutschenije pritschin utomljajemosti dispetscherow. In Letaweta, A. A., and S. A. Kosilowa: *Materialü k fisiologitscheskomu obosnowaniju trudowüch prozessow*. Moskau, Medgis, 1960, 154.

Bäumler, G.: *Statistische, experimentelle und theoretische Beiträge zur Frage der Blockierungen bei fortlaufenden Reaktionstätigkeiten.* Würzburg, Diss, 1967.

Behr, E.: *Beitrag zur Untersuchung der mentalen Leistungsfähigkeit bei definierter physischer Belastung.* München, Diss, 1970.

Bills, A. G.: Blocking: a new principle of mental fatigue. *Am J Psychol, 43*:230, 1931.

Broadbent, D. E.: The twenty dials test under quiet conditions. *Medical Research Council A.P.U. Report, 130,* 1950.

Broadbent, D. E.: A mechanical model for human attention and immediate memory. *Psychol Rev, 64*:205, 1957.

Burgess, M., and J. E. Hokanson: Effects of increased heart rate on intellectual performance. *J Abnorm Soc Psychol, 68*:85, 1964.

Courts, F. A.: Relations between experimentally induced muscular tension and memorisation. *J Exp Psychol, 25*:235, 1939.

Davis, D. R.: The disorganization of behaviour in fatigue. *J Neurol Neurosurg Psychiatry, 9*:23, 1946.

Doerr, H. O., and J. E. Hokanson: A relation between heart rate and performance in children. *J Pers Soc Psychol, 2*:70, 1965.

Düker, H.: Psychologische Untersuchungen über freie und zwangsläufige Arbeit. *Z Psychol Erg-Band, 20,* 1931.

Düker, H.: Über die Ablenkungsmöglichkeit bei freier und zwangsläufiger Arbeitsweise. *Arch f d ges Psychol, 92*:141, 1934.

Eagles, J. B., A. M. Halliday, and J. W. T. Redfearn: The effects of fatigue on tremor. In Floyd, W. F., and A. T. Welford (Eds.): *Symposium on Fatigue.* London, 1953.

Eason, R. G.: Relation between effort, tension level, skill and performance efficiency in a perceptual-motor-task. *Percept Mot Skills, 16*:297, 1963.

Eason, R. G., and C. T. White: Muscular tension, effort and tracking difficulty: Studies of parameters which affect level tension and performance efficiency. *Percept Mot Skills, 12*:331, 1961.

Eason, R. G., and J. Branks: Effect of level of activation on the quality and efficiency of performance of verbal and motor tasks. *Percept Mot Skills, 16*:525, 1963.

Graf, O.: Über lohnendste Arbeitspausen bei geistiger Arbeit. *Psychol Arbeiten, 7*:548, 1922.

Hernandez-Peon, R., H. Scherrer, and M. Jouvet: Modification of electric activity in cochlear nucleus during "Attention" in unanaesthetized cats. *Science, 123*:331, 1956.

Heumann, G.: Über die Beziehung zwischen Arbeitsdauer und Pausenwirkung. *Psychol Arbeiten, 4*:538, 1904.

Hick, E. E.: On the rate of gain of information. *Q J Exp Psychol, 4*:11, 1952.

Hylan, J. P., and E. Kraepelin: Über die Wirkung kurzer Arbeitszeiten. *Psychol Arbeiten, 4*:454, 1904.

Hyman, R.: Stimulus information as a determinant of reaction time. *J Exp Psychol, 45*: 188, 1953.

Kalsbeek, J. W. H.: Mesure objective de la surcharge mentale. *Le travail humain,* XXVIII: 121, 1965.

Kalsbeek, J. W. H.: *Mentale Belasting.* Assen, 1967.

Kalsbeek, J. W. H., and J. H. Ettema: Physiological and psychological evaluation of distraction stress. Proceedings of 2nd Intern. Congress on Ergonomics, Dortmund 1964, Supplement to *Ergonomics,* 443.

Lashley, K. S.: The experimental analysis of instinctive behavior. *Psychol Rev, 45*:445, 1938.

Merkel, J.: Die zeitlichen Verhältnisse der Willenstätigkeit. *Philos Studien, 2*:73, 1885.

Miller, J. G.: Information input overload and psychopathology. *Am J Psychiatr, 116*:695, 1960.

Miller, J. G.: Sensory overloading. In Flaherty, B. (Ed.): *Psychophysiological Aspects of Space Flight.* New York, Columbia U Pr, 1961.

Pauli R.: Der Umfang und die Enge des Bewußtseins. *Z Biol, 81*:93, 1924.

Pauli, R.: Beiträge zur Kenntnis der Arbeitskurve. *Arch ges Psychol, 97*:465, 1936.

Rivers, W. H. R., und E. Kraepelin: Über Ermüdung und Erholung. *Psychol Arbeiten 1*:627, 1896.

Schmidtke, H.: *Psychologie der Ermüdung.* Kiel, Habilitationsschrift, 1960.

Schmidtke, H.: Untersuchungen über den Erholungszeitbedarf bei psychisch beanspruchender Tätigkeit. In *Arbeitsstudien heute und morgen.* Verband für Arbeitsstudien REFA. Berlin/Köln/Frankfurt, 1963.

Schmidtke, H.: *Die Ermüdung, Symptome—Theorien—Messversuche.* Bern/Stuttgart, 1965.

Schmidtke, H.: *Leistungsbeeinflussende Faktoren im Radar-Beobachtungsdienst.* Köln-Opladen, 1966.

Schmidtke, H.: Mentale Beanspruchung. In Schmidtke, H. (Ed.): *Ergonomie I.* München, 1973.

Sherrington, C. S.: Über das Zusammenwirken der Rückenmarksreflexe und das Prinzip der gemeinsamen Endstrecke. *Ergebn Physiol, 4*:797, 1905.

Shore, M. F.: Perceptual efficiency as related to induced muscular effort and manifest anxiety. *J Exp Psychol, 55*:179, 1958.

Tyler, D. B.: Psychological changes during experimental sleep deprivation. *Dis Nerv Syst, 16*:2, 1955.

Voss, G. von: Über die Schwankungen der geistigen Arbeitsleistung. *Psychol Arbeiten, 2*:399, 1899.

Wood, C. G., and J. E. Hokanson: Effects of induced muscular tension on performance and the inverted U-function. *J Pers Soc Psychol, 1*:506, 1965.

SECTION FIVE
AGING

Introduction

ERNST SIMONSON

As was pointed out in the Introduction there is no sharp dividing line between physiological and psychological aspects of work and fatigue. Therefore, the information on psychological aspects of age trends in performance as presented in the following chapter, should be viewed in context with the much larger body of information on the effect of age on physiological functions involved in work capacity and fatigue as discussed at length in Chapter 16 and several other chapters of the preceding volume *(PWCF)*.

First of all, the decline of work capacity for moderate and heavy physical work with age is reflected in the decrease of max V_{O_2}, in the maximum attainable heart rate and cardiac stroke volume, in slower recovery after work, and in hormonal and physicochemical changes. With the decrease of max V_{O_2}, there is also a decreased reserve capacity for moderate work. However, it is unlikely that the age related deterioration of functions involved in oxygen transport will affect fatigue in light physical or mental work. In a tabulation *(PWCF*, Table 65, p. 432) summarizing the work of various authors, it was shown that decrease of performance with age occurs mainly in types of jobs with sizable physical effort largely dependent on the integrity of the cardiovascular system.

In light physical, sedentary or mental work, there are two fundamental age related processes that affect CNS functions and therefore performance: loss of neural cells and cerebral atherosclerosis. Decrease of active cell mass in the CNS is amply documented (Andrew, 1960; Brody, 1955; Ellis, 1920) and also probably extends to the retina (Simonson, et al., 1967). Coronary atherosclerosis is widespread in the clinically healthy population, increasing with age, as shown in large scale autopsy studies (Clawson, 1941; Lober, 1953). There is some evidence that asymptomatic cerebral atherosclerosis may be as common as coronary atherosclerosis with some correlation between these localizations (Simonson and McGavach, 1964).

The incidence of "ischemic" responses (S-T depression) to exercise, indicating myocardial ischemia, increases with age in apparently healthy people *(PWCF*, Chapter 12, p. 299).

There is little direct information available relating the decrease of active cell mass in CNS and skeletal muscle to age related deterioration in performance. An exception is the decrease of muscle strength with age, well documented for 150 years. In this connection, it should be pointed out that in many types of work the effect of age is minor (see *PWCF*); the deterioration of performance occurs mainly in types of strenuous physical or mental work.

Table V-I shows a striking parallelism between the decrease of the fusion frequency of flicker (FFF) and the decrease of the cerebral flow as determined with Kety's method (1955). This is not necessarily a causal relationship, but implies that decrease of the cerebral blood flow is most likely involved in the drop of the FFF, which has been used in numerous fatigue studies (see Chap. 7). It was shown earlier that the FFF is decreased in circulatory insufficiency probably due to secondary cerebral ischemia (Enzer and Simonson, 1942). Therefore, the effect of age and of fatigue on the FFF is synergistic, i.e. the FFF of an older subject in fresh condition may be similar to the FFF in a younger subject after fatigue.

The same relationship between age and fatigue applies also to other functional tests. Most of the psychological investigations of fatigue trends during work have been performed in younger subjects. From the material reviewed in the following chapter, it may be inferred that in numerous work situations the older persons start work at a lower functional level. It is not certain, however, that the functional changes during work are greater in older workers.

Simonson and Anderson (1966) compared the performance in strenuous mental work (Düker's test, level D: additions and subtractions with memorizing sub-totals) performed for an hour, in thirty-seven young, healthy men (mean age 25.1, Group A), thirty-eight older men (mean age 52.2 years, Group B) and thirty-eight ambulatory patients with coronary heart disease but without evidence of acute coronary insufficiency (mean 58.3 years, Group C). The number of correct problems in five minute periods averaged 30.1, 26.1 and 17.0 for Groups A, B, and C, respectively and the number of errors was 5.96 percent (A), 7.33 percent (B), and 11.87 percent (C). The continuum of declining performance from Group A to C is compatible with cerebral atherosclerosis, minimum in Group A, increasing with age in Group B and pronounced in Group C with documented coronary sclerosis.

TABLE V-I

CHANGES OF CEREBRAL BLOOD FLOW AND FLICKER FUSION FREQUENCY WITH AGE*

Function	Average at Age					
	20	30	40	50	60	70
Cerebral blood flow (Kety, 1955)	60.0	− 6	−10	−12	−14	−16
Flicker fusion frequency	46.0	− 1.3	− 2.8	− 4.5	− 5.8	− 9.0

* Average of various authors. Simonson, et al., 1941; Brozek and Keys, 1945; Misiak, 1947; Simonson and Brozek, 1952; Coppinger, 1955.

Abrahams and Birren (1973) compared simple and choice reaction time of twenty-four clinically healthy men (Group A, mean age 39.7 years), and twenty-four clinically healthy men, but with high coronary risk (Group B, mean age 40.7 years). The simple as well as the choice reaction time was significantly longer in Group B. Coronary risk factors have been well established in larger epidemiological studies on an international scale (as example: A. Keys, 1970). It is quite certain that asymptomatic coronary sclerosis, and most likely also cerebral atherosclerosis was more advanced in Group B. This agrees well with earlier results by Spieth (1965) who studied psychomotor performance in 600 men from 23 to 54 years, subdivided into six categories based on cardiovascular health status. Subjects with coronary heart disease (CHD) or arterial hypertension had significantly poorer scores than healthy men of the same age. More specifically, the subjects with CHD were slower in the decision phase of a complex reaction time test rather than in the movement phase. The slowing of psychomotor performance has a parallel to the slower adaptation of pulmonary cardiovascular functions in physical work (Frolkis, V. V., and Muravov, I. V., 1965; Volkov, S. M., 1965; Sokolov, K. T., 1965). Spieth suggested that the deterioration of psychomotor performance with age is probably due to disease processes (mainly atherosclerosis) related to age rather than to age itself.

If cerebral atherosclerosis is a major factor affecting work performance in older people, training in physical exercise may be beneficial for types of sedentary mental work as it is for physical work. The beneficial effect of exercise in the prevention and rehabilitation of patients is well documented but the large literature is outside the scope of this volume. In physical exercise, the systolic blood pressure increases without an increase of the diastolic blood pressure which improves the cerebral blood flow (Naumenko and Benua, 1970). Obviously, this is an area for further research of theoretical and practical interest.

In view of the decrease of physical work capacity and of neural cell mass and the increased prevalence of cerebral atherosclerosis with aging, the following chapter by Lehr and Thomae will study the question of the role of aging on altering work capacity and the experience of fatigue.

BILIOGRAPHY

Abrahams, J. P., and J. E. Birren: Reaction time as a function of age and behavioral predisposition to coronary heart disease. *J Gerontol, 28:*471, 1973.

Andrew, W.: Anatomic changes with age. In Johnson, W. J. (Ed.): *The Older Patient.* New York, Harper, 1960, pp. 8-42.

Brody, H.: Organization of the cerebral cortex. *J Comp Neurol, 102:*511, 1955.

Clawson, B. J.: Incidence of types of heart disease among 30,265 autopsies, with special reference to age and sex. *Am Heart J, 22:*607, 1941.

Ellis, R. S.: Norms for some structural changes in the human cerebellum from birth to old age. *J Comp Neurol, 32:*1, 1920.
Enzer, N., E. Simonson, and S. S. Blankstein: Fatigue of patients with circulatory insufficiency investigated by means of the fusion frequency of flicker. *Ann Intern Med, 16:*701, 1942.
Frolkis, V. V., and Muravov, I. V.: Physiological analysis of the effect of muscular activity on the aging organism. In *Fizicheskaya Kultura Istochnik Dolgoletiya* (Physical Culture—The Source of Longevity). Moscow, Fizkultura i Sport, 1965, p. 24 (Russ).
Kety, S. S., and C. F. Schmidt: N_2O method for the quantitative determination of cerebral blood flow in man. Theory, procedure and normal values. *J Clin Invest, 27:*476, 1948.
Keys, A.: Coronary heart disease in seven countries. *Am Heart Assoc Monograph Number 29,* 1970.
Lober, P. H.: Pathogenesis of coronary sclerosis. *AMA Arch Path, 55:*357, 1953.
Naumenko, A. I., and N. N. Benua: In Brozek, J., and Simonson, E. (Eds.): *The Physiological Mechanisms of Cerebral Blood Circulation.* Springfield, Thomas, 1970, pp. 123.
Simonson, E., and D. A. Anderson: Effect of age and coronary heart disease on performance and physiological responses in mental work. *7th International Congress of Gerontology,* Vienna, Austria, June 26-July 2, 1966, pp. 333-336.
Simonson, E., D. Anderson, and C. Keiper: Effect of stimulus movement on critical flicker fusion in young and older men. *J Gerontol, 22:*353, 1967.
Simonson, E., and McGavack, Th. (Eds.): *Cerebral Ischemia.* Springfield, Thomas, 1964, pp. xi-xviii.
Sokolov, K. T.: (Physiological characteristics of adaptation of pulmonary function in the aging organism.) In *Fizicheskaya Kultura Istochnik Dolgoletiya* (Physical Culture—The Source of Longevity). Moscow, Fizkultura i Sport, 1965, p. 120 (Russ).
Spieth, S.: Slowness of task performance and cardiovascular diseases. In Welford, A. T., and Birren, J. E. (Eds.): *Behavior, Aging and The Nervous System.* Springfield, Thomas, 1965.
Volkov, S. M.: Physiological analysis of adaptation to periodic endurance exercise in old age. In *Fizicheskaya Kultura Istochnik Dolgoletiya* (Physical Culture—The Source of Longevity). Moscow, Fizkultura i Sport, 1965, p. 79 (Russ).

Chapter 11

Effect of Age on Work: Psychological Aspects

URSULA LEHR and HANS THOMAE

ONE OF THE SECTIONS of the 1971 White House Conference on Aging blamed the present society for the fact that "many barriers hamper older Americans in exercising their choice in alloting time and talents and deprive our nation of the highest use of their knowledge, skills and potentialities" (1971 White House Conference on Aging, pp. 11-12).

The reason for this is defined in recommendation No. IV of this section: "Our society presently equates employability with chronological age rather than ability to perform the job" (White House Conference on Aging, p. 13).

The similarity of the situation of the older employee in most industrial countries is demonstrated by a semiofficial German publication on problems of the elderly worker commenting on OECD policies regarding this group. It compares the growing efficiency of modern machines with the decreasing ability of the elderly employee who is not able to keep abreast of the speed of innovations (Deutsche Gesellschaft für Personalführung, 1972, p. 13).

More and more management policies are guided by the opinion that flexibility in thinking is lost with 40 or even with 35 years of age (Güttich, 1969).

Actually, however, personnel managers and public policies which take a general age-bound decrease in ability for granted are not up to date as far as research on abilities in old age are concerned. The hypothesis of a general deficit in abilities with increasing age, especially in middle age (up to 65 years), had to be revised due to more careful analysis of the many factors which contribute to achievement (Koyl, 1972; Lehr, Dreher and Schmitz-Scherzer, 1970; Lehr, 1972; Nesselroade, Schaie, and Baltes, 1972; Thomae and Lehr, 1973).

MENTAL ABILITIES

The earliest psychological studies on the changes of intelligence in different age groups started in the twenties. Miles and Miles (1932), and Miles (1934), as well as Jones and Conrad (1933), concluded from their cross sectional studies that a considerable decrease in mental abilities exists even during the third decade of human life.

Since 1950, however, this age curve of mental abilities was replaced by findings pointing to the varieties of factors contributing to changes in intelligence of people of different age groups.

Schaie (1965), Baltes (1968), and others, pointed to the misleading conclusions drawn from cross sectional studies which confound age and cohort effects. One of the major cohort effects which contributes to large age differences is related to *education* and *socioeconomic* status. Many of these differences disappear or become minor if we compare persons of different age with education held constant (Granick and Friedman, 1967; Green, 1969; Nehrke, 1972). As chances for higher education were less, e.g. for the age cohorts born in 1870 to 1900 than for those born in 1930 and 1950, a high proportion of variance in the comparison of different age groups is explained by education. Birren and Morrison (1961) and Rudinger (1974) demonstrated this; the latter found in a study on 670 subjects from different social backgrounds (20-88 years of age). A variance of 23 percent of the scores of the Wechsler Intelligence Test was explained in this sample by education, compared to 11.8 percent explained by age.

Socioeconomic status (SES) defined by *occupational status* is another variable which interacts with age in the determination of differences in mental abilities. Vernon (1947) demonstrated that decline in mental ability is found especially in persons employed in routine, monotonous work. Those who were challenged by this work situation with regard to flexibility and alertness, proved to be more able than younger persons (see also Glanzer and Glaser, 1958).

Welford (1959, 1968) explains findings like these by an "occupational transfer effect" which makes knowledge and competence trained within the job, available also for the solution of other problems. Many writers formulate a "disuse hypothesis" regarding the job situation and facilities for mental training (Berkowitz and Green, 1965).

Some of the major contributions to the revision of the "age deficit model of mental abilities" came from longitudinal studies. Owens (1953, 1966) as well as Terman and Oden (1947, 1959), showed that persons with higher intelligence scores at a first test during their school or college years remain very consistent or even rise in their mental capacities. Some people believe that hereditary factors contribute to this. However, social class and educational as well as occupational factors influence this outcome to a high degree.

Health is another major factor in the determination of mental capacity (Botwinick and Birren, 1963; Rudinger and Erlemeier, 1969; Rudinger, 1971; Birren and Spieth, 1962). Healthy older people achieve the same scores as younger people, whereas sick persons show age bound decrements. Simonson and Anderson (1966) showed a close connection between coronary disease and performance in a concentration test (Düker, 1949). This test required the subject to solve arithmetical problems (addition, subtraction) for one hour. While there is a smaller difference in the scores of younger and older men, a significance difference exists between the scores of older men with and without symptoms of coronary disease. Especially from studies on institutionization, we know that the *degree of stimulation* by the environment is an important variable in the maintenance or even rehabilitation of mental capacities. From these findings we may conclude that ecological conditions of various kinds contribute to variance in intelligence scores, at least to the same degree as age (see Lehr, 1972).

As far as age related changes exist, they are related to different aspects of intelligence to a different degree. General information or vocabulary are more consistent than speed-bound performance tests. "Crystallized" intelligence (as defined by information, experience and verbal capacities) is regarded by Horn and Cattell (1966) as invariant or even increasing with age, whereas, "fluid intelligence" (as defined by flexibility and fast processing of information) shows more decline. Welford and Birren (1965) feel that this decrease in information processing should be defined as the "primary process of aging" which has to be regarded only as one of many influences on consistency and change in mental abilities during the life span.

To summarize, we may state that research on differences of mental abilities at different age levels demonstrates the multidimensional structure of consistency and change of mental abilities during the life span. Age itself contributes to these changes at a lower degree than education, SES and health.

LEARNING

One of the major complaints of elderly people and/or their families relates to losses in learning ability and memory. As far as experimental research is concerned, it could be demonstrated that older persons are less effective in learning nonsense material (e.g. nonsense syllables), whereas there exists almost no age difference in capacity of storage of meaningful and well structured material. Very often elderly persons are less able to code input, especially under conditions of limited time. Information which is too complex or presented too fast has more negative effects on older than on younger subjects. Sometimes the poorer performance of the aged in learning tests is due to insecurity and anxiety. Younger persons are more ready to take a "risk" in their responses to stimuli and to give answers even if they are not sure about their correctness (see Lehr, 1972, pp. 88-94).

Breaks during the training period result in improvement of learning in younger subjects and in impairment of learning in older subjects. This shows that learning processes in older subjects are more exposed to effects of interference. On the other hand, there are indications that part-learning is more favorable for younger subjects and learning in whole is more favorable for older subjects. Generally, however, the effects of education,

SES, occupational experience, learning motivation, and health are more important for learning than chronological age.

A summary of the various findings of experimental studies on age-learning relationships has to include at least the following items:

1. Older subjects are poorer in learning nonsense material (syllables, figures); there are minor or no differences between older and younger when learning of meaningful material is required (Preobrazhenskaya, 1966; Ruch, 1934; Korchin and Basowitz, 1957; Zaretsky and Halberstam, 1968).
2. Older subjects very often have a poorer learning technique (coding ability) which can be improved. Therefore, age decrements in learning very often can be compensated (Hulicka and Grossman, 1967; Craik, 1968).
3. If learning material is presented too quickly, older subjects are affected more than younger ones. If speed of performance is eliminated, age differences are leveled.
4. Practice increases learning in the same degree in younger and older subjects. However, the amount of learning after the first trials is greater in younger subjects; therefore, older ones need more time to attain the same level as younger ones (Roth, 1961b).
5. Very often poorer performance of older subjects in learning tasks is related to emotional problems like anxiety, rather than to ability. Feelings of insecurity can inhibit the ability to recall or verbalize (Eisdorfer, 1965).
6. Structuration and ordering of learning materials assists older people more than younger ones, especially if a higher degree of complexity is involved (Kay, 1955).
7. Breaks during the learning period are favorable for younger subjects, but unfavorable for older subjects (Downs, 1965; Roth, 1961a).
8. Very often ability rather than age is decisive for changes in learning capacity (Keevil-Rogers and Schnorre, 1969).
9. Training (continuous education) is an important factor in the maintenance of learning abilities during the years of adulthood and old age (Crovitz, 1966; Olechowsky, 1969).
10. Health is a decisive factor in the determination of consistency and change of learning abilities (Birren, Botwinick, et al., 1963; Hulicka, 1967).
11. Activity and motivational factors are major determinants of learning during the whole life span (Löwe, 1968, 1971). They are very often affected in an adverse manner by the situation of adult and aged subjects (Löwe, 1968, 1969, 1970, 1971).

PSYCHOMOTOR SKILLS

Psychomotor skills are defined by Welford (1959) as acquired patterns of integrated and coordinated movements which respond to certain stimuli or signals. Input of stimuli or information, information processing, and the response itself are the main variables involved here. According to Welford (1959, 1968), in studies on these behavioral aspects, a "primary process of aging" becomes evident, which is especially defined by decreasing speed of information processing and response. Sometimes, however, a correlation exists between slower speed and higher accuracy of the work. This leads to the formula: elderly workers perform at a slower speed but more accurately; younger subjects work faster but less accurately.

This statement is no longer valid according to some more recent findings. As in learning, degree of complexity of the task is also an important intervening variable in psychomotor tests. Greater complexity affects the performance of the older subjects in an adverse manner, whereas, this is not true for less complex tasks. If restructuring of the situation is required, time and errors increase with increasing age (Kay, 1954, 1955).

Another major intervening variable again is health. Abrahams and Birren (1973) compared simple reaction time and multiple choice reaction time of healthy men with low versus respectively high risk of later coronary disease. Both reaction times were significantly longer in the last group.

Simonson (1974) concludes that impairment of blood supply due to coronary or cerebral asymptomatic atherosclerosis is one of the main reasons for decreasing performance with increasing age, even in apparently healthy subjects.

Especially important are those findings which are related to the differentiation of pre-motor and motor time (Talland, 1964, 1968; Botwinick and Thompson, 1966, 1968). "Pre-motor time" is the period required for the cognition of the situation (from onset of signal to the start of the movement which is elicited by this signal). "Motor time" refers to the speed of movement itself. Very often pre-motor time increases with age, whereas there is no difference in motor time (see Chap. 4). If we provide an advance signal for experiments of this kind, age differences are compensated completely. The advance signal functions as a warning to be alert for the critical signal (Botwinick, et al., 1957, 1959). If the advance signal was different enough from the main signal (e.g. acoustical advance signal—visual main signal), the results were improved even more. From studies of Schneider (1969), we know of other aspects of the stimulus situation which are relevant for psychomotor performance. Personal relevance of stimulus reduces reaction time, a finding which means that the performance, especially of older subjects, can be improved by techniques for increasing the attractiveness of the stimulus. Finally, we may refer to studies on writing skills as special aspects of psychomotor performance which point to occupation as the major variable in determining consistency and change in skill with age (Simonson, 1965).

Generally, we may state that differences in psychomotor performance during life span should be defined in terms of qualitative rather than quantitative change. There are different methods to meet these changes.

AGE AND WORK PRODUCTIVITY

Studies related to changes of work productivity in older age groups are very ambiguous in their findings. One of the major obstacles in this area of research refers to problems of measurement under conditions of modern industrial production. Although empirical foundations are lacking, everybody speaks of "decreasing work productivity with increasing age." Census data of employed, unemployed and retired persons very often are used as an indirect measure for work productivity. However, many of those who retire earlier do not do so because they are, or feel they are, unable to work (Sobel, 1970, 1971). Many are forced to retire due to reorganizations in companies, cutting down production in certain areas and branches, or because older employees face discrimination and prejudice regarding their efficiency. Due to this discrimination, the chances of unemployed older workers to find a new job are less than those of younger persons (Hofbauer, Bintig and Dadzio, 1968). In any case, the different percentage of people employed in different age groups cannot be used as a measure of working capacity, as the age structure of employment is primarily determined by social and economic factors (Wolfbein, 1969; Clark and Dunne, 1956; Richardson, 1954; Murrell and Griew, 1958; Clay, 1960; Murrell, 1962).

If measured output is the criterion for work capacity, many studies do not report any age difference (Murrell and Forsaith, 1960, Breen and Spaeth, 1960; Murrell, Powesland and Forsaith, 1962). This is especially true for skills acquired in younger years (Belbin, 1966).

Apparently many factors contribute to age related changes in working productivity. Daric (1955) and Kunigk (1955) found that the amount of production decreases, while quality of production increases with age. In one of the previous studies of Belbin (1953), decrease of efficiency of elderly workers was correlated to production conditions defined by high demand of accuracy, complex instructions and detailed processing information which was partially difficult to be perceived. We may conclude, therefore, that older workers perform worse if working conditions are designed in a manner which is controversial with the most fundamental tasks of "human engineering."

On the other hand, however, older workers perform better even under conditions of heavy work, stress (dust, smoke, heat) if a high degree of responsibility is involved in the job (Belbin, 1953; Heron and Chown, 1960, 1961, 1967).

As far as existing contradictory results regarding productivity of workers from different age groups, this can be explained by different requirements of the job. Kreps (1967) believes that the pattern of change of productivity is different for semiskilled and skilled or professional work. In semiskilled workers, maximum performance rate is attained at 25 years of age and maintained at about the same level up to 55 years. According to Kreps, maximum performance in professional work is not observed before 40 and after 70 years of age. Kreps believes that these patterns of change are related to attitudes of society rather than to biological factors. Therefore, a revision of these patterns should be possible.

An alternative explanation for the decrease in efficiency in elderly workers of semiskilled status is offered by Birren (1964). He points to the fact that workers with better output are promoted with increasing age to positions of foreman, etc. Therefore, the samples of older semiskilled workers have to be regarded as selected ones which cannot be compared directly with samples of younger semiskilled workers.

This finding is supported by a study of Schmidt (1973, 1974) on the performance of workers in industrial production including automation. He analysed the age distribution of two groups differentiated by degree of qualification. This qualification was due only to performance in the job, not to education or special training.

The more qualified group (Group A) was responsible for the observation of control devices in automated production and similar complex tasks. The less qualified group (Group B) consisted of those who worked within the same job, however, with a lower degree of responsibility or in other simple jobs. The age distribution in these two groups is shown in Table 11-I. It demonstrates very clearly a rising chance of the older workers who were employed in this company to get promoted to Group A. However, the table shows, too, that beyond age 55 the percentage of older workers engaged in Group B increases again. This demonstrates that obstacles for promotion become more obvious in these age groups although generally a greater percentage of older workers is employed in more qualified work. The company belongs to a branch of the chemical industry which was in a serious economic crises during the time when the study was made. Therefore, we may conclude that the performance of the older worker was good

TABLE 11-I

AGE DISTRIBUTION OF WORKERS WITH HIGHER (GROUP A) AND LOWER (GROUP B) QUALIFICATIONS IN CHEMICAL INDUSTRY

Age Groups		Achievement Groups A %	B %
I	15-19 years	25	75
II	20-29 years	46	54
III	30-39 years	69	31
IV	40-44 years	78	22
V	45-49 years	76	24
VI	50-54 years	76	24
VII	55-59 years	69	31
VIII	60 years of age and older	64	30

From H. H. Schmidt, "Der ältere Arbeitnehmer in technischen Wandel als psychologisches Problem," thesis, University of Bonn, 1973.

enough to enable the management to maintain this age distribution although it was not due to a preferential attitude toward the older worker.

There are also studies which point to better work productivity of older workers if special attention without time pressure is required (Witte, et al., 1968). Clay (1956) studied the output of employees in printing shops. Productivity increased with age with increasing demand for attention and concentration. To find the optimal level for challenging the older worker, and to avoid stress, are the main problems in personnel management regarding older employees.

Studies from different backgrounds raise some new questions regarding problems of heavy physical work and the elderly worker. Very often physical "handicaps" which are demonstrated in experimental work can be compensated in the real life situation. The design of working plants never asks for the maximum output of efficiency (Åstrand, 1952; Eitner, et al., 1971). Very often the subjective feeling of stress in older workers is lower than in younger age groups (Schmidt, 1973).

Also, physical indicators for stress are not observed more often in older than in younger persons. According to Henschel (1969), subjects of 60 to 93 years of age did not show more symptoms of stress during work of moderate difficulty even under high temperature conditions (40°C). On the other hand, maximal oxygen consumption decreases with increasing age, pointing to increasing stress at a given submaximal level of O_2 consumption in the older age group (Simonson, 1971). However, Simonson (1974) and others point to the fact that most people never come into a situation of stress requiring maximum oxygen consumption. If older workers in heavy industry show more impairments and physical handicaps, this is not a direct outcome of their working conditions according to studies done by Eitner, Tröger and

Masius (1971) in East Germany. More important for these impairments are life history data, attitudes toward hygiene, nutrition, medical prevention and so on.

Other aspects of work productivity are related to accident rate and absenteeism. Studies with an adequate design do not support the premature expectations of a greater accident proneness and greater absenteeism in older age groups. McFarland and O'Doherty (1959) demonstrated that younger workers are more accident prone than older workers. On the other hand, they stress that older workers are more often employed in less dangerous jobs than younger workers. Speakman (1956) showed that the lowest rate of work accidents is to be found in the age range 40 to 55.

According to McFarland, Tune and Welford (1964), and Botwinick and Thompson (1966), accidents of older workers are more often due to impaired perception of, and slow reaction to danger signals, whereas those of younger workers are due more to carelessness and preference for risky behavior. This finding is supported by Lampert (1961) who found a peak in accident rate in the group of workers 15 to 30 years of age. This rise in accidents is due to risky behavior. Older workers have accidents due to carelessness due to the fact that they are used to the situation and do not anticipate unexpected events.

Although we do not include traffic problems, it might be mentioned that here, also, younger persons (up to 30 years of age) are more accident prone than older persons. However, the discrepancy between observed and expected accidents becomes smaller again after age 60. In any case, as far as accidents are concerned, older workers are not the main problem.

Summarizing, we might say that age is one of many variables also correlated to work productivity. The kind of work, the skills expected, the socioecological situation in work, the family and personal situation in work, and the family and personal situation of the employee (including health) are more important than chronological age.

BIBLIOGRAPHY

Abrahams, J. P., and J. Birren: Reaction time as a function of and behavioral predisposition to coronary heart disease. *J Gerontol, 28*:471, 1973.

Åstrand, P.-O.: *Experimental Studies of Physical Working Capacity in Relation to Sex and Age.* Copenhagen, Munksgaard, 1952.

Baltes, P. B.: Longitudinal and cross-sectional sequences in the study of age and generation effects. *Hum Dev, 11*:145, 1968.

Belbin, R. M.: Difficulties of older people in industry. *Occup Psychol, 27*:177, 1953.

Belbin, R. M.: Training methods of older workers. The employment of older workers. Paris, 1966.

Berkowitz, B., and R. E. Green: Changes in intellect with age: V. Differential changes as functions of time interval and original score. *J Genet Psychol, 53*:179, 1965.

Birren, J. E.: *The Psychology of Aging.* New York, Englewood Cliffs, 1964.
Birren, J. E., J. Botwinick, A. D. Weiss, and D. F. Morrison: Inter-relations of mental and perceptual tests given to healthy elderly men. In Birren, J. E., et al. (Ed.): *Human Aging.* PHS Publ. No. 986. Bethesda, U.S. Government Printing Office, 1963, pp. 143-156.
Birren, J. E., and D. F. Morrison: Analysis of the WAIS subtest in relation to age and education. *J Gerontol, 16*:363, 1961.
Birren, J. E., and W. Spieth: Age, response, speed and cardiovascular functions. *J Gerontol, 17*:390, 1962.
Botwinick, J., and J. E. Birren: Mental abilities and psychomotor responses in healthy aged men. In Birren, J. E. et al. (Ed.): *Human Aging.* PHS Publ. No. 986. Bethesda, U.S. Government Printing Office, 1963, pp. 97-108.
Botwinick, J., J. F. Brinley, and J. E. Birren: Sex in relation to age. *J Gerontol, 12*:300, 1957.
Botwinick, J., J. S. Robbin, and J. F. Brinley: Reorganization of perceptions with age. *J Gerontol, 14*:85, 1959.
Botwinick, J., and N. Thompson: Components of reaction time in relation to age and sex. *J Genet Psychol, 108*:175, 1966.
Botwinick, J., and N. Thompson: Age differences in reaction time: an artifact? *Gerontologist, 8*:25, 1968.
Breen, L. Z., and J. L. Spaeth: Age and productivity among workers in four Chicago companies. *J Gerontol, 15*:68, 1960.
Clark, F. L., and A. C. Dunne: *Aging in Industry.* London, Philosophical Lib, 1956.
Clay, M. H.: A study of performance in relation to age in two printing works. *J Gerontol, 11*:417, 1956.
Clay, M. H.: *The Older Worker and His Job.* London, 1960.
Craik, F. J. M.: Age differences in short term memory. In Chown, S., and Riegel, K. (Eds.): *Psychological Functioning in the Normal Aging and Senile Aged.* New York, Karger, 1968, vol. 1, pp. 44-47.
Crovitz, E.: Reversing a learning deficit in the aged. *J Gerontol, 21*:236, 1966.
Daric, J.: Survey of the employment of elderly workers in France. Old age in the modern world. Report on the *3rd International Congress of Gerontology,* London, 1955, pp. 295-299.
Downs, S.: Age in relation to part and whole learning. *J Gerontol, 20*:479, 1965.
Düker, H.: Über ein Verfahren zur Untersuchung der psychischen Leistungsfähigkeit. *Psychol Forsch, 23*:10, 1949.
Eisdorfer, C.: Verbal learning and response time in the aged. *J Genet Psychol, 107*:15, 1965.
Eitner, S., A. Tröger, and E. Masius: Schwerarbeit und Alter im mehrdimensionalen Aspekt. *Z f Alternsf, 24*:139, 1971.
Glanzer, M., and R. Glaser: Cross-sectional and longitudinal results in a study of age-related changes. Educ. Psychol. Measurement. In Birren, J. E. (Ed.): *Handbook of Aging and the Individual.* Chicago, U Chicago Pr, 1958.
Granick, S., and A. S. Friedeman: The effect of education in the decline of test performance with age. *J Gerontol, 22*:191, 1967.
Green, R. F.: Age-intelligence relationships between ages of 16 and 64: A rising trend. *Psychol, 1*:618, 1969.
Guttich, H.: Das Leben endet mit 40. *Der Arbeitgeber, 21*:102, 1969.

Henschel, A.: Age and Heat Tolerance. Report to Office of Civil Defense, 1969.
Heron, A., and S. Chown: Semi-skilled and over forty. *J Occup Psychol, 34*:264, 1960.
Heron, A., and S. Chown: Aging and the semi-skilled. *Medical Res Council Memorandum No. 40*, London, H. M. Stationery Office, 1961.
Heron, A., and S. Chown: *Age and Function*. London, Churchill, 1967.
Hofbauer, H., U. Bintig, and W. Dadzio: Materialien zur Arbeitslosigkeit älterer Arbeitnehmer in der Bundesrepublik Deutschland. *Mitteilungen des Instituts für Arbeitsmarkt- und Berufsforschung, Dez., 5*:357, 1968.
Horn, J. L., and R. B. Cattell: Age differences in primary mental ability factors. *J Gerontol, 21*:210, 1966.
Hulicka, I. M.: Short term learning-retention efficiency as a function of age and health. *J Am Geriatr Soc, 15*:285, 1967.
Hulicka, I. M.: Age changes and age differences in memory functioning. *Gerontologist, 7*:46, 1967.
Hulicka, I. M., and J. L. Grossman: Age-group comparisons for the use of mediators in paired-associate learning. *J Gerontol 22*:46, 1967.
Jones, H. E., and H. S. Conrad: The growth and decline of intelligence: A study of a homogeneous group between the ages ten and sixty. *Genet Psychol Monogr, 13*:223, 1933.
Kay, H.: The effect of position in a display upon problem solving. *Q J Exp Psychol, 6*:155, 1954.
Kay, H.: Some experiments on adult learning. In *Old Age in the Modern World*. Edinburgh, Livingstone, 1955, pp. 259-267.
Keevil-Rogers, P., and M. M. Schnore: Short term memory as a function of age in persons of above average intelligence. *J Gerontol, 24*:184, 1969.
Korchin, S. J., and H. Basowitz: Age differences in verbal learning. *J Abnorm Soc Psychol, 54*:46, 1957.
Koyl, L.: Matching the older worker to his job and his job to the worker. *Proceedings of the 9th International Congress of Gerontology*, Kiev, 2:242, 1972.
Kreps, J. M.: Job performance and job opportunity. A Note. *Gerontologist, 7*:24, 1967.
Kunigk, H.: Der ältere Mensch in Arbeit und Betrieb. In *Ber. 2. Arbeitswiss, Kongr. Dortmund, Bundesarbeitsblatt*, 1955, pp. 378-379.
Lampert, U.: Lebensalter und Unfallhäufigkeit—Beobachtungen in einem chem. Grossbetrieb. *Zbl Arb med Arteitsschutz, 11*:185, 1961.
Lehr, U.: *Psychologie des Alterns*. Heidelberg, Quelle & Meyer, 1972.
Lehr, U., G. Dreher, and R. Schmitz-Scherzer: Der ältere Arbeitnehmer im Betrieb. In Mayer, A., and Herwig, B. (Eds.): *Handbuch der Psychologie, 9, Betriebpsychologie*. Gottinger, Hogrefe, 1970, pp. 778-827.
Löwe, H.: *Der Lerneffekt in Abhängigkeit von Aktivität und Motivation. Habilitationsschrift*. Leipzig, Karl-Marx-Univ, 1968.
Löwe, H.: Aktivität und Lernerfolg bei Erwachsenen und Jugendlichen. *Probleme und Ergebnisse der Psychol, 28*:69, 1969.
Löwe, H.: *Einführung in die Lernpsychologie des Erwachsenenalters*. Berlin, VEB, 1970.
Löwe, H.: *Beiträge zur Erwachsenenqualifizierung*. Berlin, Volk und Wissen, 1971.
McFarland, R. A., and B. O'Doherty: Work and occupational skills. In Birren, J. E. (Ed.): *Handbook of Aging and the Individual*. Chicago, U Chicago Pr, 1959, pp. 452-500.

McFarland, R. A., G. S. Tune, and A. T. Welford: On the driving of automobiles by older people. *J Gerontol, 19*:190, 1964.

Miles, C. C.: The influence of speed and age on intelligence scores of adults. *J Genet Psychol, 19*:208, 1934.

Miles, C. C., and W. R. Miles: The correlation of intelligence scores and chronological age from early to late maturity. *Am J Psychol, 44*:44, 1932.

Murrell, K. F. H.: Industrial aspects of aging. *Ergonomics, 5*:147, 1962.

Murrell, K. F. H., and B. Forsaith: Age and timing in movement. *J Occup Psychol, 34*:275, 1960.

Murrell, K. F. H., and S. Griew: Age structure in the engineering industry. A study of regional effects. *J Occup Psychol, 32*:86, 1958.

Murrell, K. F. H., P. Powesland, and B. Forsaith: A study of pillar drilling in relation to age. *J Occup Psychol, 36*:45, 1962.

Nehrke, M. F.: Age, sex and educational differences in syllogistic reasoning. *J Gerontol, 27*:466, 1972.

Nesselroade, J. R., K. W. Schaie, and P. B. Baltes: Ontogenetic and generational components of structural and quantitative change in adult cognitive behavior. *J Gerontol, 27*:222, 1972.

Olechowsky, R.: *Das alternde Gedächtnis—Lernleistung und Lernmotivation Erwachsener.* Bern, Huber, 1969.

Owens, W. A.: Age and mental abilities: A longitudinal study. *Genet Psychol Monogr, 48*:3, 1953.

Owens, W. A.: Age and mental abilities: A second follow up. *J Educ Psychol, 57*:311, 1966.

Preobrazhenskaya, I., et al.: On mnemic activity in elderly persons. Symposium: Memory and action. *Proceedings International Congress Psychology*, Moscow, 1966, pp. 168.

Richardson, I. M.: Age and work: A study of 498 men in heavy industry. *Br J Industr Med, 10*:269, 1954.

Roth, E.: Lernen in verschiedenen Altersstufen. *Z Exp Angew Psychol*, 409-417, 1961a.

Roth, E.: Motorische Anpassungsfunktion und Alter. *Vita Hum, 4*:86, 1961b.

Ruch, F. L.: The differentiative effect of age upon learning. *J Genet Psychol, 31*:261, 1934.

Rudinger, G.: Determinanten der intellektuellen Leistung im höheren Alter. *Acta Gerontol, 1*:731, 1971.

Rudinger, G.: *Untersuchungen zur Methodik von Auswertung und Interpretation der Beziehungen von Persönlichkeit und Leistung im höheren Alter.* Köln-Opladen, Westdt. Verlag, 1974 (In Press).

Rudinger, G., and N. Erlemeier: Längsschnittuntersuchungen zum Problem des Zusammenhangs von Persönlichkeit und Leistung im höheren Lebensalter. *Veröffentl. Dt. Ges. Gerontol., 2*, Darmstadt, Steinkopff, 1969.

Schaie, K. W.: A general model for the study of developmental problems. *Psychol Bull, 64*:92, 1965.

Schmidt, H. H.: Der ältere Arbeitnehmer im technischen Wandel als psychologisches Problems, Thesis, Univ. Bonn, 1973.

Schmidt, H. H.: Das Problem der beruflichen Anpassung von älteren Arbeitnehmern im Bereich hochtechnischer Arbeitsplätze der industriellen Produktion. *Acta Gerntol, 4*:9, 1974.

Schneider, H.: Einfluss von Bedeutsamkeitsabstufungen innerhalb eines visuellen

Signalangebotes auf die Informationsleistung. *Probl u Ergebn d Psychol, 27/29*:7, 1969.

Simonson, E.: Performance as a function of age and cardiovascular diseases. In Welford, A. T., and Birren, J. E. (Eds.): *Behavior, Aging and the Nervous System.* Springfield, Thomas, 1965, pp. 401-431.

Simonson, E.: *Physiology of Work Capacity and Fatigue.* Springfield, Thomas, 1971.

Simonson, E.: Einfluss des Altersauf die Leistung in physiologischer Hinsicht. In Schmidtke, H. (Ed.): *Ergonomie, 2.* München, 1974.

Simonson, E., and D. A. Anderson: Effect of age and coronary heart disease on performance and physiological responses in mental work. *7th International Congress of Gerontology,* Vienna, Austria, June 26-July 2, 1966, pp. 333-336.

Simonson, E., D. Anderson, and C. Keiper: Effect of stimulus movement on critical flicker fusion in young and older men. *J Gerontol, 22*:353, 1967.

Sobel, I.: Economic changes and older workers utilization patterns. Interdiscipl. Topics. *Gerontologia, 6*:43, 1970.

Sobel, I.: Employment. Background Paper. *The White House Conference on Aging.* Washington, 1971.

Speakman, D.: Bibliography of research on changes in working capacity with age. London, Ministry of Labour and National Service, 1956.

Talland, G. A.: The effect of warning signals on reaction time in youth and old age. *J Gerontol, 19*:31, 1964.

Talland, G. A.: *Human Aging and Behavior.* New York, London, Acad Pr, 1968.

Terman, L. M., and M. H. Oden: *Genetic Studies of Genius.* Stanford, Stanford U Pr, 1947, Vol. 4.

Terman, L. M., and M. H. Oden: *The Gifted Group at Mid-Life.* Stanford, Stanford U Pr, 1959.

Thomae, H., and U. Lehr: *Berufliche Leistungsfähigkeit im mittleren und höheren Erwachsenenalter.* Göttingen, Schwartz, 1973.

Vernon, P. E.: The variation of intelligence with occupation, age, and locality. *Br J Psychol, 1/2*:52-63, 1947.

Welford, A. T.: *Aging and Human Skill.* London, Oxford U Pr, 1958.

Welford, A. T.: Psychomotor performance. In Birren, J. E. (Ed.): *Handbook of Aging and the Individual.* Chicago, U Chicago Pr, 1959, pp. 562-613.

Welford, A. T.: Industrial work suitable for older people: Some British studies. In Thomae, H., and Lehr, U. (Eds.): *Altern-Probleme und Tatsachen.* Frankfurt, Akad. Verlagsanstalt, 1968, pp. 269-283.

Welford, A. T., and J. E. Birren: *Behavior, Aging and the Nervous System.* Springfield, Thomas, 1965.

White House Conference on Aging: *A Report to the Delegates from the Conference Sections on Special Concern Sessions.* Washington, D.C., 1971.

Witte, N. D., E. Stehenskaja, W. W. Kryshanowskaja, and L. Gawrila: Veränderungen der beruflichen Arbeitsfähigkeit im Zusammenhang mit Alter und Arbeitsbedingungen. In Thomae, H., and Lehr, U. (Eds.): *Altern—Probleme und Tatsachen.* Frankfurt, Akad, Reihe, 1968.

Wolfbein, S. L.: Work force and retirement trends in older population. *Proceedings of the 8th International Congress of Gerontology,* Washington, D.C., *1*:314, 1969.

Zaretzky, H. H., and J. I. Halberstam: Age differences in paired-associate-learning. *J Gerontol, 23*:165, 1968.

Chapter 12

The Older Driver

ERNST SIMONSON

Driving an automobile is one of the most universal types of activity in the United States and, to a somewhat lesser degree, in Western European countries. It involves a greater risk of injury (or death) than most other activities in industry or sports. Nevertheless, there is a surprising lack of information on driving performance in respect to age, quite in contrast to the substantial number of investigations of industrial jobs. To the best of my knowledge, no comparison of driving performance of older and younger drivers on the road, with quantitative comparison of driver's input, i.e. steering wheel movements, brake and gas pedal use, speed, acceleration and distance traveled, such as Platt's studies (1964) in younger drivers, has been reported, or even laboratory studies with sophisticated driving simulators, such as Drew's, et al. (1960) study on the effect of alcohol. Therefore, conclusions about the effect of age on driving performance and the psychophysiological stress involved must be mainly inferred from laboratory studies of various psychological functions presumably pertinent for driving performance.

Driving is a complex psychophysiological stress situation involving vigilance, short term memory, reaction times, sensory functions, hormonal changes (essentially catecholamine output), cardiovascular responses, etc. Most of these functions are affected by age.

ACCIDENT STATISTICS

Impairment of older drivers is not revealed by accident statistics because of changing driving habits with age, and the dropout with age of poor or injury prone drivers, or drivers with some other handicaps (McFarland, et al., 1964). Another factor ameliorating the accident rate of older drivers is the utilization of driving experience. The percentage of drivers involved in accidents and who were held at fault is at a minimum in middle age (40-49 years), increasing at both ends (McFarland, et al., 1964—based on data from Great Britain, 1953; Connecticut, 1955; California, 1958). This U-shaped distribution applies also if exposure, i.e. accident rate per distance, is taken into consideration: it is highest in the 18 to 23 age group, second highest in the older age group, and lowest in middle age. In contrast, according to Lauer (1952), the average number of automobile accidents of licensed male drivers in the U.S. per 100,000 miles over a two year period shows a peak at age 20, and drops with progressing age, reaching a plateau at 50 years. In the same study, the accident rate which was not adjusted to distance, shows the U-form as earlier studies, with a peak at 20 years, a low plateau from 35 to 65 years, rising again after 65 years, but still far below the peak at 20 years.

The most recent information has been provided by J. Rozeske (personal communication, 1974): automobile accidents of 2,200,000 licensed drivers in Minnesota during 1973. Figure 12-1 shows the total rate of accidents (with and without injury) in percent of licensed drivers by age (six age groups) and time of the day (eight time intervals). At all times the peak of the total accident rate is at age 15 to 24 years, dropping with age from midnight to 8 A.M. and also from 3 P.M. to midnight. There is a slight increase in the oldest age group from 9 A.M. to 3 P.M. The very low accident rate in drivers over 65 years from midnight to 5 A.M. must be due to restriction of driving during darkness. The totals across age columns (right part of Fig. 12-1) show a continuous drop from the youngest to the oldest age group. The distribution of accidents resulting in injury by age and time of the day is quite similar. However, the cause of accidents in young and old-

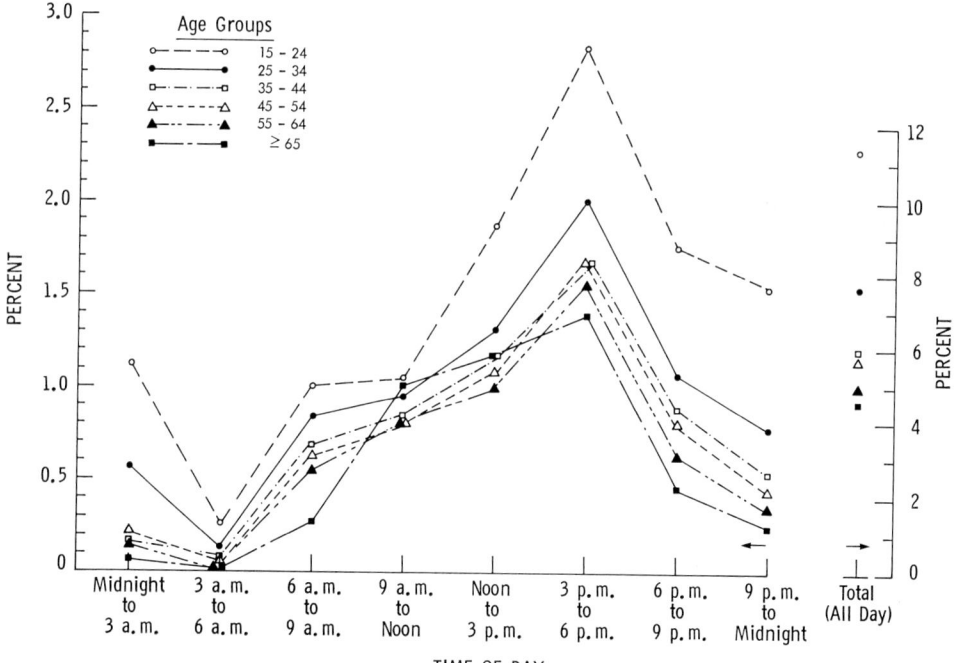

Figure 12-1. Total automobile accident rate (with and without injury) in percent of licensed drivers by age and time of day (State of Minnesota, 1973).

er drivers is different: speeding, driving on the wrong side of the road, and faulty equipment predominated in the age group under 25; failure to give right of way, improper turning, improper starting, and ignoring stop signs occurred more in the older age group.

In summary, psychophysiological handicaps of the older driver are not revealed by accident statistics, i.e. they appear to be fully compensated by their change of driving habits. However, it should be pointed out that the effect of more extreme handicaps may not show up in the very large population sample of licensed drivers. Of potential pertinence is the presence of asymptomatic disease such as arterial hypertension, coronary and cerebral atherosclerosis, and diabetes, which is wide spread in apparently healthy populations and increases with age.

Some degree of coronary atherosclerosis, occasionally quite advanced, has been demonstrated in autopsy material in Minnesota population even in absence of clinical heart disease (Clawson, 1941; Lober, 1973). This accounts for the increasing frequency of "ischemic" response of the electrocardiogram (ECG) to the physical effort with age (reviewed in *PWCF*, Chap. 12). According to Waller (1964), drivers with pathological conditions had 30 percent more accidents than healthy drivers and 10 to 20 percent of the driving population has a medical condition of potential significance for driving. Hoffmann (1963) compared changes of heart rate, blood pressure and electrocardiogram (ECG) in 600 healthy drivers and 58 ambulatory drivers with coronary heart disease under three different conditions: a. highway driving with low traffic density, b. urban driving with high traffic density, and c. critical traffic situations (overtaking, sudden stops, etc.). The percentage of "abnormal" ECG changes (ST depression and/or flattening or inversion of T wave) in healthy drivers was: a. 0.0%, b. 15.75%, c. 23.75%, and striking in drivers with coronary disease: a. 11.5%, b. 46.1%, c. 61.5%. It is of interest that significant ECG changes were found in a minority of healthy drivers, but they occurred more frequently in drivers with coronary arterial heart disease (CHD) (without acute coronary insufficiency during the test). In three healthy young drivers, we found significant T wave changes in long distance driving, dependent on road events (Simonson, et al., 1968). The heart rate increased by 20 to 25 beats in city driving: nearly identical for driver and passenger, which is not surprising since the passenger shares the emotional impact of critical situations. Collins and associates (1965) compared the heart rate of a 30-year-old woman as a driver and as a passenger. As a passenger, the heart rate was 20 bpm higher than as a driver. Hoffmann found similar increases of heart rate, but little difference between healthy drivers and drivers with CHD. In dense, fast moving traffic, the heart rate of healthy drivers increased up to 140 bpm (Taggart and Gibbons, 1967).

The results demonstrate clearly that cardiovascular stress is involved in the complex stress situation of driving an automobile. Due to a higher prevalence of coronary atherosclerosis, either clinically silent or overt, the older driver is more vulnerable to the cardiovascular stress of driving an automobile. Cardiovascular changes may secondarily affect psychological functions. Bellet (1967) found ST-T depression during a 150 minute daytime drive in 8 of 46 patients with coronary heart disease in confirmation of Hoffmann's (1963) findings, but failed to find changes in healthy drivers as observed by Hoffmann and in our experiments (Simonson, et al., 1968).

It is unlikely that the ECG changes in young healthy drivers are due to coronary insufficiency, as assumed by Hoffmann, but they may well be in older drivers. Coronary insufficiency may be a contributing factor to accidents, but valid statistical evidence is lacking, although several cases of cardiac death during driving have been reported. Of 60 drivers who succumbed to sudden cardiac death, in 11 the fatal attack occurred during driving, a rather high incidence (Hoffmann). However, in the large majority a heart attack during driving is not fatal. Out of 82,000 reported automobile accidents in 1965 involving 140,000 drivers in Minnesota only in 159 cases was illness listed as a contributory cause (C. Staffeld and G. Oster: Personal communication, 1967). On the basis of distribution of CHD, assuming one hour of average duration of driving per day (a conservative estimate), approximately 700 heart attacks should be expected to occur during driving in male drivers of 40 years or older and 1,000 for male and female drivers over 40 in Minnesota, which is substantial as a potential accident risk (Simonson, et al., 1968). This estimate is based on a prevalence of CHD alone. Arterial hypertension and diabetes also have a high prevalence in older populations adding to the risk. This estimate shows that only a very small minority of heart attacks or other illness during driving is reported.

VISION

Of all sensory functions, vision is the most important one for driving an automobile. There is a strong correlation between age and the increase of visual thresholds during dark adaptation, mathematically formulated by McFarland (1960). Table 12-I shows a condensation of his results based on investigation of 240 male subjects from 16 to 89 years.

The rate of dark adaptation is not affected by age, but the visual thresholds are higher with age at any time during the whole course (40 min.) of dark adaptation. In all age groups the transition point from photopic (cones) to scotopic (rods), dark adaptation occurred at 5 min. dark adaptation. This point is of particular importance, because at lower levels color discrimination is impossible and visual acuity is impaired. Table 12-I

TABLE 12-I

MEAN DARK ADAPTATION THRESHOLDS AT DIFFERENT AGES

Age	16-19	30-39	50-59	70-79
Time				
0-30 sec.	6.42	6.37	6.87	7.16
5 min.	5.58	5.07	6.17	6.49
10 min.	4.17	4.17	4.77	5.71
40 min.	2.34	2.75	3.32	4.11

Condensed from R. A. McFarland, et al., "Dark Adaptation as a Function of Age: A Statistical Analysis," *Journal of Gerontology,* 15:149, 1960.

shows that in older subjects, this critical point is reached at a significantly higher level of illumination. The effect of age is more pronounced at the terminal level of dark adaptation, i.e. after 30 to 40 min. than it is in the early phase. On the average, the just noticeable light stimulus after 40 min. dark adaptation is about 239 times greater in the oldest age group than it is in the teenage group. Immediately after a bright light exposure during the first minutes of dark adaptation, it becomes about five times greater. Therefore, there is a definite handicap of the older driver for night driving; it would take a much longer time to attain the sensitivity for light perception at a given level of low illumination. This implies also the recognition levels for objects in the dark, i.e. a visibility level. At the same time the sensitivity to glare is increased (AAA Report No. 4, 1939). After glare exposure by headlights of oncoming cars, the older driver will be slower to adapt to a low illumination level. It should be noted, however, that there is considerable individual variability. However, Bransford (1939) and Cobb (1939) found no significant correlation between resistance to glare and accident rate per year or per mile.

In the study of the Eno Foundation (1948) in Connecticut and Michigan on 186 and 200 drivers, respectively, without consideration of age, there was no significant correlation between dark adaptation and accident rates. However, the samples were small for valid accident statistics.

There is also some impairment for daylight driving with age. Figure 12-2 shows the visibility level of well printed 6 point type for four levels of illumination (Guth, 1957) at age 19 to 63 years. There is a parallel decrease at the four illumination levels, accelerating with age, i.e. most pronounced from 55 to 63 years and probably beyond. However, to a certain degree, the decline of visibility can be compensated by a higher illumination level. For instance, at 50 footcandles the visibility at age 63 would be nearly identical to that at age 36 years and 30 footcandles.

According to L. Goldstein's review (1961), the effect of visual acuity on automobile driving has been studied quite extensively, but the effect of age was never considered. The results were not uniform. There was no significant effect of visual acuity on the accident rate in the comparatively small sample of the Eno Foundation Project; while in Cobb's study on larger samples of 2,200 and 3,000 drivers, the correlation varied from not significant to a low level of significance (0.065), too low for any reliable prediction. Similar results were obtained by Lauer, et al. (1952) in the Camp Lee and Fort Knox studies in army drivers (1941, 1942) with rating of driving performance as criterion. The correlations were too low for any prediction of driving performance from visual acuity measurements.

There is a significant increase with age of the exposure time needed for identification of pictures in a tachistoscope (Wallace, 1956). This may be relevant in the reaction to critical traffic situations.

Auditory thresholds also increase with age particularly at higher frequency. However, the increase of visual thresholds is far more important for

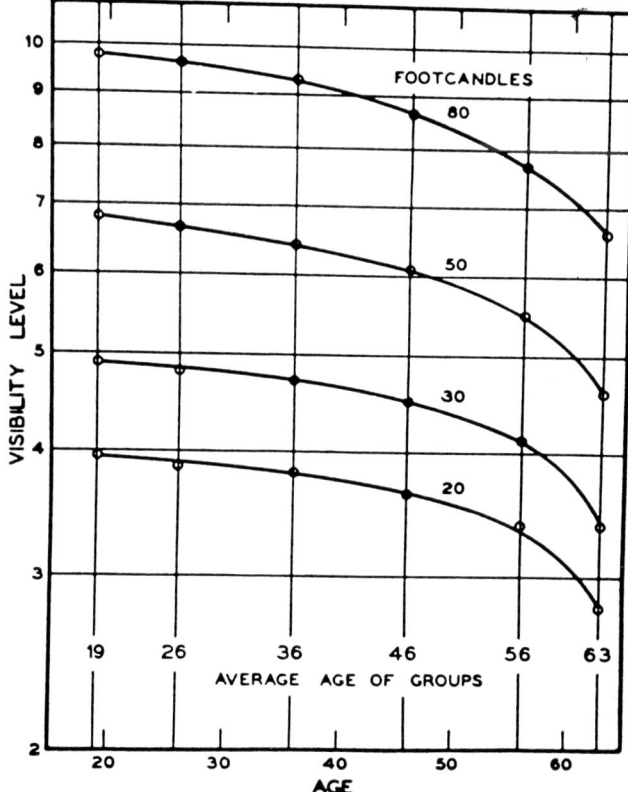

Figure 12-2. Illustration of the decrease in visibility level of well-printed 6-point type with increasing age for several levels of illumination (Reproduced from S. K. Guth, A. A. Eastman, and J. F. McNelis, *Illuminating Engineering*, 51(10):656-660, 1956, Fig. 1).

driving an automobile. In general, acoustic signals in traffic are far above the threshold level even for the average older driver. In four tests of auditory acuity (Cobb, 1939), the correlation to the accident rate per year varied from -0.022 (not significant) to -0.054 (significant, but too low for any individual or even group prediction).

REACTION TIMES AND INFORMATION UTILIZATION

While reaction times decrease with age (Welford, 1958), the age differences (in fractions of a second) are small and of questionable significance for driving performance. As pointed out by McFarland, "The essence of driving skill is not to react quickly to definite known signals, for example, in some driver-testing devices by pressing a brake pedal when a red signal flashes on the dashboard, but to be able to appraise the constant flux of traffic conditions quickly and accurately. Driving skill does not depend upon speed of action as much as on the speed and accuracy of perception and judgment to identify the situation in response to which action is required."

In studies without consideration of age, Cobb found no correlation between simple reaction time and accidents/year in 2,200 drivers, while in a more specific test of braking reaction time the correlation of $r = 0.052$ was significant but very low. In the Camp Lee study (1942), there was a significant but low correlation in 718 army drivers between simple reaction time and road test rating. Lauer, et al. (1952) found no correlation between the means of a choice reaction time and rated driver performance, but there was a significant, but quite low correlation ($r = 0.17$) to the errors in performance. It may be mentioned that there is no significant effect of fatigue on reaction time (Chap. 4, Hayes).

Speed and accuracy in the acquisition and processing of information which also involves short term memory is relevant for driving performance. Deterioration of these functions, as well as the ability to discriminate between critical, noncritical and neutral signals in fatigue, discussed in Chapters 8 through 10 by H. Schmidtke, is a potential source of accidents. Chapter 10 gives an impressive example for failure of these functions in fatigue resulting in a critical traffic situation.

In Cobb's investigations, the correlation of the Harvard Vigilance Test to accidents/year was low but significant ($r = 0.065$) while the correlation to eight measures of a driving simulator was extremely variable, between $+.022$ and $-.079$ for 3,000 subjects. It is possible that age has a depressing effect on these functions, particularly in combination with fatigue. Unfortunately, the bulk of experiments has been performed on younger subjects, and no precise information on age differences is yet available.

Two-hand coordination also failed to be a reliable predictor for rated driving performance in army drivers (Goldstein, et al., 1952; Lauer, et al., 1952).

In summary the reliability of visual tests, reaction times, or motor co-ordination for prediction of accidents or driving performance is poor in studies without consideration of age. It may be implied that the effect of age on these functions does not permit a clear evaluation of the accident proneness or driving performance of the older driver. This may be due to driving performance being too complex to be related to isolated components in relatively simple laboratory tests.

However, there is information that short term memory declines significantly with age (Welford, 1959). This function is of particular importance when a situation requires keeping some information in memory for a short time while doing something else or watching other signals (Kirchner, 1958; Suci, Dowduff and Braun, 1962). This applies to the situation of driving with a continuously changing display of various types of signals requiring differential response. Broadbent and Heron (1962) found that older subjects performed poorer than younger subjects in such situations in laboratory tests. McFarland concludes from his experiences of industrial and agricultural accidents that slower operation is, in general, the main reason for the accident risk of older drivers.

The handicaps of the older driver, however, can be largely compensated by a change in driving habits. Particularly, slower driving speed is important since it decreases the flux of signals and allows more time for reaction thus reducing the probability of critical situations. In general, the average older driver is aware of his handicaps and drives slower over shorter distances, avoids driving in darkness and bad weather, and is involved in alcohol intoxication less frequently (R. Provost: Personal communication, 1974). The reduction of the speed limit in the United States from 70 to 55 mph mainly benefits the older driver, thus reducing age differences in driving performance.

The question of possible age restriction in driver licensing has been discussed by McFarland (1964). Due to the great individual variability of all functions involved, any age restriction would result in gross injustice to individual drivers. Many older persons are better drivers than many younger drivers. Driving tests which require the driver to express his actions in words are shown to be inadequate. Similarly, the failure of older people to answer questions in examinations for a drivers license has little bearing in actual driving performance.

In conclusion, there is a lack of pertinent information on the older driver, in obvious contrast to the general importance of the problem. More research on driving performance of the older driver in the various traffic situations is needed, preferably road tests with automated equipment or with sophisticated driving simulators.

BIBLIOGRAPHY

Bellet, S.: Driving stress and coronary patients: a major problem. *JAMA, 200:*33, 1967.

Bransford, T.: *Relation of Performance on Drivers' Tests to Automobile Accidents and Violations of Traffic Regulations in the District of Columbia,* Unpublished Ph.D. dissertation, American University, 1939.

Broadbent, D. E., and A. Heron: Effects of a subsidiary task on performances involving immediate memory by younger and older men. *Br J Psychol, 53:*189, 1962.

Clawson, B. J.: Incidence of types of heart disease among 30,265 autopsies, with special reference to age and sex. *Am Heart J, 22:*607, 1941.

Cobb, P. W.: *Report to the Highway Research Board on the Automobile Driver Tests Administered to 3663 Persons in Connecticut, 1936-7, and the Relation of the Test Scores to the Accidents Sustained.* Unpublished report to Highway Research Board, Washington, D.C., 1939, pp. 72.

Collins, V. P., W. D. West, W. G. McTaggart, and A. R. Maxwell: *Telemetry in a Driving Safety Study.* Proc. Nat. Telem. Conf. 1965, pp. 1241.

Drew, G. C., W. P. Colguhoun, and H. A. Long: Effect of small doses of alcohol on a skill resembling driving. *Res Council Memorandum No. 38.* London, H. M. Stationery Office, 1960, pp. 1-108.

Eno Foundation for Highway Traffic Control: *Personal Characteristics of Traffic Accident Repeaters,* Saugatuck, Conn., 1948.

Goldstein, L. G.: Research of human variables in safe motor vehicle operation: a correlation summary of predictor variables and criterion measures. In *The Driver Behavior Research Project Report,* Washington, George Washington Univ., 1961, p. 72.

Goldstein, L. G., and J. N. Mosel: A factor study of drivers' attitudes with further study on driver aggression. *Highway Research Board Bulletin 172, NAS-NRC Publication 532,* Washington, D.C., U.S. Government Printing Office, 1956.

Guth, S. K., A. A. Eastman, and J. F. McNelis: *Lighting requirements for older workers.* Lamp Divn., General Eelectric Co., Preprint No. 22, 1957, 16 pp.

Hoffmann, H.: Herzkranke an Steur von Kraftfahrzeugen. *Münch med Wochenschr, 105:* 1790, 1963.

Kirchner, W.: Age differences in short-term retention of rapidly changing information. *J Exp Psychol, 55:*352, 1958.

Lauer, A. R.: Age and Sex in Relation to Accidents. *Highway Research Board, Iowa, Bulletin 60,* 1952, pp. 25-35.

Lauer, A. R., et al.: Aptitude tests for army motor vehicle operators. *Personnel Research Section, TAGO, Report 981,* Washington, D.C., Department of the Army, 1952.

Lober, P. H.: Pathogenesis of coronary sclerosis. *Arch Pathol, 55:*357, 1973.

McFarland, R. A., R. G. Doney, A. B. Bertrand, and D. C. Ward: Dark adaptation as a function of age: A statistical analysis. *J Gerontol, 15:*149, 1960.

McFarland, R. A., G. S. Tune, and A. T. Welford: On the driving of automobiles by older people. *J Gerontol, 19:*190, 1964.

Platt, F. N.: Objective measurements of individual driver behavior. *Society of Automot Engineers,* 1964, p. 809A.

Report No. 178: Summary of Fort Knox driver study. *Personnel Research Section, TAGO,* Department of the Army, 1941.
Report No. 318: The relation of psychophysical tests, driving experience and driver information to truck driving performance at Camp Lee, Va. *Personnel Research Section, TAGO,* Department of the Army, 1942.
Simonson, E., Ch. Baker, N. Burns, Ch. Keiper, O. H. Schmitt, and S. Stackhause: Cardiovascular stress (electrocardiographic changes) produced by driving an automobile. *Am Heart J, 75:*125, 1968.
Suci, G. J., M. D. Dowduff, and J. C. Braun: Interference in short-term retention as a function of age. In Tribbins, C., and Donahue, W. (Eds.): *Social and Psychological Aspects of Aging.* New York. Columbia U Pr, 1962, pp. 701-708.
Taggart, P., and D. Gibbons: Motorcar driving and the heart rate. *Br Med J, 1:*411, 1967.
Wallace, J. G.: Some studies of perception in relation to age. *Br J Psychol, 47:*283, 1956.
Waller, J. A.: Driver, accident link reported. *AMA News,* Sept. 28, 1964, p. 13.
Welford, A. T.: *Aging and Human Skill.* London, Oxford U Pr, 1958.
Welford, A. T.: Psychomotor performance. In Birren, J. E. (Ed.): *Handbook of Aging and the Individual.* Chicago, Chicago U Pr. 1959, pp. 562-613.

SECTION SIX
INTROSPECTIVE ASPECTS OF WORK AND FATIGUE

Chapter 13

Motivation, Values, and Chronobehavioral Aspects of Fatigue

HANS W. WENDT and PATRICIA R. PALMERTON

HISTORICAL NOTE: CONCERN WITH FATIGUE AS A POTENTIALLY MOTIVATIONAL PROBLEM

WHILE THE PHENOMENA encountered in this field are as ancient as human organized activity, systematic concern with "fatigue" in any sense approaching modern usage actually dates to the stage of major industrialization in Western countries in the late 19th century. This historical observation is directly relevant for the problems taken up in this chapter because it seems to us that neither the type of concern nor the concepts employed have made advances at a rate comparable to the progress in other fields. While this may sound like an indictment of an entire discipline—and a sophisticated one—the difficulty has little to do with level of sophistication and is more fundamental in nature. Indeed, the individuals investing often a lifetime of effort in this sector, cannot be faulted. Rather, we believe that the reasons have a great deal more to do with our inability to perceive the underlying theoretical (indeed philosophical) basis of our entire occupation with fatigue; with the values, frequently unexamined ones, of a feverishly active and production oriented society and their ramifications; and incidentally the difficulty of communication between the "product" or machine oriented researcher on the one hand, and the clinician on the other. As in other behavioral sciences, one result has been that what should be looked upon as a network or system, has rarely been modelled in this fashion. These observations become less trivial only by virtue of the finding that systems thinking has meanwhile entered many other fields. Fortunately, it is gradually beginning to enter fatigue research as well, as several chapters in this volume and the preceding one attest, if not always explicitly.

Historically it is interesting that even the very earliest "fatigue" studies show about the same concern with the multiplicity of the phenomena encountered as do contemporary ones. One might point to the examples of Burnham (1908), Kraepelin (cf. Rivers and Kraepelin, 1896), Mosso (1892), Münsterberg (1912) and Thorndike (1900) on the one hand, as well as to the contributions made by moderns, such as Bartley and Chute (1947), Bartenwerfer (1969, 1970), Bornemann (1952), von Bracken

(1951, 1952), Grandjean (1970), Kinsman and Weiser (cf. Chapter 14 in this volume), Rüssel (1968), Schaefer (1970), Schmidtke (1965), Simonson (cf. 1935 and numerous studies since) and several others. Indeed, all of the above share a considerable awareness of one aspect of performance and fatigue that has proven particularly intractable in practical work and yet whose existence has been denied by no one—the complex of motivational parameters.

This has led to a curious situation. As far as the interaction of motivation with fatigue is concerned there have been, throughout the history of this research, sophisticated pointers from many quarters. Sometimes motivation has almost served as a fundamental notion underlying all of "fatigue," as in some of Thorndike's thinking; sometimes motivation has been one component explicitly mentioned as part of the whole performance network. At other times it has served a much more poorly defined function—and criticized accordingly by psychophysiologists (e.g. Lindsley, 1957)—becoming something like a general purpose "black box" type of variable that is produced whenever results are hard to explain otherwise. Thus it has been a combination of a *post hoc* explanation and a stumbling block, an uncomfortable but necessary variable with which to contend. Since many of us are guilty of this lapse, we may refrain from pinning any names on specific schools of research (and are asking the reader's indulgence in this omission). Suffice it to say that many a study conducted in and outside the work environment has found little relationship between say, the duration or demand characteristics of the work and any performance changes, or fatigue ratings for that matter; and in order to help explain what seemed to be a violation of simpler mechanistic principles, "motivation" was a convenient *spiritus ex machina*. Actually, motivational variables could have lent themselves to consideration by way of analysis of covariance and other statistical devices. However, even the intent to proceed along these lines, in the obvious interest of improved prediction, for a long time tended to be handicapped by the lack of motivation measures that were reliable, let alone valid and generalizable. Leaving aside certain physiological criteria—and in particular some activation or arousal measures from that domain which are treated elsewhere in these volumes—tangible improvements in psychological methodology may be traced to the early 1950's. As an important example, the work on "achievement motivation" (McClelland, et al., 1953, 1961) has been instrumental. Among other things its methodology (1) had its roots in both the clinical and experimental approaches to the study of personality; (2) led to beginnings of a quantification that we believe to be useful for our present framework; (3) demonstrated to researchers the potential fruitfulness for motivation study of measures based on imagery or projection in one sense or another. It also made clear that "respondent" measures like questionnaires, many rating scales etc., apparently play a different role in prediction.

Inasmuch as fatigue research has been a viable undertaking for three generations, we would summarize this activity somewhat as follows: during the first generation, the fundamental importance of motivation in the network was clearly recognized and even specially emphasized, but left behind little empirical knowledge; during the second generation, much of the original thinking along these lines was dormant in both research and its applications, while tools for motivational measurement were being developed elsewhere; finally in the present generation, we see a revival of interest both in terms of theory and the beginnings of a methodology that would give motivation an empirical status commensurate with other fatigue parameters which already have a long and respectable experimental history. Perhaps even more important, during this third phase (beginning after the second world war) psychologists are beginning to acknowledge something else still: viz., that the motivational domain is nearly impossible to separate from the underlying societal values, last not least those of an "achieving society," just as it cannot ignore its technological state of development and its attendant ways of thinking. Nor is such an examination a Marxist prerogative. The point we would make is that ultimately, the *models of man* which we entertain and which enter our behavior have a great deal to do with our assessment of "fatigue" (whatever that shall be) and even our very research of the subject. Certainly, the inside of the "black boxes" found in research need *not* simply hold more of the "energy" or "reservoir" types of factors that had governed so much of the general and mechanical enterprise of the 19th century; and, anticipating the concluding notes below, second generation fatigue research, just as other areas of psychology, appears to have taken much of its presumed utility and many even of its procedures from modelling the First Law of thermodynamics—perhaps too much so in view of what we have learned since.

SOME DEFINITIONAL ISSUES

When writing about a concept, the definition of that concept is of primary importance—preferably a definition which is clear, concise, operational and which has all the other things we like definitions to have. This is clearly not the case with either of the concepts of "fatigue" or "motivation." Much of the research on fatigue seems to be plagued with a vagueness about what is really being researched, the term being applied to many states from muscular exhaustion to emotional satiation or frustration.

Part of the problem appears to be related to what is often referred to as the "subjective" aspect of fatigue. Bartley (1964; cf. also his comments in Chap. 15) defines this as a "self-recognizable state in which the individual feels inadequate for his task, based on bodily experience of discomfort, weakness, slowness, etc., and also upon other cognitive criteria such as feelings of futility, etc.," and points out that it is necessary to relate an organism to its surroundings, to take into account the sensory inputs being experienced by and having an effect upon the organism. In spite of the importance of this subjective state in relation to performance, it has long been avoided, especially in academic psychology, as research emphasized behavior rather than experience—behavior being measurable and observable and more easily empiricized. Research has been aimed at studying performance decrement, with the "subjective" feelings being a side issue. Only recently has there been an acknowledged return to the more cognitive, perceptual and experiential phenomena (Kinsman and Weiser, Chap. 14; McClelland, 1955), the behavioristic approach seeming to leave too many questions unsatisfactorily answered, if answered at all.

But there is still, ". . . a lurking belief that something called fatigue underlies work output and work decrement, and that such studies" (i.e. those studying work output and work decrement) "will help to discover what fatigue really is" (Bartley, 1964). In doing so, one may be taking the chance of masking what fatigue is by putting the concept within the framework of "work output" rather than viewing "work output" and "fatigue" as two mutually independent clusters of variables which sometimes interact. It seems important, therefore, to emphasize that fatigue studies in which work, effort, performance, etc., are the dependent variables tend to look at one aspect of fatigue, but not at the conceptual domain as a whole. The above author, for example, calls for the phenomena of fatigue to be approached in an organizational way, understanding being reached by finding the patterns of underlying conditions rather than quantifying input and output. Fatigue is not something describable of a body part, but deals with the organism as a whole and expresses its overall relation to the environment, not the least of which involves its approach and avoidance pattern, observable or not. Phenomena that seem to be a part of the organism's overall condition even when it is fatigued *are* not in themselves fatigue. The two interact; but impairment of performance can occur without fatigue, and fatigue can occur without impairment.

Bartlett (1953) had defined fatigue as "a term used to cover all those determinable changes in the expression of an activity which can be traced to the continuing exercise of that activity under its normal operational conditions, and which can be shown to lead, either immediately or after delay, to deterioration in the expression of that activity, or more simply, to results within the activity that are not wanted." Of course, one problem is, "not wanted" by whom? (cf. our comments below on the sociocultural aspects of this issue). He also offered several suggestions for studying fatigue: to separate for study the various successive stages of the operation involved. Thus, changes in the smoothness of the responses may be taken to signal the beginning of a measurable fatigue reaction; the irregularity of responses reacts against the "display field" within which the organism is acting, and the field begins to disintegrate with the consequence that the "right" actions are done at the "wrong" time, and the disintegration continues, etc. This reference to the coordination of subunits (such as small muscles, etc.) and certain temporal aspects has been anticipated in some degree by earlier investigators, e.g. Bills (1931) and Münsterberg (1912).

Bartlett and his associates' definition and suggestions encompass much of the research which has been done on fatigue, and it covers an important measurable part of the phenomena; yet it does not take into account that all those "determinable changes" may not necessarily be due to fatigue, as well as the possibility that those changes may be tempered by other factors within the organism, and in the organism's environment; but the latter is rarely examined at all. As pointed out by Browne (1953), and representing the views of others including authors of the present two volumes, a decrease in performance may easily be masked by a greater effort being made to achieve the same results. Welford (1953) notes that the intrusion of other stimuli during the performance of a task can cause the disruption of the performance of the task, which in turn leads to further disturbance. In addition, the awareness that his performance is falling short may induce anxiety within a subject about whether he will carry out his task to a successful conclusion, further increasing the disruption (cf. our notes below on stress and anxiety effects). Here is a performance decrement or impairment—is fatigue the cause of the decrement? Or is fatigue the description of the decrement? Or is fatigue the description of the cause of the decrement? On the one hand, these questions exemplify some of the confusion we face in studying fatigue as work or performance decrement or *vice versa*. On the other, they imply that a systems approach might capture essentials that currently are hard to bring into view. An adequate, if temporary, designation of the way in which the term "fatigue" is used would be especially important when looking at fatigue as it interacts with motivation—ideally the two concepts should be kept separate, to avoid assuming that "unmotivated" is "fatigued" or *vice versa*, or to avoid masking what fatigue may be by not recognizing the possibility that motivation may be playing a part in the demonstrated performance. Nonetheless, we recognize that what is desirable in theory may not be feasible in practice. And even on the empirical level our discussion of the role of the motivational component throughout this chapter is in itself ample proof that even "desirable" operational definitions frequently either do not fit the questions we should really be asking, or lead us back to the same unproductive circle. Significantly, although we may be a little more successful with the motivational concepts, it is the very definition of fatigue as will become evident, which demonstrably brings in factors from an "outside" and, in any case, much larger domain.

DETERMINANTS OF FATIGUE FROM OUTSIDE THE TASK SETTING

An Excursion Into Achievement Motivation

Throughout this chapter we are referring to hypothesized as well as empirically noted effects of achievement concerns, drives, values, or some of their connotations. A brief overview of what kinds of behavior are involved in such a construct may, therefore, be of interest. One widespread approach to the definition of achievement motivation in the past 20 years (originally following Murray, 1938) has made use of controlled fantasies or imagery (McClelland, et al., 1953, 1955; Atkinson, 1958; Heckhausen, 1967). In one of the better known methodologies, a person produces an imaginative story centering on a number of ambiguous stimulus pictures shown for a few seconds. McClelland, et al. consider this an analogy to the sampling of numerous physiological processes where the total universe of data is clearly unavailable, such as in blood sampling, etc., and in fact, literally speak of "thought samples." After applying certain "gating" criteria, the measure of achievement (or affiliative, or power, or other) concerns is obtained by totalling up some ten different types of content, all of which are either theoretically or empirically related to what is meant by achievement concern (or, in their usual inference, achievement motivation, n (need) Achievement). If a person shows no such content (whose scoring incidentally is highly reliable and has been computerized with fair success) he or she is classified as low in n Ach. The more of the critical categories generated and tallied, the higher the achievement drive; etc. This comparatively simple procedure (and criticized in part on those very grounds and often on others, cf. Klinger and McNelly, 1969) has yielded various relationships with actual behavior, both in task settings of interest in our context and elsewhere (McClelland, 1953, 1961). Some examples must suffice here. Thus, correlations are found with behaviors such as these: performance, so long as there are no outside pressures on the person; the level of risk a person will choose, other things equal; the kinds of work associates preferred; the magnitude of the Zeigarnik effect, that is, how well a task is remembered which the person had been unable to complete; the speed or readiness with which success or failure related words are recognized, or how ambiguous words are interpreted; and a variety of other measures both on the individual and the societal level.

The above summary has been based primarily on the imagery method and thus, a projective test (cf. Heckhausen, 1963; Fisch, et al., 1970). However, there are other approaches to this domain which for one reason or another employ questionnaires and rating scales. While these yield interesting and "achievement relevant" materials in themselves, a number of investigators have concluded that the several types of approach probably do not measure the same things and sometimes have to be carefully distinguished. For example, one of them may be tapping more of the dynamics of "motivating," the other more cognitive aspects of "values."

In the present chapter we are not making a particularly systematic distinction other than occasional references to the type of assessment used in a given context. For a summary of the various approaches, results and critique, Atkinson (1958), McClelland (1961) and Heckhausen (1967) are still among the most comprehensive sources.

A body of related research attempts to track the origins of this general disposition—whether it is called a motive, value, or something else—to early socialization in the home, for example, the stress upon independence in male children. It is this social psychological network in particular which gave impetus to several of the fatigue studies discussed below: obviously, socialization practices are linked to cultural expectations at large, as well as to the underlying philosophies of subcultures or entire societies. This will include a number of sociological variables such as economic status, sex roles, mobility, religion, ethnicity and others. Thus, ultimately, when a person "thinks" achievement and behaves as an "achiever," a host of other factors are brought in by way of supplementary cognitions, expectancies, symbols, fears, hopes, habits, and so forth. It is not surprising that many authors have been interested in this syndrome. Perhaps more interesting still in a larger context, some have gone on to link the motivation and personality dynamics to societal events like the Protestant, Capitalist or Socialist movements. Since we are not engaged in a sociological or political treatise we can merely allude to this area, which has been explored since (and even before) Max Weber (1904) and by other social theorists.

Cultural-Religious Influences and Values

If a measure of "fatigue" is to be defined and correlated with "motivation," problems will arise which concern not only the technicalities of such a device but extend to other nontrivial issues having to do with the overall significance of work, fatigue, effort, etc., in a given cultural environment. For example, both the study of the work process and the study of fatigue, including measures of the latter, may pay more, or less, attention to energetic components such as physiological exhaustion, etc. (cf. Vol. I of this series). On the other hand, they may focus more, or less, on the attitudinal and motivational components. There are now some promising approaches to capture the experiential side of all of these, as shown in the exhaustive studies reviewed and conducted by Kinsman and Weiser (1973; and in this volume). The point is that the very kind of emphasis in one's subjective experience *and* in research, is related to the extent to which the given subculture has internalized such things as say, the work philosophies of the Protestant or even Socialist revolutions; both of those appear to have generated (in some of their outcomes) somewhat comparable kinds of work ethic. A statement such as, "I want to do my best" may be followed further along in the task sequence by one of several options. At one extreme there may be "I want to go on, but I am too exhausted." Or else, "I don't care, or don't want to go on even though I could." Depending which of these is in evidence the consequences will also vary insofar as further activity itself is concerned, as well as what kind of measure could *predict* performance, etc., from here on.

It seems a plausible hypothesis that in achievement oriented cultures an emphasis upon exhaustion, energy, capability, reservoir models, etc., may well have particular adjustment value for the individual. Indeed, an emphasis on negative motivation (much as it had impressed students of fatigue as far back as Thorndike!) may well be heavily sanctioned. In any case, the "exhaustion" interpretation probably involves the lesser degree of cognitive dissonance (Festinger, 1957). Yet, even in such environments, motivational factors could actually account for as much behavioral variance as the "capacity" measures. Observations of this nature, of course, run through a good bit of fatigue research, as already noted. We would argue, however, that 1. they seem to have become less prominent after Thorndike's time, and 2. their recognition has rarely been put into the societal context of values, norms and roles in such a way that empirical study was facilitated.

A related problem is posed by the cultural background of the very people who make the study of fatigue their concern: fatigue research *per se*, appears to be primarily found with those cultural groups and in environments which are themselves achievement oriented. Given this background, can we really expect much else but emphasis on performance, limits of capability, and widespread disregard or even ignorance of motivational variables?

It is instructive to look at some findings which show the relevance of one's overall value background for the experience of fatigue. Thus a value questionnaire was administered to 83 male German high school seniors (Wendt, 1956) asking them to respond to such items as "I cannot really enjoy a break until I have successfully completed a substantial piece of work"; or, "I work like a slave at everything I undertake until I am satisfied with the results"; etc. The overall score was regarded as a respondent type measure of achievement orientation, or "v Achievement," which differs from "n Achievement" (deCharms, 1955). The same subjects (Ss) were tested after 3 to 5 hours of strenuous school work at the end of which they had, in addition, performed a complex arithmetic task (Düker, 1949). The Ss then rated themselves on several graphic scales including two that are relevant in the present context: 1. the degree of avoidance motive present ("opposed to working any longer") and 2. degree of exhaustion present ("exhausted and spent, worn out"). As Figure 13-1 shows the ratings on the avoidance scale reflect the expected effect of what might also be called "achievement" socialization. The exhaustion measure, too, suggests a certain amount of denial as a function of achievement values, but the trend is weak and/or not significant. Incidentally, the prior perform-

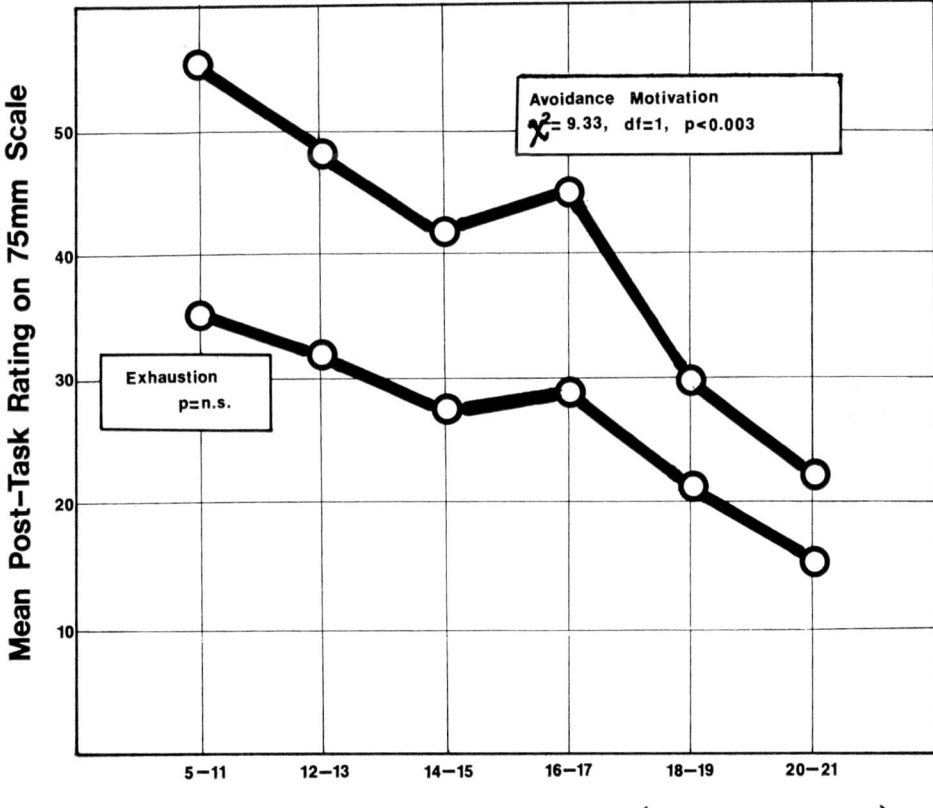

Figure 13-1. Achievement orientation scores vs. mean post-task rating. Description—see text.

TABLE 13-I

	In Oneself	In "Others"
Partial correlation, "Exhausted, spent" vs. "Opposed to continue work"	−0.02	0.66

ance on the arithmetic task did not correlate with either of the above measures. With the same Ss there is a significant effect of something like "projection" in the sense of clinical psychology. There are several indicators of this, and one piece of evidence is as follows.

First, we partialled out the common correlation with a subjective arousal rating ("Alert" vs. "Dulled/inattentive"). We then find (Table 13-I) the following relationships among the individual's own rating space in comparison with how he perceives the fatigue domain of anonymous "others" working under supposedly comparable conditions.

The latter relationship as well as the difference in correlations are, of course, highly significant for the N in question. Evidently, at the projective "distance"—which may be less threatening to the self-image of an achievement oriented person—the fatigue/exhaustion syndrome is readily likened to avoidance (with 44% predictor variance), something that is not recognized or not verbalized in one's own experience after several hours of demanding work. Another finding from the same study is somewhat of a corollary. When we remove, again by partial correlation, the common contribution of the exhaustion variable from the correlation of the other two examined here, we note a sizeable difference in the interpretation of the motivational versus the subjective *arousal* component (Table 13-II).

The difference is again statistically significant although less easily interpreted than in the analysis above. In fact, whether we are really dealing with a projection mechanism of the clinical type (also put in question by Rüssel, 1964), or with influences operating at a primarily semantic or surface structure level cannot be determined from the information at hand. Incidentally, the correlation between "exhaustion" and "inattention" is essentially the same for "self" and "other" ratings, with 0.41 and 0.48 respectively. It is in any event clear that several components of the fatigue experience are strongly influenced, or even defined, by work related *attitudes* of the individual. It would be instructive to replicate this kind of study using the

TABLE 13-II

	In Oneself	In "Others"
Partial correlation, "Opposed to continue work" vs. "Dulled, inattentive"	0.53	−0.34

more purified adjective clusters of the recent Kinsman and Weiser experiments, especially if those materials were available in the form of factor scores.

Research on fatigue and vigilance (cf. Schmidtke's chapter in this volume) and industrial performance generally has long been aware of nonlinear effects. That is, intermediate work loads may be accompanied by improvements in performance or feeling whereas very light work or else work near exhaustion can lead to a substantially different outcome, something to which we will return below. This point raises another question: could it be that the fatigue described will *eventually* emphasize an avoidance motive component provided the individual is approaching objective exhaustion? In a way such a demonstration would be particularly instructive. Some might argue the tangible evidence of one's actual capacity limits must lead, if anything, to a greater prominence of such physiological, etc., descriptions. However, we reasoned that any "shielding effect" that ordinarily intervenes between achievement values and the recognition of the negative motive component, might break down under high work loads: this then would lead to an even greater rather than lesser awareness of avoidance. As a partial test, 50 female student Ss at a highly competitive American Eastern college were asked for their *definitions* of "fatigue," choosing from word lists offering seven different categories and under two load conditions: 1. at the beginning of final exam preparations and 2. after 10 to 14 hours of essentially continuous study. The following Table 13-III (modified from Wendt, 1955) shows the outcome for the two sets of criteria of interest here, omitting those few Ss who used neither of them.

Thus, in the absence of considerable work load, negative motivation and avoidance components in the Ss' perception are practically absent, but they increase substantially as objective exhaustion presumably is *more* plainly felt. Possibly then, additional stress at least partially interferes with one's awareness of achievement values and the cognitive elaboration that would be in keeping with such norms. While there is some ambiguity in the above result in that time of day entered into the Ss' ratings, we do not consider this a major distortion in this particular case.

Earlier we had implied that the Protestant or comparable work ethics might not only have an impact upon achievement motivation but would also color people's very experience of many task situations. The former as-

TABLE 13-III

Percent of Ss Choosing	Before Exam Period	After 10-14 Hours Study
Exhaustion and physiological criteria	95.1	73.5
Avoidance and other negative motivation	4.9	26.5

pect has been explored in a number of investigations, often quantitatively (e.g. McClelland, et al., 1955; 1961). Occasionally there have been attempts to relate the religio-cultural environment more explicitly to the fatigue domain. Thus as part of a larger study on Canadian university Ss ($N = 339$) directed at the perception of behavior as to its supposed morality (Fabrycky and Wendt, 1968), Ss were also asked to define the fatigue experience by choosing the "most valid" 10 from among 20 randomly arranged terms. The latter had been selected on the basis of pilot experiments so as to tap both the criteria of exhaustion and those of negative motivation. Examples of the former included drained, exhausted, incapacitated, unable, weary, etc. The latter group was made up of terms such as disgusted, disinterested, lazy, unambitious, unwilling, etc. A score was based on the relative frequency of the "motivation" vs. the "exhaustion" definitions, and then related to a variety of other measures.

We shall focus mostly on the average weight given the avoidance descriptions by several groups of Ss who had undergone presumably different socializations in terms of their religion as well as birth order. In this context, the latter variable is to function primarily as a replication, thus lending more stability to data some of which are based on small N's. In order to interpret the figures below, it may be useful to give the following range of equivalences. A weight or scale value of 1 was assigned to fatigue definitions which included no or only one avoidance motive term out of ten chosen; a weight of 2, to definitions including 2 or 3 such terms; a weight of 3, to 4 or 5 motive terms; and a weight of 4, where from 6 to the maximum 10 terms came from the motivation domain as defined. Since the materials were given out in a class environment as a "take home" assignment, to remove special pressure upon the Ss, it is not surprising that, generally, the "exhaustion" definitions predominate—in fact, the 70 to 80 percent usage here is similar to the earlier study with the pre-exam task setting referred to above. The interesting finding is, however, that the stated definitions of at least the male Ss show a fairly conspicuous relationship with the socioreligious cluster. That is, the Protestant Ss are least inclined to define fatigue in motivational terms (less than 10% usage), while the Roman Catholic Ss are relatively most ready to do so (about 25%). In addition, they show the *least* interindividual variability despite the higher means, contrary to what might be expected statistically. It should be noted that because of their very similar trend, the few identifiable Jewish Ss have been included with the Protestants. With these qualifications, the results for the male Ss are given in the following Table 13-IV.

Among the females the picture is less clear. A direct comparison is not possible since special selection factors operating in the Canadian university scene of the mid-60's would tend to affect the very entrance of women and

TABLE 13-IV

Mean Scale Value Assigned Negative Motivational Terms in Fatigue	Firstborn	Later Born	Weighted Mean	Total N
Protestant	1.39	1.35	1.37	126
Anglican	1.68	1.16	1.43	37
Catholic	2.18	2.00	2.09	21

therefore, the degree of representativeness. Not implausibly, however, first born women (from all three subcultures) were relatively more likely to emphasize "exhaustion" terms in their definitions than did their male counterparts. In a general way such findings might corroborate data from other studies which have demonstrated differences in the fatigue and negative motivation components in the subjective experiences of men and women (cf. Pierson and Lockhart, 1964).

A number of orthogonal factor analyses were carried out on the correlation matrices in 12 subgroups defined by Ss' sex, religion and birth order. While the outcomes were frequently complex, a few results may shed additional light on the kinds of motivational issues raised here. The most obvious finding is that the fatigue definition (*qua* motivational variable) loads on virtually none of five factors extracted for the male and female *Protestant* subgroups; the largest coefficients found are 0.26 and 0.29 respectively and are statistically inconsequential. On the other hand, the fatigue definition variable does load (and about four times as strongly in terms of the respective r^2) on at least one each of the several factors identified among the Anglican and Catholic subgroups, with loadings from 0.46 to 0.61. At the same time, the composition of these factors differs to some extent across populations. Generally, then, not only is the relative *emphasis* on the motivational aspect different, but also, in terms of the factor analysis, the fatigue definition of the Protestant Ss is clearly embedded in a different *context*. Complex though this higher order effect may appear, it does suggest that the sociocultural dimension is of much greater importance than we would have suspected. Somehow then, fatigue research had better concern itself with a domain of behavior that up to now seemed safely within the purview of social philosophers, psychologists, and other "outsiders."

Emotional and Personal History Factors

Using a kind of energy reservoir model in reverse, Grandjean (1968)—despite his emphasis upon its constituent seven or more dimensions—once compared fatigue to the level of liquid in a container. Different sources add to this "liquid," analogous to the accumulation of effects contributing to the everyday experience of fatigue. Recovery, the outflow from the container, is a process which takes place during sleep, with the occurrence of recovery approximately compensating for the stresses to the organism which had contributed to the fatigue. Physical exertion and sleep deficit obviously add to fatigue, but in addition, an important source is the organism's emotional state.

The discussion and awareness of "emotional fatigue," those subjective feelings of tiredness, lethargy, etc., has given rise to varying ideas, some of which regard emotional fatigue as a sort of symbolic expression of, or as a defense against, consciously disowned needs or wishes. It has also been viewed as occurring as a result of the expenditure of energy due to other psychological conflicts. The outward demonstration of fatigue and sleep may then become an escape mechanism, signifying retreat from an anxiety producing conflict. Furthermore, expressed fatigue may serve as a substitute expression for anger, as in Freud's Fräulein Elisabeth (Freud, 1952; see also Laughlin, 1967).

Chronic subjective fatigue seems often to be a manifestation of such fatigue associated with emotional phenomena—pronounced tiredness throughout the day, irritability, depression, listlessness or apathy, sometimes including a complaint of "I just don't have any motivation," which of course is interesting for this very discussion. Many persons chronically fatigued are sometimes considered "functionally" ill, with anxiety states and/or depression as an accompaniment. People suffering from certain psychoneuroses do exhibit fatigue more readily: for example, female depressives given a task of lifting a 2 kg weight with a middle finger, reported "subjective" fatigue more rapidly. They also quit the task more quickly than patients with anxiety or other neurotic traits (Hemphill, et al., 1952; cf. also Gross and Bartley, 1951).

The term "neurasthenia" is sometimes used to designate chronic or subjective fatigue as an emotional reaction, one "characterized particularly by symptoms of . . . weakness, fatigability, feelings of inadequacy, irritability, poor concentration, and by the presence of a variety of other lesser physical, psychologic, and emotional features" (Laughlin, 1967). The subjective feelings, in turn, may be accompanied by performance decrements and seeming decreases in capability. Neurasthenics perform less well under stress, often become symptomatic after psychic trauma, and have low working capacities.[1]

As clinicians are aware, the definition of neurasthenia has been fairly unstable, from being the "garbage can of medicine" (Chatel and Peele, 1970, citing Fore), or the catch-all of most neuroses, to being primarily descriptive of a fatigue state, whether subjective or manifested by decreased

---

1. The differences in capacity to exercise may, in turn, conceivably be linked to the neurasthenic's excessive lactate production during standard exercise (Taylor, et al., 1970).

work capacity. The term first arose to deal with nonpsychotic yet psychiatric conditions, and is viewed as having opened up the way to the use of psychotherapy (Mora, 1970). The discussion concerning definitions has been revived recently, and neurasthenia has been suggested as descriptive of complaints of chronic weakness, tiredness, and exhaustion, in order to separate these symptoms from "depressive neurosis."[2]

Over the years many ways have been proposed to deal with neurasthenia: thus at one time, the presumed relationship of food to intellectual capacity, proposed by George Miller Beard in the late 1800's, became an essential basis for the treatment of the neurasthenic. Many patients then were "required to consume extracts of animal brain to replenish the molecular constitution of his exhausted brain" (Haller, 1970). Our society is still charmed with the offers to take care of "tired blood," with cures promised by vitamins and minerals, hormones, travel ("Get Away from It All!") to help us rid ourselves of our "unexplainable" fatigue.

Be this as it may, the subjective fatigue experienced, whether termed neurasthenia, emotional fatigue or other, is related to the overall psychological state of the individual, is of widespread concern, and does have an undeniable effect upon our attitudes, judgments, willingness and ability to perform. Laughlin (1967) even speaks of an incentive-fatigue ratio, an *"inverse-relation between the amount of incentive which is present, and the amount of fatigue which is experienced. The more incentive, the less fatigue."* So far this relationship, which is certainly suggestive of a motivational criterion, is not yet well documented. It *has* been found that sleep deprivation reduced what was termed "motivation" (Engles, et al., 1953). We are presenting some empirical evidence along similar lines later in this chapter in the context of performance.

Emotional fatigue, however, may itself have some antecedents in the framework of motivation. It has been shown "that persons with affective disorders (neurasthenia or dysthymia) typically set extremely high levels of aspiration . . . 'atypical' changes in aspiration following success and failure are associated with 'atypical' levels of aspiration" (Atkinson, 1964). In the latter author's framework, where a person's motive to achieve success (M_S) is greater than his motive to avoid failure (M_{AF}), his level of aspiration will be pretty realistic. However, when that relationship is reversed (i.e. where $M_{AF} > M_S$ the level of aspiration will reflect a protective strategy—either being very low, where success is guaranteed, or very high, where failure is not the individual's fault: either case of course represents an avoidance of more realistic goals. Moreover, according to several

---

2. In the United States, the term "neurasthenia" had not been used as an official classification for many years, until 1968 when it was again introduced for the sake of international consistency. There is still much controversy about its precise definition—in this chapter it is used to describe a generalized state characterized by chronic subjective fatigue.

studies, persons with $M_S > M_{AF}$ perform at a higher level than those with $M_{AF} > M_S$ (Atkinson, 1964; Heckhausen, 1963, 1968).

Technically, the motive to achieve success and the motive to avoid failure are often understood as personality dispositions. In any case, an individual's pre-experimental motivation level—either as a facet of his personality or as affected by his current environment—has been suggested as a significant variable affecting actual performance such as in industry (Fleishman, 1958; Vroom, 1964). In addition, it affects the degree to which a certain level of arousal can be produced by instructions within the experimental situation (French, 1955).

Individual differences are also seen in the reactions which arise from certain test conditions. In a study by Davis (1947), RAF pilots were carrying out an exercise in instrument flying in the Cambridge Cockpit testing device. This situation involved skilled activity and prolonged effort at a difficult task. There were two distinct reactions: in one group of Ss, all parts of the task were affected, errors more frequent and overcorrected. The pilots felt under strain, and there were signs of emotionality. In the other group, some parts of work were affected more than others, errors were less frequent but the correction was slow and larger. Interest decreased, and the Ss became apathetic and discouraged. In all cases there was a performance decrement (the task was assumed "fatiguing"—let us just say that the results confirm the expected disorganization of the activity).

Feelings of monotony, in addition, are related not just to the task being performed, but also to more general factors in workers, the individual perception helping to determine how monotonous repetitive work may be (cf. Bartenwerfer, 1970). There is a tendency for personality variables to be important. For example susceptible workers seem to be less satisfied with their personal lives and with the plant situation even in aspects not directly concerned with the repetitiveness (Smith, 1955). A person's own ego-involvement in the situation in turn seems to be related to the tiredness which he reports and the adequacy of his work (Bartley, 1957; Meltzer and Ludwig, 1967).

We must recognize then that neurasthenia, emotional fatigue, personality dispositions, motivation, individual variation, are all inextricably bound up in the study of fatigue effects. A person will always carry some of these determinants into the task situation with him; some of these are more demonstrable than others, making it easier to identify and account for their influence. We are undoubtedly completely unaware of some of these factors, which makes it imperative to deal at least with those of which we *are* aware, or rather, which we can make accessible to research. This may include the systematic exploration of the subjective experience (e.g. Kinsman and Weiser's chapter in this volume; Wolf, 1967), as well as some other ways which are emphasized in the present chapter.

Circadian and Other Chronobehavioral Factors

Extensive work in recent years has identified numerous physiological and behavioral variables which are subject to periodicities. The most widely researched of these concern circadian phenomena, i.e. changes following some regular pattern over the course of approximately 24 hours. Whether in a given instance we are dealing with analogs of "built-in" clocks in the organism, as is argued (cf. Hastings, 1970) or whether all such rhythms are caused or at least *re*synchronized by the environment (cf. Brown, 1970), is outside the present scope of discussion. In any case, the many periodicities so far discovered now suggest that systematic fluctuations also occur in the domain of exhaustion feelings and motivation, along with arousal and vigilance (both of the latter having seen a great deal more documentation). For comprehensive surveys of relevant periodicities in humans, Aschoff (1965), Bünning (1964), Halberg (1969), Hildebrandt (1971), Kanabrocki, et al. (1974), Luce (1970), Orme (1969), and Reinberg (1971), among others, may be consulted.

Some new materials more directly pertinent to the present topic were obtained from a pilot study (Moen, 1973) where student Ss charted their feeling states and various physiological functions, using standard procedures of self-measurement (autorhythmometry; cf. Halberg, et al., 1972). The psychological state measures included eighty adjectives with instructions to check the five most applicable nine times daily over the course of several days. For this preliminary purpose we tallied the occurrence of states connoting avoidance feelings or negative motivation, as well as states connoting fatigue of the "exhaustion" type as already discussed. In this particular study neither kind of description was particularly common as the Ss paid more attention to social feelings and behaviors. The first group (24 usable tallies in all) consisted of terms such as bored, disgusted, lazy, unmotivated; the second group (29 tallies) of beat, exhausted, lethargic, weak and weary. It may be noted that in terms of the recent dimensional analyses by Kinsman and Weiser (e.g. 1973) this grouping was probably not optimal. In any case, a score of relative "motivation" emphasis was then defined as simply the percentage of the former terms in the total, and plotted over the course of two days. This is an unsophisticated procedure but it does have the advantage of staying close to the data base. Despite the irregularities due to the small N's, the "relative avoidance" score shows a steep upward trend about noon, rapidly stabilizing near 50 percent values and with a minor peak in late evening at 2100 hrs (after which avoidance references again decrease towards their early morning lows of 10% or less).

This finding is at least partially in keeping with an observation made earlier. In other words, despite the—presumable—greater subjective "nearness" of actual physiological exhaustion at the end of a working day, this aspect is not necessarily reflected in the individual's experience. Because of the limited number of observations available for the ratings, it was not practical to subject the proportion measure to a periodicity analysis such as least squares cosine fitting (Cosinor; cf. Halberg, et al., 1967). In this context, incidentally, we are ignoring the theoretical problem whether a cosine fit is actually doing justice to the underlying mechanism, a point made by Wever (1973) and others. For example, the dependent variable scores may contain a mix of lower or higher order derivatives or integrals of the underlying response system (cf. Schmitt, 1974).

In a subsequent investigation, student Ss were taking a larger number of measures on themselves including several physiological tests, with readings and notations six times a day for 13 days. All variables were subjected to a spectral analysis of the time series and the cosine fitting procedure mentioned. This provides estimates of the peaks ("acrophases") of the various functions under the assumption that an exact 24-hour rhythm underlies some observed variability, as well as estimates and confidence limits for other preselected periods. (The international glossary by Halberg and Katinas provides definitions for the terms used here and elsewhere.) In this case, the iteration covered the entire 20 to 28-hour spectral window, which proved to be informative as will be seen later. Some of the data from this study seem to illuminate the distinction between "exhaustion" and "motivation" type reports during the course of the day, with Ss undergoing greater or lesser task involvement during the two-week period studied. Nearly complete chronobehavioral and physiological analyses were actually available on eleven female Ss. Six male Ss, whose protocols were analyzed in part, did not appear to react substantially differently. The feeling states reported by the Ss were classified by fatigue type as experienced, based on prior hypotheses. There were forty-two predetermined and one open (i.e. write-in) state descriptions. Specifically, references to drained, exhausted, unable, weak, and worn out, were considered fatigue statements close to the "exhaustion" cluster, and assumed to involve one particular kind of physiological/chemical base. On the other hand, terms such as avoiding, disgusted, indifferent, lazy, or unmotivated were defined as negative motivation indicators which, presumably, involve a different network as far as the neuophysiological substratum is concerned.

The most general finding for the present purpose is that the exhaustion type descriptions show a fairly clear rhythm with well-defined peak or acrophase. In this sample the medians of the fitted peaks of virtually all such terms are seen after midnight, with Table 13-V providing the two most in-

TABLE 13-V

Term Chosen as Descriptive	Median Interpolated Acrophase, Hours	Range of Computed Acrophases, Hours
Drained	0159	2019...0743
Exhausted	0245	1924...0812

teresting examples. The range of the eleven individually computed peak functions—more meaningful here than the standard deviation—is also indicated.

By contrast, the motivation (avoidance) states show a very different pattern. For one thing, about half of the Ss exhibit a well-defined and statistically significant circadian variability as such. That is, individual Ss show distinctive peaks; however, at the same time, their location is idiosyncratic. In our limited sample of cases, this is most apparent for two terms which are also probably the most unambiguous descriptors of avoidance tendencies. Thus for "unmotivated" we find circadian rhythms with individual Ss' acrophases throughout the entire 24-hour day, from 0142 hrs to 2304 hrs. For "disgusted" the actual acrophases (whether significant or not within a given S, cf. above) likewise range from 0054 hrs through 1723 hrs. It may be incidentally relevant that two other kinds of fatigue have also been distinguished on the basis of differential circadian criteria (Reinberg, et al., 1973).

Several observations are *à propos* in reporting these findings. For one thing, they may help explain a result noted earlier that otherwise might seem almost contradictory: we had found a seemingly *stable* preference for "motivation" descriptions in another rhythmometric experiment for the afternoon to evening statements. However, the measure there had been defined as a proportion out of the totality of both exhaustion and motivation terms used. Possibly then, the observed constancy was contributed or at least augmented by the fairly stable exhaustion component—this would generate a discernible time pattern for the ratio measure even where the other component shows considerable randomness.

The Ss were also asked to perform some psychomotor tasks, first at a "comfortable" or "most natural" rate (with *no* motivational implications, as it was explained), and subsequently at their maximum possible speed. Presumably the second type of instruction brings in the element of effort and motivation, whereas the first kind might be more indicative of the transient arousal at that time. The question is, would we again find that the motivation related inputs 1. are compatible with the presence of stable circadian rhythms, yet 2. their peaks show more interindividual variability than is found for the exhaustion *or* arousal components of the performance in question? As an example, we may look at a finger dexterity task employed in this context. According to the instructions the S would touch and count fingers with the thumbs of both hands but going in opposite directions for 20 rounds; this is difficult for some people and usually requires good concentration. Over the two-week period, this test too was performed under instructions of both "leisurely or comfortable" and "as fast as possible without making an error." Portions of the instructions seem to resemble a study by Wotzka and Grandjean (1968) on thirty air traffic controllers. (However, their parameters were different in other respects, and no specific chronobehavioral or spectral analysis seems to have been conducted there.) Both for our sample as a whole and on an individual basis, statistically significant circadians were detected in the spectral analysis. However, under the "comfortable" condition the median performance peak, that is, fastest finger counting was computed at 1638 hrs from the cosine fit. The individual acrophases ranged from 1400 to 1905, thus showing good population stability, since S.D. $\leq$ 60 min. There is an interesting corollary in the finding of a similar arousal peak as measured by critical flicker frequency (CFF), near 1600 hrs as graphically estimated from one of the published curves on the air traffic controllers (Grandjean, 1970). Now again, in the present study, when instructions are calling for *maximum* effort anything like a mean or "typical" acrophase is impossible to define, and the peaks are found throughout the day: individual Ss do show circadian rhythms, with about half statistically significant as such, but the range of peaks is from 0520 hrs through 2108 hrs, with only one apparent gap near the normal mid-sleep span. The result is the more convincing in that speed scores under the two conditions (comfortable vs. maximum performance) are positively correlated as one would expect: if anything this fact would obscure the *difference* in the distributions here noted. However, there was no practical method, given the kinds of data, to correct for the confounding.

A review of other work reveals a curious similarity between the erratic time pattern of the motivational peaks vs. the relative stability of the exhaustion peaks in our human Ss and some results obtained in other mammals. For example, in mice and rats, a number of functions that are presumably central in the physiology of capacity and exhaustion, exhibit well-defined acrophases which are individually significant, highly stable and similar in phase throughout the species. Instances may be seen in the circadian function of liver glycogen, adrenal or serum corticosterone, survival time and resistance to various toxins, temperature regulation, and a number of others (cf. Halberg, 1969; Kleitman, 1967; Luce, 1970). At the same time highly "idiosyncratic"—though again individually stable—behavioral characteristics have been noted in rodents regarding their preferred *distribution* of effort (drive, or motivation?) throughout the day (cf. Richter, 1958; 1967). We do not wish to enter into an idle speculation on the similarities of mice and men. However, it may be well to point out that where this is meaningful at all, the discussion might profit from considering chronobehavioral data, since the methodology is now reasonably accessible following the development of practical algorithms and computerization.

Further analysis of our data revealed an apparent phase lag (within a given individual) involving the state descriptions studied here. Thus, on an individual level, the references to "exhaustion" are generally lagging the references to "drained" feeling states. Of the 11 Ss studied systematically, 9 follow this pattern, and the average lag over all 11 Ss is 74.4 min. (S.D. 130.7 min.). In turn, and despite the striking randomness of the avoidance motive maxima as recorded over the 24-hour span, those references are at least roughly in phase with the "exhaustion" criteria, lagging the latter by 100 min. (with S.D. 297.3 min., however). Relationships of this type can be uncovered by appropriate fitting procedures but would not be readily accessible from even a detailed examination of the data universe by more standard psychological methods.

Finally, spectral analysis suggests the presence of interesting differences in period length. All of the above discussion had been based on the model of an exact 24-hour rhythm. However, the Cosinor program used here (Tong, et al., 1973) can, of course, be adapted to other periods as well. In the present case, optimal fits were computed for the entire 20 to 28-hour spectral window, with the result that for many of the state references the "logical" 24-hour period assumption is not the optimal one. In other words, the fit improves when other periods are admitted into the model. In part such a result is a statistical artifact since even a basically stable 24-hour rhythm would be subject to some randomness as far as the behavioral correlates are concerned. Therefore, purely accidental deviations, too, within the dimension of the dependent variables might be interpreted by the regression program as indicative of a "better" fit at, say, 24.2 rather than 24.0 hours, etc. Indeed, as a general rule we should expect higher statistical significances for individual cosine fits as we open up the spectral analysis so that periods increasingly below and above 24 hours (truly *circa*dian in other words!) are accepted. Our data bear this out in many instances, and no comment is necessary where "precision" is obtained by, in fact, capitalizing on chance—a problem that, of course, plagues statistical analyses nearly everywhere. The situation is not so easily resolved where a fit to, say, a 20.5-hour period, or to 27.7 hours, etc., yields high statistical significance while the 24-hour fit suggests virtual randomness. There is no space here to list in detail all such instances in the above data. Nevertheless, one general observation provides suggestions for later work. This is the fact that with "exhaustion" type descriptions, better fits are more common (at least in our sample) when the regressions are calculated on a 27 to 28-hour model or possibly still longer periods. By contrast, better statistical fits are frequently obtained for the "motivation" terms when the iteration focuses on periods near 20 hours (or probably, shorter periods still, that is ultradian rhythms). For technical reasons, we cannot document this observation in a rigorous format, but it does seem to suggest a mechanism that bears further study.

In sum, we have some evidence that the motivational component in the fatigue experience has statistical and distribution characteristics over time that are at variance with some other aspects of fatigue. At the very least, it is more idiosyncratic. In itself, the claim that motives are interindividually variable is a commonplace observation in much of psychology—indeed, it is implied in much of the fatigue literature as well, even though terms descriptive of motivational factors in Ss' experience do not always fall into an identifiable cluster (cf. Kinsman and Weiser, Chap. 14 in this volume). However, we have also seen that such a statement has some nontrivial aspects in the chronobehavioral context. It is not easy to explain why the interindividual variability extends to the timing of the peaks in the presence of statistically stable circadian rhythms as such. It raises some complex neurophysiological issues which we are not in a position to tackle at present but some of whose ramifications have been taken up, if not in the above context, by Simonson and others in the first volume of this series (cf. also Grandjean, 1970; Schaefer, 1970).

Conceivably there may also be a relationship between the primarily "clinical" domain of specific fatigue manifestations on the one hand, which was reviewed in the last section, and some chronobehavioral patterns on the other. More specifically, a diagnosed chronic fatigue syndrome might affect people's *free-running* cycles. It is well-known that in the absence of external synchronizers such as in caves or bunkers etc. Ss' activity and physiological cycles will free-run and stabilize at periods of approximately 25 hours or more (but compare the discussion by Wever, 1973). The possible role of greater or lesser degrees of "chronic" or clinically relevant fatigue states in such periodicities is presently unclear. It is tempting—though admittedly simple-minded—to speculate about particularly long circadian cycles in such syndromes. Conversely, if significant extensions were found, we would gain an interesting diagnostic or at least research tool for following up such cases, comparing different types of therapy etc., by measuring Ss' free-running cycles for several days at a time. It might be noted that this hypothesis is independent of those proposals which regard complex desynchronizations of several physiological rhythms in respect to one another, as correlates of mental illness generally (Halberg, 1968).

Besides short-term circadian or even shorter ultradian rhythms, there is some general evidence pointing to motivational and probably other fatigue related changes over longer periods of time. Changes of performance and (often indirectly presumed) motive states as well as feeling tone through the course of the day and week have often been noted in industrial environments and controlled studies (cf. Colqohoun, 1971; Kleitman, 1967; Rüssel, 1968; McCormick and Tiffin, 1974). The menstrual cycle in females as well as other circatrigintan phenomena, and possibly effects in males of a comparable nature, have been investigated for their relationship to subjective fatigue states as well as various kinds of overt behavior indicative of possible motivational fluctuations (Garron and Shekelle, 1973; Procacci, et al., 1974). It is fair to point out, however, that the motive changes underlying some of the monthly variability have more often been implied or observed clinically rather than subjected to rigorous psychometric assessment of other kinds, admittedly a difficult problem where continuous measures are desired (Kinsman and Weiser, Chap. 14). Compromise possibilities for methodology may be seen in the studies of Wessman and Ricks (1966), as well as in such approaches as those of Fiske and Maddi (e.g. Maddi, 1961; cf. Appley, 1971; Schönpflug and Wicker, 1971). Still other methods, and occasionally findings, would assist in the purpose of studying fatigue and motivation over time, for example the variant of factor analysis identified as P-technique. In fact, in one such application (Cattell, 1966), long-term changes were studied (in a single individual) over several months. An inspection of the time trends published of what the author defines as "dynamic source traits" reveals an interesting cyclicity of approximately 6.3—but not 7—days duration for a cluster of attitudes and behaviors seen as indicative of fatigue. Presumably the measures tap a motive component as well, as has been the case in a number of industrial studies.

Still longer cycles can be studied. Thus motivational, arousal and other fatigue related states may vary throughout the course of the year. Such (circannual) phenomena include several kinds of activation components (cf. Halberg, 1969; Hildebrandt, 1971). In some studies the circannual activation is hard to separate from the psychological or behavioral outcomes themselves. Some recent findings which may become relevant for fatigue or motivation research in the area of mother-infant interactions (and apparently their long range effects on later behavior) have been reported elsewhere (Wendt, 1974). At the other end of the scale, this kind of work may eventually complement those long range "phase" studies of human behavior where the periods in question are many years in duration (cf. Thomae and Lehr, 1973).

MOTIVATION AND ITS EFFECTS UPON PERFORMANCE, FATIGUE AND AROUSAL
Suggestion, Expectancy, and Incentive

It has long been known that suggestion is a very powerful force, and that what a person believes to be true about himself and his ability to do will have a great influence upon the resultant behavior. The reality of a person's perception about a situation and of his expectations likewise contributes to his performance of the task and his subsequent responses (such as further approach, or perhaps avoidance) to his success or failure at the task. Suggestions and expectancies are an integral part of everyday life, and we constantly seek support and confirmation, encouragement and reassurance. We seek information when confronted with ambiguities, whether the sources be "expert" opinions, religion, peer relationships, astrology, or a systematic study of behavior, for that matter. Just how suggestion and expectancy affect behavior and performance has been the subject of much research, some of which is relevant to this chapter. Actually, the topic of expectancy is a very broad one, and our notes here cannot adequately cover even the role played by expectancy in the concept of motivation proper, where there are numerous ramifications.

A person's expectancy about the task or performance situation usually has a substantial effect upon how that person performs but also, upon the degree of fatigue which he reports. In particular, the perception of the probability of success at a certain task is an important variable in evaluating a person's performance. According to certain motivational theories, this expectancy interacts with the individual motivation to influence performance, with the difficulty of the task, the probability level at which the person will optimally perform, and the amount of persistence with which the person will pursue the task (Klinger and McNelly, 1969; Feather, 1961; cf. Vroom, 1964). How a person perceives that task to begin with is also relevant. Ash (1964) provided an early example of research by his finding that performance on an ergograph could be increased by lightening the weight, *and* by leading the S to *believe* that the weight had been lightened. Similarly, Jarrard (1960) transferred people from one weight to another identical (actual) weight but smaller in size, thus eliciting the well-known size-weight illusion (the smaller one appears heavier other things equal); in this case, they would make fewer lifts before becoming "exhausted" than people lifting the same size weight throughout the task. In turn, those who transferred from the small weight to a similar one but larger in size (which therefore appeared lighter) made more lifts.

Besides being associated with perceptions of necessary exertion, performance and feelings of fatigue are related to how long a person expects to have to work. With a group of Ss given a series of tasks assumed "fatiguing," some were led to believe that their assignment was virtually done after a certain number had been completed, while some expected that they must continue for a longer period of time. Those who believed that they were near completion reported a greater increase in fatigue than those who expected to continue (Walster and Aronson, 1967; cf. also Snyder, et al., 1974).

Some of the work dealing with the effects of suggestion in performance has been in the context of studying hypnotic effects. Barber (1966), among others, offers a critical evaluation of various experimental studies related to hypnosis she finds that "hypnotic induction" which does not include suggestions for improved performance, also does not significantly enhance either strength, endurance or performance. In addition, "motivational suggestions," whether given under the hypnotic state *or* in a waking condition, will raise people's output on many tests of strength and endurance. Indeed, hypnosis alone does not affect either strength or endurance—"motivational suggestions" are needed. Orne (1959), for example, found that, compared with a weight-holding task of endurance which actually was an entirely hallucinatory exercise under hypnosis, Ss had a much greater endurance in a waking condition supplemented by suggestions than they had while in trance. In a similar study, the Ss—half of whom had been assessed to be highly susceptible to hypnotic procedures and half of whom evidently were not, were tested for hand strength and weight-holding endurance in a counterbalanced design involving hypnotic and waking treatments. All were urged at some point under both treatments to perform their best. The "motivation suggestions" were indeed effective, but they proved just as effective when given under waking conditions as when given under the hypnotic condition; moreover, in this latter study at least, the performance of the "nonsusceptible" Ss was actually superior throughout the sessions (London and Fuhrer, 1961). Both of these studies demonstrate the effectiveness of "motivational suggestion" upon performance. In practice such suggestions can vary from offering a tangible reinforcer (e.g. money) for better performance to mainly verbal encouragement for the subject to do his best. It is fair to point out, however, that other evidence is not as clearcut, and some of it points to observable physiological and perceptual changes which interact in complex ways with performance, for example muscular exertion (cf. Morgan, et al., 1971).

According to Barber, Hull had suggested early that the person turning out better performance under hypnosis may not have been motivated under the waking condition to begin with. In other words, any actual differences between the hypnotic and waking performances might be explained by the *low* or depressed performance in a waking state rather than a greatly increased performance in a hypnotic state. We would think that such an explanation, where valid, would apply to rather special populations or conditions but, at any rate, the argument does again demonstrate the importance of the suggestion and motivated states.

At the same time, the difficulty in measuring the effects of the hypnotic state because of intervening motivational variables becomes apparent; such difficulties have also been observed by Simonson in regard to static work (1971): in measuring static work, one must measure strength and endurance which, he points out, will apparently vary with motivation. Ss who seem to have high motivation show low coefficients of variation for endurance; however, Ss average in motivation are more influenced by outside stimuli, hypnosis, etc. (i.e. if one is poorly motivated, he is more easily distracted), leading to contradictory results. Also, statistically speaking there may be ceiling effects operating in the former group but not in the latter. "On balance, it seems that hypnosis, pain-relieving procedures or other stimuli improve the maximum contraction" (in static work) "or duration of submaximum performance particularly in poorly motivated subjects by removing some sort of inhibition, while highly motivated subjects can produce their maximum effort and sustain submaximum tensions to the point of fatigue without artifice . . . in experiments where the subjects can be chosen for their good motivation, the individual variation is fairly small; when no such choice can be made, the variation is greater" (Simonson, 1971).

Suggestions that are considered motivational influences in the situation plausibly interact with level of ability. People classified as "high ability" who received verbal encouragement and who were urged to perform produced a significant difference in their performance in a self-paced task; those who were classified as "low ability" did not produce such a difference (Fleishman, 1958). Other studies corroborate this interaction between low and high ability Ss (Locke, 1965).

Within the framework of the studies concerning hypnosis, one could see the results as conscious versus unconscious intention to perform in a certain way, the "intention" being a part of the motivated state. Welford (1968) notes the variations in ergographic records and the occurrence of partial recoveries during a performance decline. He suggests that these fluctuations are more than random, that some probably correspond to periods of special effort and that these "recoveries" can be produced by urging the subject to "try harder." In addition, "fatigue effects are to some extent under voluntary control, in the sense, perhaps, that the subject sets levels of effort he is willing to make and of discomfort he is prepared to bear." In studies primarily directed towards the relationship between intent and level of performance, it has been suggested that intent interacts with performance in a significantly linear way—higher level of intention is directly related to higher level of performance (Locke, 1966). One might view this in terms of expectancy, with the level of intention relating to the level of expectancy held by the individual, but so far this is hypothetical.

The intention of a person to act in a particular way has also been associated with the existence of an "incentive" within the acting situation. The presence of an incentive and the addition of an incentive is discussed in many studies concerned with "motivating" individuals.

Actually the term "incentive" is usually given a rather more rigorous meaning in psychological, particularly motivational theory. Thus for Atkinson (e.g. 1964), incentive is defined strictly as a function—in his approach a linear one—of the individual's subjective probability of success in a specific task. The product of the incentive parameter and probability of success should then maximize at 50 percent probability of success although factually it tends to peak more often between 25 and 40 percent. "Motivation," for example achievement motivation, enters simply as an outside multiplier so that, again in theory, the product of motivation and incentive predicts performance. Conversely, what is often termed "incentive" in industrial studies of fatigue etc., would largely be envisioned within the theoretical framework of "reinforcers." On the other hand, when the psychological theorist (let us say one of the operant conditioning persuasion) is referring to "reinforcement" schedules and their planned adjustment with the objective of changing behavior, industrial researchers might not necessarily term this a change of "incentive." Some might classify such procedures as "motivating," etc. There is considerable confusion, but is it nearly impossible to legislate complete consistency by *fiat* such as by systematically rephrasing the terminology of all the research (much of it applied in nature) that is the basis for our brief review here. Thus with the present use of terminology, we will continue with terminology that is fairly loose, hoping that the reader will interpret the meaning in proper context.

Whatever the definition of incentive in detail, individuals are affected differently by these factors, ranging from performance at a much higher level to having their performance completely deteriorate. Schwab (1953) gives a simple example of a reinforcement or incentive affecting the level of performance, and the order of magnitude: individuals were required to hang from a horizontal bar for as long as possible, and the length of time Ss would hang on the bar was measured under three different motivational conditions: 1. where the person was under his characteristic or momentary level of motivation; 2. with the addition of strong suggestion and urging, or at times supplemented by hypnosis; and 3. with a reward of $5 if the S would increase his "bar time." Individuals hung on longer under the second condition than under the first, and almost twice as long under the third condition as under the first. Unfortunately in such an experiment the very definition of the improvement measure—here nearly 100 percent (and thus indirectly of our conclusions in respect to fatigue effects!)—is heavily dependent upon the effort under the minimum, "normal" or resting condition, etc. Obviously this poses a major problem of operationalization in itself.

The individual motivational orientation as it interacts with conditions of reinforcement has been the focus of interest for a certain amount of work here. For example, in working with institutionalized retardates, Haywood and Weaver (1967) found that Ss who seemed to work simply because there was a task (i.e. were intrinsically motivated) performed more efficiently when presented with a task type incentive, that is, were promised another task to do. On the other hand, Ss not so inclined (and assumed to be extrinsically motivated), performed better with a monetary incentive. Apparently higher order interactions and individual variations are responsible for different results in the two groups. This individual orientation has been investigated in many respects including achievement or affiliation motivation. The personality dispositions involved might be viewed as contributing to the amount of incentive which is present for a person in a particular situation by determining the aspects of the situation which would be reinforcing for a particular individual. As an example, an individual's status and what that implies also has been shown to affect his performance—individuals' status and its changes within their peer group affect people differently. People often maintain performance levels "congruent" with their status: when the performance of a worker who has initially had high status in a group is made to appear to decrease, his actual performance will improve; however, after his status has been lowered by appropriate techniques, his actual performance declines. At this point, when the performance is made to appear to be better, his performance declines further. A rise in status then results in improved performance, etc. (Burnstein and Zajonc, 1965). One explanation is that Ss with low status have little incentive to perform to begin with, since their performance counts for very little. Another interpretation suggests that a person's previous experience with social controls and roles implies certain role expectations; thus he may have learned to associate greater incentives with being congruent with those role expectations than with being disparate (Klinger and McNelly, 1969).

The kind of performance and its context make a difference, and the achievement or avoidance of certain *goals* are affected by such factors as status effects and varying motivational orientations. The ascertainment of specific goals for performance, and how clear the task is, have been shown to be related to performance, and, more relevant here, are related to self-reports of tiredness (Bartley, 1957; Locke and Bryan, 1966). Having a definite goal toward which to strive perhaps serves to direct the attention of the individual, channeling his energies in that direction. The introduction of "incentives" or reinforcers discriminately may accomplish the same. As an example, by adding incentives to conflicting tasks, one a tracking task and the other of memorizing nonsense syllables, Eason and Branks (1963) successfully manipulated the amount of attention and effort as well as its direction. The relationship between tension level (presumably reflecting the amount of effort exerted) and performance was shown to be dependent upon which task a person was primarily giving his attention, determined by the incentives associated with the tasks. Tension level, irrelevant muscular activity, stress, have all been associated with improved performance (e.g. Courts, 1942; Eason and Branks, 1963; Shaw, 1956; Welford, 1968). Physical measurements of muscular tension and electromyographic gradient slopes have received attention as criteria for the amount of effort exerted during a task, or even as a measure of motivation—the assumption being made that if one is more motivated, he will exert more in performing a task, which in turn improves his performance (Bartoshuk, 1955; Mücher, et al., 1957).

Throughout the preceding discussion, the *primary* emphasis has been upon the effects of various "motivational" phenomena in performance with only incidental references to reported fatigue or exhaustion. Where does this leave us as far as "fatigue" is concerned? We have quoted some studies demonstrating many different effects of the interaction between motivation and *performance*—yet, this is only a beginning in looking at the interaction between motivation and *fatigue*. The study of effects of reward or incentives and associated tension levels brings another interesting aspect to the fore—the tension level of particular muscles during the task activity as a possible measure of the exertion or the quantity of effort put into the task (Bartenwerfer, 1969, 1970; Eason and Branks, 1963; Locke and Bryan, 1966). This would seem to relate directly to the eventual accumulation of factors contributing to fatigue, both objective and subjective.

If tension level is associated with improved performance, this is so only up to a certain point; apparently there is always an optimal degree of tension at which performance is at its best. Beyond this point, performance deteriorates, following an inverted U-relationship. Quantitative studies of this phenomenon are largely lacking, a state of affairs, we feel, that contributes to one of *the* fundamental problems in a great deal of fatigue and motivational research, *viz.* that of specifying the *location* of the peak of optimal performance and the amount of associated stimuli which either lead to that peak or beyond it to the point of deterioration. A relationship of that general nature has long been postulated in arousal theory: as level of arousal increases so does performance, up to an optimum level beyond which a further increase in activation causes a decrement or fatigue (e.g. Fischbein, et al., 1968; Thorndike, 1912; Welford, 1968). However, it seems to us that neither psychologists nor neurophysiologists have been able to provide the theory with generally applicable parameters (cf. Bartenwerfer, 1969; Bartley's note in this volume; Grandjean, 1970; Schaefer, 1970). Overall, however, and in a very general way the connection between the addition of incentives in EMG or in muscular tension levels certainly supports the assumption that "incentive" and "motivational" conditions lead to increased arousal. We will return to this problem below.

Vigilance studies, aside from their importance in their own right (cf. Schmidtke, chapter in this volume), provide us with additional perspectives regarding the effects of incentives and motivation. Manipulation of Ss' apparent "motivation" by means of money, for example, can mitigate the common and well-known rapid decline in vigilance performance, at least on a short-term basis; on the other hand, withdrawal of such incentives results in an extensive depressive effect (Bergum and Lehr, 1964). Highly "selected" Ss (who may possibly be regarded as more highly motivated) will also detect signals more easily, as found in Mackworth's vigilance studies (after Broadbent, 1953). Level of performance is to some extent dependent upon the S's expectations about the nature of the vigilance task (Welford, 1968). For example, people led to believe that a vigilance task will be challenging will perform at a higher level than people led to believe that the task will be boring to begin with. This again shows the importance of task perception upon the associated performance (Lucaccini, et al., 1968). At the same time, the performance decrement observed in vigilance situations is probably quite different from that observed in situations generally considered "fatiguing"; for example its time trend is usually different. The explanation is frequently offered that the latter seem to be the result of "overload" and the former the result of "underload" (Welford, 1968).

Generally, a motivation theory of vigilance along the lines of a theory of activation does seem viable and relevant for fatigue research. An increase in motivation "will tend to offset any fall of activation during a prolonged watch" in a vigilance situation (Welford, 1968). Finally, observations that electric shock for example, added to a vigilance task, will result in a higher subjective and autonomic arousal and a slower performance decrement, give support to the arousal theory (Dureman and Bodén, 1972). The work by Grandjean (1969), Schaefer (1970), and several other investigators point in a similar direction.

Stress and Anxiety

The interaction of fatigue and anxiety is well known in clinical psychology, and some kinds of "fatigue" are manifested by clinical descriptions (or complaints) of tiredness, lethargy, or simply by acting it out in sleeping a great deal. Some clinicians have gone so far as to say that fatigue is mainly a matter of the emotions, excepting the case of objective muscular fatigue (e.g. Hornstra, 1955). Prolonged physical or psychological exertion in a highly stressful situation contributes to mistakes and misjudgements following the initial stress, which can be alleviated by having another person take over the responsibility for decisions (Laughlin, 1967). And, in the laboratory, induced stress through warning of failure at a task which would be followed by an electric shock in case of further failure, was followed by significant decrement in continuous performance (Davidson, et al., 1956).

It has been postulated that anxiety contributes to the generalized drive state or state of arousal, hence fitting into the well-researched inverted U-relationship between arousal level and performance. (Many psychologists regard anxiety as a drive—see Atkinson, 1964; we follow a fairly common convention when we treat it similarly, but do not wish to make a theoretical commitment here). The relationship is demonstrated in studies with relatively uncomplicated tasks which in themselves would not invoke anxiety about performance. In these cases, Ss with a higher tested anxiety tend to perform better than Ss low in anxiety. However, with more complex tasks, highly anxious Ss perform more poorly (Spence, et al., 1956). Impairment of performance is also seen in people high in affiliative anxiety who were required to act in the presence of an audience (Quarter and Marcus, 1971). Generally in situations which are "ego-involving," individuals low in anxiety accomplish more—and may show less observable fatigue—than highly anxious ones. On the other hand, in task-oriented conditions, both high and low anxious persons may perform quite similarly (Nicholson, 1958).

The above findings point out the importance of the stimulus situation, at least in terms of an individual's involvement, in its interaction with anxiety level. Davis (1953) suggested that the anticipation of psychological danger will have the same effect upon performance as the increase or decrease of a drive: "As the anticipation of danger increases, the lower becomes the intensity of a stimulus necessary to evoke a response, and the less specific does the stimulus have to be. At the same time, the responses become more frequent, more rapid and more vigorous; new modes of response are more readily acquired and unrewarded modes suppressed. Conversely, responsiveness declines as the anticipation of danger declines." After the initial reaction of more frequent responses, etc., if the anxiety is not alleviated the activity declines, and the individuals become inactive altogether. If anxiety or anticipation of failure as in this case is acting as an arousing mechanism, this kind of pattern would be expected—an increment in performance until such a point is reached that the increased arousal no longer facilitates but hinders performance.

Ego-involvement and instructions generally considered "motivating" can interact with trait anxiety in a number of ways. In fact, the interaction effects are frequently more conspicuous than the main effects, statistically speaking. For example instruction that is more "hope" than "fear" oriented will raise the need for achievement (by some kinds of measures) of people low in anxiety, while instruction that is more "fear" oriented will add to the motivation of highly anxious individuals. Thus Sarason (1956) found the interaction between anxiety and motivation significant, low and middle anxious Ss performing better under highly motivating instructions, highly anxious Ss clearly doing worse. The interaction between success and failure with motivation measures is also significant: Ss under conditions of high motivation who have failed perform at a higher level upon their return to the task situation than those Ss under conditions of low motivation. Additionally, the highly motivated Ss who had not failed perform at a lower level than the low motivation/nonfailed Ss. In terms of arousal, the motivating instructions may increase the generalized level of arousal which in turn acts in a facilitative way with the Ss low in trait anxiety, but serves to increase the arousal to a debilitating level in highly anxious Ss.

The anticipation of performance falling short as well as the actual occurrence of such a contingency further increases the activation—to a mild degree helping to organize performance, but eventually contributing to the disorganization phenomena of fatigue (von Bracken, 1952, 1956). To quote Welford (1968) ". . . If activation and arousal outlast the circumstances giving rise to them, they will be liable to build up progressively during performance unless time is allowed for them to die away."

Cognitive Aspects

The concept of arousal or activation, however, again only serves to explain one aspect of the interaction between the occurrence of stimulation and the following changes in performance and in self-reports of alertness, feelings of stress, or fatigue. At least in discussing the neurophysiological aspects of fatigue it has become necessary to include the fact that not all "stimulation" will contribute to the increase in level of activation. Among other things, level of arousal is certainly not related in any obvious way to some overall (physical?) level of stimulation to which the individual is subjected (cf. Schaefer, 1970). Rather, the information which the stimuli carry and the individually specific significance of that information play a necessary and imposing part in the resultant activation.

Grandjean (1968) lucidly discussed this kind of situation and the role of the inhibitory-activating neurophysiological system. Neural pathways from the cortex, the regions associated with consciousness, perception, and thinking, lead impulses to this activating system: its stimulation in turn maintains the cortex (and behavior) in a state of functional arousal. The entire system, therefore, can be stimulated by the environment, and subsequently by the information which the environment is conveying to the organism. Some of us, however, are left here with the question of just how does this information act to "stimulate," and the feeling that we are getting into the long shunned area of cognitive aspects of psychology. The addition of "incentives," "motivating conditions," manipulation of the valence of a goal—making it more or less desirable—its significance for the individual ... all of these have an effect upon a person's performance. And all, in some aspect of their functioning, point to the presence of cognitive processes as contributing to the changes in activation and some fatigue phenomena at least indirectly. In a discussion of cognitive aspects of motivation, Dember (1974) summarizes this more recent kind of concern: "Emotional impact of autonomic arousal is highly dependent on the context in which the arousal occurs—context provided by manipulations that clearly are mediated by cognitive processes.... Too many issues are skirted" (by the arousal model). "Psychologists do care about what people perceive and why, for example, certain events are arousing for some people at some times. It may be that ultimately these various psychological processes do all pass through a single blender ("arousal") and come out undifferential glop at the other end, but what they were like before becoming homogenized may still be worth asking." The informational value of events is important, and so too is the way in which an individual processes that "information." The term should be understood here to include both the meaning given it by information theory and processes so high in complexity that even sophisticated computer modelling, in our opinion, has as yet shown only limited promise in leading towards parametric research, let alone ultimate understanding.

PREDICTING EFFECTS OF PERFORMANCE UPON FATIGUE

A number of studies have put in question one of the more classical notions to the effect that performance would somehow relate—perhaps even in a linear fashion—to fatigue levels. It is not that this notion is an unreasonable one in itself especially if one considers some of the neurophysiological concomitants, as several authors have done, and some of whose implications were reviewed above. Moreover, some like Grandjean (1968) explicitly include "decrease of motivation" in their fatigue frameworks, and we have been interested in some other approaches that seem compatible with our own work.

Of course, arousal parameters in particular are involved in virtually all work situations although their effects may become most tangible in those which can be modelled after a signal detection paradigm. The best-explored of these situations occur in vigilance studies proper, a number of which are reviewed elsewhere in this book. But even in other, less well-defined conditions of work the very presence of arousal functions—no matter how covert—suggests complex interactions which will lead to overt fatigue symptoms (or their absence) in a variety of dimensions. Clearly, despite many of the theoretically oriented studies in this area, we are still largely in the dark about the optimal model that would somehow tie the motivational, exhaustion, and arousal dimensions together in a comprehensive fashion. Nor can we offer any such model, especially one that would capture (and in manageable statistical format) the intricacies of a host of nonlinear relationships: as stated before, the latter problem in particular seems to be one of the two major reasons why so much of fatigue research has often gone around in circles. Occasionally, however, some study attempts to relate the motivational or arousal antecedents to the output and its consequences. And occasionally, also, several of the variables mentioned can be shown to fit into a network that lends itself to meaningful interpretations, or at least suggests hypotheses for further study. As one example we shall review an earlier experiment that addressed itself to the motivation and arousal dimensions, along with some explicit concern regarding certain traditional fatigue variables. This particular study involved thirty-eight male high school seniors, and was conducted in a generally neutral school task setting (Wendt, 1955). The relevant variables are as follows:

1. The focal dimension for theoretical reasons is "need for achievement" as then defined by McClelland, et al. (1953). Presumably, among other things, the inter-individual variability seen here is related to various cultural factors which make for different socialization pressures, including values, religion, ethnicity and so forth, which had been recognized as important earlier in this chapter.

2. An arousal measure was defined by the *changes* in critical flicker fusion frequency (CFF) recorded over the course of the task session. The semi-automated electronic device used here lends itself to group administration, thereby eliminating some of the usual error variance found in the traditional individual sessions (Mücher and Wendt, 1951; Wendt, 1953). Overall, of course, the approach bears much resemblance to the pioneering

work by Brozek and Keys (1944), Simonson and Enzer (1941, 1959), and others. The comprehensive overview offered by Landis (1953), while now dated in particulars, is still informative about the background of these measures and the nearly 2,000 applications up to that time. Some of these, of course, would seem to bear out criticism to the effect that in the fatigue context, the method can easily be overrated or even be grossly misleading (cf. the more recent commentary by Schaefer, 1970).

3. Performance on the Düker (1949) arithmetic task, by number of problem units attempted; along with

4. The attendant accuracy, expressed by error percentages. Finally, the sessions included instructions for

5. Subjects' graphic ratings of "interest" in the arithmetic task after completing a 50 min. session;

6. Subjects' ratings of "boredom"; as well as

7. Subjects' ratings of "fatigue" following completion. Fatigue was not further defined here; however, given the option of expressing a motivational component via both the "boredom" *and* "interest" dimensions, our general experience suggests that Ss' definitions would then focus on the subjective experience of physiological or exhaustion phenomena.

A network of results (Fig. 13-2) summarizes the outcome somewhat more

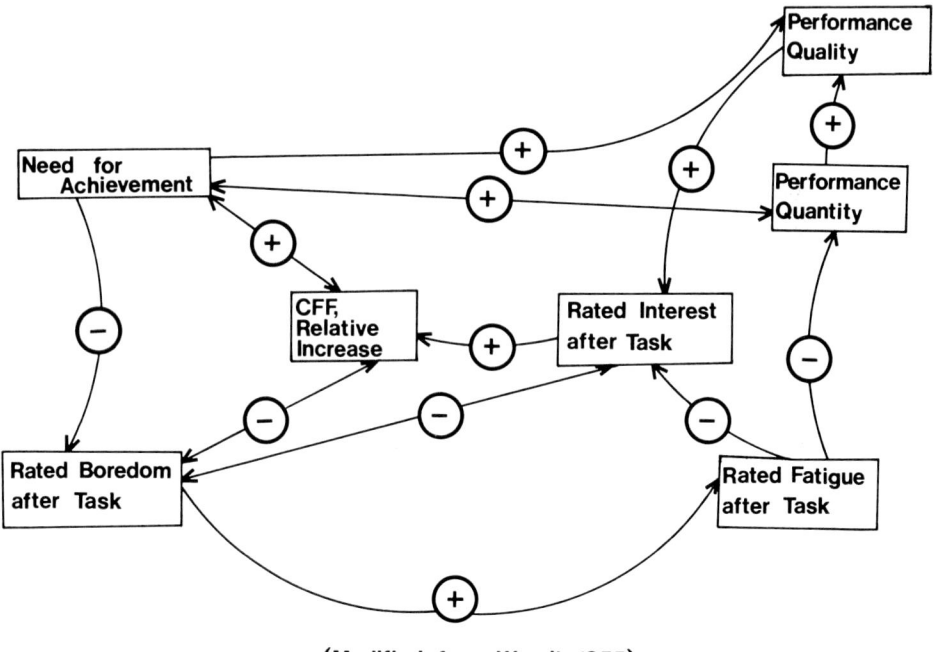

(Modified from Wendt, 1955)

Figure 13-2. Schematic diagram of relationship between performance, fatigue, boredom and CFF changes. Description—see text.

succinctly than the more customary table of correlations. The direction of the relationships is shown by + and − signs, respectively. Also, a crude indication of linearity is provided by double-headed arrows. Curved single arrows in turn show the direction of most successful prediction via t-tests of sub-group means where there is (significant or merely suggestive) nonlinearity.

In the above experimental situation, the work is of the nature of a clerical task requiring high concentration although not vigilance in the sense usually studied. Generally, it may be regarded as "intermediate" in overall effort. The latter may be stressed here in view of the interesting results of Ehlers (1965) and Hashimoto, et al. (1964, 1967) which would lead us to expect different results as a function of degree of overall stress.

The following findings appear worth noting in the context of this section:

1. Achievement motivation is directly predictive of output, of the CFF measure, and of boredom ratings afterwards, with low to intermediate correlation coefficients of approximately 0.30 to 0.60 (not shown).

2. The arousal measure in turn occupies a central position in that it shares variance with the Ss' interest ratings, achievement motivation, and boredom ratings (all in meaningful directions; cf. also Grandjean, 1970).

3. The fatigue assessments are related to the concurrent boredom and interest ratings but also, to the preceding performance level. We note that the more the Ss worked—quantitatively though not qualitatively—the less fatigued they claim to be. At the same time, the attendant effort or arousal that might account for some of this effect, is entering the system indirectly, primarily via the n Achievement.

4. The "motivational" dimension of interest (approach tendency) appears to be an observable outcome of the task performance as such, at least of its quality, while the negative characteristics of boredom and fatigue are not. The latter variables are mediated by the presumably more stable personality characteristics of achievement motivation, in conjunction with situation specific changes in the CFF or arousal indicator. Over and above these notes, the graph may speak for itself; it may be noted that a replication on fourteen college student Ss was on the whole compatible with the results shown.

The comparatively small number of variables and the statistical situation within this particular network would make a factor analysis unprofitable. For one thing, a one-factor (bipolar) solution would be one of the more defensible outcomes, but, of course, any solution is partially distorted by the nonlinearities indicated. For another, this kind of reductionist approach might well obscure whatever logic the observer would otherwise perceive, or want to follow up, in the interrelations (cf. also Kalveram,

1970, for another relevant critique). First and second order partial correlations could be explanatory assists for some of the variables; however, we feel this method, too, would only be a substitute. Specifically, a path analysis (cf. Wright, 1960) should be suitable for testing the viability of the perhaps two or three more obvious causal hypotheses regarding the underlying processes. However, the raw data needed for such a procedure are inaccessible at this time.

CLOSING THE CIRCLE
Some Notes Regarding the Logic of Potential Fatigue Indicators

Previous discussion and, we believe, the conclusions of several chapters in this book illustrate some of the problems that psychological fatigue research continues to face, and at the same time may have suggested some avenues for future work in this field. For one thing it may have become clear that a given state of exhaustion—whether subjectively defined or approximated by some of the neurophysiological measures now becoming available—will not necessarily correlate with previous performance, or in the "expected" direction. It may not even relate to other observable behaviors at the time of that measurement. Whether under such circumstances any of our measures, including subjective assessments, should still be regarded as "fatigue indications" is moot. It depends on the use we wish to make of such an indicator or, perhaps more correctly, of an optimally weighted combination of such measures. One of the ancient conclusions from the work of the World War I Industrial Fatigue Research Board had been the pessimistic observation that anything like a "fatigue test" was impossible to construct (Muscio, 1921). Other authors have argued that the impossibility had its roots more in the kinds of questions asked by the researcher than in the substance of the problem. At the beginning of this chapter we noted that indeed, the "questions" asked in such a context—both by the researcher and in the final analysis by any working individual of his or her own state—are partially dependent upon cultural and other variables some of which enter from well outside the task environment as such. Apparently all of us, researcher and worker alike, "walk in the door" with idiosyncratic notions and frameworks as to what fatigue is, what its implications are, what one should look for in this domain, and by implication, how "it" might be measured. Faced with this state of affairs (recognized or not) some investigators have suggested changes in the measurement approach. Thus one of us in earlier work has offered some arguments which run counter to a number of conventional assumptions. For example we claimed that a fatigue test—like any sort of assessment device—was necessarily measuring best whatever it was validated against in the first place. Moreover, since a great deal of validation had undeniably involved *duration* of previous work, it was argued (not entirely tongue-in-check) that the usual "fatigue test" was really the equivalent of a clock telling the investigator or industrial supervisor how many hours into the work session it was, albeit not very accurately (Wendt, 1956, 1958). Also, difficulties were pointed out which result purely from the statistical properties of a network of the variables often thought relevant. Suppose that we are in fact concerned with the predictive validity of a fatigue test in terms of subsequent performance—a claim we felt to be one of the more defensible if not the only logical possibility. In such a case the efficacy of the test is a function of the external validation criterion as well as the magnitude of the (minimally three) correlations involved. For example, let the fatigue test correlate with a desired or validating criterion (e.g. duration of previous work, EMG, 17-ketosteroid output, or whatever else) at a respectable $r = 0.80$; also, let that criterion correlate with, say, the actual performance to be predicted at $r = 0.50$. From a trival theorem governing three-variable relationships, it will then follow that the "fatigue test" can correlate with the performance throughout an entire numerical range of -0.12 ("negative" validity!) to $+.92$. Nor can anything like a "most probable" value within this range be estimated without making additional (and possibly quite tenuous) assumptions. The prediction stabilizes substantially in cases where one of the partial correlations in the system should be accessible. On the other hand, it is difficult to see how the investigator would normally tap this additional information. (Or can his "intuition" be construed, perhaps, as a statement that is in the logical nature of a first order partial correlation?)

Now, the above reasoning is not without problems of its own, and several authors have taken issue with one or another of the arguments put forward, such as Bartenwerfer (1965), Rüssel (1964), Schmidtke (1965) and others. Certainly the critique showed that the situation we had assumed to exist was frequently mitigated by other factors if nothing else. Yet overall, the discussion served to highlight in its own way some of the very issues that have tended to perplex many of the authors whose work has been reviewed here.

Furthermore, in balance, improvements in fatigue research should come from a reorientation in its logic as well. The exploration and multidimensional study of arousal parameters, physiological concomitants, or subjective experiences under stress, are all necessary and productive enterprises in their own right. At the same time, we would suggest that for a good many present-day applications, it is equally fruitful to focus upon the prediction of *performance* more explicitly. The question, then, is what avenues would promise advances along those lines—which of the numerous manifestations of fatigue can serve in some sort of predictor function? It will have become obvious from the discussion in this chapter that we are expecting some gains towards this objective from motivational indicators. The following section is therefore directed at a brief exploration of such possibilities.

Predicting Future Performance From Motivational Components of Fatigue

In view of the cultural, psychodynamic and other influences that operate on our internal processing of cognitive data it is evident that such processes —in order to have prediction value—cannot easily be tapped directly or overtly. However, there are circumstances where a more clinically oriented approach may be fruitful. One of the better known precedents for such an approach is the Thematic Apperception Test of Morgan and Murray, already introduced. In fact, the seven-variable network discussed in the previous section suggests that motivational changes in the task situation might be reflected in changes of some aspects of achievement imagery, for example; the latter might in turn be used to predict performance quantity or quality. In practice, such a method is in any case time consuming; it might also be poorly received among the people in a workaday environment or by supervisory staff (several investigators' experiences in industry would point in that direction). Theoretically more important, that particular version of a projective method for assessing motive states is not well suited to repeated application because of the difficulty in designing parallel forms. Moreover, it has been plagued by technical problems on other counts such as low reliability, erratic validity, and some others for which the evaluations by Atkinson and collaborators (cf. Atkinson, 1958) or critiques such as Klinger's (1969) may be consulted. An additional problem in the fatigue context—though poorly explored to date—may be that this kind of test is largely constructed around approach parameters (one is almost justified in speaking of a whole approach motive philosophy!). Even the possibility of scoring it for "fear of failure" etc. (Birney, et al., 1969; Heckhausen, 1963, 1967) is in some ways only the other side of the coin. Certainly the designers of the several variants of the technique were not particularly interested in studying "avoidance" phenomena other than certain underlying fear dynamics. Yet in the fatigue domain, much does argue for the common presence of avoidance components, recognized or not, in addition to diminished approach tendencies. Moreover, some of the evidence now suggests that the two may well be orthogonal rather than opposites. For the above and related reasons, some authors have again begun to work with greatly simplified rating scales which can be made reasonably projective in nature, and which may focus on approach as well as avoidance aspects, along with other elements in the fatigue experience. The projective characteristic would help circumvent some of the kinds of modifiers from the sociocultural or clinical domain which may block off the components we would hope to study. The simplicity of such devices on the other hand makes for flexibility of application and for easier scoring. Rating scales when used in clinical or experimental assessment have ambiguities and validity problems of their own which are frequently disregarded (cf. McClelland, 1951). However, such issues would eventually have to be resolved on an empirical level. We should certainly explore such scales for what they might have to offer fatigue research for the specific purpose of performance prediction. Some limited examples, drawn in part from research already referenced, may serve to round out this discussion.

In one preliminary study (Antoni, et al., 1955) five male student Ss were working for 150 min. on the Pauli test of continuous one-digit addition and subtraction. At the end of the period they were asked to rate on a 75 mm graphic scale, the degree of "willingness" or "unwillingness" of comparable "others" in the task situation to go on with this kind of work. It should be noted that a simple "bipolar" model was implied here. The ratings were plotted against the Ss' own further performance during the subsequent 50 min. testing period. While the N is too small for a trend analysis, there was a relationship between the avoidance ratings assigned to anonymous others and the Ss' own later performance, with a rank correlation tau $= 0.80$ ($P < 0.05$, one-tailed test). There was no significant correlation between these Ss' own stated "exhaustion" or "unwillingness to continue," and their performance.

A similar study was conducted in a business environment. The participants were two groups of women inspectors ($N = 22$ and 38, respectively) of soccer pool betting tickets. This work could not be automated at the time and had to be done at night. Since the profits of the organization were heavily dependent on getting the materials scored correctly by morning, a piece rate system was in effect, and the work environment by all accounts was high pressure in nature. There was a 10-min. break every two hours. Three graphic scales were designed and pre-tested, (1) Willing/ambitious vs. Unwilling/opposed to continue work; (2) Alert/attentive vs. Dulled/inattentive; (3) No symptoms of exhaustion vs. Exhausted/various physical symptoms. The scales were handed out during the breaks, and with two sets of instructions: one requested the inspector to check her own momentary state, the other, to describe the state of the typical "other" person in the work bay. The various ratings were then plotted against the Ss' own performance (number of tickets scored and sorted) during the *following* two-hour work span. Several results are worth noting. For one, in the "self" rating condition—but even in their assessment of "others"—the Ss rarely checked scale positions near the negative pole, especially for "unwillingness"; most of their motive statements were in the center or towards the positive end of the scale. However, even with the avoidance pole largely shunned, a relationship emerged between the perception of the motive state of "others" and worker's own performance level. Figure 13-3 illustrates one of the findings; it is seen that the results in one group were much clearer than in the other. Since the two groups had been tested at different times and under somewhat different circumstances, separate analyses of variance along with analyses of covariance were performed. This allowed for the fact that overall averages during the shift varied substantially from one individual to another. The major results were significant and in the expected direction. While the curvilinearity is not readily explained, it suggests that the overall strength of the relationship can best be expressed by a correlation ratio; the appropriate values amount to $eta_{xy} = 0.55$ and 0.52, respectively. More to the point in the present context, the Ss' ratings of their own remaining motivation did not (significantly) predict their subsequent performance levels. Furthermore, a relationship is totally lacking with exhaustion and physical symptoms whether experienced by the worker herself or symptoms assumed in "others" among her colleagues. The category of Alert vs. Dulled occu-

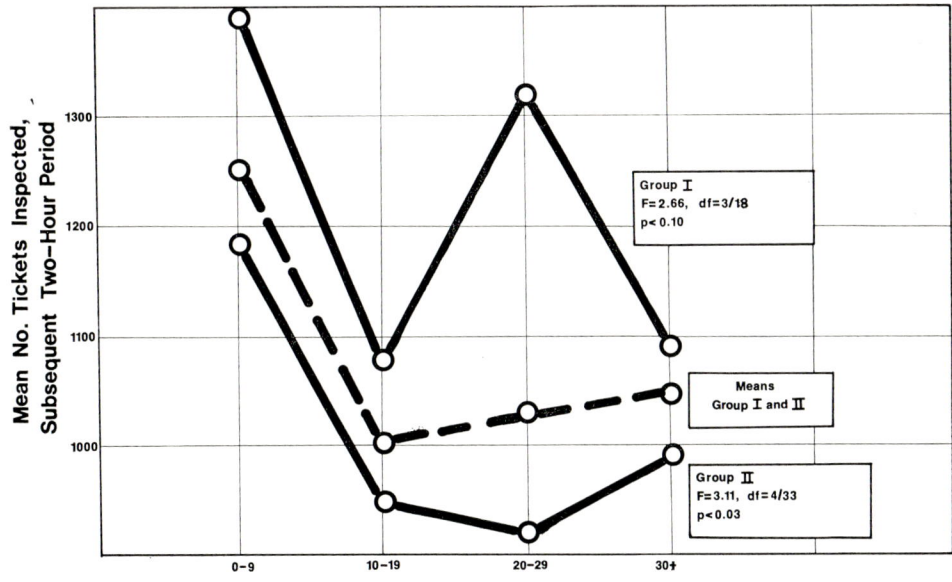

Figure 13-3. Relationship between ratings of task avoidance (abscissa) vs. performance (number of tickets inspected).

pies an intermediate position. None of its linear or nonlinear correlations are significant, however, there is a trend such that the rating of others' alertness (rather than self-evaluation) is somewhat more indicative of the person's own later performance. The implication may be that the investigators were tapping an arousal parameter which, of course, has already been found fruitful in other studies. The particular work environment of the investigation just summarized did not permit to follow up on this angle by a manageable physiological procedure. Six male workers occupied with a similar task in this setting were also tested. Their results point roughly in the same direction as for the women, however, the small N makes a discussion of the (largely nonsignificant) statistics tenuous.

Several later studies attempted to replicate portions of the above results, or were directed at some of their implications. Thus Bartenwerfer (1960) was able to show that different levels of prior work load will have a special impact on the assessment of "others" and will in general affect ratings in dimensions similar to the ones employed in the above study. His attempt to replicate the predictive component of these mechanisms seems to have been less positive, and he has increasingly worked with physiological indicators such as heart rate change, electroencephalographic criteria, and electrodermal responses.

Other authors have specifically focused on the distinction between "self" and "other" assessments, or have investigated the crude projection hypothesis (Haider, 1961; Rüssel, 1962, 1964). The work of Rüssel and his collaborators has been particularly detailed and aimed at new information in this complex area which obviously overlaps the clinical (or psychodynamic) as well as the experimental sectors. There is not space here to review all of his findings and qualifications. However, one of the more interesting outcomes to us is some support for his hypothesis that in situations of the kind studied by Wendt (e.g. 1956) we may be dealing with a *contrast* phenomenon between the self and other rating, rather than—or in addition to—something along the lines of the "projection" believed to take place. The work there did not specifically include the impact of the value and achievement framework in the worker's experiences, or for the fatigue researcher for that matter. Overall we feel, in any case, that future attempts to use motive components of the fatigue state for prediction purposes—including the option of "projected" approach or avoidance—must take into account those more recent empirical results and theoretical critiques.

Finally, some results are available concerning the time trend of such ratings (Rüssel, 1962). These could have been reviewed in our section on chronobehavioral factors in the fatigue experience; however, one of the findings more properly belongs with our conclusions here. The author does not report regression data and was not concerned with spectral analysis or curve fits based on a cosine, exponential or some other mathematical model. Nonetheless, the results there suggest that work stress is accompanied by a kind of disintegration process over time by the criterion of a gradually decreasing intercorrelation *among* various experiential and probably also behavioral indicators. In statistical terms, it would appear that the factor structure of the fatigue domain becomes more diffuse, less organized, as work progresses. This is hardly a trivial result, and future research may well profit from a more systematic study of those variables which enter into the "disintegration" process (cf. also von Bracken, 1956) that is observed at the level of the behavioral interfaces of the fatigue syndrome.

The following block diagram (Fig. 13-4) summarizes clusters of variables discussed in this chapter (and in one aspect anticipates the concluding note below). As has become obvious before, the approach to the fatigue domain proposed here takes many of its cues from *outside* the immediate task setting. This approach and more specifically its emphasis on motivational and chronobehavioral factors sets it apart from more traditional investigations. While we recognize the complexity of the interactions, we have not tried to identify even the more obvious feedback loops (as Schaefer and some others have done for the physiological domain, cf. above). Nor has there been an attempt to give specific meaning to the numerous 'black boxes"—many of these no doubt involve second order differential equations whose parameters are beyond our reach at this time.

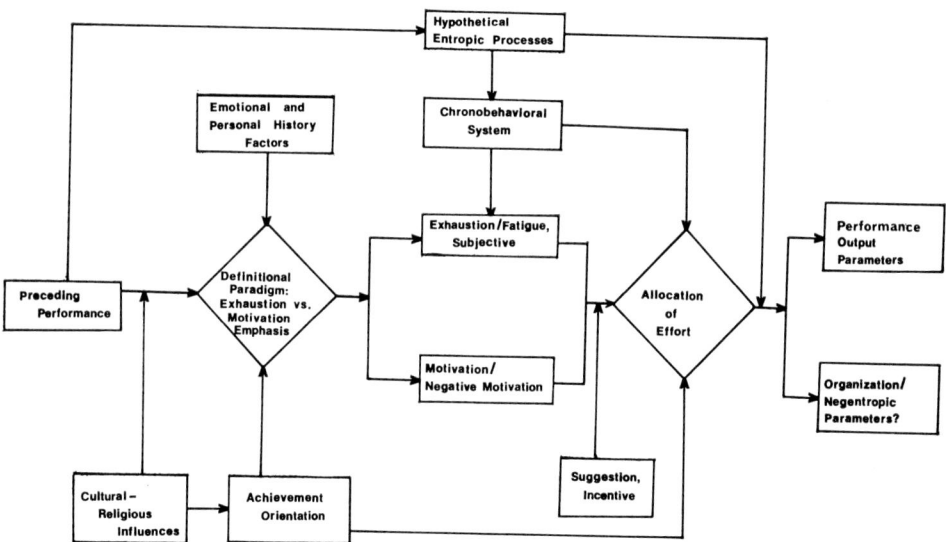

Figure 13-4. Schematic diagram of interrelation (multiple feed back) between performance, subjective fatigue, motivation and other internal and external factors.

For these reasons, the diagram as it stands can hardly represent statements about an actual or even hypothesized psychophysiological "system," desirable though this would be. Its scope is necessarily more modest, and at most it can serve as a prescription for doing more research along the various paths sketched here.

A SPECULATIVE CONCLUSION

Over the years and almost periodically, the study of fatigue has led investigators and the directly concerned or "experiencing" individuals alike away from the criteria of simple work decrements. Time and again, as we see it, sophisticated analysis of people's behavior and experiences has pointed instead to changes of dimensionality, integration and disintegration of activity, or generally speaking to the need for models that are more properly placed in an information theoretical context than belonging with the analogy of mechanical stress, the dynamics of forces and other vectorial phenomena. This seems to us hardly accidental. Perhaps what we will ultimately recognize as central in the fatigue phenomena is the manifestation of general *entropic* processes, and of the natural trend towards disorder, states of higher statistical probability within an overall system which can, however, be compensated or temporarily reversed by the organism. If this notion should develop into a useful model, then even the apparently "undesirable" changes of arousal and motivation patterns might all correspond to entropic mechanisms in the sense of statistical thermodynamics. On the other hand, "motivation" in the sense of approach, arousal and correlated performance *increments* might reflect *negentropic* processes of some sort. Both of these processes, and the latter kind in particular, are becoming increasingly relevant for the life sciences as reviewed (after precedents such as Schroedinger's) by Allport (1955), Bateson (1972), von Bertalanfafy (1967), Klix (1971), or Prigogine, et al. (1973). They have also been speculatively introduced in other more limited behavioral contexts (cf. Wendt, 1974).

Is it too far-fetched to think that eventually, we may develop tools for the realistic study of negentropic mechanisms—that is, order generating and regenerating psychobiological processes in the organism for which the motivational or even chronobehavioral aspects of "fatigue" are perhaps significant expressions? It seems to us that in this case the psychology of fatigue and motivation would have progressed from a model that seemed rather firmly grounded in the First Law of thermodynamics, to another approach that would somehow be anchored to the implications of the Second Law—but then, unavoidably also, would have to cope with the kinds of problems already faced in such contexts by other, fundamental life sciences.

BIBLIOGRAPHY

Allport, F. H.: *Theories of Perception and the Concept of Structure.* New York, Wiley, 1955.

Antoni, W., Rosemarie Petruschkat, and H. W. Wendt: Antrieb, Aufmerksamkeit und Erschöpfung als Ermüdungskriterien in der Selbst- und Fremdeinstufung, *Unpublished Ms,* Univ. of Mainz, 1955.

Appley, M. H. (Ed.): *Adaptation-level Theory.* New York, Acad Pr, 1971.

Aschoff, J. (Ed.): *Circadian clocks.* Amsterdam, North-Holland, 1965.

Ash, I. E.: Fatigue and its effects upon control. *Arch Psychol, 4,* No. 31, 1914.

Atkinson, J. W. (Ed.): *Motives in Fantasy, Action, and Society.* Princeton, Van Nostrand, 1958.

Atkinson, J. W.: *An Introduction to Motivation.* Princeton, Van Nostrand, 1964.

Barber, T. X.: The effects of "hypnosis" and motivation suggestions on strength and endurance: a critical review of research studies. *Br J Soc Clin Psychol, 5:*42-50, 1966.

Bartlett, F. C.: Psychological criteria of fatigue. In Floyd, W. F., and A. T. Welford (Eds.): *Symposium on Fatigue.* London, 1953.

Bartley, S. H., and Eloise Chute: *Fatigue and Impairment in Man.* New York, McGraw-Hill, 1947.

Bartley, S. H.: Fatigue and inadequacy. *Physiol Rev, 37:*301-324, 1957.

Bartley, S. H.: Some things to realize about fatigue. *J Sports Med Phys Fitness, 4:*153-157, 1964.

Bartley, S. H.: Definitional note: what shall we call fatigue? *This volume,* Chap. 15.

Bartoshuk, A. K.: EMG gradients as indicants of motivation. *Can J Psychol, 9:*215-230, 1955.

Bartenwerfer, H.: Herzrhythmik-Merkmale als Indikatoren psychischer Anspannung. *Psychol Beiträge, 4:*7-25, 1960.

Bartenwerfer, H.: Beiträge zum Problem der psychischen Beanspruchung. *I. Forschungsbericht, Nordrhein-Westfalen,* Nr. 808.—Köln & Opladen, 1960.

Bartenwerfer, H. G.: Über Beanspruchung und Ermüdung bei psychischer Aktivität. *Habil-Schrift,* Univ. of Marburg, 1965.

Bartenwerfer, H.: Einige praktische Konsequenzen aus der Aktivierungstheorie. *Zschr exper angew Psychol, 16:*195-222, 1969.

Bartenwerfer, H.: Psychische Beanspruchung und Ermüdung. In Mayer, A., and Herwig, B. (Eds.): *Handbuch der Psychologie.* Göttingen, Hogrefe, 1970, Vol. 9.

Bateson, G.: *Steps to an Ecology of Mind. Collected Essays.* New York, Chandler, Ballantine, 1972.

Bergum, B. O., and D. J. Lehr: Monetary incentives and vigilance. *J Exp Psychol, 67:*197-198, 1964.

Bertalanffy, L. von: *Robots, Men and Minds.* New York, Braziller, 1967.

Bills, A. G.: Blocking, a new principle of mental fatigue. *Am J Psychol, 43:*230-245, 1931.

Birney, R. C., H. Burdick, and R. C. Teevan: *Fear of Failure.* Princeton, Van Nostrand, 1969.

Bornemann, E. (Ed.): *Ermüdung, ihre Erscheinungsformen und Verhütung.* Lüneburg, Kinau, 1952.

Bracken, H. von: Ermüdungsforschung und Erziehungswissenschaft. *Bildung und Erziehung, 4:*348, 1951.

Bracken, H. von: Zur Psychopathologie der Ermüdung. In Bornemann, E. (Ed.): *Ermüdung, ihre Erscheinungsformen und Verhütung*. Lüneburg, Kinau, 1952.
Bracken, H. von: Paradoxien der Ermüdung. *Zbl f Arbeitswiss, 10*:177-179, 1956.
Broadbent, D. E.: Neglect of the surroundings in relation to fatigue decrements in output. In Floyd, W. F., and A. T. Welford (Eds.): *Symposium on Fatigue*. London, 1953.
Brown, F. A., Jr.: Hypothesis of environmental timing of the clock. In Brown, F. A., Hastings, J. W., and Palmer, J. D. (Eds.): *The Biological Clock: Two Views*. New York, Acad Pr, 1970.
Browne, R. C.: Fatigue, fact or fiction? In Floyd, W. F., and A. T. Welford (Eds.): *Symposium on Fatigue*. London, 1953.
Brozek, J., and A. Keys: Flicker fusion frequency as a test of fatigue. *J Industry Hyg, 26*:169-174, 1944.
Bünning, E.: *The Physiological Clock*. Berlin, Springer, 1964.
Burnham, W. H.: The problem of fatigue. *Am J Psychol, 19*:385-399, 1908.
Burnstein, E., and R. B. Zajonc: Individual task performance in a changing social structure. *Sociometry, 28*:16-29, 1965.
Cattell, R. B.: *The Scientific Analysis of Personality*. Chicago, Aldine, 1966.
Chatel, J. C., and R. Peele: A centennial review of neurasthenia. *Am J Psychiatry, 126*: 1404-1413, 1970.
Colquhoun, W. P. (Ed.): *Biological Rhythms and Human Performance*. New York, Acad Pr, 1971.
Courts, F. A.: Dynamogenic effect of muscle tension. *J Exp Psychol, 30*:504-510, 1942.
Davidson, W. Z., J. A. Andrews, and S. Ross: Effects of stress and anxiety on continuous high speed color naming. *J Exp Psychol, 52*:13-17, 1956.
Davis, D. R.: The disorganization of behavior in fatigue. *J Neurol Psychiatry, 9*:23-29, 1947.
Davis, D. R.: Satiation and frustration as determinants of fatigue. In Floyd, W. F., and A. T. Welford (Eds.): *Symposium on Fatigue*. London, 1953.
deCharms, R., H. W. Morrison, W. Reitman, and D. C. McClelland: Behavioral correlates of directly and indirectly measured achievement motivation. In McClelland, D. C. (Ed.): *Studies in Motivation*. New York, Appleton-Century, 1955.
Dember, W. N.: Motivation and the cognitive revolution. *Am Psychol, 29*:161-168, 1974.
Düker, H.: Über ein Verfahren zur Untersuchung der psychischen Leistungsfähigkeit. *Psychol Forschung, 23*:10-24, 1949.
Dureman, E. I., and Ch. Bodén: Fatigue in simulated car driving. *Ergonomics, 15*:299-308, 1972.
Eason, R. G., and J. Branks: Effect of level of activation on the quality and efficiency of performance of verbal and motor tasks. *Percept Mot Skills, 15*:525-543, 1963.
Ehlers, Th.: Alkoholbedingte Motivationsänderungen und Unfallgefährdung. *Berichte aus dem Institut f. Psychologie*, Univ. Marburg/Lahn, Nr. 3, 1965.
Engles, J. B., A. M. Halliday, and J. W. T. Redfearn: Effects of fatigue on tremor. In Floyd, W. F., and A. T. Welford (Eds.): *Symposium on Fatigue*. London, 1953.
Fabrycky, J., and H. W. Wendt: Values, motives and the perception of code violation, as a function of religious background, sex, and ordinal position in Canadian students. Univ. of Victoria, B.C., *Unpublished multivariate analysis*, 1968.
Feather, N. T.: Persistence in relation to achievement motivation, anxiety about failure, and task difficulty, *Dissertation Abstracts, 21*:2378, 1961.
Festinger, L.: *A Theory of Cognitive Dissonance*. New York, Row, Peterson, 1957.

Fisch, R., H. D. Schmalt, and Helga Fisch: Ein Messverfahren zur Bestimmung der Intensität und Extensität der Leistungsmotivation. *Bericht, Psychologisches Institut der Univ. des Saarlandes,* Saarbrücken, 1970.

Fischbein, E., I. Pampu, and I. Mînzat: Distribution of efforts in case of fatigue, under the influence of motivation. *Revue Roumaine des Sciences Sociales: Série de Psycologie, 12:*3-13, 1968.

Fleishman, E. A.: A relationship between incentive motivation and ability level in psychomotor performance. *J Exp Psychol, 56:*78-81, 1958.

Floyd, W. F., and A. T. Welford (Eds.): *Symposium on Fatigue.* London, Lewis, 1953.

French, Elizabeth G.: Some characteristics of achievement motivation. *J Exp Psychol, 50:*232-236, 1955.

Freud, S.: *Gesammelte Werke, Band 1.* London, Imago, 1952.

Garron, D. C., and R. B. Shekelle: Mood, personality, and the menstrual cycle. *Paper, 53rd Annual Convention, Western Psychol Association,* Anaheim, 1973.

Grandjean, E. P.: Fatigue, its physiological and psychological significance. *Ergonomics, 11:*427-436, 1968.

Grandjean, E. P.: Fatigue. Yant Memorial Lectures. *Am Industr Hygiene Assoc J, 31:* 401, 1970.

Gross, I. H., and S. H. Bartley: Fatigue in house care. *J Appl Psychol, 35:*205-207, 1951.

Haider, M.: *Ermüdung, Beanspruchung und Leistung. Eine Einführung in die Ermüdungs- und Monotonieforschung.* Wien, Deuticke, 1962.

Halberg, F.: Physiologic considerations underlying rhythmometry, with special reference to emotional illness. In *Symposium Bell-Air III.* Geneva, Masson, 1968.

Halberg, F.: Chronobiology. *Am Rev Physiol, 31:*675-725, 1969.

Halberg, F., G. S. Katinas, et al.: *Chronobiologic Glossary of the International Society for the Study of Biological Rhythms.* U of Minnesota, ca. 1971.

Halberg, F., Y. L. Tong, and E. A. Johnson: Circadian system phase—an aspect of temporal morphology; procedures and illustrative examples. In H. von Mayersbach (Ed.): *The Cellular Aspects of Biorhythms.* New York/Berlin, Springer, 1967.

Halberg, F., E. A. Johnson, W. Nelson, W. Runge, and R. Sothern: Autorhythmometry —procedures for physiologic self-measurements and their analysis. *Physiology Teacher, Am Physiol Society, 1:*1-11, 1972.

Haller, J. S.: Neurasthenia, medical profession and urban "blahs." *NY J Med, 70:*2489-2497, 1970.

Hashimoto, K.: Estimation of the driver's work load in high speed electric car operation on the new Tokaido line in Japan. *Ergonomics, Supplement: Proceed 2nd Internat Congress of Ergonomics (Dortmund),* 1964, pp. 463-469.

Hashimoto, K., K. Kogi, et al.: Physiological strain of high speed bus driving on the Mei-Shin Expressway and the effects of moderation of speed restrictions. *J Railway Lab Sci, 20:*1, 1967.

Hastings, J. W.: Cellular-biochemical clock hypothesis. In Brown, F. A., Hastings, J. W., and Palmer, J. D. (Eds.): *The Biological Clock: Two Views.* New York, Acad Pr, 1970.

Haywood, H. C., and S. J. Weaver: Differential effects of motivational orientations and incentive conditions on motor performance in institutionalized retardates. *Am J Ment Defic, 72:*459-467, 1967.

Heckhausen, H.: *Hoffnung und Furcht in der Leistungsmotivation.* Meisenheim a. Glan, Hain, 1963.

Heckhausen, H.: *The Anatomy of Achievement Motivation.* New York, Acad Pr, 1967.

Hemphill, R. E., K. R. L. Hall, and T. G. Crooker: A preliminary report on fatigue and pain tolerance in depressive and psychoneurotic patients. *J Ment Sci, 98*:433-440, 1952.

Hildebrandt, G.: Spontan-rhythmische Schwankungen der Leistungsfähigkeit beim Menschen. *Die Mediz Welt, 22*:640-648, 1971.

Hornstra, L.: Over de vermoeiheid, II. *Mens en Onderneming, 9*:250-259, 1955.

Jarrard, L. E.: The role of visual cues in the performance of ergographic work. *J Exp Psychol, 60*:57-63, 1960.

Kalveram, K. T.: Über Faktorenanalyse. Kritik eines theoretischen Konzepts und seine mathematische Neuformulierung. *Archiv f. Psychologie, 122*:92-118, 1970.

Kanabrocki, E. L., L. E. Scheving, F. Halberg, R. L. Brewer, and T. L. Bird: Circadian variation in presumably healthy young soldiers. *U.S. Dept of Commerce, National Tech. Info. Service*, Document No. PB 228427, Springfield, P.O.B. 1553. Ca. 1974.

Kinsman, R. A., P. C. Weiser, and D. A. Stamper: Multidimensional analysis of subjective symptomatology during prolonged strenuous exercize. *Ergonomics, 16*:211-241, 1973.

Kinsman, R. A., and P. C. Weiser: Subjective symptomatology during work and fatigue. *This Volume*, Chap. 14.

Kleitman, N.: *Sleep and Wakefulness.* (Rev. Ed.) Chicago, U of Chicago Pr, 1967.

Klinger, E., and F. W. McNelly, Jr.: Fantasy need achievement and performance: a role analysis. *Psychol Rev, 76*:574-591, 1969.

Klix, F.: *Information und Verhalten. Kybernetische Aspekte der organismischen Informationsverarbeitung.* Berlin, VEB Dtsch. Verlag der Wissensch., 1971.

Landis, C.: An annotated bibliography of flicker fusion phenomena, covering the period 1740-1952. *Armed Forces National Research Council,* Vision Committee Secretariat. Ann Arbor, U of Michigan, 1953.

Laughlin, H. P.: The fatigue reactions. In *The Neuroses.* Washington, Butterworths, 1967.

Lindsley, D. B.: Psychophysiology and motivation. In Jones, M. R. (Ed.): *Nebraska Symposium of Motivation.* Lincoln, U of Nebraska Pr, 1957.

Locke, E. A.: Interaction of ability and motivation in performance. *Percept Mot Skills, 21*:719-725, 1965.

Locke, E.: The relationship of intentions to level of performance. *J Appl Psychol, 50:* 60-66, 1966.

Locke, E. A., and J. F. Bryan: Cognitive aspects of psychomotor performance: the effects of performance goals on level of performance. *J Appl Psychol, 50*:286-291, 1966.

London, P., and M. Fuhrer: Hypnosis, motivation, and performance. *J Pers, 29*:321-333, 1961.

Lucaccini, L. F., A. Freedy, and J. Lyman: Motivational factors in vigilance: effects of instructions on performance in a complex vigilance task. *Percep Mot Skills, 26*:783, 786, 1968.

Luce, Gay G.: *Biological Rhythms in Psychiatry and Medicine.* U.S. Dept. of Health, Education and Welfare, National Institute of Mental Health, Publ. No. 2088. Chevy Chase, Publ. Health Service Doc., 1970.

Maddi, S. R.: Affective tone during environmental regularity and change. *J Abnorm Soc Psychol, 62*:338-345, 1961.

McClelland, D. C., J. W. Atkinson, R. A. Clark, and E. L. Lowell: *The Achievement Motive.* New York, Appleton-Century, 1953.

McClelland, D. C. (Ed.): *Studies in Motivation.* New York, Appleton-Century, 1955.
McClelland, D. C.: The psychology of mental content reconsidered. *Psych Rev, 62*:297-302, 1955.
McClelland, D. C.: *Personality.* New York, Sloane, 1951, 1960.
McClelland, D. C.: *The Achieving Society.* Princeton, Van Nostrand, 1961.
McCormick, E. J., and J. Tiffin: *Industrial Psychology,* 6th ed. Englewood Cliffs, Prentice-Hall, 1974.
Meltzer, H., and D. Ludwig: Memory dynamics and work motivation. *Proceedings of the 75th Annual Convention of the APA, 2*:271-272, 1967.
Moen, Patricia: Investigation of circadian and other fluctuations of socially relevant mood states in women. *Unpubl. Ms,* Macalester College, 1973.
Mora, G.: Antecedent to neurosis. *Int J Psychiatry, 9*:57-60, 1970-71.
Morgan, W. P., P. B. Raven, Barbara L. Drinkwater, and S. M. Horvath: Perceptual and metabolic responsivity to standard bicycle ergometry following various hypnotic suggestions. *Paper, Canadian Association of Sports Sciences and the American College of Sports Medicine,* Toronto, 1971.
Mosso, A.: *Die Ermüdung.* Leipzig, 1892.
Mücher, H., et al.: *Psychische und physiologische Wirkungen des Wetters.* Aulendorf, Württemberg, Editio Cantor, 1957.
Mücher, H., and H. W. Wendt: Gruppenversuch zur Bestimmung der kritischen Verschmelzungsfrequenz beim binokularen Sehen: Änderungen unter Koffein und nach normaler Tagesarbeit. *Arch Exp Pathol Pharmakol, 214*:29-37, 1951.
Münsterberg, H.: *Psychologie und Wirtschaftsleben.* Leipzig, 1912.
Murray, H. A.: *Explorations in Personality.* New York, Oxford U Pr, 1938.
Muscio, B.: Is a fatigue test possible? *Br J Psychol, 12*:31-46, 1921.
Nicholson, W. M.: The influence of anxiety upon learning: interference or drive increment? *J Pers, 26*:303-319, 1958.
Orme, J. E.: *Time, Experience and Behavior.* London, Iliffe Books; New York, American Elsevier, 1969.
Orne, M. T.: The nature of hypnosis: artifact and essence. *J Abnorm Soc Psychol, 58*:277-299, 1959.
Pierson, W. R., and A. Lockhart: Fatigue, work decrement and endurance of women in a simple repetitive task. *Aerospace Med, 35*:724, 1964.
Prigogine, I., G. Nicholis, and A. Babloyantz: Nonequilibrium problems in biological phenomena. *Ann NY Acad Sci, 231*:99-100, 1973.
Procacci, P., Michelle della Corte, M. Zoppi, and M. Maresca: Rhythmic changes of the cutaneous pain threshold in man. A general review. *Chronobiologia, 1*:77-96, 1974.
Quarter, J., and A. Marcus: Drive level and audience effect: a test of Zajonc's theory. *J Soc Psychol, 83*:99-105, 1971.
Reinberg, A.: Les rhythmes biologiques. *La Recherche, 2*:241-250, 1971.
Reinberg, A., et al.: Changes in circadian temporal structure (including sleep) of 20 shift-workers (8-hour shift—weekly rotation). A field study with autorhythmometry, *Paper, XIth Internat. Conference, International Society for Chronobiology.* Hannover, Med. Hochschule, 1973.
Richter, C. P.: Abnormal but regular cycles in behavior and metabolism in rats and catatonic-schizophrenics. In Reiss, M. (Ed.): *Psychoendocrinology.* New York, Grune & Stratton, 1958.

Richter, C. P.: A hitherto unrecognized difference between man and other primates. *Science, 154:*427, 1966.

Rivers, W. H. R., and E. Kraepelin: Über Ermüdung und Erholung. *Psychol Arbeiten, 1:*627-678, 1896.

Rüssel, A.: Belastung und Ermüdung an unterschiedlichen Arbeitsplätzen. *Zschr exper angew Psychol, 9:*12-54, 1962.

Rüssel, A.: Selbst- und Fremdeinstufungen des Befindens bei der Arbeit. *Zschr exper angew Psychol, 11:*95-129, 1964.

Rüssel, A.: *Das Befinden des Menschen bei der Arbeit. Eine Utersuchung an berufstätigen Frauen.* Frechen/Köln, Bartmann, 1968.

Sarason, I. G.: Effect of anxiety, motivational instructions, and failure on serial learning. *J Exp Psychol, 51:*253-260, 1956.

Schaefer, H.: Ermüdung und Müdigkeit. In Baust, W. (Ed.): *Ermüdung, Schlaf und Traum.* Stuttgart, Wissenschaftl, Verlagsgesellsch, 1970.

Schaefer, H.: Epilogue. *This volume.*

Schmidtke, H.: *Die Ermüdung. Symptome, Theorien, Messversuche.* Bern & Stuttgart, Huber, 1965.

Schmidtke, H.: Vigilance. *This volume,* Chap. 8.

Schmidtke, H.: Disturbances of information processing. *This volume,* Chap. 10.

Schmitt, O. H.: Chronobiophysics. *Chronobiologia, 1:*28-37, 1974.

Schönpflug, W., and G. Wicker: Psychische Prozesse beim psychologischen Skalieren. VI. Aktiviertheit bei der Verwendung verschiedener Skalierungsmethoden. *Psychol Beiträge, 13:*431-439, 1971.

Schwab, R. S.: Motivation in measurements of fatigue. In Floyd, W. F., and Welford, A. T. (Eds.): *Symposium on Fatigue.* London, 1953.

Shaw, W. A.: Facilitating effects of induced tension upon the perception span for digits. *J Exp Psychol, 51:*113-117, 1956.

Simonson, E.: Der heutige Stand der Theorie der Ermüdung. *Erg Physiol, 37:*299, 1935.

Simonson, E.: The fusion frequency of flicker as a criterion of central nervous system fatigue. *Am J Ophtalmol, 47:*556, 1959.

Simonson, E. (Ed.): *Physiology of Work Capacity and Fatigue.* Springfield, Thomas, 1971.

Simonson, E., and V. Enzer: Measurement of fusion frequency of flicker as a test for fatigue of the central nervous system. *J Industr Hyg Toxicol, 23:*83-89, 1941.

Smith, Patricia C.: The prediction of individual differences in susceptibility to industrial monotony. *J Appl Psychol, 39:*322-329, 1955.

Snyder, M., R. Schulz, and E. E. Jones: Expectancy and apparent duration as determinants of fatigue. *J Pers Soc Psychol, 29:*426, 1974.

Spence, K. W., I. E. Faber, and H. H. McFann: The relations of anxiety (drive) level to performance in competitional and non-competitional paired associates learning. *J Exp Psychol, 52:*296-305, 1956.

Taylor, M. A., et al.: Neurasthenia in the seventies. *Am J Psychiatry, 127:*390-391, 1970.

Thomae, H., and Ursula Lehr (w/ G. Dreher and W. Opgenoorth): Berufliche Leistungsfähigkeit im mittleren und höheren Erwachsenenalter. Eine Analyse des Forschungsstandes. Göttingen, Schwartz, 1973.

Thorndike, E.: Mental fatigue I. II. Mental fatigue in school children. *Psych Rev. 7:*547-572, 1900.

Thorndike, E.: The curve of work. *Psychol Rev, 19:*165-194, 1912.

Tong, Y. L., J. Lee, and F. Halberg: Mean number-weighted cosinor technique resolves phase- and frequency-synchronized rhythms with differing mesors and amplitudes. *Paper, XIth International Conference, International Society for Chronobiology.* Hannover, Med. Hochschule, 1973.

Vroom, V. H.: *Work and Motivation.* New York, Wiley, 1964.

Walster, B., and E. Aaronson: Effect of expectancy of task duration on the experience of fatigue. *J Exp Soc Psychol, 3:*41-46, 1967.

Weber, M.: *Die protestantische Ethik und der Geist des Kapitalismus.* Tübingen, Mohr, 1904, 1920.

Welford, A. T.: The psychologist's problem in measuring fatigue. In Floyd, W. F., and A. T. Welford (Eds.): *Symposium on Fatigue.* London, 1953.

Welford, A. T.: *Fundamentals of Skill.* New York, Barnes & Noble, 1968.

Wendt, H. W.: Über zwei Methoden zur Bestimmung der binokularen kritischen Verschmelzungsfrequenz im Gruppenversch. In *Bericht, 17. und 18. Kongress der Dtsch Gesellsch f Psychol.* Göttingen, Verl f Psych, 1953.

Wendt, H. W.: Ermüdungsindikatoren: ihre Logik, Abhängigkeit von Werthaltungen, und die Vorhersage der Belastungsleistung. In *Bericht, 20. Kongress der Dtsch Gesellsch f Psychol.* Göttingen, Verl f Psych, 1955.

Wendt, H. W.: Motivation, effort, and performance. In McClelland, D. C. (Ed.): *Studies in Motivation.* New York, Appleton-Century, 1955.

Wendt, H. W.: Über Ermüdungsindikatoren. *Psychologie und Praxis, 2:*129-146, 1956.

Wendt, H. W.: On fatigue and/or motivation. *Percept Mot Skills, 8:*121-122, 1958.

Wendt, H. W.: Early circannual rhythms and adult human behaviour. *Int J Chronobiology, 2:*57-86, 1974.

Wessman, A. E., and D. F. Ricks: *Mood and Personality.* New York, Holt, 1966.

Wever, R.: Hat der Mensch nur *eine* 'innere Uhr'? *Umschau in Wissenschaft und Technik, 73:*551-558, 1973.

Wolf, G.: Construct validation of measures of three kinds of experiential fatigue. *Percept Mot Skills, 24:*1067-1076, 1967.

Wotzka, G., and E. Grandjean: Physiologische und psychologische Ermüdungsmessungen bei Flugverkehrsleitern. *Zschr f Präventivmedizin, 13:*204-206, 1968.

Wright, S.: Path coefficients and path regressions: alternative or complementary concepts? *Biometrics, 16:*189-202, 1960.

Chapter 14

Subjective Symptomatology During Work and Fatigue

ROBERT A. KINSMAN and PHILIP C. WEISER

The concern of this chapter centers around what has been called "subjective fatigue"—the feeling states experienced during the performance of work. Changes in these feeling states often may be related to work tolerance and performance. For example, individuals engaged in sports or any type of physical activity involving prolonged, strenuous exercise must continually determine their level of energy expenditure and the length of time they are willing to continue work. In general, the point at which a person quits may correspond to when he "feels very tired" or "worn out."

Welford (1965), however, has noted that the symptoms commonly associated with subjective fatigue have been viewed as difficult to measure adequately. Consequently, until recently they have been neglected by most investigators in favor of more directly observable physiological, neurological, or behavioral events. Indeed, a search of the literature in this area quickly reveals many inadequacies in methodology and a paucity of well directed and systematic investigations of subjective symptomatology during work. Fortunately, as will be seen, there are also some promising experimental approaches which have recently appeared in the literature.

It is certainly true that subjective symptoms cannot be measured directly. By definition, a symptom is a privately experienced event made public only when the experience is *reported* to an observer. The measurement of these symptoms is, therefore, necessarily indirect, depending on reliable self-report techniques. Furthermore, it is important to realize that the subjective symptoms most of us usually associate with fatigue *per se,* such as tiredness, lack of energy, or feeling worn out, probably encompass only a few of the many types of subjective symptoms that might be reported during work performance. Other subjective qualities as diverse as pain, thermal sensations, or boredom often occur during work. It is important to differentiate between these subjective qualities as Welford (1965) has pointed out. In recent years, there has been renewed effort to develop self-report techniques to measure such subjective qualities accompanying work performance.

It has frequently been assumed that subjective symptoms must inevitably

---

This chapter was supported in part by NIH Grants MH24222-01 and HL14985-02.

be related to work performance under any task condition. Some authors have suggested that the opposite is true, that is, that subjective symptoms are not related to work performance (e.g. Pierson, 1963a). As with many extreme positions in science, both statements are overgeneralizations. Frequently there have been work situations where no relationship between symptomatology and performance have been reported or would be expected. While this lack of relationship could result from the selection of the method of measurement or the specific quality measured, it may adequately reflect the real situation.

The objectives of this chapter are first to review and evaluate studies of the various subjective qualities reported during work, and second, to propose a model permitting a more appropriate conceptualization of subjective fatigue. The review section, comprising roughly the first three-fourths of the chapter, is not exhaustive but serves to exemplify the methods of measurement used and the subjective qualities studied. The reader is forewarned that the review often involves detailed discussion of individual studies since an adequate, critical overview of this area does not appear to exist. We hope the persistence of the interested reader will be rewarded by the novel conceptual organization of the area provided in the last quarter of the chapter.

THE MEASUREMENT OF SUBJECTIVE QUALITIES

Subjective symptoms represent one level of measurement during work performance in a matrix (the organism) which consists of a diversity of organizational levels. Questions should be asked about relationships within as well as between levels of biological organization during work performance: What *are* the subjective symptoms experienced during work? How do these differ between tasks? How do these change during the course of work? What are their relationships to physiological, and especially neurological, levels of organization? When are they related to work performance and work tolerance? When are they not related? None of these questions presume a specific answer, but the answers are bound to be informationally rich. If the first order of business in studies of subjective symptoms during work—measurement—is handled adequately, the answers to such questions as these will be interesting in their own right.

Scaling Techniques

There are a variety of solutions to the problem of *adequate* measurement that are available from the areas of psychophysics (e.g. see S. S. Stevens, 1957), psychological assessment (e.g. see Jackson and Messick, 1967), and, in particular, psychometric scaling (e.g. Guilford, 1954). Recent developments in scaling techniques have been reviewed by Cliff (1973) in an article containing over 200 references for the period 1968 to 1972 alone. The available scaling techniques have been used only recently in a *systematic* program of research in the area of work performance.

S. S. Stevens (1960) has discussed the numerical properties of various types of scales. Before proceeding further, it may be useful to review the characteristics of scales. A scale simply refers to the assignment of numbers to objects or events in order to differentiate between them. *Nominal* scales are the simplest means of numerical assignment providing only a substitute name for the purposes of identification. Social Security numbers, automobile license plates, and the numbers given to football players are all examples of nominal scaling. No information is provided about the magnitude of some quality of the objects to which numbers are assigned. The automobile with a license plate AL-4516 may either be a Volkswagen sedan or a Cadillac Eldorado according to nominal scaling.

In an *ordinal* scale, numbers are assigned according to the order of magnitude for some attribute which objects or events possess. For example, a compulsive psychometrician may ask his wife to rate how hungry she is on a 5-point scale before deciding on the restaurant for dinner. He may say "suppose a 5 is the hungriest you've ever been and 1 is the least hungry you've ever been. How hungry are you on a scale of 1 to 5?" If she's willing to put up with this nonsense, she may reply 4 indicating that she's very hungry, but not as "hungry as she's ever been." The scale thus allows a rough quantification of a subjective quality, hunger, and the psychometrician can use this information in making his choice of restaurants for dinner. In such an ordinal scale, however, there is no true zero point representing the complete absence of hunger, nor are the intervals on the scale necessarily equidistant. The difference between 4 and 5 or 1 and 2 on the "hunger scale" may both be 1 scale point, but may not represent equal differences in the magnitude of the subjective quality measured. Nevertheless, most applications of scaling techniques to measure subjective feelings during work performance have used rating scales with ordinal properties. As we will see, the shortcomings of ordinal scales, absence of a "true" zero point and equal intervals, can largely be overcome in most applications.

Interval scales possess all the attributes of ordinal scales, but the intervals between adjacent categories are equal. A thermometer is the most familiar interval scale with degrees indicating the magnitude of the difference between points on the scale. However, like ordinal scales, the interval scale lacks a true zero point. The zero on a Centigrade or Fahrenheit thermometer does *not* correspond to the "absence of heat." Interval scales can be constructed to measure subjective qualities, but require the use of rather lengthy psychometric techniques such as the method of equal appearing intervals (Thurstone and Chave, 1929; also see Niven, 1953; Guilford, 1950,

1954). In the measurement of subjective qualities during work performance, interval scaling is best exemplified by the studies of Pearson and Byars (1956) and of McNelly (1957), both of which will be discussed in some detail.

Only the *ratio* scales have a true zero point representing the absence of the attribute measured while also providing magnitude measurement by equal intervals in the units of measurement. Psychophysical techniques are used to obtain ratio scales for subjective qualities.

Most attempts to quantify subjective qualities during work have used *ordinal* rating scales. The inherent shortcomings of the ordinal scales can largely be overcome in most applications. The intervals between ordinal scale points often can be made to *appear* equidistant by careful selection of the verbal descriptions accompanying each scale point, physically representing the verbal descriptions at equal intervals, and by indicating equal intervals in the numbering of scale points, e.g. values of 0, 1, . . . , 4. Furthermore, a zero point can be provided by anchoring the first category with "not present" indicating complete absence of the subjective quality. Such ordinal scales have often been treated statistically as if they were true equal-interval scales. Overall and Klett (1972) have noted that equal-appearing interval scales "have frequently been demonstrated to be linearly related to Thurstone type equal-interval scales except in the extreme categories." Such scales are among the simplest to construct and to use; therefore, they have enjoyed the widest application in studies of subjective fatigue to be discussed.

TYPES OF MEASUREMENT OF SUBJECTIVE QUALITIES

In this section the techniques available to measure subjective qualities during work performance will be reviewed and evaluated. Measurement has relied primarily on two general methodologies: (1) psychophysical techniques and (2) rating scales. Psychophysical techniques produce ratio scales which although more precise in describing relationships between stimulus levels and perceptions, are less useful in most work situations. Rating scales have enjoyed a wider application largely because of the ease with which the ordinal or interval scales may be used. Most recently, a third general methodology involving multivariate statistical procedures has been used to identify categories or dimensions of symptomatology related to work performance.

Psychophysical Studies

There has been renewed interest in the application of psychophysical techniques to relate subjective qualities to certain parameters of work performance (see Table 14-I). These techniques provide a *ratio scaling* that relates stimulus level to the perception of the stimulus. Application of psychophysics to the area of work performance provides rather precise answers to questions regarding how the perception of effort increases as physical activity increases.

Classical psychophysics has a long history extending back to the 19th century and the work of Weber (1834), Fechner (1877), and Plateau (1872). Detailed discussions of the development of psychophysics have been presented by S. S. Stevens (1957, 1960). Psychophysics involves the description of the relationship between *perceived* change in a physical stimulus, the psychological dimension, and change in the objective intensity or quality of the stimulus measured in physical units, the physical dimension. For many years, it was assumed that Fechner had accurately described the relationship between perception and levels of a physical stimulus as a logarithmic function:

$$\Psi = k \log \Phi \qquad (1)$$

where Ψ is the subjective unit of the psychological scale, k is a constant and Φ is the level of the physical stimulus.

Since the 1930's, however, under the influence of modern psychophysicists such as S. S. Stevens and Ekman, this relationship is generally agreed to be better approximated by a power function:

$$\Psi = k \ (\Phi)^m \qquad (2)$$

where m is an exponent defining the power function fitting the shape of the curve.

The value of the constant threshold, i.e. the minimum stimulus level which the individual can perceive may also be included in the power function as a constant:

$$\Psi = k \ (\Phi - a)^m \qquad (3)$$

where a is an additive constant included to bring the zero point of the physical scale in line with the zero of the psychological scale. Inclusion of this constant in the equation will generally result in a rescaling of stimulus values corresponding to the range of perception. According to S. S. Stevens (1960), it was Luce (1959) who noted that "the use of an additive constant to bring the zero of the physical scale into coincidence with the zero of the psychological scale is a proper generalization of the power law."

This power function has been found to be applicable to subjective judgments covering a wide range of stimulus modalities including brightness, pitch, loudness, taste, odor, and heaviness (S. S. Stevens, 1957) as well as the perception of force exerted during work performance (Borg, 1962; Schmale, Schmidtke, and Vukovich, 1963; and Bernyer, 1967), and fatigue (Bujas, Pavlina, Sremec, Vidaček, and Vodanović, 1966). An example of a power function relating perception of exertion ("Anstrengung") to load level expressed as percentage of maximum load is shown in Figure 14-1.

Various psychophysical methods are used to derive the power functions. These have been described in detail in numerous sources (e.g. see Stevens, 1957, 1960; and Ekman, 1958, 1959). It is beyond the scope of this chapter to discuss in detail the many issues and methods in the area of psychophysics. However, it may be worthwhile to describe two of the more useful psychophysical methods of ratio scaling: the *estimation* and *production* methods, both of which have been applied to the perception of force exerted during work.

In general, *estimation* methods require the subject either to estimate the relative magnitude (magnitude estimation) of physical stimuli by assigning numerical values (e.g. 105, 120, etc.) to a series of comparative stimuli in reference to a standard stimulus of a given numerical magnitude (e.g. 100); or, to estimate the percentage magnitude (ratio estimation) of the comparative stimuli in relation to the standard. The *production* methods, in contrast, require the subject to *produce* a stimulus that is either a multiple of (ratio production) or a specified magnitude (magnitude production) of a standard stimulus of given intensity. In work situations, the stimulus dimension in a psychophysical study might typically be work load (e.g. kpm/min. on ergometer tasks), weight lifted, and grade or walking speed on a treadmill. By these psychophysical methods, ratio units of perceptual values may be obtained based on the judgments associated with the sequence of comparative stimuli presented in relation to the standard stimuli used. The psychophysical relationship between perceptual values and values of the physical stimuli can frequently be described by equation 2 or 3 above. When this function is plotted on log-log coordinates, the exponent of the power function (m) defines the slope of a straight line, permitting direct comparisons between perception-stimulus relationships for different stimulus modalities. In general, a high exponent indicates that the perception of the stimulus changes rapidly with respect to changes in the physical stimulus; in contrast, a low exponent indicates that the perception changes relatively more slowly with respect to the physical dimension. For example, exponents of the power function for loudness have been found to be about .6 indicating that the perception of loudness grows slowly relative to changes in sound intensities. In contrast, the exponent for electric shock has been observed to be 3.5, indicating that perception changes rapidly with respect to shock intensity.

Table 14-I presents a summary of specific psychophysical studies relating to physical work, indicating the task and psychophysical method used, the subject population studied, the subjective quality measured, and the exponent of the power function obtained. In an initial study, Borg and Dahlstrom (1960) investigated perception of force exerted (pedal resistance) on a bicycle ergometer using four subjects. The ratio estimation technique

TABLE 14-I
PSYCHOPHYSICAL STUDIES DURING WORK PERFORMANCE

Subjective Quality	Physical Modality	Task	Subjects	Exponent of Power Function	Studies
Force exerted	Work load (kpm/min)	Bicycle ergometer	Young males (n = 4)	1.6	See Borg (1962)
Force exerted	Work load (kpm/min)	Bicycle ergometer	Young males (n = 12)	1.6	See Borg (1962)
Force exerted	Work load (kpm/min)	Bicycle ergometer	Young male students (n = 12)	1.8	See Borg (1962)
Force exerted	Force of pressure (lbs)	A. Stationary foot pedal B. Hand grip	Young males and females (n = 12)	A. 1.65 B. 1.65	Eisler (1962)
Force exerted	Work load (kpm/sec)	Arm and leg ergometer	Young males and females (n = 20)	1.4	Schmale, Schmidtke, and Vukovich (1963)
Force exerted	Work load (kpm/sec)	Wrist-curling	Young males and females (n = 6)	1.9	Schmale, Schmidtke, and Vukovich (1963)
Force exerted	Weight (kp)	Weight-holding	Young males and females (n = 10)	3.1	Schmale, Schmidtke, and Vukovich (1963)
Force exerted	Weight (grams)	Lifting weights by manually pressing levers	Young males (n = 3)	1.8 to 2.5	Bernyer (1967)
Force exerted	Force of pressure (newtons)	Hand grip	Males (n = 18)	1.7	Stevens and Cain (1970); also see Stevens and Mack (1959) and Cain and Stevens (1971)
General feeling of fatigue	Duration of effort (secs)	Weight-holding	Males (n = 5)	1.5	Bujas, Pauling, Sremec, and Vidachek (1966)

was used with power levels measured in kpm/min. This study resulted in the power function with an exponent of 1.6 and having a high test-retest reliability (r = .95). In subsequent pilot work, Borg (1962) determined that length of the work period, varied systematically between 5 and 100 sec, affected the perception of force exerted: longer work periods resulted in higher perceived force exerted for the same task.

Subsequently, twelve male subjects were studied using the ratio production method. Five standard load levels, presented for five seconds, were used: 500, 700, 900, 1,000, and 1,300 kpm/min. On each trial, the subject was required to establish (i.e. produce) a load level equal to one half of the standard. The derived power function had an exponent identical to the earlier preliminary study. An estimate of test-retest reliability for this data was exceptionally high: r = .96. Perceived force exerted was also studied in a group of twenty-two male subjects using the ratio production method wherein one power level (800 kpm/min.) was halved 10 times by ascending (5 trials) or descending (5 trials) to the perceived mid-point. Calculations indicated that the resulting power function had an exponent between 1.39 and 1.73.

Using ratio estimation, as opposed to the production method described above, Borg (1962) derived the power function for perceived force exerted using twelve male subjects between 20 and 30 years of age. In this study, load-levels of 300, 600, 900, and 1,200 kpm/min. were presented in pairs, one immediately after another, for 20 seconds each. The task for the subject was to estimate the intensity of the lower load level of each pair as a percentage of the higher. Each trial was separated by a 30-second rest period. Six of the twelve pairs were in ascending order, and six in descending order; order of presentation was random. After completion of this experimental sequence, the same subjects were rerun with the pairs presented in ascending order, so that within each pair and across trials, higher stimulus intensities followed lower stimulus intensities. This latter condition was designed to correspond with the stimulus sequence often used in work tests. The obtained power functions had exponents of 1.8 and 1.2 for the random and ascending series, respectively. An ascending series thus appears to lead to a higher absolute threshold for force exerted (300 vs. 200 kpm/ min.) and to a less rapid increase in perceived force exerted relative to load level. This effect upon the exponent of the power function has been labeled "hysteresis" (S. S. Stevens, 1957).

Borg's studies suggest that the exponent for perceived force exerted during cycling is 1.4 to 1.8, corresponding quite well to that obtained for other work modalities. For example, perceived force of handgrip was found to have an exponent of 1.7 (J. C. Stevens and Mack, 1959), perceived heaviness of lifted weights has been found to have an exponent of approximately 1.45

using both production and estimation techniques (S. S. Stevens and Galanter, 1957), and the perception of respiratory sensations—pressure, lung volume, and ventilatory volume—have been found to have exponents of 1.5, 1.3, and 1.9, respectively (Bakers and Tenney, 1970).

Eisler (1962) derived a ratio scaling of subjective force exerted for a mixed group of men and women using magnitude production and estimation techniques. The principal interest of this study was to evaluate the exponent of the power function for force exerted when large muscle groups were used. Additionally, Eisler inquired about the correspondence between the exponent for work involving large muscle groups, i.e. exerting a force in a horizontal direction against a foot pedal, and work involving small muscle groups, i.e. squeezing a handgrip. For the foot pedal task, the exponent of the power function for force exerted was found to be approximately 1.6, in excellent agreement with the findings of Borg (1962a) who had used the bicycle ergometer. To compare the exponents of the two work tasks, Eisler used two matching tasks: (a) the subject was required to squeeze a hand grip to match the force previously exerted against the foot pedal, and (b) vice versa. If the perception of force exerted changed with the physical force exerted in the same way for both hand grip and foot pedal tasks, the slope of a plot of force exerted for the hand grip vs. foot pedal matching tasks would equal unity. Results confirmed that, in fact, the slope of both lines (hand grip vs. foot pedal and foot pedal vs. hand grip) were unity. Thus, these results suggest that the perception of force exerted changes with the actual physical force exerted similarly for both large and small muscle groups, with power functions having exponents of approximately 1.6.

Schmale, Schmidtke, and Vukovich (1963) have summarized their own substantial psychophysical studies of work, reporting on a variety of tasks ranging from dynamic work (arm and leg bicycle ergometer tasks, and wrist curling) to static work (holding up a weight). For each of the dynamic work tasks, the production method was used to derive the power function. For the bicycle ergometer tasks, a linear relationship was found between "Anstrengung" (perceived exertion) for both leg and arm work. This linear relationship permitted derivation of a common power function for both arm and leg work relating "Anstrengung" to load level defined in percent of maximum load (P): $\Psi = (P + 2.44)^{1.4}$. The exponent agrees with that reported subsequently by Borg (1962) for dynamic work on the bicycle ergometer. For static work involving holding up weights suspended from the wrist, the power function relating "Anstrengung" to weight expressed as a percent of maximum weight that could be held (P) was: $\Psi = .000008 \, (P + 42.1)^{3.1}$. A graph of this power function is presented in Figure 14-1. In summary, the exponent of the power function for dynamic

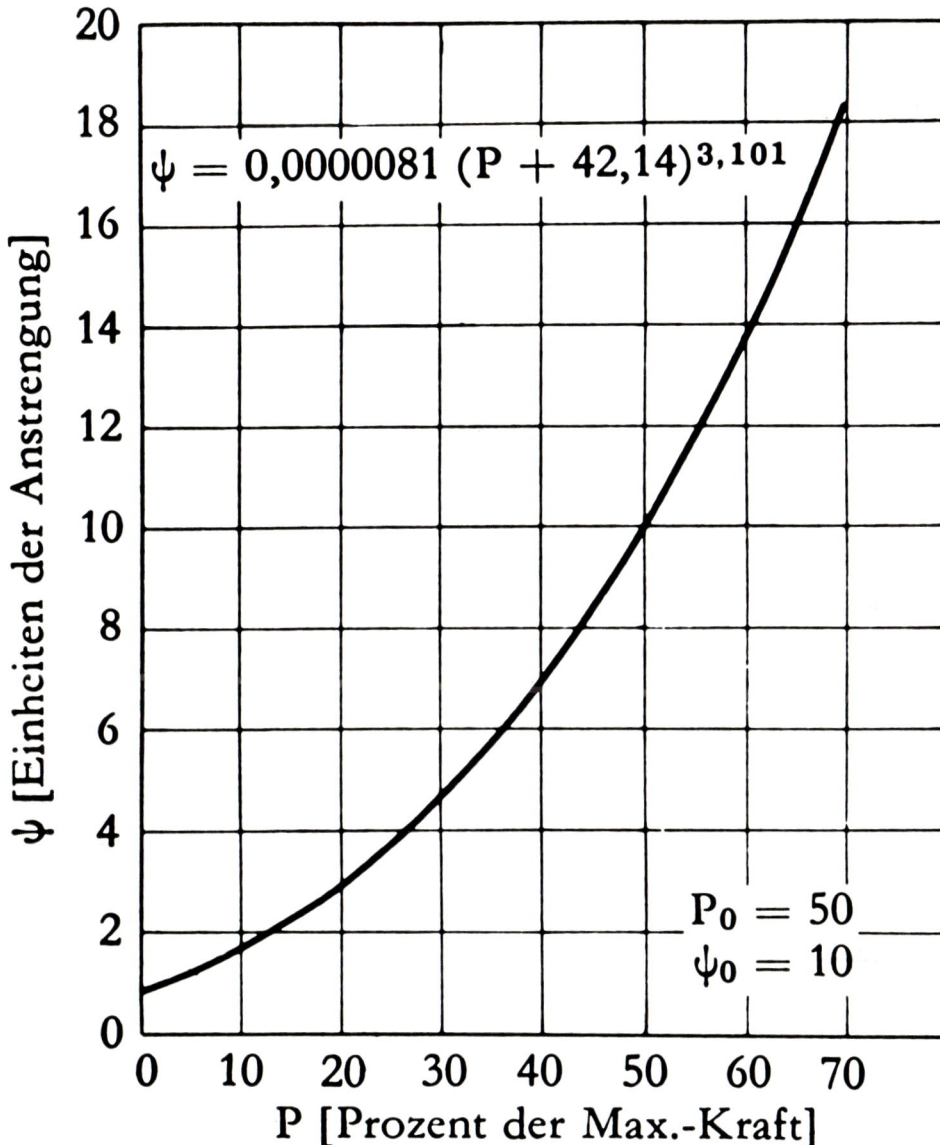

Figure 14-1. Power function relating "Anstrengung" (effort) to weight as a percentage of maximum strength (From H. Schmale, H. Schmidtke, and A. Vukovich, "Untersuchungen über den Grad der subjektiv gegebenen Beanspruchung bei Körperlicher Arbeit, *Forschungsbericht des Landes Nordrhein-Westfalen, Nr* 1261, 1963).

work was between 1.4 to 1.9 whether the work involved arms, legs, or wrist curling. However, the exponent obtained for static work, 3.1, was considerably higher.

Bernyer (1967) has demonstrated that production methods (e.g. the method of bisections) may result in different mathematical functions for perceived heaviness of lifted weights depending on whether the test series presented was in ascending or descending order. For ascending order, a power function with exponents ranging from 1.8 to 2.5 describes the positively accelerated perception-stimulus relationship adequately; for a descending series, a negatively accelerated function is produced, apparently described more adequately by a Fechnerian log function, shown in equation 1 above. The actual relationship derived by psychophysical techniques has been shown to be substantially influenced by task requirements. Among the factors affecting the obtained psychophysical relationships are, as previously noted, the direction of the series presented (e.g. ascending or descending) and time-order errors related to order of presentation of the stimuli in a series (S. S. Stevens, 1957).

Hosman (1967) studied the time-course for the "feeling of exhaustion" in 5 subjects during three prolonged static work tasks. Using cross-modality matching against white noise, 9 of the 15 total responses showed a linear growth function. In 2 trials the increase was negatively accelerated, while in only 4 trials did the time-course show a positive acceleration. However, since the subjective response was reported as an average of 10 sessions at each task, the linear response might partially represent a timing bias that could have developed after several sessions (see p. 370). More detailed and sophisticated psychophysical analysis of the time course for fatigue during prolonged static work has been reported by J. C. Stevens and Cain.

J. C. Stevens and Cain (1970) explored the more complex interaction that the effects of force and duration have upon perceived force of handgrip using 18 male subjects. In an initial study, magnitude estimation was used to obtain a ratio scaling of perceived force relative to handgrip squeezes at forces between 22 and 220 newtons (5 to 50 lbs) for durations of 4 to 60 secs. Power functions were derived separately for force and duration. For force, the exponent was 1.4. However, they noted that because of the tendency for subjects to attenuate the range of numbers used in magnitude estimation (i.e., regression bias; see S. S. Stevens and Greenbaum, 1966), the value of the exponent was depressed and actually closer to 1.7. The latter is also the exponent found experimentally in the earlier study by J. C. Stevens and Mack (1959). Perceived effort also increased with duration, having an exponent of 0.57 (i.e., 0.70 when adjusted for regression bias). One equation could then describe the combination of force and duration which "produces the same terminal perceived force, Ψ_c: $\Psi_c = K\Phi^{1.7}t^{.7}$ where Ψ represents force in newtons, this time in seconds, and K is the constant level of perceived force at the limit of endurance. Rearrangement of this equation yields a simplified, one-exponent equation: $\Psi_c = K\Phi^{2.43}t$ which is independent of regression bias, being obtainable from either the biased or unbiased independent estimates for force and duration. Based on these findings, they suggested that subjects instructed to maintain a constant perceived effort would demonstrate diminishing force exerted over time, a result obtained earlier by Eason (1959).

In a subsequent study, Cain and J. C. Stevens (1971) explored these implications using a unique constant effort task. First, for a group of 12 male subjects, the earlier magnitude estimation study was replicated for phasic squeezes at seven forces between 88 and 429 newtons (19.8 to 96.4 lbs). The obtained power function had an exponent within the expected range. Next, for each of the forces, the subjects were asked to maintain their *effort* on the handgrip task *constant* for 2.5 min. Results indicated that actual force exerted typically dropped off rapidly for the first 20 secs, with a much slower decline in force thereafter. A single exception to this generality was for the lowest force squeeze, 88 newtons (19.8 lbs) for which a consistent, slow decline was observed throughout the 2.5 min duration. A two-exponent equation could describe the initially rapid, then slower decline in force across time. On the basis of these results, it was predicted that "two different constant-effort contractions may arouse the same degree of fatigue when the areas under their respective force versus duration curves are equal." A subsequent study impressively supported this prediction.

Since two components were involved in the force-duration curves of Cain and J. C. Stevens (1971) for the constant-effort contractions, a fast then slow decline, it was suggested that two separate physiological processes may be involved in the perception of effort: "(the fast) one—representing activity of mechanoreceptors in the tendons or the skin, and the (slow) term the activity of receptors sensitive to noxious metabolites produced by muscular activity." At least one alternative explanation may be proposed: the fast decline in force may have been due to derecruitment of glycolytic, fast twitch fibers in favor of less rapidly fatiguing oxidative, slow twitch fibers.

Their subsequent studies of surface electromyography (Cain and J. C. Stevens, 1973) indicated the EMG activity in the forearm initially did decrease rapidly similar to force in constant-effort handgrip tasks but tended to asymptote at a point where force was still declining. Their two-process model could also be explained by the alternative explanation noted above. In summary, in a series of elegant psychophysical studies on constant-effort tasks, J. C. Stevens and Cain attempted to relate perceived effort to physiological processes and acknowledged that perceived effort is founded on more than a single underlying physiological process.

In the psychophysical studies described above, perception of force exerted or "Anstrengung" (exertion) was related to stimulus intensity for fixed, brief work periods. Bujas, Paulina, Sremec, Vidacek, and Vodanovic (1966) noted that the research of J. C. Stevens and Mack (1959) and Borg (1962), and presumably Schmale, et al. (1963) and Bernyer (1967), do not present psychophysical power functions relating the perception of "fatigue" to *duration* of effort. They pointed out that brief effort or momentary exertion, used in the above studies, may not lead to "fatigue" although the effort expended may be relatively high. Bujas, et al. present information about the psychophysical relationship for the feeling of fatigue *per se* during periods differing in the duration of static work. Using well-trained subjects a steady tension was exerted by holding a 7.17 kg weight with the arm upright and the elbow supported. Durations of 30, 60, 90, 120, 150, and 180 sec. were used and the psychophysical function relating the perception of fatigue to duration of effort was derived using the magnitude estimation method. Fatigue ratings were obtained 30 and 60 sec. after termination of each trial. The subjects were told to include feelings of "tightness, numbness, increase in muscle sensitivity through pain, weight" and so on in their judgments of "fatigue." The obtained power function for the overall group was $\Psi = .0048 \, (\Phi - 30'')^{1.54}$ for the mid-range of the curve relating perception of fatigue to task duration. In a subsequent experiment, the identical procedure was repeated while integrated EMG amplitude from four muscle groups of the arm was recorded. A power function for the mid-range of the curve relating integrated EMG levels to task duration was almost identical to the psychophysical function: $\Sigma EMG = .0051 \, (\Phi - 30'')^{1.51}$ indicating impressively high correspondence between the growth of fatigue in static work and EMG activity. It is also of interest that the exponent of the power function for both fatigue and EMG activity in this study falls within the range of exponents observed for force exerted in the studies described above.

These psychophysical studies provide important information about the relationships between perception of effort and load levels during various types of work performance. In general, for positive (i.e. concentric) work, the exponents of the power functions for force exerted and fatigue in a variety of situations fall within a limited range (1.4 to 1.9), indicating that the perceptions increase at a moderate rate relative to changes in the physical work stimulus. An interesting contrast existed for the exponent (3.1) of the weight-holding task of Schmale, et al. (1963) which may be related to the negative (eccentric) nature of the task. However, psychophysical techniques are currently limited in regard to application for the evaluation of subjective fatigue on a longitudinal basis. With the exception of Bujas, et al. (1966), most of these studies relate a subjective quality (e.g. perception of intensity) to the actual intensity of an *external* physical stimulus. Subjective fatigue can be conceived as arising from a different source; specifically, the cues defining subjective fatigue may derive from the *internal* physiological processes activated by work. There is thus no easy way to identify *intensity* of the "physical" stimulus when in fact precise *origins* of these physiological cues are not well understood. Presently, there is no clear way to derive the power function describing such relationships. Furthermore, none of the available psychophysical techniques are readily applicable to measurement of subjective qualities during work performance on an ongoing basis. Future applications of psychophysical methods may prove to overcome these difficulties, but changes in methodology will be required.

Alternative scaling techniques discussed in the following sections have been applied more frequently to the measurement of subjective qualities or symptoms during work primarily because of their applicability to prolonged work situations. These techniques may be roughly grouped into (1) nondimensional, single point measures, (2) unidimensional rating scale techniques, and (3) multidimensional rating scale techniques.

Nondimensional, Single Point Measures

In Table 14-II, studies using nondimensional, single point measurement of subjective qualities in work are shown. These studies have employed the simplest methods of measurement which generally require a single verbal report during work performance. Most often an attempt is made to identify factors displacing the "fatigue" point toward or away from the initiation of work. Inspection of the table reveals little consistency between the studies in regard to the subjective qualities measured (tiredness and undifferentiated fatigue), tasks used, or subject populations selected. It is worth noting that just such inconsistency has hampered the development of a meaningful overview of research concerning subjective fatigue.

In a study by McGrath, Wittkower, and Cleghorn (1954), the undifferentiated (i.e. global) feeling of fatigue was regarded as an all-or-none event, characteristic of single point measurement. Specifically, ratings of various factors which were regarded as "causing fatigue" during long distance flights were obtained from aircraft crews. The crews studied consisted of Canadian pilots, co-pilots, navigators, and radio officers who flew DC 6's in the Tokyo Airlift. The three legs of the flight were 10 to 18 hours each separated by 48-hour layovers. Group discussions and individual interviews were used to identify factors which the crewmen believed to cause fatigue. The specific factors chosen for inclusion in a questionnaire were identified during these preliminary group discussions and interviews. Each of the thirty-four factors were arranged on a 4-point ordinal scale to permit rating from "no importance" (1) in causing fatigue to "great importance" (4). However, the quantitative data available from the questionnaire was not summarized in the report. Conclusions were based principally on the nonquantitative information derived from the interviews and group discussions.

TABLE 14-II
NONDIMENSIONAL MEASUREMENT OF SUBJECTIVE FATIGUE

Subjective Quality Measured	Task	Subjects	Studies
"Undifferentiated fatigue"	Airplane flights	Male aircarft crews (n = 100)	McGrath, Wittkower, and Cleghorn (1954)
"Undifferentiated fatigue"	Reaction time task	Male medical students (n = 26) Female P.E. students (n = 15)	Pierson (1963), Pierson and Lockhart (1964)
Tiredness	Manual and office work	Male manual and office workers (n = 379)	Griffith, Kerr, Mayo, and Topal (1950)
Tiredness	Isometric weight lifting	Female psychiatric patients (n = 42)	Hemphill, Hall, and Crookes (1952)

Members of the crews tended to report boredom, but only minimal fatigue, during the first six hours of a flight. From six to 10 hours, the crewmen reported becoming tired, sleepy, and irritable. Causes of fatigue were grouped into three categories: (1) *General Factors,* such as length of flight, delayed flights and false starts, details prior to takeoff, reliability of radio communications and navigational aids, bad weather, monotony and boredom of familiar routes, number of intermediate stops, and drinking the night before the flight; (2) *Specific Factors,* associated with problems peculiar to the DC 6 aircraft (including noise and vibration, design of the flight deck and instrument panels, and uncomfortably fitting oxygen masks), and problems peculiar to the route (including post-flight conditions, recreational facilities at stopover points, and irregular hours); and (3) *Personal Factors,* such as inexperience and tension within the crew, relative burden of responsibility, relationships with higher authorities, and domestic worries.

In this study, no information was obtained to quantify fatigue or performance during the course of flights. The authors were well aware of this basic limitation in their study. They note that the "method used in this investigation might be criticized on the grounds that information gathered was of a purely subjective nature and was given in retrospect." Continuing to discuss these limitations, they clearly indicate the two ingredients minimally necessary to conduct research evaluating the role of subjective fatigue longitudinally during work performance: (1) An adequate *measure of subjective fatigue* for which "no satisfactory objective tests [had] as yet been designed" and (2) *Performance measures* to evaluate "the subject's performance under normal operating [or working] conditions."

Pierson (1963a) attempted to relate the occurrence of "fatigue" in twenty-six male medical students to performance on a reaction time task using an apparatus described by Pierson and Rasch (1959). On each trial, an auditory preparatory signal was given approximtely one second before presentation of a light stimulus which cued the response. Each subject was required to release a telegraph key and move their hand 11 in. forward through a light beam when the light stimulus appeared. Reaction time (RT) was measured as the latency between presentation of the light and the release of the key, while movement time (MT) was measured from the release of the key to the breaking of the light beam. Trials were presented at intervals of approximately 10 seconds with the task continuing until the subject indicated that he could no longer proceed. During the task, the subject was required to indicate when he "believed his responses were becoming slower." The trial on which this report was given was defined as the "fatigue" point. Subjects were also asked to indicate the point at which they became bored with the task.

A significant relationship (r = .47) was found between RT latency and the trial on which the "fatigue" report was given. This relationship means that slower RT's tended to be associated with later fatigue points, while early fatigue points were more often concomitant with faster RT's. More importantly, no differences in RT or MT were found between five baseline trials, selected near the beginning of the task, five trials following the fatigue point, and the last five trials preceding voluntary termination. Furthermore, no relationship (r = .02) was found between the "fatigue" trial and total trials performed before voluntary termination. Pierson (1963b) reported that measures of unspecified isometric strength for these same subjects were found to be unrelated either to RT and MT decrement or the trial defined as the fatigue point. He concluded that "subjective impressions of performance bear little relationship to actual performance" and that the "subjective experience of fatigue is not a valid criterion for the ability to perform speed or endurance type muscular work."

In regard to Pierson's conclusions, it should be noted first that a study subsequently reported by Pierson and Rich (1967) found a steady O_2 consumption during this task. Performance of the task required only slightly greater O_2 uptake than baseline measures obtained while the subjects were sitting quietly (330 ml/min. vs. 280 ml/min.). Therefore, generalization of these results to "speed or endurance type muscular work" appears unjustified. At best, the results may be generalized to sedentary type tasks. Additionally, RT and MT performance decrement was measured as the slowest block of five trials within a sequence averaging 174 trials for the group of subjects. In tasks of this kind, random variations in performance across trials would be expected due to momentary fluctuations in motivation, concentration, and so on. As the measure of performance decrement, selection of the slowest block of five trials may therefore reflect nothing more than random changes in performance. In fact, since there was no systematic trend toward deteriorating performance across trials, as the data indicates, it is hardly conceivable that "the subjective experience of fatigue" would be related to RT or MT decrements in this study. In a word, Pierson's conclusions seem unfounded.

A subsequent study (Pierson and Lockhart, 1964) did qualify the earlier conclusions of Pierson (1963a). Using fifteen female physical education majors with a mean age of 19.6 years, an attempt to replicate the earlier study was made. This time, the principal finding was a *significant* relationship (r = .59) between the trial on which "fatigue" was reported and the total number of trials performed. The "fatigue" point for male medical students had been found to be clearly unrelated to endurance (r = .02). One might suggest that these conflicting findings may be explained by differences in motivation and cooperation with task requirements. For example, those medical students who reported "boredom" (7 of 26) did so at a mean trial of 70.4 while those female subjects reporting boredom (4 of 15) did not do so until trial 102.4 even though females quit earlier (an average of 171 total trials for the males vs. 151 for the females). The male subjects evidently quit performing for reasons unrelated to "fatigue," while the female subjects seemed to be more highly motivated, quitting for reasons more related to "fatigue." All other findings in this study were generally consistent with Pierson (1963a). Obviously, there are problems related to replicability as the contrasting principal findings between the studies indicate, and specifically require qualification of the earlier conclusions concerning the relationship between subjective report of fatigue and performance factors.

A study by Griffith, Kerr, Mayo, and Topal (1950) is another example of a single point measurement technique. They employed a simple "tear ballot" used previously by Kerr (1943) to determine the hour during each half of an eight-hour shift when manual workers, foremen, and office workers reported feeling "most rested" or "most tired." To indicate the hour of each half-shift, the subjects simply tore the appropriate corner off the ballot. Data for the study were reduced to percentages reporting "most tired" and "most rested" during each four-hour period. Findings were remarkably uniform for all types of work and are schematized in Figure 14-2. There was a tendency for workers to report feeling "most tired" during the first and fourth hour of the morning and the last hour of the afternoon. Manual workers more than 36 years old reported feeling "most tired" more often during the last hour of the morning and afternoon periods than did younger manual workers. Information about the consistency of this technique is sketchy, although it is reported that "repeat-test reliability coefficients for small groups ranged from .69 to .92." No information was available concerning validity of the self-report since no other measures of work performance were obtained. Information provided by this study is limited, since only a single point of "most tired" was reported, it was impossible to evaluate relative *levels* of fatigue on an hourly basis across the work shifts. By focusing on *percentages* of workers reporting "most tired," an erroneous conclusion was also drawn, i.e. "Older workers report significantly greater variation of such feelings ('most tired' and 'most rested') than do employees under the age of 36." This conclusion may be correct for workers as a whole, but since the relative *degree* of tiredness was not measured, no conclusion can be made concerning the variability in tiredness reported by workers in different age groups.

Hemphill, Hall, and Crookes (1952) also used a single point measurement technique within a simple weight-holding task. Using the middle finger of the right hand, female psychiatric patients classified as endoge-

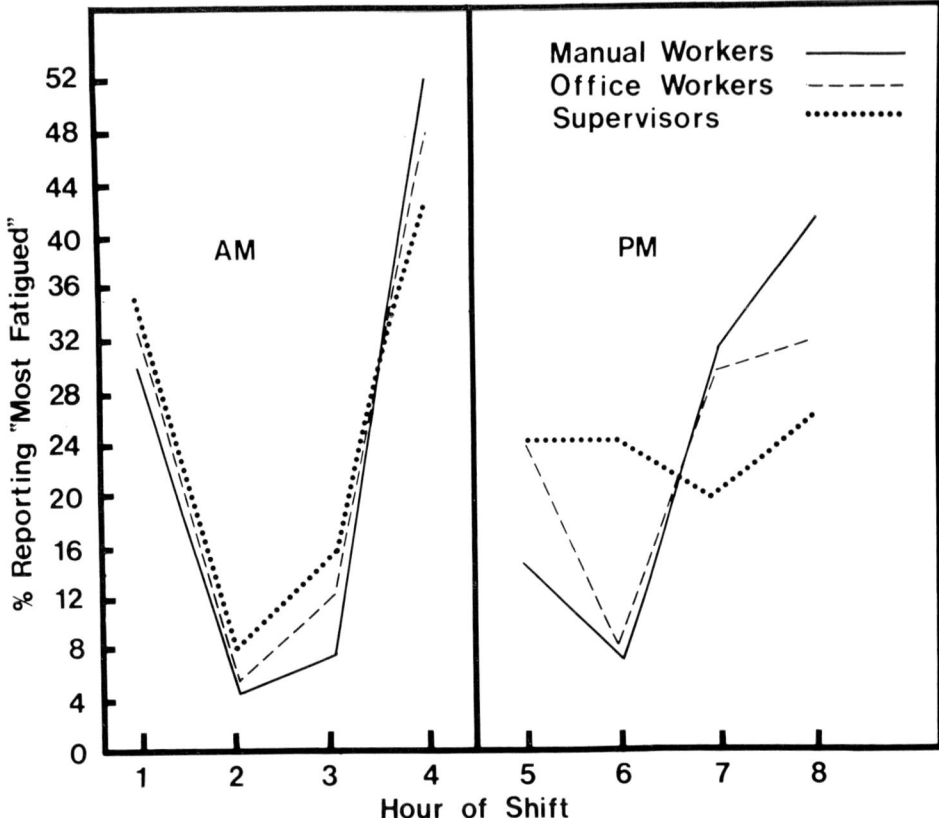

Figure 14-2. Percentage of workers reporting feeling "most fatigued" during the morning (AM) and afternoon (PM) halves of an eight-hour shift (From J. W. Griffith, et al, "Changes in Subjective Fatigue and Readiness for Work During the Eight-Hour Shift," *Journal of Applied Psychology*, 34:163, 1950).

nous depressives and anxiety neurotics were instructed to lift a small weight (2 kg) for as long as possible. They were asked to report when they "began to feel tired." The results indicated that the "endogenous depressive" patients reported feeling tired more rapidly and quit sooner after reporting tiredness than patients classified as anxiety neurotics. The results suggest that endogenous depressive patients, who are characteristically "fatigued" and with minimal energy reserves, became tired more readily during static work. Anxiety neurotics, on the other hand, are frequently characterized by an agitated, aroused kind of depression which may actually serve to reduce the degree of tiredness during activity or static work.

Single point, nondimensional measures of fatigue are open to criticism. "Fatigue" is conceptualized in these studies as an all-or-none event: either the individual is experiencing a certain "degree" of fatigue, or he is not.

It is hard to defend such a notion, either conceptually or psychometrically. First, experience suggests that, in general, one can report a variety of intensities of subjective qualities—one has, at different times, felt fresh, somewhat tired or extremely worn out. It would seem more logical that the symptoms would increase quantitatively, in some fashion, the longer one performs work. Measurement should be designed to quantify at least ordinal levels of the subjective experience.

Second, from the standpoint of measurement, good psychometrics also suggests that some arrangement be made to measure quantitative *levels* of fatigue. Without this possibility, the relationship between subjective fatigue and work decrement or endurance cannot be clearly specified. It takes at least three points to define a function, and theoretically a subjective event varying in intensity such as subjective fatigue, can be measured on more than three points. Additionally, reliability is known to increase, up to some limit, as the range of scores increases. Single point measures can thus be expected to be less reliable than multi-point, or dimensional, measures of subjective fatigue.

Unidimensional Rating Scales

Studies using unidimensional rating scales to evaluate subjective qualities during work are summarized in Table 14-III. An example of an early study attempting to dimensionally quantify a single subjective quality, i.e. "feeling tone," is provided by Foltz, Jung, and Cisler (1944). They had seven male subjects ride a bicycle ergometer at 1235 kpm/min. while pedalling at 54 rpm's until unable to maintain the required level of performance. This work of about 2.8 L/min. V_{O_2} would be approximately 85 percent max V_{O_2} of nearly 3.3 L/min. for an "average" young male. All subjects rode twice daily with the rides separated by a 10-minute rest period until a total of 378 rides were obtained over 27 days. Ratings of "feeling tone" were obtained *before* each ride using a 15-point rating scale ranging from "the worse I have ever felt in my life" (1) to "the best I have ever felt in my life" (15) while the midpoint (8) required the response "the way I usually feel." Ride duration was the measure of performance and ranged from 2 to 22 min. The study was designed to test the hypothesis that work performance is influenced by how an individual feels before beginning work. Results indicated that the relationship between ride duration and prework "feeling tone" was negligible and, in fact, slightly opposite from predicted. The authors suggested that work performance was unrelated to prework subjective feeling states.

The approach used by Foltz, et al. represents one of the early systematic efforts to relate a subjective quality (prework "feeling tone") to performance in a laboratory work situation. However, this study again exemplifies

TABLE 14-III

RATING SCALES IN THE MEASUREMENT OF SUBJECTIVE FATIGUE

Subjective Quality Measured	Scale Point Range	Task	Subjects	Studies
"Feeling tone"	15	Bicycle ergometer	Healthy males	Foltz, Jung, and Cisler (1944)
"Undifferentiated fatigue"	4	Housework	Healthy females; housewives	Gross and Bartley (1951)
"Undifferentiated fatigue"	9	Bicycle ergometer; normal conditions	Healthy males	Nunney (1963)
Tiredness	5	Mental work: Verbal and qualitative	Healthy males	Poffenberger (1928)
Tiredness	20	Psychomotor tasks; drug states	Healthy males; US Air Force enlisted men	Pearson and Byars (1956); Pearson (1957)
Tiredness	20	Prolonged aircraft flights	Healthy males; aircraft crews	Buckley and Hartman (1969); Hartman, et al. (1974a, b)
Tiredness	9	Psychomotor task	Males and females; college students	McNelly (1957)
Tiredness	5	Factory workers	Healthy males; butchers	Bujas, Sremeg, and Vidachek (1965)
Tiredness	10	Portages	Healthy males	Strauss and Carlock (1966)
Tiredness	7	Bicycle ergometer	Healthy males	Heuting and Sarphati (1966)
Tiredness	13.5	Psychomotor task; visual threshold	Healthy males; college students	Walster and Aronson (1967)
Perceived effort	15	Bicycle ergometer; normal conditions	Healthy males	Borg (1961a); Borg (1962); Borg and Linderholm (1967); Frankenhauser, Post, Nordhader, and Sjolberg (1969); Kay, and Shephard (1969); Bar-Or, et al. (1972); Skinner, et al. (1969; 1973b); Morgan (1973)

Perceived effort	15	Bicycle ergometer; normal conditions	Male cardiac patients	Borg, and Linderholm (1970)
Perceived effort	15	Bicycle ergometer; hypoxic conditions	Healthy males	Gerben, House, and Winsman (1972) Weiser, et al. (unpublished observation)
Perceived effort	15	Bicycle ergometer; dynamic weight lifting; wheelbarrow pushing	Healthy males	Gamberale (1972)
Perceived effort	15	Bicycle ergometer; concentric and eccentric work	Healthy males and females	Henrikson, Knuttgen, and Bonde-Petersen (1972)
Perceived effort	15	Treadmill walking and running	Healthy males	Noble, et al. (1973)
Perceived effort expended	5	Treadmill walking	Healthy males	Lloyd and McClaskey (1971)
Perceived effort expended	5 and 10	Isometric contraction; hand dynamometer	Healthy males	Caldwell and Smith (1967); Caldwell (1967)
Pain intensity	5	Isometric contraction; hand dynamometer and arm pull	Healthy males	Caldwell and Smith (1966); Caldwell and Smith (1967); Menzer, Smith, and Caldwell (1969); Lloyd, Voor, and Thieman (1970); Lloyd (1971); Lloyd (1972)
Discomfort	4	Bicycle ergometer	Healthy males	Gagge, Stolwijk, and Saltin (1969)
Thermal sensation	7			

the caution required in design and interpretation of research in this area. First, no attempt was made to equate work levels for the individual subjects. While information was not presented regarding individual differences in such factors as max V_{O_2} or heart rate response to specific work levels, almost surely there were differences in working capacity between the individual subjects. These individual differences in working capacity, while not well known at that time (Simonson and Enzer, 1942), would greatly influence ride duration. Failure to equate work levels during exercise, however, would lead to a substantial attenuation of the relationship between "feeling tone" before work and subsequent work performance.

Second, it would appear that performance data for all 378 rides and subjective ratings for the seven subjects were grouped across subjects to obtain the correlation between ride duration and prework "feeling tone." Grouping data in this way violates an assumption of independence of the pairs of observations for correlational analysis and could further attenuate any potential relationship in the data. Therefore, on the basis of this study, little can be concluded regarding the relationship between pre-work "feeling tone" and subsequent work output due to these inherent design and methodological problems. In addition, since subjective symptomatology *during* work, or produced by work, was not measured, the implications for the area of subjective fatigue are limited. However, studies of this sort could lead the unsuspecting reviewer to conclude that "research has indicated" that subjective symptoms are unrelated to work performance.

In contrast to Foltz, et al., the remaining studies described in this section measure subjective qualities *during* work performance. These have focused upon five types of subjective qualities during work: undifferentiated fatigue, tiredness, effort, pain, and thermal discomfort.

Undifferentiated Fatigue

A study by Gross and Bartley (1951) provides an example of the use of a simple rating scale to measure undifferentiated fatigue. A four-point rating scale (Great, Moderate, Little, None) was employed. A group of twenty women rated their level of fatigue at 30-minute intervals at the beginning and throughout a two-hour period of housework. Records were maintained concerning the quality and quantity of work performed. Those reporting the most fatigue cleaned fewer rooms than those moderately fatigued, but more than those reporting little or no fatigue. The women reporting the most fatigue also received the lowest ratings for quality of housework performed. Additionally, it was found that the rating of fatigue for some women tended to peak at the middle of the work period even though there was no intervening rest. The latter observation was regarded as support for the notion that subjective fatigue is not consistently related to the amount of energy expended. Examination of the individual protocols suggests that some subjects may have been timing the work period, reporting less fatigue as the end of the period neared. In contrast, most reported increased fatigue toward the end of the work period. This is an occasional observation when work periods are of a fixed duration, and appears related to expectations about the length of a dull, nonrewarding task. Walster and Aronson (1967; see p. 365) found an increase in fatigue reports toward completion of a monotonous task of fixed duration. Additionally, Gross and Bartley noted that there was a "lack of distinction in the minds of the subjects between localized muscle discomfort from stooping, etc., and the overall personal experimental (sic) state we identify as fatigue." Recently, a task specific category of subjective qualities experienced during work, including those related to localized muscle discomfort, have been identified statistically within a larger set of fatigue symptoms (Weiser, Kinsman and Stamper, 1973).

Nunney (1963) used a nine-point rating scale to evaluate subjective fatigue in eighty male college students. The testing program encompassed six test sessions of five min. given on alternate days. The subjects were divided into five groups: A control group; two groups who bicycled on an ergometer, either with no load or a seven-lb load; and two groups who ran on a treadmill at 6 mph, either on a 0 percent or on a 25 percent grade. The rating scale ranged from No Fatigue (1) to Extreme Fatigue (9) and was given 15 sec. after cessation of work. Pulse rate was measured before, at the end of the work task, and after 10 min. of recovery. If the mean testing pulse rate was 80 bpm (the actual value was not reported), then the mean pulse rate was 91 and 137 bpm for the 0 and seven-lb bicycle work tasks and 141 and 181 bpm for the 0 percent and 25 percent treadmill work. This indicates that the work loads were progressively heavier, with the two middle tasks nearly the same and the heaviest nearly 100 percent max Vo_2. We note that Nunney, similar to Foltz, et al. (1944) did not control for individual differences in the ability to do aerobic work as measured by max Vo_2. The fatigue scale scores at the end of work were 1, 4, 4, and 6 for the respective work loads. The *group means* for pulse rate changes and fatigue scale scores correlated highly ($r = .99$), suggesting that for tasks demanding a larger circulatory adaptation there is a corresponding increase in subjective fatigue. Intratask variability was large for fatigue scale scores, but these scores were not significantly correlated to pulse rate changes. Considering the relationships between pulse rate and subjective fatigue ratings for a single work load on a task, the correlations were low (r's ranging from $-.03$ to $+.37$). These low correlations would be expected when the range of work loads relative to max Vo_2 within tasks are attenuated relative to the range represented across all tasks and work loads. While

Nunney concludes "that physiological changes are not directly related to fatigue," his data actually support a direct relationship between fatigue measures and work as indicated by heart rate changes when there is a sufficiently high range in work loads.

Tiredness

As early as 1928, Poffenberger reported the use of a simple rating scale to evaluate the feeling of tiredness during prolonged *mental* work. Ten subjects performed up to fourteen consecutive trials on each of four tasks: continuous addition, sentence completion, judging of written compositions and various independent forms of a rather lengthy intelligence test. In the case of the composition judging, 10 specimen compositions were rated on each trial. For the other tasks, each trial required 20 to 30 minutes of continuous performance. Performance was measured on each trial, and ratings of tiredness were obtained using a seven-point *ordinal* scale, given immediately before the first trial and after each trial of a task. The rating scale ranged from "extremely good" (1) to "extremely tired" (7) with a midpoint defined as "medium" (4). Results indicated that the mean rating of tiredness increased across trials in a fairly linear manner for all tasks, although overall performance remained (1) unchanged—for sentence completion or composition judging, (2) improved—for intelligence testing, or (3) deteriorated—for addition. Due to improvement in the tasks resulting from practice, the relationship between mental work and the feeling of tiredness may have been masked for all of the tasks except addition. Presumably, addition is a highly learned task, the performance of which would not be expected to improve with additional practice. Thus, the relationship between the subjective quality "tiredness" and performance would be most clearly manifest for the addition task. Subjects showing the greatest performance decrement for each task reported a large increase in tiredness; those showing the least performance decrement reported substantially less tiredness across trials. Poffenberger's results thus indicate a fairly clear relationship between "tiredness" and performance in prolonged mental work.

Pearson and Byars (1956) and Pearson (1957) reported the development of a 10-item unidimensional scale measuring the subjective quality of tiredness. Their *interval* scale represents the most thorough effort to devise a measure of subjective fatigue as a unidimensional feeling of tiredness. Procedures for scale construction recommended by Edwards and Kilpatrick (1948) were followed. The problem was to select a set of adjectives that could be arranged in a continuum, with *equidistant* adjacent items, so that the subject could report his level of tiredness by pinpointing a position along this continuum. An initial set of 500 adjectives were selected. All ambiguous items were eliminated, and the remaining ninety-two items were scaled using Thurstone's method of equal appearing intervals (see Guilford, 1954). Briefly, independent judges sorted each item into nine categories ranging from extreme well being (1) to extreme fatigue (9). All forty-eight items showing low interjudge agreement were eliminated. The forty-four remaining items were arranged in a checklist and provided with choices of "better than," "same as," or "worse than" allowing an individual to place himself on a continuum of subjective tiredness. A developmental study involving a lengthy psychomotor task (Multidimensional Pursuit Test; Hauty and Payne, 1956) was used to further eliminate those items with low validity and internal consistency. Finally, two equivalent forms (A and B) of the checklist were constructed. The item composition of one form (Form A) of the checklist is shown below:

Item	Order No.
1. Like I'm bursting with energy	(2)
2. Extremely peppy	(6)
3. Very lively	(12)
4. Very refreshed	(9)
5. Quite fresh	(4)
6. Somewhat fresh	(7)
7. Slightly tired	(1)
8. Slightly pooped	(5)
9. Fairly well pooped	(11)
10. Petered out	(8)
11. Very tired	(13)
12. Extremely tired	(3)
13. Ready to drop	(10)

In application, the items were arranged in a random order as indicated in the right-hand column. The colloquial content of the checklist ("petered out," "ready to drop," "fairly well pooped") is apparent.

A validation study using the same psychomotor task showed that equivalent forms of the checklist intercorrelated highly ($r = .92$) both for 100 experimentally fatigued and for 100 control subjects. The scores for experimentally fatigued subjects were significantly increased from pre- to post-task. Additionally, the checklist clearly differentiated between experimentally fatigued and control subjects. Subsequently, the checklist was shown to differentiate between subjects given analeptic (5 mg of dextro-amphetamine sulfate) and depressant (.65 mg hyoscine hydrobromide mixed with 50 mg of diphenhydramine hydrochloride) drugs in a single-blind study. As a unidimensional measure of tiredness, Pearson's interval scale is unsurpassed since it was constructed systematically according to sound psychometric principles.

Unfortunately, application of the checklist beyond the original validating studies has been limited although the authors suggest that its applicability should be general. Its widest application has been to evaluate changes in fatigue during aeromedical studies by Hartman and his coworkers. In a study by Buckley and Hartman (1969), Pearson's checklist was used to evaluate changes in subjective tiredness during a 32-hour transatlantic helicopter flight. The flight was accompanied by loss of usual sleeping patterns, decreased food intake, continuous vibration, and flicker illumination common to rotary wing aircraft. Ratings on tiredness showed an almost linear increase throughout the flight, with an interesting recovery spurt during fly-by in a Paris airshow even though no rest periods intervened. During this fly-by, which occurred at the end of the flight, tiredness ratings decreased to a point reported 14 to 16 hours earlier. Such a recovery phenomenon may occur in tasks of fixed duration in which there is high expectation of personal reward upon successful completion. Such a phenomenon may be related to the Hullian goal-gradient (Hull, 1943; 1952). Similar application of this scale have been made to the study of the in-flight fatigue of FB-111 crews (Hartman, Hale and Johnson, 1974) and C5 jet transport crews (Hartman, Hale, Harris, and Stanford, 1974).

McNelly (1954) also used Thurstone scaling techniques to develop a 9-point rating scale of tiredness. Again, an attempt was made to construct an *interval* scale with adjacent scale points of equidistance. One form of McNelly's scale is shown below:

Item	Mean Scale Point
About to fall over	1.1
Fagged	2.2
Let down	3.2
A little tired	3.8
Average	5.0
Fairly well	5.9
In gear	7.0
Very good	7.9
Terrific	8.9

Preliminary Thurstone scaling was performed on 123 adjective items or phrases by 10 judges. The judges sorted each item into categories according to increasing degree of tiredness, establishing a preliminary mean scale point value for each item. Sixty (60) adjective items or phrases with the least variability were retained, and rescaled by the same judges. The second scaling had a high correlation ($r = .95$) with the first scaling. Of these 60 items, two groups of nine items each were selected on the basis of (1) having low variability and (2) being approximately one scale point apart. The mean scale values for one set of nine items are shown above.

The validity of the scale was tested on eighty male and female undergraduates using a block turning task with heavy (11 ounces) or light (.4 ounces) blocks either with massed practice (without rest) or spaced practice (rest after each trial). Each trial consisted of turning twenty blocks as rapidly as possible. The interval scale was administered before and after

1,000 trials. As expected, spaced practice produced both less work decrement and lower "tiredness" scores than did massed practice. Ratings of tiredness showed a significant change pre- to post-work, although the relationship between the subjective ratings and work decrement was quite low ($r = .30$). While McNelly's scale has frequently been cited, to the best of our knowledge it has not been used in any other studies reported in the literature. Its validity in other work situations is essentially unknown. Similar to the Pearson and Byars' scale (1956; Pearson, 1957) the composition of McNelly's scale includes colloquial items (e.g. fagged, in gear, etc.) which appear to be unique in regard to culture, time, and geographic location.

Bujas, Sremeg, and Vidachek (1965) comprehensively investigated the relationships between the subjective quality of tiredness and other variables in 115 butchers from the same factory after an eight-hour work shift. A five-point scale was used to obtain ratings of tiredness. The scale ranged from "Generally I am not tired" (1) to "I feel very tired" (5). Only 4.4 percent of the workers reported that they were generally *not* tired after work, while 26.5, 49.6, 12.4, and 7.1 percent reported feeling "slightly," "moderately," "quite," or "very" tired, respectively. Ratings of tiredness were independent of estimates of the workers productivity made by the foremen and plant supervisors. However, the authors note that productivity ratings tended to be uniformly high for all workers so that no discrimination in productivity was achieved by the supervisors' ratings. It is interesting to note that the tired workers reported having less satisfaction with their work, sleeping less well at night, less appetite, generally feeling less healthy, and more often being in a worse mood at and away from work than their less tired co-workers. This study is similar in many ways to that of McGrath, et al. (1954) in that the emphasis was upon identification of factors *contributing* to the subjective feelings of tiredness or fatigue that occur during occupational activities.

Strauss and Carlock (1966) measured subjective tiredness during portages with various loads using an 11-point rating scale developed by Psychometric Affiliates (1954). This rating scale ranged from "worn out, too tired to do anything" (1) to "not tired at all, fresh enough to start a full day" (11). Ten male subjects ranging in age from 18 to 35 years carried weights of 10 to 34 lbs during three walks over a two-mile course performed at two-hour intervals. Two portage modalities were used for each weight condition: comfortable, i.e. weights carried on the back, and uncomfortable, i.e. weights carried by hand. Performance on a battery of perceptual and psychomotor tests and ratings of tiredness were obtained before and after each portage. Walking time did not differ between light and heavy portages and was found to be unrelated to tiredness scores. However, the most uncomfortable portage modality was associated with reports of more tiredness. Task performance was significantly related to ratings of tiredness for each of the tests administered, with correlations ranging from −.62 (for perceptual speed and accuracy) to −.89 (for locating and marking identical pairs of names within a list).

Heuting and Sarphati (1966) noted that subjective ratings obtained during work performance could be subject to Tichener's "stimulus error." Specifically, the *load* levels on an ergometer may be presented in such a way as to provide the subjects with *external* information capable of altering their judgments about subjective tiredness. Thus, a subject given information about the load level at which he is performing will be apt to base his subjective rating of tiredness, in part, on that external information. Heuting and Sarphati had their subjects perform on a bicycle ergometer for 11 minutes on 13 successive days. The terminal load level for each daily session was selected as one of seven equal increments between 1050 and 1950 kpm/min. For each session, the initial work load was 45 kpm/min; it was increased by 10 percent of the final load level for each minute thereafter. Previous studies (Heuting, 1964; Heuting and Visser, 1960) indicated that the work load appeared to increase equally for each of these graded work schedules. Thus, estimates of tiredness could be obtained that were less affected by external information. Tiredness was rated in three ways: (1) during each minute of work the subjects positioned a potentiometer pointer along a blank scale to a location between horizontal and vertical corresponding to their level of tiredness; (2) immediately post-work the subjects adjusted the volume of a white noise source to match their level of tiredness; and (3) immediately post-work, the subjects indicated their level of tiredness on a seven-point scale ranging from "feeling fit, rested" (1) to "feeling extremely tired, exhausted" (7).

Average correlations between the terminal work load and post-work tiredness ratings ranged from .71, for the pointer, to .49 for both the white noise and seven-point rating scale. *Individual* correlations generally ranged from .54 to .93. The regression lines between work load and individual post-work ratings of tiredness were clearly linear. The study indicates the feasibility of measuring subjective status during work performance by rating scale techniques. Additionally, the potentiometer method showed the highest post-work relationship to work level. This result may have been due to the subjects' familiarity with this rating technique since it was used more frequently than the other two methods. Thus, there is the suggestion that *experience* with the rating technique may improve the relationship between subjective status and work load.

Janssen and Docter (1973) explored the change in fatigue during static work and recovery using Heuting's method (1968) of "fatigue" assessment. They had six well-trained male subjects exert pulls with the forearm at

25, 35, and 45 percent of their voluntary maximal capacity for intervals of 2.5 min., followed by 2 min. of recovery. Fatigue measures were obtained at rest and at 30 sec. intervals throughout the static work task and recovery. An essentially linear growth of fatigue was observed, more rapid for the higher work loads, with the expected steeper decline during recovery. Reproducibility was very high, and similar results were obtained for the left and right arm. Predictably, heart rate changes in this static work task were less impressively related to the course of work and recovery than the fatigue ratings (see Chap. 11 "Physiology of Work Capacity and Fatigue"). The impressive linearity may have been partially a result of timing during this relatively brief, fixed duration task.

While Heuting and Sarphati (1966) noted that external information about the work load level during exercise could influence reports of subjective tiredness, they did not directly test the effects of such external information on subjective reports. A more direct test of the effects of task information on subjective report was made by Walster and Aronson (1967). They reasoned that reports of tiredness would depend on time perceived to be remaining in the task: after the same duration on a task, a report of "very tired" would be incompatible with information that considerably more time is required. In contrast, such a report would be more compatible with information that the task is near completion. Two groups of 10 subjects were told that they would be required to complete either three (short expectancy) or five (long expectancy) trials during the study. Each trial involved two tasks: (1) marking X's on graph paper squares at the rate of one/second for 10 minutes, and (2) obtaining the visual threshold to white light which required approximately 10 additional minutes. Ratings of tiredness were obtained on each trial after the X-marking task. A rating scale ranging from "as fresh as I have ever been" (1) to "as tired as I have ever been" (13.5) was used. Only data from the first three trials were used in making the comparison between groups. Results indicated that the subjects in the three-trial condition reported a sudden increase in tiredness on trial three, while subjects in the five-trial condition did not report a corresponding increase. These results support the notion that information about task duration can influence subjective report. As yet, there have been no studies testing this effect for tasks involving physical work. This could be done by manipulating external information about such variables as load level and task duration. It would also be of interest to explore the possibility that motivational factors would differentially affect the subjective reports near the end of the task.

Subjective reports of fatigue may well be affected by the relationship between external (e.g. apparent task duration) and internal physiological cues as described by Snyder, Schulz, and Jones (1974). Briefly, their hypothesis was that when an internal standard of subjective fatigue is lacking, individuals believing that they have worked longer durations demonstrate more behavioral fatigue than those believing they have worked shorter durations, even though both groups work equally long. However, when clear, physiological cues are present, the effect of *apparent* duration may well be reversed since it conflicts with the predominant internal standard. A study using brief psychomotor tasks appeared to support this hypothesis. Studies such as these deriving from attribution theory (see Jones, Kanouse, Kelley, Nisbett, Valins, and Weiner, 1972) could contribute substantively to subjective fatigue and its behavioral correlates. Unfortunately, very little has yet been accomplished in this regard, and more adequate subjective rating techniques need to be employed together with improved physiological measures and work performance tasks.

Exertion

During work performance, rating scale techniques have been used to evaluate *perceived effort* by Borg (1962) and his co-workers while *perceived effort expended* has been studied by Lloyd and McClaskey (1971). Both will be discussed below.

EFFORT. In a recent review, Borg (1973) has traced the development of a rating scale of perceived effort (RPE) specifically designed for use during bicycle ergometer work. Initially (Borg, 1962) the scale consisted of 21 points with odd points, 3 through 19, anchored by verbal phrases: 3, extremely light; 5, very light; 7, light; 9, fairly light; 11, neither light nor laborious; 13, fairly laborious; 15, laborious; 17, very laborious; and 19, extremely laborious. On the basis of several initial studies, the scale was revised to include 15 points, 6 through 20, as follows:

6	
7	Very, very light
8	
9	Very light
10	
11	Fairly light
12	
13	Somewhat hard
14	
15	Hard
16	
17	Very hard
18	
19	Very, very hard
20	

The scale was presented in quarto fashion, with equal intervals between adjacent scale points, so that the full scale could be seen by the subject when making his ratings of perceived effort. The RPE scale is currently "so constructed that the heart rate (HR) of a normal, healthy middle-aged man can be predicted if the RPE value is multiplied by 10; thus RPE × 10 = HR" (Borg, 1971). Borg cautions, however, that this equation should not be taken too literally since deviations from the equation result from "difficulties in rating, lack of motivation, and disease." Specific circumstances in which the relationship between HR and RPE can be altered will be discussed below.

The load level giving a heart rate of 170 beats/min. can be obtained to define the Physical Working Capacity$_{170}$ (PWC$_{170}$; Wahlung, 1948). At a work level corresponding to PWC$_{170}$, an RPE of 16.5 was obtained and defined as PWC$_R$ (Borg, 1962a). The correlation between PWC$_{170}$ and PWC$_R$ was .61 indicating that, in general, the higher the work load for PWC$_{170}$, the higher the PWC$_R$. For an overall work test, RPE tended to grow as a negatively accelerated function of the work load. The correlation between HR and RPE across several work loads was .85, indicating exceptionally high validity. The high validity suggests that the reliability of the rating scale would also be high since, as a general rule, validity cannot exceed the square root of reliability (Cronbach, 1960). This is to be expected since the linear work load-heart rate relationship for individuals has been shown to be highly reliable (Rowell, 1969).

In a validation study, PWC$_R$ and PWC$_{170}$ were compared to wage rates among forestry workers (Borg, 1962a). The PWC$_{170}$ correlated at a low level ($r = .24$) to wage rates, while PWC$_R$, the subjective estimate, was considerably higher ($r = .54$). Borg suggests that the PWC$_R$ takes into account motivational components not inherent to PWC$_{170}$ but which affect on-the-job performance considerably.

Gamberale (1972) has compared RPE on other tasks with that obtained during bicycling. He noted that the RPE scale was constructed to reflect heart rate (HR) increments of 10 beats between successive scale points. According to this basis, a rating of seven on the RPE scale ("Very, very light") would correspond approximately to a heart rate of 70 beats/min. Twelve male subjects (20 to 35 years of age) performed three tasks: (1) bicycling at work loads of 300, 600, and 900 kpm/min; (2) repetitive lifting of 1.35, 3.35, and 5.35 kg weights 25 cm above a shoulder height starting point; and (3) pushing a wheel barrow loaded with 36, 66, and 96 kg at 100 m/min. In general, these tasks have different muscle mass requirements. The bicycle ergometer task may be characterized as dynamic work requiring a large muscle mass, while the weightlifting involved work using a small muscle mass. The wheel barrow task was a combination of static work (load on the arms) and dynamic work (walking).

The range in heart rates and RPE ratings was greatest for the bicycle ergometer task (approximately from 100 to 185 beats/min), and least for the wheel barrow task (from 100 to 130 beats/min). The weight lifting produced an intermediate heart rate response (from 110 to 140 beats/min). Mean RPE and HR values were linearly related for all tasks with the RPE close to 1/10 of HR. However, RPE correlated most highly with HR for the bicycle ergometer task ($r = .94$), least for the wheel barrow task ($r = .42$), and at an intermediate level for the weight lifting task ($r = .64$). In general, instructions to rate the overall perception of effort, as opposed to rate specifically the perception of efforts in arms or legs, resulted in a higher relationship between the mean HR and RPE. Nevertheless, differences were observed in the relationships between RPE and HR with specific and overall instructions. As might be expected, for the weight lifting task, specific instructions resulted in a closer relationship between RPE and HR. This suggests that caution should be observed when instructing subjects to employ the RPE scale for different tasks.

Gamberale noted that "it proved beyond the scope and the possibility of the present investigation to provide a satisfactory estimate of the level of correlation between heart rate and RPE." On a statistical basis, assuming equivalent variability in the measure of RPE and heart rate, it could be expected that a reduction in range of heart rate, as in the wheel barrow and weight lifting task, would lead to an attentuation of the correlation between heart rate and ratings on the RPE scale. It would be worthwhile to evaluate the relationship between RPE and heart rate on tasks differing in the degree of dynamic work and muscle mass involvement while employing equivalently sizeable ranges in heart rates produced across levels of each task.

As will be discussed (see p. 391), within the past decade a substantial international literature has become available concerning the systematic measurement of a specific subjective quality, perceived effort, in carefully controlled work conditions (also see Table 14-III).

EFFORT EXPENDED. Another aspect of subjective effort is the perceived amount of total available effort expended during work performance. In a study by Lloyd and McClaskey (1971), eighteen male subjects with an average age of approximately 21 years rated perceived effort expended during performance on a motor-driven treadmill using a unique five-point scale. The rating technique had been developed earlier by Caldwell (1967) for use on an isometric handgrip task (see p. 370). Each subject was asked to respond when he perceived that successive 1/5's of his total available effort had been expended. The first response during work (1) was defined as the point where 1/5 of his total available effort had been expended; the response (5) defined the point at which he had expended *all* of his effort. Thus, the rating procedure can be described as a self-paced technique in that ratings were volunteered by the subject rather than requested at selected points by the experimenter. By prior agreement, performance terminated when the subject called out "5". During the task, all subjects walked on the treadmill at 0 percent grade at 75 percent of their maximum walking speed. Maximum walking speed was determined by noting the points at which the subject broke into a jog during three preliminary trials with increasing treadmill speed and the point at which he started walking after jogging during subsequent deceleration. Eight daily walks at 75 percent maximum walking speed were obtained for each subject during which he called out the points indicating when successive 1/5's of his total available effort had been expended. All subjects were instructed to continue walking as long as possible.

As shown in Figure 14-3, results indicated a highly linear relationship between subjective judgments of the amount of effort expended and mean time on the task. Endurance times tended to increase through the third session, and showed a slight decrease on subsequent sessions. This increase in walk duration may have been due to the effects of practice. The degree of linearity between subjective ratings and mean task time generally increased across the eight sessions, with the last five sessions showing remarkable linearity. In view of these results, Lloyd and McClaskey suggest that subjects "have both the capacity to attend to psychological and physiological cues and to report, on a psychological continuum, their judgments of increasing difficulty of the task or their diminishing capacity to perform."

While the degree of linearity in the relationship between perceived ef-

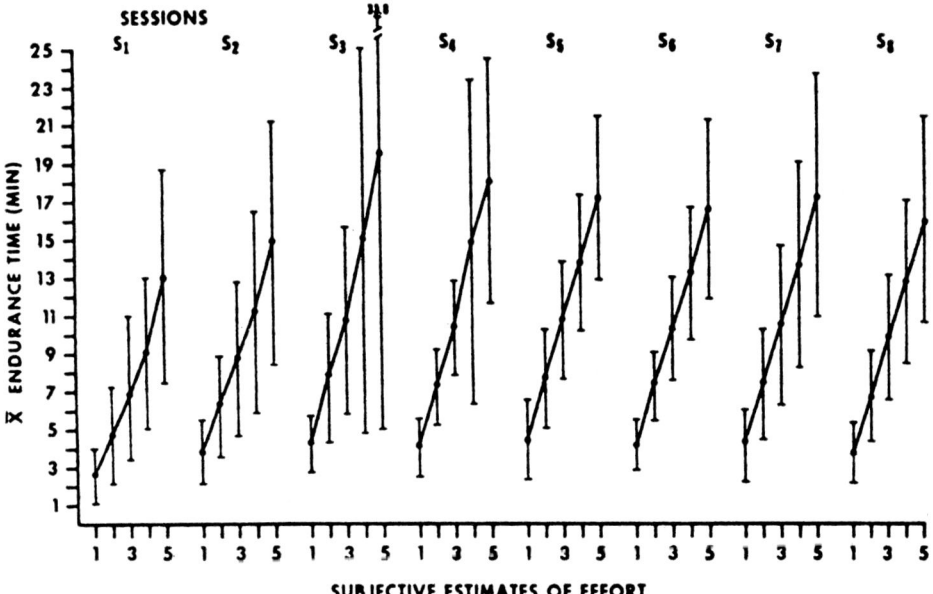

Figure 14-3. Subjective estimates of effort related to mean endurance time during treadmill performance (From A. J. Lloyd, and E. B. McClaskey, "Subjective Assessment of Effort in Dynamic Work," *Journal of Motor Behavior*, 3:49, 1971).

fort expended and task time is impressive, the study raises several interesting questions. First, considerable variability was represented in the data. Standard deviations shown in Figure 14-3 indicate a very broad range of endurance times. In addition, average endurance times (approximately 13 to 19 min.) seem short for such a treadmill task. Were the subjects really performing near the limits of their endurance capacities? In fact, Lloyd and McClaskey note that on session three, which had the greatest variability, two subjects were able to walk 41 and 69 minutes. This raises the possibility that having subjects perform at a given percentage of maximum walking speed might not effectively place each subject at the same relative work load. In other words, 75 percent maximum walking speed may be a physiologically "empty" variable for normalizing endurance capacity compared to maximum aerobic power or other physiological variables such as heart rate. Unfortunately, no data is available in the literature examining the relationship between percent maximum walking speed and measures of endurance capacity. Second, to what degree would the observed linearity found for the subjects as a group exist for individual subjects? No data is presented in this regard. Third, to what degree does this task represent an exercise in timing? The possibility of a timing artifact can be raised almost everytime the self-paced rating technique is used. While the authors clearly regard the data as a demonstration that perceived effort expended is being measured, it is quite possible that each subject was simply *timing* successive fifths of the total duration he was *willing* to spend on the task. Stevens (1957) has discussed categorical and magnitude estimation of time durations which humans can learn to do quite well. No doubt perceived effort expended was being measured in some way, but it is difficult to separate the degree to which effort expended contributed to these results apart from judgments of elapsed time. Additional comment will be offered in the following section regarding timing artifacts in the self-paced rating techniques.

Pain

Pain is another subjective quality experienced during work performance. Caldwell (1967) and Caldwell and Smith (1967) have found a linear relationship between time on an isometric task and ratings of both pain intensity and perceived effort expended. In both of these studies, the subject was required to hold a hand dynamometer at submaximal levels until it became necessary, in the subject's own judgment, to stop. Subjects were required to indicate when pain intensity attained values of 1 to 5 in the same self-paced fashion as that used by Lloyd and McClaskey (1971) for ratings of perceived effort expended. Under these conditions, ratings of pain intensity could be influenced by the subjects' ability to time successive intervals, as has been discussed. If, with practice, a subject could call out successive ratings of pain intensity at intervals matched on the time dimension, the relationship between ratings of pain intensity and time on the isometric task would attain a spurious linearity. As noted above, this is a problem also relevant to the interpretation of the Lloyd and McClaskey (1971) study.

Menzer, Smith, and Caldwell (1969) addressed the problem of the possible timing artifact directly. In this study, using the same isometric task, pain ratings by the self-paced technique were compared to those obtained by an irregular report technique adapted from Beecher (1966) and Smith, Egbert, Markowitz, Mosteller, and Beecher (1966). As in previous studies, the subjects were required to sustain a submaximal handgrip, either 25 or 40 percent of maximum, until they judged it necessary to stop. One group of subjects used the self-paced technique calling out the numbers "1" through "5" as these subjective intensities were reached, terminating performance at the highest rating of pain intensity, "5." A second group of subjects were required to select a rating of from "1" to "5" at the request of the experimenter made at random, irregular intervals during the task. All subjects were practiced on *both* rating procedures *before* the experiment began. Their notion was straightforward: if timing of the intervals accounted for the linearity observed in previous studies, the irregular report ratings would be expected to be less linear than the self-paced technique. The results, however, clearly indicated that for subjects practiced on both techniques, the self-paced and irregular ratings produced equally linear relationships with time on the isometric task for average values of perceived pain for the group as a whole.

Nevertheless, these results do not eliminate the possibility that self-paced ratings of perceived *effort expended* used by Lloyd and McClaskey (1971) contained a timing artifact. In the latter study, each rating scale point referred to the estimated proportion of total available effort expended. This may be worthwhile reviewing in some detail. A rating of "1" meant that 1/5 of the subject's total effort was expended; when the subject called out "5" this meant, by definition, that *all* his available effort was expended and he stopped performing the treadmill task. Such a procedure is virtually identical to having the subject state when he is one-fifth through the task, two-fifths through the task, and so on, making the successive ratings highly dependent on the subject's ability to estimate and match successive intervals.

In an excellent study by Lloyd, Voor, and Thieman (1970) ratings of pain were obtained during an isometric hand dynamometer task of either 25 or 50 percent of maximum grip strength. During each of two trials, the forty male subjects reported their ratings of pain intensity using the self-paced technique. The two trials were separated by a rest period of 15 minutes. The results of the study are depicted in Figure 14-4, showing the re-

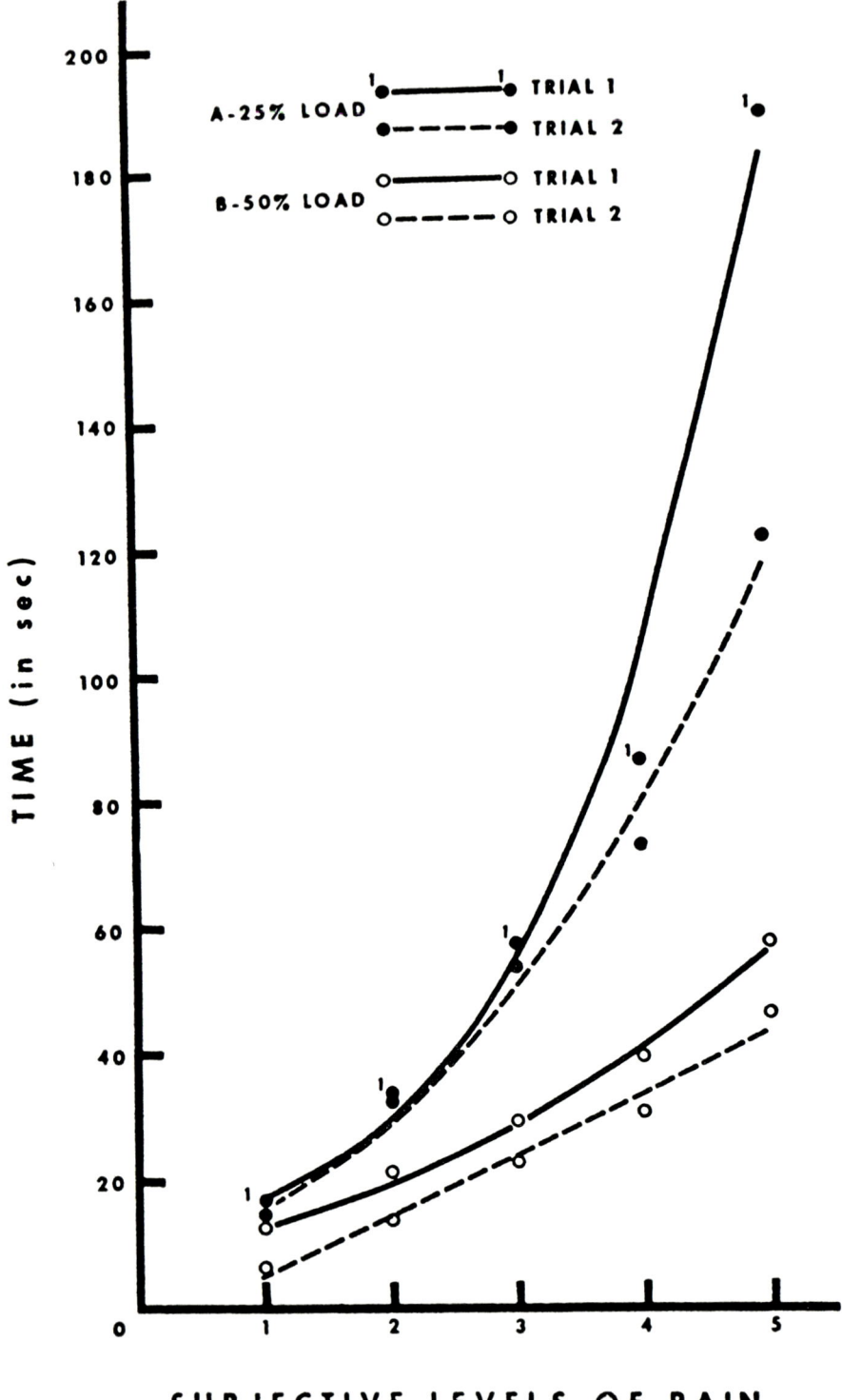

Figure 14-4. Subjective estimates of pain related to endurance time during isometric hand dynamometer tasks (From A. J. Lloyd, J. H. Voor, and T. J. Thieman, "Subjective and Electromyographic Assessment of Isometric Muscle Contractions," *Ergonomics, 13:* 685, 1970).

lationship between pain intensity ratings and average time on the isometric task. From the figure, it can be seen that ratings of pain increased regularly across time on the task, in a generally quadratic fashion, particularly for the 25 percent load level. Ratings for the 50 percent load level were much more linear for both trials. It is interesting that Trial 2 was more linear in appearance than Trial 1 for *both* load levels, although the decrease in average task duration for the 25 percent load level on Trial 2 was more pronounced. A decrease in the average task duration for the 25 percent load level may reflect a learned timing effect inherent to the self-paced ratings of pain. This effect due to timing of successive intervals, was not observed by Menzer, Smith, and Caldwell (1969), an apparent paradox which may be resolved by the fact that the latter's subjects were already *well practiced before* the experimental trials began.

Thus, even for self-paced ratings of pain, the issue of a timing artifact does not appear resolved. Examining the two functions for the 25 percent load level, the successive intervals in Trial 1 were approximately 16, 18, 24, 27, and 105 sec. while for Trial 2 the intervals between ratings were somewhat more equal, approximately 13, 19, 21, 21, and 50 sec. Since Menzer, Smith, and Caldwell (1969) note that their subjects were given practice on both self-paced and irregular rating procedures before the experimental trials were initiated, interval timing may have been learned during practice with the self-paced procedure and *transferred* to the irregular rating procedure during the experimental sessions. Whether this transfer phenomenon does happen or not is an empirical question which should be resolved by further research. Also, the Menzer, et al. subjects had a much lower average task duration than Lloyd, et al. (approximately 65-96 sec. vs. 120-190 sec.) for the same 25 percent load level. This suggests that, in general, the briefer the task duration, the more equal the intervals will be between successive self-paced ratings of pain. Perhaps this difference exists since it is easier to divide a short interval into equal subdivisions than a longer one. While these comments have been offered critically to evaluate the self-paced rating technique, the ability to time work duration could turn out to be an actual phenomenon representing an important parameter used to "pace" work performance.

Thermal Discomfort

Gagge, Stolwijk, and Saltin (1969) used rating scales to relate thermal sensation and discomfort to the level of work being performed. Four male subjects rode at work loads of 25, 50, and 75 percent max Vo_2 on a bicycle ergometer under conditions of different ambient temperature (10°, 20°, and 30°C). A four-point scale of discomfort was used ranging from "comfortable" (1) to "very uncomfortable" (4). Thermal sensation was measured on a seven-point scale ranging from cold (1) to hot (7). Physiological measurements including rectal, muscle (quadriceps), and average skin temperature were also obtained along with measures of sweat loss and heat conductance. Each subject rode for periods of 40 min. at each work level and ambient temperature. Results indicated that at the start of exercise changes in both thermal and comfort sensations were related to the rise in mean body temperature. However, after 30 to 40 min. of exercise, the sensation of "warm discomfort" (obtained by deleting ratings of slightly cool or below) related most highly to skin sweating ($r = .66$), although relatively high relationships were also found for skin conductance ($r = .56$), rectal temperature ($r = .55$), and metabolic rate ($r = .53$). When one highly trained subject was excluded from the data, the correlation between skin sweating increased substantially (to $r = .84$). Thermal sensations, from cold to hot (as opposed to "warm discomfort") were principally related to ambient air temperature ($r = .72$) and skin temperature ($r = .73$). The lower boundary for a comfort zone during steady exercise appeared to be determined by exercise levels and ambient temperatures at which there was no sweating. The upper boundary for the comfort zone during steady exercise was found to be associated with "skin sweat rate equivalent to an evaporative heat loss of 150 kcal/m^2/hour or approximately 65 percent wetness of the skin" provided "the percentage of maximum oxygen uptake [does not] exceed 50 percent." This study illustrates the power of subjective qualities, combined with measurement of appropriate physiological parameters, in adding to an understanding of the adaptive responses to work performance.

By confining attention to one subjective quality, many of the above studies have yielded considerable valuable insights regarding the nature of individual subjective symptoms during work performance. However, subjective symptomatology during work, as Bartley and Chute (1947) have noted, is probably more *complex* than a single subjective quality is able to encompass. During work performance a variety of categories of subjective symptoms may be experienced, each of which may be related to work performance in some way. By focusing on only one subjective quality, the essential complexity of the range in subjective qualities is ignored. Attempts to dimensionally quantify a number of subjective qualities during work will be described in the following section.

Multidimensional Analysis of Subjective Qualities

By now it should be clear that a variety of subjective qualities have been measured preceding or during work performance. These have included "feeling tone" (Foltz, et al., 1944), undifferentiated fatigue (Nunney, 1963; Pierson, 1963a; Bujas, et al., 1966), tiredness (Poffenberger, 1928; Griffith, et al., 1950; Pearson and Byars, 1956; McNelly, 1957), perceived force exerted (Borg and Dahlstrom, 1960; Eisler, 1962; Schmale, Schmidtke, and Vukovich, 1963; Bernyer, 1967), perceived effort (Borg, 1962a; Gamberale, 1972), perceived effort expended (Caldwell, 1967; Lloyd and McClaskey, 1971), pain intensity (Caldwell and Smith, 1967; Caldwell, 1967; Menzer, et al., 1969; Lloyd, et al., 1970), and thermal discomfort (Gagge, et al., 1969) [See Tables 14-I through 14-III]. Since a variety of subjective qualities occur and can be measured during work performance, another approach might begin by first inquiring what the categories of subjective symptoms are and how they are interrelated during work performance. Studies such as these may also aid in the conceptual organization of the melange of different subjective qualities measured during work.

The rationale for the application of multidimensional techniques to work performance derives from the reasoning that work produces changes in a variety of subjective qualities (symptoms). As noted by Bartley and Chute (1947), certain of these subjective symptoms occurring during work should be considered conceptually discrete from others. Prolonged exercise may produce subjective symptoms such as boredom or an aversion to the physical activity which may also be significantly related to work tolerance. Therefore, subjective symptomatology may be conceived as a set of conceptually clear, discrete symptoms which increase together during work performance (Kinsman, Weiser, and Stamper, 1973). Multidimensional analysis, such as factor analysis or key cluster analysis, provide means to identify sets of symptoms that group together to form such symptom categories. Table 14-IV presents an outline of studies relevant to the multidimensional analysis of subjective symptomatology during work performance and fatigue.

Although Wotzka and Grandjean (1968) did not specifically use multidimensional techniques, they did give a battery of ten 7-point rating scales as well as measured critical flicker fusion (CFF) and two tapping tests to sixty-eight air traffic controllers throughout their work day. They found a common trend between the mean values of the self-rating of "refreshed-tired" and CFF, grid tapping, and ordinary tapping tests. The ratings and performances were high during the day and low during the night. Regardless of the actual starting hour, the mean values of the self-rating scales, "strong-weak," "refreshed-tired," "vigorous-exhausted," and "awake-sleep" gradually changed concurrently toward the direction of fatigue. After the time that these ratings exceeded the neutral point (4), between the 5th and 7th hour of work, there was also a rapid drop in the mean values for CFF, tapping, and grid tapping. Since there are significant correlations (from $r = .26$ to .32) between the changes in "refreshed-tired" scores, CFF, and grid tapping, Wotzka and Grandjean suggested that subjects with a marked decrease of CFF or grid tapping performance also had a greater deviation toward being

TABLE 14-IV
MULTIDIMENSIONAL STUDIES OF SUBJECTIVE QUALITIES DURING WORK

Subjective Dimensions	Development	Task	Subjects	Studies
....	Key cluster analysis	Various tests of mental work	? (n = 49)	Bujas, Petz, Krkovic, and Sorokin (1960)
Nervous; drowsy; and exhaustion	Factor analysis	Reporting a fatiguing situation	College students (n = 150)	Wolf (1967)
High activation, 12 factors; moderate activation, 9 factors; low activation, 5 factors (see text)	Factor analysis	Reporting a situation	College students (n = 315)	Wijting, Wollack, and Smith (1970)
Physical; mental and neuro-sensory	....	....	....	Industrial Fatigue Research Committee of the Japanese Association of Industrial Health (1954)
Drowsiness and dullness; difficulty in concentration; and projection of physical disintegration	Factor analysis	Various jobs	Workers (n = 9,575)	Saito, Kogi, and Kashiwagi (1970)
Motivation; task aversion; fatigue (general and leg)	Key cluster analysis	Bicycle ergometer (56% max VO_2)	Young males (n = 63)	Kinsman, Weiser, and Stamper (1973) Weiser, Kinsman, and Stamper (1973)

"tired." On the basis of this finding, they hypothesized that the changes in these measures indicate a *common* state that Wotzka and Grandjean would label "fatigue." Their contribution to conceptualizing fatigue lies in the acknowledgement that a variety of subjective and behavioral measures, rather than any single variable, show change during prolonged work.

As early as 1960, Bujas, Petz, Krkovic, and Sorokin had reported application of multidimensional techniques (i.e. key cluster analysis) to evaluate relationships between individual mental tests (e.g. tests of reasoning, perception, numerical ability, etc.) under normal control conditions and "fatigue" induced by a 24-hour period of sleeplessness followed by a 10 kilometer walk. While subjective symptoms were not measured in this study, Bujas, et al. did find that following induced "fatigue," the *relationships* between various psychological tests were altered. They suggest that fatigue may be understood as a disintegration or disorganization of the psychological and physiological processes that existed during *nonfatigued* performance of work. Examples of these changes in the adaptative responses to work during fatigue have been discussed in detail in Chapter 1. The multidimensional approach to subjective symptomatology during work is implicit in this study since pattern-like changes in discrete subjective symptom categories may be inferred to occur along with alterations in other psychophysiological processes.

Using a varimax factor analysis, Wolf (1967) identified three fatigue categories within a set of thirty adjectives given to a group of 150 subjects in the preliminary study. The subjects were instructed to check those adjectives associated with an imagined "fatiguing situation." The selection of the situation was left up to the subject. No details were provided concerning how the original set of adjectives were originally selected or arranged within the checklist for rating. The three categories identified were labeled *Exhaustion* (Physically Tired, Aching Muscles, Exhausted, Easily Distracted, No Energy and Perspiring); *Drowsy* (Mentally Sluggish, Want to Fall Asleep, Lazy, Drowsy, Feel Sleepy, and Tired; and *Nervous* (Tense, Jumpy, Keyed Up, Head Tightness, Feel Dizzy, and Irritable).

A speed of tapping task of one minute duration, and two pursuit-rotor tracking tasks given for five, 30-second trials, were used to test the validity of these categories. Validation data was limited since no decrement in performance was observed for 35 to 65 percent of the subjects on the tasks. Thus, the tasks, which were brief and easily accomplished, seemed inadequate to induce a significant level of fatigue. In fact, the relationships between performance decrement across trials, for those showing a decrement, and scores on each of the fatigue categories were found to be negligible.

Wolf also measured subjective effort immediately after task performance by the inclusion of two unspecified "effort" items rated as being either present, indeterminate, or absent. He noted that some of the subjects who reported a feeling of increased effort also reported higher post-task scores on the three fatigue categories. On this basis, he suggested that "fatigue is a product of *motivation,* not task" [author's italics]. This assumes that the categories are sufficiently generalizable to alternative work situations; however, the tasks on which he based his conclusions, as noted above, appeared inadequate to induce fatigue. In addition, it was also assumed that reports of effort are indicative of motivational level. Subjective effort has already been discussed above as one subjective quality commonly *experienced* during work, and having relationships to work capacity and endurance. Subjective effort should not be assumed *also* to be a measure of *motivational* level. The value of Wolf's study lies largely in the identification of subjective qualities reported to be experienced during imaginary fatiguing situations which group on a *connotative* basis (i.e. share a common meaning).

In a subsequent study by Wijting, Wollack and Smith (1970), Wolf's findings were substantiated and extended in regard to the factorial organization of subjective qualities: three hundred and fifteen subjects were asked to indicate which of 132 selected subjective qualities printed on a checklist were experienced during *imaginal* states of "high activation" (e.g. "being awakened by a loud noise"), "moderate activation" (e.g. "playing a card game"), or "low activation" (e.g. "sunbathing"). Varimax factor analysis of the checklist protocols identified twelve, nine, and five subjective factors for the high, moderate, and low imaginal states of activation, respectively. For imaginal "high activation," Wolf's *Exhaustion* factor was essentially replicated, while his *Nervous* and *Drowsy* factors emerged in the "low activation" condition. More interestingly, a *General Fatigue* factor, consisting of twenty-four subjective items, emerged for the imaginal "moderate activation" condition. The General Fatigue factor consisted of subjective items such as "drowsy," "tired," "dull," "slow," "physically tired," "sluggish," "no energy," and so on. No validation data is presented in which measures of subjective symptoms were obtained in actual situations. Neither Wolf (1967) nor Wijting, et al. (1970) have used their subjective symptom factors to measure fatigue in real or adequately fatiguing work situations.

As early as 1949, Kirihara urged that subjective factors be studied in investigations directly dealing with industrial fatigue in Japan. Subsequently, under the auspices of the Japanese Industrial Fatigue Research Committee (1954), 30 symptoms of subjective fatigue were listed in an "Inventory for the Subjective Symptoms of Fatigue." The initial inventory included three symptom categories labeled Physical, Mental, and Neurosensory Fatigue arranged in a checklist so that an individual could indicate the presence or absence of each symptom. The initial inventory was formulated on a conceptual, rather than empirical grouping, of items within the symptom categories. During the period 1965 to 1967, the items of this inventory were used to develop a Fatigue Scale by factor analytic techniques (Kogi, et al., 1970). This Fatigue Scale is shown in Table 14-V. It consists of three factors: *Drowsiness, Difficulty in Concentration,* and *Projection of Physical Disintegration,* the latter similar to the *Nervous* factor of Wolf (1967). A description of the empirical approach leading to the derivation of the 1967 Fatigue Scale is presented by Saito, Kogi, and Kashiwagi (1970). They empirically derived the factorial structure using protocols of 9,575 workers occupied in eighteen different industrial jobs. Scores for the three fatigue factors showed increasing frequency of report during the course of work for most occupations, although certain differences occurred between occupations in the manner with which the symptoms grouped empirically.

Kogi, Saito, and Mitsuihashi (1970) validated the fatigue scale shown in Table 14-V using protocols for railway yard workers (n = 309), iron foundry workers (n = 181), and railroad engine drivers (n = 365) before, during, and after an eight-hour work shift. The factorial structure of the inventory *changed* pre- to post-work, and differed between industrial jobs, suggesting that the appropriate fatigue scale to be used might be tailored to the characteristics of each job situation. For example, clerical workers may not complain of the *same* physical symptoms as workers in an iron foundry who are engaged in a more highly physical occupation. There were clear differences in the frequency of reported symptoms for the jobs in the Kogi, et al. study: most iron workers reported feeling thirsty post work (82%), having

TABLE 14-V

1967 FATIGUE SCALE OF THE INDUSTRIAL FATIGUE RESEARCH COMMITTEE OF JAPAN

Drowsiness	Difficulty in Concentrating	Bodily Complaints
1. Feel heavy in the head*	11. Difficulty thinking*	21. Headache*
2. Feel tired in the whole body*	12. Become weary while talking	22. Stiffness in the shoulders
3. Tired legs*	13. Irritable	23. Low back pain
4. Yawning*	14. Unable to concentrate*	24. Constrained in breathing
5. Feel confused*	15. No interest in things	25. Thirsty
6. Become drowsy*	16. Apt to forget things*	26. Husky voice*
7. Eye strain*	17. Apt to make mistakes	27. Dizzy
8. Become rigid or clumsy when moving	18. Anxious about things	28. Eyelid spasms*
9. Feel unsteady while standing	19. Unable to maintain a straight posture*	29. Limb tremors*
10. Want to lie down*	20. No energy*	30. Feel ill*

* Symptom items validated within the symptom categories of the 1967 Fatigue Scale by K. Kogi, et al., "Validity of Three Components of Subjective Fatigue Feelings," *Journal of Science of Labour,* 46:251, 1970; and Y. Saito, et al., "Factors Underlying Subjective Feelings of Fatigue," *Journal of Science of Labour,* 46:205, 1970.

heavy legs (91%), and being generally tired (67%); in contrast, engine drivers, engaged in a physically less demanding job, reported only infrequently experiencing these symptoms post work (27%, 28%, and 24% for thirsty, heavy legs, and general tiredness, respectively). Such differences affect the derived factorial structure of the fatigue scale. Thus, specific symptoms and symptom categories may not apply in the evaluation of "fatigue" in certain work situations.

Additionally, the derivation of the symptom factors of this fatigue scale has been based on the *frequency* with which groups of workers check the occurrence of the symptoms during or post work. Yoshitake (1969, 1971) has found that the reported *frequency* of symptoms on the 1967 Fatigue Scale have a "high correlation" between ratings of *severity* of undifferentiated fatigue for office workers.

Recently, the multidimensional analysis of subjective symptomatology has been applied to a standard work situation on the bicycle ergometer in controlled laboratory conditions (Kinsman, Weiser, and Stamper, 1973). In this study, four stages were involved in the development of a Physical Activity Questionnaire (PAQ) designed to describe *categories* of subjective symptoms experienced as a result of prolonged bicycle riding. First, a wide range of adjective items, potentially descriptive of subjective changes experienced from rest to the end of prolonged physical work were selected for inclusion in an Initial Adjective Checklist (IAC). These items, shown

TABLE 14-VI
ITEMS PRESENTED IN THE INITIAL ADJECTIVE LIST*

1. Perspiring	22. Determined	43. Happy
2. Short of Breath	23. Comfortable	44. Headache
3. Muscle Tremors	24. Leg Cramps	45. Pleased
4. Test Attention	25. Working Hard	46. Distracted
5. Weak	26. Hard to Breathe	47. Head Tightening
6. Easy to Think	27. Easy to Concentrate	48. Nauseated
7. Physically Tired	28. Leg Twitching	49. Meter Attention
8. Leg Aches	29. Drive	50. Jumpy
9. Lively	30. Heart Pounding	51. Dizzy
10. Weary	31. Refreshed	52. Listless
11. Out of Gas	32. Tired	53. Satisfied
12. Rather Quit	33. Weak Legs	54. Depressed
13. Aching Muscles	34. Drained	55. Abdominal Cramps
14. Lazy	35. Do Something Else	56. Tense
15. Bored	36. Shaky Legs	57. Irritable
16. Sore from Sitting	37. Hard to Keep Going	58. Backache
17. Heavy Legs	38. Vigorous	59. Angry
18. Numb	39. Dry Mouth	60. Fidgety
19. Easygoing	40. Panting	61. Active
20. Worn Out	41. Sweating	62. Worried
21. Thirsty	42. Fed Up	63. Drowsy

*Items 1 to 41 inclusive were retained for the Modified Adjective List (From Kinsman, Weiser, and Stamper, 1973).

PHYSICAL ACTIVITY QUESTIONNAIRE DERIVED BY KEY CLUSTER ANALYSIS*

Item No.†	Symptom Category‡				
1	C2	Perspiring severely	Perspiring badly	Perspiring some	Perspiring a little	Not perspiring at all
2	C1	Severely short of breath	Quite short of breath	Some shortness of breath	A little short of breath	Not at all short of breath
9	C3	Very lively	A little lively	About as lively as usual	Less lively than usual	Not at all lively
13	C1	Severely aching muscles	Badly aching muscles	Muscles aching some	Muscles aching a little	No aching muscles at all
20	C1	Severely worn out	Badly worn out	Worn out some	A little worn out	Not at all worn out
22	C3	Very determined	A little determined	About usual determination	Less determined than usual	Not at all determined
23	C2	Very comfortable	A little comfortable	About usual comfort	Less comfortable than usual	Not at all comfortable
26	C1	Very hard to breathe	Quite hard to breathe	Some difficulty in breathing	A little difficulty in breathing	Not at all difficult to breathe
29	C3	A lot of drive	A little drive	About average drive	Less drive than usual	No drive at all
30	C1	Severe heart pounding	Bad heart pounding	Some heart pounding	A little heart pounding	No heart pounding at all
33	C1	Severely weak legs	Quite weak legs	Some leg weakness	A little leg weakness	No leg weakness at all
34	C1	Severely drained	Quite drained	Drained some	A little drained	Not drained at all
35	C2	Want to do something else very much	Want to do something else a little	Want to do something else as much as usual	Want to do something else less than usual	Do not want to do something else at all
36	C1	Severely shaky legs	Quite shaky legs	Some leg shakiness	A little leg shakiness	No leg shakiness at all
38	C3	Very vigorous	A little vigorous	About usual vigor	Less vigorous than usual	Not at all vigorous
39	C1	A severely dry mouth	A badly dry mouth	Some dryness in the mouth	A little dryness in the mouth	No dryness in the mouth at all
40	C1	Panting severely	Panting badly	Panting some	Panting a little	Not panting at all
41	C2	Severely sweating	Badly sweating	Some sweating	A little sweating	Not sweating at all

* According to order of appearance in the standard form of the Initial Adjective List. (From Kinsman, Weiser and Stamper, 1973).
† Items 9, 22, 23, 29, and 38 were scaled from 1 (absent) to 5 (severe) while the remainder were scaled from 5 (severe) to 1 (absent).
‡ C1 = Fatigue; C2 = Task Aversion; C3 = Motivation.

in Table 14-VI, were assembled from previously reported measures of fatigue (Pearson and Byars, 1956; Wolf, 1967), the General High Altitude Questionnaire (Evans, 1966; Stamper, Kinsman, and Evans, 1970; Stamper, Sterner, and Kinsman, 1971), as well as additional items suggested by the research team. Second, each descriptive item was arranged along a five-point ordinal scale of severity by using appropriate modifiers according to procedures adapted from Nowlis and Nowlis (1956). Examples of the scaled items as they appeared in the six-page IAC are shown in Table 14-VII. In practice, the subject could rate the level of his subjective experience by circling the applicable descriptive phrase defining a point along the five-point scale for each item. Third, sixty-four subjects, on two occasions at least three days apart, rode the bicycle ergometer at a work load approximating 56 percent max Vo_2. Before each ride, subjects were given explicit instructions to continue pedalling until they became so discomforted that it was necessary to stop. Immediately before Ride 1, the IAC was completed twice to provide experience with the use of the instrument. The end-of-ride IAC was completed while sitting on the bicycle ergometer, with instructions to describe the subjective experiences while riding just before terminating the ride. Identical pre- and end-of-ride IAC administrations were given for Ride 2. Fourth, those items that were either redundant in meaning or showed less than a 10 percent mean change from pre- to the end-of-ride for both rides were eliminated. For the remaining forty-one items which comprised the Modified Adjective Checklist (MAC), the mean pre- to end-of-ride increase ranged from 10 to 84 percent.

Key cluster analysis (Tryon and Bailey, 1970) was then performed on the end-of-ride MAC protocols to empirically identify nonredundant categories of items describing unique aspects of subjective change. In brief, these categories were empirically grouped by key cluster analysis according to the following three criteria: (1) high collinearity between items within a category, i.e. the items within a category shared a similar pattern of correlation across all other items of the MAC, (2) maximum independence between all categories, and (3) maximum accountability by the smallest number of categories of the total variability within the score space. These empirically derived categories may be regarded as subscales whose scores are obtained by adding individual member item values.

Accordingly, it was assured that only those items reasonably expected to show change were studied. Furthermore, key cluster analysis was performed on only those items actually showing change on an empirical basis, thereby building validity into the selection procedure. Finally, analyses were performed on the end-of-ride scores, thereby identifying symptom categories that group together near the end-point of work tolerance.

Three symptom categories common to both rides, were identified and labeled on a conceptual basis: *Fatigue* (panting, short of breath, worn out, drained, legs weak, heart pounding, difficult to breathe, shaky legs, aching muscles, and dry mouth); *Task Aversion* (sweating, perspiring, uncomfortable, want to do something else); and *Motivation* (drive, vigorous, determined, lively). In Figure 14-5, the geometrical organization of these categories is shown on a Spherical Analysis (SPAN) diagram for the Ride 2 data. In the SPAN diagram, the loci of the categories (clusters) are shaded and located on the surface of a three-dimensional sphere. The boxes labeled I, II and III are the termini of *orthogonal,* i.e. independent, axes which are located by the factoring process and pass through the origin of the sphere to form the orthogonal factor structure. Similar to coordinates on a map, the orthogonal structure primarily serves as a frame of reference to locate the *oblique* categories, the shaded areas labeled C1, C2 and C3. The oblique structure represented in the diagram depicts the actual relationships between the categories. For a detailed discussion of the SPAN diagram, see Tryon and Bailey (1970).

While all symptom categories form distinct groupings, Fatigue appears to be the most dense and tightly packed, indicating that the relationships between items within this category are high. In fact, internal consistency reliabilities were generally high for all categories ranging from .94 for Fatigue to .77 for Motivation. The symptom categories were quite independent from one another: intercorrelations among the category scores ranged from .34 to .17 for Ride 2. Since two rides were performed, it was possible to evaluate stability of the *amount* of *change* from pre- to end-of-ride for the categories. Stability measures were respectably high for Fatigue and Task Aversion ($r = .83$ and .65); however, the Motivation category had a low stability of change ($r = .38$). Individual category scores changed significantly from pre- to end-of-ride for both rides: 95, 58, and 11 percent for Ride 1 and 105, 80, and 21 percent for Ride 2 for Fatigue, Task Aversion and Motivation.

The *Fatigue* category appears to be composed of those subjective symptoms describing *bodily feeling states* associated with prolonged exercise (Kinsman, Weiser, and Stamper, 1973). In a subsequent study (Weiser, et al., 1973) two subcategories of *Fatigue* were identified and labeled General Fatigue (worn out, weary, tired, out of energy) and Leg Fatigue (leg aches, leg cramps, muscle aches, muscle tremors, leg twitch, heavy legs, shaky legs). Only a moderate relationship existed between these two subcategories ($r = .58$) indicating a maximum of 34 percent overlap in the common variability of both Fatigue components. The symptom items of General Fatigue group largely on a connotative basis and agree in composition with the comparable categories previously identified by Wolf (1967) and Wijting, et al. (1970) as discussed above. The composition also agrees with

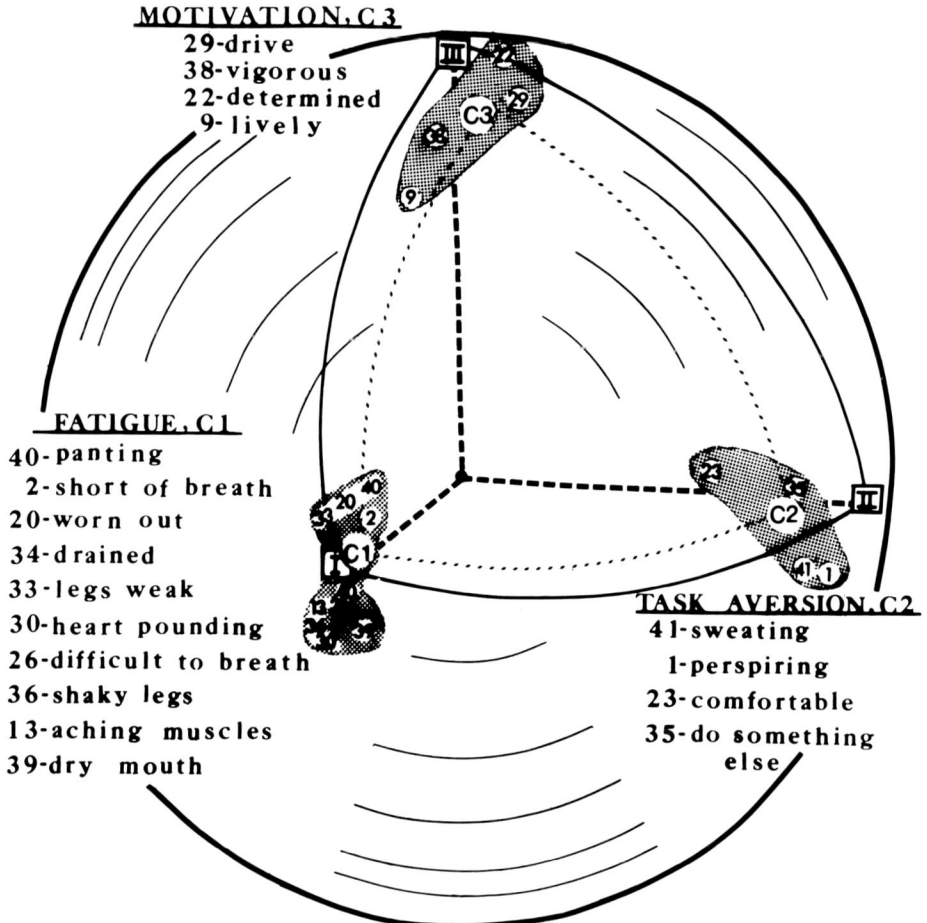

Figure 14-5. Spherical Analysis (SPAN) diagram showing the organization and structure of three symptom categories identified at the end of bicycle ergometry work. For explanation, see text (From R. A. Kinsman, P. C. Weiser, and D. A. Stamper, "Multidimensional Analysis of Subjective Sympotomatology During Prolonged Strenuous Exercise," *Ergonomics, 16*:211, 1973).

comparable categories identified by Kinsman, Luparello, et al. (1973) in studies of asthma symptomatology, and Stamper, et al. (1970, 1971) in studies of the symptomatology of acute mountain sickness. Thus, it seems to represent a truly *general* type of subjective fatigue, common to different tasks, environmental conditions, and pathology. On the other hand, Leg Fatigue is a symptom subcategory apparently *specific* to tasks that are highly leg dependent such as bicycle riding. A variety of physiological changes occurring during bicycling (e.g. increased input from muscle spindles and Golgi tendon organs) feed back to higher nervous centers as internal physiological cues which may contribute to the self-report of the Leg Fatigue symptoms. A group of cardiopulmonary symptoms within the overall Fatigue symptom cluster (short of breath, panting, difficult to breathe, and heart pounding) also appeared as a distinguishable subcategory more closely associated with Leg Fatigue than with General Fatigue (Weiser, et al., 1973).

Task Aversion, the second symptom cluster, appears to measure a general level of *discomfort* and a disinclination to continue the task (Kinsman, Weiser and Stamper, 1973). The inclusion of the doublet symptom set, "perspiring" and "sweating" in conjunction with the level of discomfort ("comfort") appears reasonable in view of the study by Gagge, et al. (1969) which indicated that the sensation of thermal *discomfort* during bicycling was principally related to sweating.

Motivation, although conceptually clear, has a low stability as noted above and shows a relatively minimal change during exercise as compared to *Fatigue* (and its subcategories) or to *Task Aversion.* This does not necessarily minimize the value of the *Motivation* category but suggests that motivational level may fluctuate on a daily basis, while being relatively *constant* throughout a single work session.

Finally, it should be noted that ride durations varied substantially in this study, ranging from 1½ min. to 98 min. In spite of this extraordinary range, the test-retest reliability between Rides 1 and 2 was high: $r = .80$. This range occurred even though subjects performed at 55.6 ± 2.8 percent estimated max V_{O_2}. Thus, other factors in addition to aerobic capacity are obviously required to account for differences in work tolerance during strenuous exercise. One of these may be the relative heart rate increment during exercise. In general, subjects having a high heart rate increment early in the exercise period chose to discontinue riding sooner than subjects with lower heart rate increments (Weiser, Stamper, Kinsman, and Hannon, 1971). Motivational factors, personality differences and performance expectations deriving from prior athletic or work history, may also be importantly involved. There needs to be more information in this regard since these factors may also influence subjective report.

In summary, results of these studies indicate that a complex set of symptoms are experienced during physical work. Nonetheless, these symptoms may be organized meaningfully (i.e. empirically and conceptually) into categories. Dimensional analysis of subjective symptomatology during work may clarify the meaning of terms such as subjective fatigue. This approach also implies that differences may exist between identifiable types of individuals in regard to their *pattern* of changes across various categories of subjective symptomatology. For example, during a given task, one type of individual may tend to terminate work in response to an increase in the subjective symptoms labeled Fatigue, while another type may quit because of flagging motivation together with a rising aversion to the task associated with increased discomfort. It is also likely that the relevant symptom *categories* may differ between tasks, just as the patterns of symptomatology may differ between individuals. Thus, these studies suggest that while the use of simple unidimensional scales of a single subjective quality may provide useful information, they may well be limited in regard to the representative richness of the subjective experience during work. Without adequate caution, complex patterning of subjective changes could obscure any direct relationships between a single subjective quality, work tolerance, and the underlying substrata of physiological factors.

OBSERVATIONS ON THE ROLE OF SYMPTOMATOLOGY DURING WORK AND FATIGUE

Subjective fatigue has often been discussed as if it were a simple self-explanatory concept. However, the research applications reviewed have frequently either avoided the use of a global report of undifferentiated fatigue in favor of discrete, objectively definable subjective qualities, or have used reports of undifferentiated fatigue to relatively little advantage.

In our estimation only one study (Bujas, et al., 1966) has used reports of undifferentiated fatigue in which clear relationships have been shown between the subjective rating and physiological parameters, i.e. EMG activity during work. In this study the subjects were clearly informed about the composite, discrete subjective qualities that should enter into their judgments of fatigue during an isometric weight-holding task. Specifically, they were told to attend to feelings of "tightness, numbness," and to an "increase in muscle sensitivity to pain, weight, and so on" in their judgments of fatigue.

Herein lies a clue that may help to define what is meant by a report of undifferentiated fatigue. Specifically, undifferentiated fatigue might best be regarded as a superordinate feeling state into which is focused a set of discrete subjective qualities arising during work. The composite subjective qualities focused into such a superordinate report will depend on a variety of factors such as the nature of the task. This is why a person doing prolonged *mental* arithmetic can finally describe himself as feeling fatigued, just as a bicycle rider, performing strenuous *physical* work, can do likewise. But the meaning of the report of "fatigue" in terms of the underlying discrete symptoms and physiological factors involved is necessarily quite different for the two tasks. Thus, the report of undifferentiated fatigue might best be regarded as a superordinate subjective state into which is funneled discrete subjective symptoms.

The above provides a starting point for a conceptualization of subjective fatigue. The following will serve as a summary statement for this chapter. Specifically, three ingredients will be involved in this conceptualization: (1) the report of subjective symptomatology, including undifferentiated fatigue, categories of symptoms, and discrete symptoms; (2) the physiological substrata which is importantly altered during work; and (3) the relationship between physiological factors and symptomatology during work.

Subjective Symptomatology

The full range of individual subjective qualities studied during work is extensive enough to provide some difficulty in developing an organizational schema. In the order presented earlier in this chapter, these include force exerted, undifferentiated fatigue, tiredness, perceived effort and effort expended, pain intensity, thermal discomfort, and thermal sensations. At least one study (Foltz, Jung, and Cisler, 1944) obtained pre-work reports of a vague state called "feeling tone." At this time, the available multidimensional studies of subjective qualities are few but demonstrate that wide ranges of discrete symptoms can be organized meaningfully into more limited, but conceptually clear categories. Of these multidimensional studies, at the time of this writing, only two have identified categories of symptoms using a controlled laboratory situation and a standard work task, i.e. the bicycle ergometer (Kinsman, Weiser, and Stamper, 1973; Weiser, Kinsman, and Stamper, 1973). These studies provide an opportunity for some comparisons between unidimensional and multidimensional studies employing bicycle ergometry. Additionally, as noted earlier, they help to clarify the meaning of subjective fatigue.

In general, the connotatively similar subjective qualities of "weak," "worn out," "no energy," "tired," "weary," "exhausted," and "fatigued" tend to cluster in a wide variety of situations including imaginal states of activation or fatigue (Wolf, 1967; Wijting, et al., 1970), exposure to high terrestial altitude (Stamper et al., 1970; Stamper, et al., 1971), acute asthmatic attacks (Kinsman, Luparello, et al., 1973; Kinsman, O'Banion, et al., 1973) and during bicycle work (Kinsman, Weiser, and Stamper, 1973; Weiser, Kinsman, and Stamper, 1973). Together, they can be described as composite items of a subordinate category which we have labeled General Fatigue (Weiser, Kinsman, and Stamper, 1973).

But what is meant by such a category labeled General Fatigue? One way of answering this question is to locate its position within the larger set of subjective symptoms experienced during work. Figure 14-6 presents a pyramidal schema, including General Fatigue, which comprises several levels of subjective report during bicycle riding. This schema is an outgrowth of the multidimensional studies of symptomatology during prolonged bicycle riding (Kinsman, Weiser, and Stamper, 1973; Weiser, Kinsman, and Stamper,

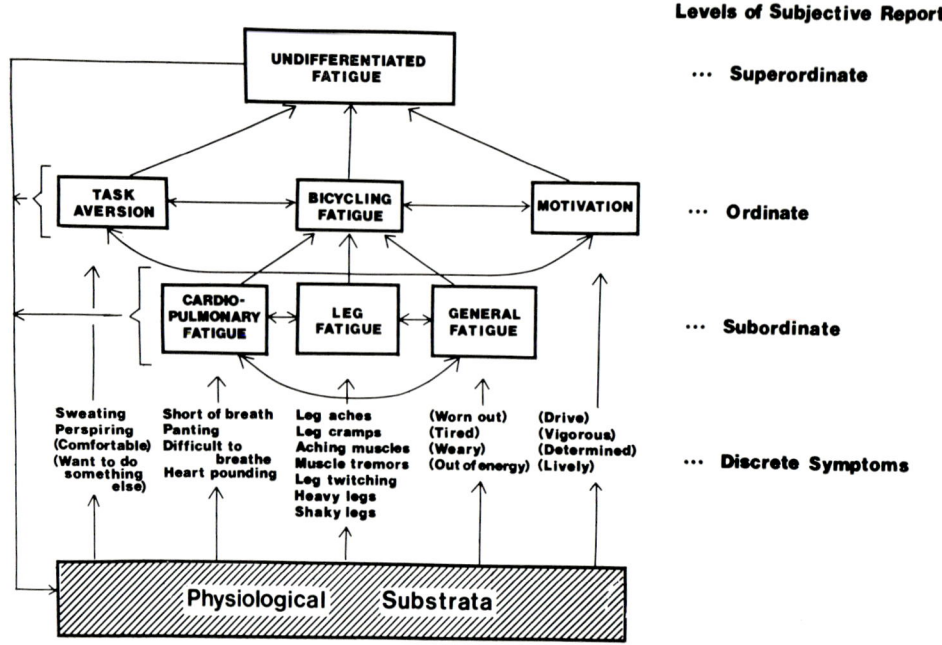

Figure 14-6. Pyramidal schema describing levels of subjective report during bicycle ergometer work. For explanation, see text.

1973). The basic framework would be applicable to the performance of *any* task although the specific symptoms and symptom categories may changes substantially between tasks.

In Figure 14-6, the levels of subjective report are labeled in the right hand margin. At the most basic level, the assumption is made that discrete symptoms have their genesis in known or as yet unidentified physiological changes occurring during work, i.e. within the Physiological Substrata.[1] On a statistical basis, these discrete symptoms have been shown to organize into meaningful groups. At the lowest level of organization, these groupings of discrete symptoms have been labeled Subordinate. The Subordinate level of organization includes three component subcategories; i.e. Cardiopulmonary, Leg, and General Fatigue, of a Bicycling Fatigue category shown in the middle level labeled Ordinate. Also at the Ordinate level are two additional categories of symptoms labeled Task Aversion and Motivation each comprised of a set of discrete symptoms. In turn, the symptom categories at the Ordinate level funnel into the highest level of subjective report. At

---

1. In Figure 14-6, the discrete symptoms indicated in parentheses are not clearly a simple, *direct* function of changes in the physiological substrata.

this superordinate level occur such global reports as Undifferentiated Fatigue.

In general, the arrows between and within levels represent relationships between symptom categories which may be defined empirically. First, the *vertical* arrows indicate that subjective report at a higher level is assumed to be dependent upon physiological events and/or subjective report occurring at a lower level. Second, the *horizontal* arrows indicate that relationships are assumed to exist between the subjective report occurring within any level.

Within this schema, a single *superordinate* report of Undifferentiated Fatigue is composed of discrete symptoms occurring at lower levels. Therefore, this level of subjective report is the most remote from the physiological events that serve to generate discrete symptoms during work. Obviously, the relationships between such a superordinate report and a particular physiological event can be expected to be very difficult to define adequately since mediating symptoms and physiological events intercede.

This pyramidal schema should serve two important functions: first, it provides a way of analyzing what is meant by subjective report during work. By indicating that discrete symptoms may organize into related yet unique categories, and at different levels, it should encourage more precise definition of what is meant by terms such as subjective fatigue: what are people being asked to rate in studies involving subjective fatigue and how can other subjective events affect the ratings obtained? Second, it suggests that the relationships between subjective ratings and specific physiological events during work can be most *precisely* defined at the level of the discrete symptoms and most *imprecisely* at the level of Undifferentiated Fatigue, i.e. the Superordinate level.

In summary, progress in the area of the psychophysiological aspects of fatigue involving subjective symptomatology can best be achieved if the degree of "differentiation," i.e. discreteness, of the subjective report used can be specified clearly.

Psychophysiological Aspects of Subjective Symptomatology

A number of studies, some already reviewed, also have examined changes in subjective qualities during work together with changes in certain physiological parameters, including heart rate, skin and body temperature and heat conductance, sweating, heat loss from the skin, electromyographic (EMG) activity and catecholamine excretion. All of the studies provide some information about the physiological substrata affected during work performance and about the relationship of physiological factors to the genesis of subjective changes experienced.

Fatigue

Several studies have investigated the changes of heart rate and EMG in relation to reports of several forms of fatigue as illustrated in the schema described above (Fig. 14-6). Nunney (1963) obtained global reports of undifferentiated fatigue during physical work. Heart rate was significantly related to the work load and to a global report of undifferentiated fatigue. The most obvious, and also the most probable, conclusion would be the *more work* that one is doing, the *more fatigue* in a global sense one will report. This relationship between HR and ratings of undifferentiated fatigue is difficult to explain in more detail. An explanation of this is suggested in the above schema: undifferentiated fatigue is distant from the ongoing cardiovascular functioning and integrates many intervening, and as yet unspecified, discrete symptom qualities.

A psychophysical study of Bujas, et al. (1966), relating undifferentiated fatigue to isometric work has already been reviewed. They reported a remarkable similarity between the psychophysical power functions for both the perception of undifferentiated fatigue and the integrated EMG amplitude recorded midway through the task. One should note that the subjects were instructed to attend to specific subjective qualities and to give their estimates of fatigue so that the reports were closer to physiological events than the undifferentiated global report utilized by Nunney (1963). Consequently, it would be of interest to explore the relation between the growth of muscle electrical activity and the growth of fatigue reported as a consequence of isometric work.

Symptomatology categories representing more differentiated aspects of subjective fatigue belong to the ordinate and subordinate levels of subjective report (i.e. those described by Kinsman, Weiser, and Stamper, 1973 and Weiser, et al., 1973) and have not yet been related to changes in the physiological substrata. Changes in *motor unit* EMG activity could become synchronized during prolonged exercise with an increased amplitude as has been observed by Lloyd and his co-workers who studied the relationship between reports of pain and EMG activity during isometric work. Lloyd (1971) has shown that EMG changes are associated with a shift to higher amplitude, lower frequency motor unit activity. Since impulse frequency is proportional to motoneuron size (Ruch and Patton, 1967) this would correspond to a change from motor units having larger motoneurons, i.e. white muscle fibers (see Chap. 1), to less fatiguable red muscle motor units with smaller motoneurons. Within the muscle fibers, an altered sodium-potassium balance could produce muscle cell membrane hyperpolarization, while central nervous influences could increase motoneuron inhibition (see Åstrand and Rodahl, 1970).

In addition, Kogi and Hakamada (according to Åstrand and Rodahl, 1970) have reported decreased proprioceptive afferent impulses from muscle spindles during isometric-isotonic contractions. This suggests that *mechanoceptors* such as muscle spindles and Golgi tendon organs must be considered in any physiological explanations of changes in the Leg Fatigue symptom category. Moreover, *joint pain receptors* have been suggested by Basmajian (1967) to play a role in the local fatigue reported by subjects passively holding weights. This suggests that pain receptors in leg articular capsules and ligaments may be responsible for certain discrete symptoms of Leg Fatigue, e.g. Aching Legs. Also, compression of muscle blood vessels during exercise could lead to the release of potassium or bradykinin (Ruch and Patton, 1967), thereby activating leg *chemoreceptors*. Such changes are also associated with reports of an aching pain. Further research could proceed to evaluate the relationship(s) of symptomatology changes to the underlying physiological processes such as those mentioned above.

Perceived Effort

Scales of perceived effort are the best studied of the scales used for rating subjective qualities during work. By now, there has been sufficient research to demonstrate the validity, reliability, and replicability of the findings relating Borg's RPE scales, in particular, to various work levels and physiological parameters during standard work situations to recommend application in appropriate studies. Evidence suggests that the RPE scale may be *more* useful than physiological indices of working capacity in real-life situations (e.g. Borg, 1962) since it may merge both motivational factors and physiological cues in a single index. Additionally, its clinical application shows promise in some areas (e.g. Borg and Linderholm, 1970). For the first time, an active international research interest in the application of a single rating technique to a specific subjective quality has developed which has already begun to demonstrate utility.

The development of the RPE scale has been described in detail. Briefly, RPE was shown by Borg (1962) to increase generally in a linear fashion with an increase in work load on a bicycle ergometer. This observation has consistently been confirmed by others (Borg and Linderholm, 1967; Frankenhaeuser, et al., 1969; Skinner, et al., 1969; Kay and Shepherd, 1969; Ekblom and Goldbarg, 1971; Edwards, et al., 1972; Pandolf, et al., 1972; Bar-Or, et al., 1972; Gamberale, 1972; Henriksson, et al., 1972; Gerben, et al., 1972; Skinner, et al., 1973a, b; Noble, et al. 1973; Pandolf and Noble, 1973; Morgan, 1973; Weiser, et al., unpublished observations).

After four to six min. of work on a bicycle ergometer, RPE was also found by Borg (1962) to be elevated along with an increase in heart rate. In fact, as was reviewed earlier, RPE and HR were shown to be highly correlated. Borg (1973) has pointed out in a recent review that the scaling of RPE has been changed so that a new relationship, RPE = HR/10, could be obtained during standard bicycle work. He has suggested the RPE "can be of great help in the assessment of physical working capacity for work on the bicycle ergometer" (Borg, 1962, p. 41). Again, many reports have confirmed the RPE-HR relationship (see the references cited above). It is important to note that Borg limits this relationship to work on a bicycle ergometer in a thermoneutral environment (i.e. 24°C).

The question now arises concerning whether the RPE-HR relationship is true in general over all tasks and work situations. In the following discussion, this relationship will be shown to be highly dependent upon the task being performed. First HR during work in heat is increased about 1 pbm for every 1°C increase in environmental temperature (Kamon and Belding, 1969) and should be associated with a higher RPE. Skinner, et al. (1973b) found that for "lean" men walking on a treadmill in a progressively increasing work task at 32°C, the RPE scores were greater than the values obtained at 24°C. HR was elevated about 10 bpm in the heat. In contrast, Pandolf, et al. (1972) studied the effects of heat on the RPE-HR relationship during a prolonged bicycling task at about 40 percent max V_{O_2}, but in an environment having air moving past the subject at 30 meters per min. They found no differences between the RPE values obtained at 24°, 44°, or 54°C. HR was elevated about 20 bpm and 30 bpm at 47° and 54°C. In this situation, consequently, they concluded that "under the stress of heat, [HR] may not be the stimulus utilized for arriving at rated perceived exertion."

Second, working continuously on a bicycle ergometer at the same power, e.g. 1000 kpm/min., but at different pedalling rates produces the same HR response and should give similar RPE values. Henriksson, et al. (1972), however, found that pedalling at 30 rpm resulted in higher RPE scores than at 60 rpm, and Pandolf and Noble (1973) have reported higher values at 40 rpm than at 60 or 80 rpm. Both found similar heart rates at the equivalent power outputs, and both concluded that sensory input from mechanoreceptors may be another source of cues, in addition to HR, integrated via feedback loops into the report of perceived effort.

Finally, Ekblom and Goldbarg (1971) used autonomic blocking drugs elegantly to dissociate RPE from the HR response to bicycling. To block the sympathetic control of HR increase, propranolol was injected, while atropine was injected to block parasympathetic control. Neither drug altered max V_{O_2}, but propranolol decreased and atropine elevated HR at a given submaximal work load. However, *neither* drug changed the report of RPE at *any* given workload. Ekblom and Goldbarg conclude that "it is quite clear that tachycardia as such is not a primary factor for the [report] of RPE during work." They propose, furthermore, that a "local factor," i.e. the feeling of strain in the working muscles "is an important factor in [the report of] RPE."

RPE also does not seem to arise *per se* from the work load expressed in absolute terms or in terms of percent max V_{O_2}. That is, in the studies that investigated the influence of pedalling speed (Henriksson, et al., 1972; Pandolf and Noble, 1973), the higher RPE scores at lower rpm's were associated with oxygen uptakes that did not differ from the other pedalling rates. Also, Edwards, et al. (1971) compared an intermittent bicycle work task with continuous work at an equivalent power output and found higher RPE values for intermittent work that had the same oxygen uptake as a continuous work task. These observations suggest that RPE would be the result of motor system feedback and, consequently, might be highly dependent upon the task being performed.

That the RPE report is strongly affected by the work task becomes quite evident when one compares running or walking to cycling, arm to leg work, and eccentric (negative) to concentric (positive) work. Many studies have compared running to cycling (Ekblom and Goldbarg, 1971; Bar-Or, et al., 1972; Skinner, et al., 1973b), and all have found that at a given oxygen uptake, RPE was *greater* for bicycle work. However, Ekblom and Goldbarg (1971), Skinner, et al. (1927b), and others have found that max V_{O_2} was reduced when the work task was switched from running to cycling. Expressed in relative terms, i.e. as percent max V_{O_2}, RPE reports become similar for the two tasks (Ekblom and Goldbarg, 1971 and Skinner, et al., 1973b). Ekblom and Goldbarg (1971) have suggested that since there is more pronounced static work in cycling "the higher RPE scoring for a given submaximal work on the bicycle may be caused by the higher local muscular strain [associated with a] higher blood lactate concentration."

For walking, Noble, et al. (1973) observed that HR was less than running at velocities below 4.9 mph. At 4.9 mph, the HR values for walking and running intersected, i.e. were equal. Above 4.9 mph, walking gave HR's greater than running. RPE followed the same pattern, but the point at which RPE and velocity values for running and walking intersected was significantly lower (4.3 mph). Also at the same HR, RPE was higher for walking than for running. Noble, et al. concluded that the difference appeared to be due to the differing influence of the "local factor" proposed by Ekblom and Goldbarg (1971), i.e. strain in the working muscles.

Second, arm work is similar to cycling in that it gives higher RPE scores at the same HR (Gamberale, 1972; Ekblom and Goldbarg, 1971). RPE is also higher for armwork at the same oxygen uptake. However, changes in

RPE were associated with similar increases in blood lactate concentration. Gamberale (1972) suggested the following hypothesis: "the higher the blood lactate concentration an excercise produces as compared to oxygen uptake, the higher will be the level of the overall perception of exertion. . . ." Ekblom and Goldbarg (1971) further emphasized that "RPE . . . seems to be related to the size of the muscle mass involved.

Finally, Henriksson, et al. (1972) have shown that negative work done eccentrically on a bicycle ergometer is associated with higher RPE scores than positive concentric work at the same HR or oxygen uptake. They point out "that different types of information or sensory input are being integrated in various combinations or under different weightings in the two exercise conditions. In addition, the forced stretch placed on the muscle in eccentric exercise might result in an increase in Golgi tendon organ activity and, thereby, in an inhibition upon motor neurons [and could result in], greater numbers of motor impulses . . . to recruit the appropriate number of [motor units]. This may result in [an] increased exertion perception and would help explain the greater exertion perception in eccentric exercise at similar levels of metabolism and circulatory and ventilatory stress."

Additional evidence for motor systems feedback as the basis for perceived effort comes from studies on training, hypoxia, and prolonged work. Docktor and Sharkey (1971) found that training on a treadmill task (walking at 3.5 mph with the grade raised 1% per min.) showed no change in RPE for a work load that gave a HR of 150 bpm, although this workload had increased during training. Ekblom and Goldbarg (1971) tested men on a bicycle ergometer before and after eight weeks of cross-country running. Max V_{O_2} increased from 2.90 to 3.35 L/min, yet RPE scores were the same for relative workloads expressed as a percentage of max V_{O_2}. However, for the same absolute work load, RPE was decreased after training. Ekblom and Goldbarg suggested that the explanation "can be found in both the lesser strain on the cardio-respiratory systems and in the improved function of the working muscles, which is reflected in the lower oxygen deficit and blood lactate concentration." Chapter 2 points out that the adaptation to training results in muscle hypertrophy and enhancement of the capacity of the muscle to produce energy for contraction, along with an increase in capillaries especially around high-oxidative slow-twitch fibers. Thus after training, work at a given load level could be the result of fewer motor units contracting with the decreased motor units' recruitment. If so, this reduction in recruitment, via feedback pathways, would result in a lower perception of effort.

Hypoxia produces an effect opposite to that of training. Max V_{O_2} is decreased some 20 to 25 percent at 14,000 ft (see Chapters 13 and 14, Vol. 1). Gerben, et al. (1972) found that an hypoxic environment of 12 percent O_2 (approx. 15,000 ft altitude) significantly increased RPE for a given work task. Weiser, et al. (unpublished observations) studied six men working at about 30, 60, and 100 percent max V_{O_2} in Denver, Colorado (5,300 ft altitude) and on Pikes Peak (14,110 ft altitude). They observed that RPE was the same at both locations although the workloads were decreased at high altitude to match the Denver percent max V_{O_2} load levels. It is tempting to speculate that due to the altered oxygen gradient between muscle fibers and capillaries in the working muscles, more motor units were recruited to do the same relative work. Hence, motor activity would be increased and would be reflected by the increased RPE.

With prolonged work, Pandoff, et al. (1972), Morgan (1973), and Weiser, et al. (unpublished observations) have observed a gradual increase of RPE from the fifth min. of work to the end of the task. A speculation similar to that offered for hypoxia, i.e. increased recruitment of motor units, could be a partial explanation for these observations.

Thus, RPE has become widely accepted as a valid and reliable scaling tool for measuring perceived effort. In terms of the proposed model, RPE probably belongs to the superordinate level of subjective symptoms, and consequently is the result of the integration of many discrete cues having different weights, as Henriksson, et al. (1972) have suggested. If RPE is a superordinate quality, then it is not "close to" the physiological substrata. Of all the symptoms reported in this review, Borg's RPE has been best characterized, and two conclusions can now be drawn. First, as emphasized in Chapter 1 (see Figs. 1-1 and 1-6), perceived effort forms part of the overall feedback system that enables us to perform work. Much evidence now suggests that the information concerning perceived effort feeds back from the motor system. However, the direct neuronal linkage from the motor centers and the role of peripheral proprioceptive feedback loops are not known. Second, the relationship between RPE has been shown in the studies discussed above to be directly related to HR only under standard conditions, as Borg (1962) emphasized. Specifically, deviations from cycling in a thermoneutral environment and the use of autonomic nervous system blocking agents clearly demonstrate that RPE can be dissociated from cardiac frequency.

Pain

In a study reviewed previously, Lloyd, Voor, and Thieman (1970) also measured EMG changes along with pain ratings in an isometric hand dynamometer task using either 25, or 50 percent of maximum grip strength. This task involved the self-paced rating technique in which each subject was required to call out "1" when he first noticed perceptible pain, and so on while a final call of "5" was defined as intolerable pain corresponding to task termination. In general, average EMG amplitude of the biceps increased with time and with successively higher pain ratings. One of the more intriguing observations made by Lloyd, et al. (1970) was that EMG amplitude tended to increase rather abruptly toward the latter part of the task, closely associated with the onset of muscle tremors. It is interesting to note that Weiser, et al. (1973) also found a subjective symptom, Muscle Tremors, that was significantly increased during prolonged bicycle work. This increase in EMG amplitude was interpreted as the time corresponding to muscle fatigue, while the additional time that the subject persisted beyond this point was suggested to be due to psychological factors associated with motivational level.

Also, Lloyd (1971) had ten male subjects perform an isometric task involving sustained contraction of the elbow flexors at 30, 50, and 70 percent of their maximum level. EMG activity in the biceps, triceps, deltoid, and contralateral triceps were monitored throughout the task. As in previous studies by Lloyd, subjects were instructed to continue for as long as possible and to rate the level of pain intensity on a five-point scale using the self-paced technique. All subjects were run three times at each load level during nine sessions. Ratings of pain intensity were related quadratically with time on the task for the 30 and 70 percent load levels and linerally for the 50 percent load level. There were striking differences in the rate in which subjective pain intensity increased between load levels, increasing much more rapidly for the higher load levels (also see Menzer, Smith, and Caldwell, 1969; Lloyd and McClaskey, 1971; Lloyd, Voor, and Thieman, 1970). Mean EMG amplitude for the biceps at each of the ratings of subjective pain showed a clear increase for all load levels as ratings of pain intensity increased. Increases in EMG activity in the triceps, deltoid, and contralateral triceps also increased with pain ratings, although the contralateral triceps increased only for the high ratings of pain intensity (4 and 5) for the 70 percent load only. One of the outstanding features of this study involved frequency analysis of the EMG for each of the ratings of pain intensity. For each load level, but more so for the two higher load levels, as the rating of pain intensity increased there was a marked *increase* in amplitude in EMG amplitude for the lower frequencies and a lesser *decrease* in amplitude for the higher EMG frequencies. Lloyd suggested that with increasing pain intensity during isometric tasks, there is a recruitment of higher threshold motor units firing at a low frequency. An alternative concept specifying an increased *rate* of firing during increased fatigue received no support from Lloyd's data. This study stands as an excellent demonstration of the payoff potential in relating subjective report during work performance to physiological variables.

Lloyd (1972) has subsequently demonstrated that when an auditory bioelectric feedback signal (biofeedback) proportional to EMG amplitude was provided to subjects doing isometric tasks similar to that used by Lloyd (1971), the level of muscle activity (mean EMG amplitude) required to maintain contraction was significantly reduced across all ratings of pain intensity. These differences were obtained in spite of the fact that mean endurance times and average times for successive self-paced ratings was not different for subjects provided and not provided EMG feedback. These results indicate that biofeedback improves efficiency of isometric performance without affecting total endurance time or the points at which various ratings of pain intensity are given. Since it may require a number of training sessions before significant improvement in performance is noted using biofeedback, it would be interesting to determine how biofeedback would affect endurance time and self-paced ratings of pain intensity across repetitive training trials during isometric work.

Thermal Discomfort

Changes in both the subjective qualities, Thermal Sensation and Discomfort, have been related by Gagge, et al. (1969) to physiological variables associated with thermoregulation; this study has been reviewed in detail. Briefly, the sensation of "warm discomfort" after 30 to 40 min. of work was related to metabolic rate, rectal temperature, skin conductance, and most highly to sweating rate ($r = .66$). In contrast, perception of thermal sensations were principally related to the ambient air temperature and to the skin temperature.

SUMMARY AND CONCLUSIONS

Many different subjective qualities have been measured during work representing different aspects of multidimensionally organized subjective symptomatology. These qualities have been measured either by using psychophysical methods (see Table 14-I) or rating scales (see Tables 14-II through 14-IV). A model has been proposed in this review (see Fig. 14-6) that stratifies these qualities into different levels of subjective report beginning with the discrete symptoms, forming categories of symptoms at intermediate levels, and finally converging into a global, superordinate level of report typified by Undifferentiated Fatigue. All levels of symptomatology are presumed to be linked by feedback loops to the underlying physiological substrata. Cues from changes in the physiological substrata during work give rise to the reported symptoms. In turn, the symptomatology experienced can affect work performance.

In the model, the concept of the ordinate and subordinate levels of subjective report also emphasizes that the significant subjective qualities experienced are highly dependent on the work task performed. First, the amount of muscle mass utilized, e.g. arm or leg work, will alter the discrete subjective qualities and the manner in which they group at the ordinate or subordinate levels. Second, the intensity of work relative to the maximal aerobic power obtainable for any task will determine the intensity of subjective symptoms experienced.

Viewed according to a classic division, work can be divided roughly into categories according to the predominant energy requirements of the task: mental, sedentary, and strenuous. In tasks studied to date wherein subjective fatigue has been measured, these divisions have not always been clear cut. Nevertheless, the object of the brief summary which follows is simply to show that the subjective qualities composing what is termed subjective fatigue differ according to task requirements.

A. As early as 1928, Poffenberger showed that a global report of undifferentiated fatigue increased in association with the amount of mental work performed and was related to performance decrement. The pattern of discrete symptom qualities involved in mental work and sedentary, light submaximal work appears to differ from those tasks that require a higher energy expenditure. Specifically, Kogi, et al. (1970) have found that individuals such as hospital pharmacists generally report experiencing infrequent discrete symptoms although about 25 to 37 percent of these complained of eye strain, shoulder stiffness, and heavy legs at the end of work. Engine drivers, engaged in a form of sedentary, light submaximal work, also complained of these symptoms most often. In contrast to factory workers engaged in heavy physical work, all symptoms reported were infrequent for the pharmacists and engine drivers while factor analysis indicated that the organization of the same set of symptoms into *categories* differed widely between these occupations. Any global rating of Undifferentiated Fatigue used would likely integrate numerous such discrete symptom qualities. In fact, it has been demonstrated that global reports of Undifferentiated Fatigue change, as expected, during housework (Gross and Bartley, 1951), operation of aircraft (Pearson and Byars, 1956; Buckley and Hartman, 1969), and formal psychomotor tasks (McNelley, 1957). The difficulty in interpreting all of these latter studies has simply been due to Undifferentiated Fatigue being a composite of discrete symptoms. The specification of the discrete symptom qualities involved in fatigue during mental and light submaximal work and the manner in which they group, is a useful area for further research.

B. Subjective symptomatology observed during moderate or heavy work tasks can be grouped into two major categories: perceived fatigue and perceived effort. Other symptoms studied have been perceived effort expended, pain, discomfort, and thermal sensations.

1. During these types of tasks, a definite grouping of discrete symptoms

has been identified (Wolf, 1967; Kinsman, Weiser and Stamper, 1973) and labeled simply Fatigue.

   a. Reported qualities composing the Fatigue category are clearly dependent on the types of tasks being performed. Weiser, et al. (1973) have found that a distinct Leg Fatigue grouping of items could be separated from items descriptive of General Fatigue for subjects performing prolonged strenuous bicycle work. Again, Kogi, et al. (1970) have found that persons employed on differing physical tasks, such as iron foundry workers, report different frequencies of symptoms experienced and, in turn, demonstrate different organizational groupings of symptom qualities to form symptom categories.

   b. As the work load is increased on the bicycle ergometer, scores increase for Leg Fatigue, Cardiopulmonary, and General Fatigue categories reported after five min. of work (Weiser, unpublished observation). Nunney (1963) has found that the report for a global measure of fatigue increased with increasing work along with the expected increase of HR. Heuting and Sarphati (1966) also observed a greater rating of undifferentiated fatigue for a bicycle task that finished in a higher work load.

   c. Finally, throughout the duration of a prolonged work task, Weiser, et al. (unpublished observations) have observed increased scores for the Fatigue, Cardiopulmonary Fatigue, and General Fatigue categories. Buckley and Hartman (1969) found that the rating of global fatigue (Pearson and Byars, 1956) increased throughout a transatlantic helicopter flight, but decreased during the "flyby" staged in Paris at the end of the flight.

2. Borg's Rating of Perceived Effort (RPE) has become recognized as a valid and reliable scale, although the discrete symptoms integrated by RPE remain to be defined more completely.

   a. RPE scores are highly dependent upon the work task. Running produces a different RPE score when compared to cycling at a given heart rate (Ekblom and Goldbarg, 1971; Bar-Or, et al., 1972; Skinner, et al., 1973b) or to walking (Noble, et al., 1973). Arm work gives a higher RPE at a given heart rate than does cycling (Ekblom and Goldbarg, 1971; Gamberale, 1972). Negative, eccentric work also produces a higher RPE score at a given heart rate than does positive, concentric work (Henriksson, et al., 1972). In fact, for equivalent power outputs, subjects pedalling at 60 rpm have reported lower RPE scores than when pedalling at 30 rpm (Henriksson, et al., 1972) or at 40 rpm (Pandolf and Noble, 1973).

   b. When work is expressed as being a percent of maximal performance, the variability in RPE becomes markedly reduced. For example, the differences between cycling and running (Ekblom and Goldbarg, 1971; Bar-Or, et al., 1972; Skinner, et al., 1973b), cycling during normoxic and hypoxic environment (Gerben, et al., 1972; Weiser, et al., unpublished observations), and cycling before and after training (Ekblom and Goldbarg, 1971) can be explained by the changes in maximal aerobic power produced by these situations. Also, Schmale, et al. (1963) have observed that the effort involved in holding a weight measured by a psychophysical technique was similar for men and women if perceived effort was related to relative weight held, i.e. weight held divided by maximal weight that could be held.

c. RPE increases throughout the course of bicycle work at a fixed load level (Pandolf, et al., 1972; Morgan, 1973; Weiser, et al., unpublished observations).

d. In view of the observations presented, RPE appears to reflect the state of activity of the motor system. RPE is correlated to cardiopulmonary responses when different work loads are compared under standard work conditions, e.g. on a bicycle ergometer, a point clearly emphasized by Borg (1962).

3. A rating of perceived effort expended was found by Lloyd and McClaskey (1971) to increase linearly throughout a prolonged walking task, with the most pronounced linearity occurring only after several trials on the task.

4. Likewise, with practiced subjects ratings of pain and perceived effort expended have been shown to increase linearly during exhausting prolonged isometric work (Caldwell and Smith, 1967; Lloyd, et al., 1970).

5. The sensation of "warm discomfort" after 30 to 40 min. of work was found by Gagge, et al. (1969) to be related to metabolic rate, rectal temperature, skin conductance, and most highly to sweating rate. In contrast, they observed that the perception of thermal sensations were principally related to the ambient air temperature and to the skin temperature.

BIBLIOGRAPHY

Åstrand, P.-O., and K. Rodahl: *Textbook of Work Physiology*. New York, McGraw-Hill, 1970.

Bakers, J. H., and S. M. Tenney: The perception of some sensations associated with breathing. *Respir Physiol, 10*:85, 1970.

Bar-Or, O., J. S. Skinner, E. R. Buskirk, and G. Borg: Physiological and perceptual indicators of physical stress in 41- to 60-year-old men who vary in conditioning level and in body fatness. *Med Sci Sports, 4*:96, 1972.

Bartley, S. H., and E. Chute: *Fatigue and Impairment in Man*. New York, McGraw-Hill, 1947.

Basmajian, J. V.: *Muscles Alive. Their Functions Revealed by Electromyography.* Baltimore, Williams & Wilkins, 1967.
Beecher, H. K.: Pain: one mystery solved. *Science, 151*:840, 1966.
Bernyer, G.: Une échelle de sensation d'effort musculaire. *Annee Psychologique, 67*:23, 1967.
Borg, G.: Perceived exertion in relation to physical work load and pulse rate. *Kungl Fysiogr Sallsk i Lund Forh, 11*:105, 1961a.
Borg, G.: Interindividual scaling and the perception of muscular force. *Kungl Fysiograf Sallsk i Lund Forh, 31*:117, 1961b.
Borg, G.: *Physical Performance and Perceived Exertion.* Gleerups, Lund, 1962.
Borg, G.: The perception of physical performance. In Shepherd, R. J. (Ed.): *Frontiers of Physical Fitness.* Springfield, Thomas, 1971.
Borg, G.: Perceived exertion: a note on "history" and methods. *Med Sci Sports, 5*:90, 1972.
Borg, G., and H. Dahlström: The perception of muscular work. *Umea Vetenskapliga Bibliotek Skriftserie, 5*:1, 1960.
Borg, G., and H. Linderholm: Perceived exertion and pulse rate during graded exercise in various age groups. *Acta Med Scand, Suppl, 472*:194, 1967.
Borg, G., and H. Linderholm: Exercise performance and perceived exertion in patients with coronary insufficiency, arterial hypertension and vasoregulatory asthenia. *Acta Med Scand, 187*:17, 1970.
Buckley, C. J., and B. O. Hartman: Aeromedical aspects of the first nonstop transatlantic helicopter flight: 1. General mission overview and subjective fatigue analyses. *Aerospace Med, 710,* 1969.
Bujas, Z., Ž. Pavlina, B. Sremec, S. Vidaček, and M. Vodanović: Subjecktivno procjenjivanje umora. *Archiv Hig Rada, 17*:275, 1966.
Bujas, Z., B. Petz, A. Krković, and B. Sorokin: Faktorska analiza intelektualnog rada u stanju svježine i u stanju umora. *Archiv Hig Rada, 11*:206, 1960.
Bujas, Z., B. Sremec, and S. Vidacek: Doževljaj umora i njegove asocijacije s nekim drugim varij ablama. *Archiv Hig Rada, 16*:111, 1965.
Cain, W. S., and J. C. Stevens: Effort in sustained and phasic handgrip contractions. *Am J Psychol, 84*:52, 1971.
Cain, W. S., and J. C. Stevens: Constant-effort contractions related to the electromyogram. *Med Sci Sports, 5*:121, 1973.
Caldwell, L. S.: The scaling of effort produced by strenuous isometric muscle contractions. *USAMRL Report No. 749,* 1967.
Caldwell, L. S., and R. P. Smith: Subjective estimation of effort, reserve, and ischemic pain. *USAMRL No. 730,* 1967.
Cliff, N.: Scaling. In Mussen, P. H., and Rosenweig, M. R. (Eds.): *Annual Review of Psychology.* Palo Alto, Annual Reviews, 1973.
Cronbach, L. J.: *Essentials of Psychological Testing.* New York, Harper, 1960.
Dirken, J. M.: Industrial shift work: decrease in well-being and specific effects. *Ergonomics, 9*:115, 1966.
Docktor, R., and B. J. Sharkey: Note on some physiological and subjective reactions to exercise and training. *Percept Mot Skills, 32*:233, 1971.
Eason, R. G.: The surface electromyogram (EMG) gauges subjective effort. *Percept Mot Skills, 9*:359, 1959.
Edwards, A. L., and F. P. Kilpatrick: A technique for the construction of attitude scales. *J Appl Psychol, 32*:374, 1948.

Edwards, R. H. T., A. Melcher, C. M. Hesser, O. Wigertz, and L.-G. Ekelund: Physiological correlates of perceived exertion in continuous and intermittent exercise with the same average power output. *Eur J Clin Invest, 2:*108, 1972.

Eisler, H.: Subjective scale of force for a large muscle group. *J Exp Psychol, 64:*253, 1962.

Ekblom, B., and A. N. Goldbarg: The influence of physical training and other factors on the subjective rating of perceived exertion. *Acta Physiol Scand, 83:*399, 1971.

Ekman, G.: Two generalized ratio scaling methods. *J Psychol, 45:*287, 1958.

Ekman, G.: Weber's law and related functions. *J Psychol, 47:*343, 1959.

Evans, W. O.: Measurement of subjective symptomatology of acute high altitude sickness. *Psychol Rep, 19:*815, 1966.

Fechner, G. T.: *In Sachen der Psychophysik.* Leipzig, 1877.

Foltz, E. E., F. T. Jung, and L. E. Cisler: The effect of some internal factors on human work output and recovery. *Am J Physiol, 141:*641, 1944.

Frankenhaeuser, M., B. Post, B. Nordheden, and H. Sjoeberg: Physiological and subjective reactions to different physical work loads. *Percept Mot Skills, 28:*343, 1969.

Gagge, A. P., J. A. J. Stolwijk, and B. Saltin: Comfort and thermal sensations and associated physiological responses during exercise at various ambient temperatures. *Environ Res, 2:*209, 1969.

Gamberale, F.: Perceived exertion, heart rate, oxygen uptake and blood lactate in different work operations. *Ergonomics, 15:*545, 1972.

Gerben, J. J., J. L. House, and F. R. Winsmann: Self-paced ergometer performance: effects of pedal resistance, motivational contingency and inspired oxygen concentration. *Percept Mot Skills, 34:*875, 1972.

Griffith, J. W., W. A. Kerr, T. B. Mayo, Jr., and J. R. Topal: Changes in subjective fatigue and readiness for work during the eight-hour shift. *J Appl Psychol, 34:*163, 1950.

Gross, I. H., and S. Bartley: Fatigue in house care. *J Appl Psychol, 35:*205, 1951.

Guilford, J. P.: *Fundamental Statistics in Psychology and Education.* New York, McGraw-Hill, 1950.

Guilford, J. P.: *Psychometric Methods,* 2nd ed. New York, McGraw-Hill, 1954.

Hartman, B. O., H. B. Hale, and W. A. Johnson: Fatigue in FB-111 crew members. *Aerospace Med, 45:*1026, 1974.

Hartman, B. O., H. B. Hale, D. A. Harris, and J. F. Sanford III: Psychobiologic aspects of double-crew long-duration missions in C-5 aircraft. *Aerospace Med, 45:*1149, 1974.

Hauty, G. T., and R. B. Payne: Fatigue and the perceptual field of work. *J. Appl Psychol, 40:*40, 1956.

Hemphill, R. E., K. R. L. Hall, and T. G. Crookes: A preliminary report on fatigue and pain tolerance in depressive and psychoneurotic patients. *J Ment Sci, 98:*433, 1952.

Henriksson, J., H. G. Knuttgen, and F. Bonde-Petersen: Perceived exertion during exercise with concentric and eccentric muscle contractions. *Ergonomics, 15:*537, 1972.

Heuting, J. E.: Relationships between some physiological and psychological variables with regard to physical exercise. *Acta Physiol Pharmacol Heerlandia, 13:*198, 1964.

Heuting, J. E., and H. R. Sarphati: Measuring fatigue. *J Appl Psychol, 50:*535, 1966.

Heuting, J. E., and P. Visser: Une contribution au probleme des relations entre les phenomenes subjectifs et objectifs de la fatigue. *Arch Int Physiol, 68:*860, 1960.

Hosman, J.: Adaptation to muscular effort. *Reports from the Psychological Laboratories,* University of Stockholm, 1967.

Hull, C. L.: *Principles of Behavior.* New York, Appleton, 1943.

Hull, C. L.: *A Behavior System*. New Haven, Yale U Pr, 1952.
Jackson, D., and S. Messick (Eds.): *Problems in Human Assessment*. New York, McGraw-Hill, 1967.
Janssen, C. G. C., and H. J. Docter: Quantitative subjective assessment of fatigue in static muscle effort. *Europ J Appl Physiol, 32*:81, 1973.
Jones, E. E., D. Kanouse, H. H. Kelley, R. E. Nisbett, S. Valins, and B. Weiner: *Attribution: Perceiving the Causes of Behavior*. Morristown, N.J., General Learning Pr, 1972.
Kamon, E., and H. S. Belding: Comparison of heart rate changes when measured during physical activity and in the heat. Cited by Pandolf, et al., 1972.
Kay, C., and R. J. Shepherd: On muscle strength and the threshold of anaerobic work. *Int Z Angew Physiol, 27*:311, 1969.
Kerr, W. A.: Where they like to work; work place preference of 228 electrical workers in terms of music. *J Appl Psychol, 27*:438, 1943.
Kinsman, R. A., T. Luparello, K. O'Banion, and S. Spector: Multidimensional analysis of the subjective symptomatology of asthma. *Psychosom Med, 35*:250, 1973.
Kinsman, R. A., K. O'Banion, P. Resnikoff, T. J. Luparello, and S. L. Spector: Subjective symptoms of acute asthma within a heterogeneous sample of asthmatics. *J Allergy Clin Immunol, 52*:284, 1973.
Kinsman, R. A., P. C. Weiser, and D. A. Stamper: Multidimensional analysis of subjective symptomatology during prolonged strenuous exercise. *Ergonomics, 16*:211, 1973.
Kirihara, S.: Reality of industrial fatigue. *Journal of Science of Labour, 25*:209, 1949.
Kogi, K., Y. Saito, and T. Mitsuhashi: Validity of three components of subjective fatigue feelings. *Journal of Science of Labour, 46*:251, 1970.
Lloyd, A. J.: Surface electromyography during sustained isometric contractions. *J Appl Physiol, 30*:713, 1971.
Lloyd, A. J.: Auditory EMG feedback during a sustained submaximum isometric contraction. *Res Quart, 43*:39, 1972.
Lloyd, A. J., and E. B. McClaskey: Subjective assessment of effort in dynamic work. *J Mot Behav, 3*:49, 1971.
Lloyd, A. J., J. H. Voor, and T. J. Thieman: Subjective and electromyographic assessment of isometric muscle contractions. *Ergonomics, 13*:685, 1970.
Luce, R. D.: On the possible psychophysical laws. *Psychol Rev, 66*:81, 1959.
McGrath, S. D., E. D. Wittkower, and R. A. Cleghorn: Some observations on airscrew fatigue in the RCAF—Tokyo airlift. *J Aviat Med, 25*:23, 1954.
McNelly, G.: The development and laboratory validation of a subjective fatigue scale, Ph.D. Thesis, Purdue University, 1954.
Menzer, J., P. Smith, and L. S. Caldwell: Self-paced and irregular methods of subjective estimation of pain. *Psychon Sci, 15*:287, 1969.
Morgan, W. P.: Psychological factors influencing perceived exertion. *Med Sci Sports, 5*:97, 1973.
Niven, J. R.: A comparison of two attitude scaling techniques. *Educ Psychol Meas, 13*:65, 1953.
Noble, B. J., K. F. Metz, K. B. Pandolf, C. W. Bell, E. Cafarelli, and W. E. Sime: Perceived exertion during walking and running. *Med Sci Sports, 5*:116, 1973.
Nowlis, V., and H. Nowlis: The description and analysis of mood. *Ann NY Acad Sci, 65*:245, 1956.

Nunney, D. N.: Fatigue, impairment, and psycho-motor learning. *Percept Mot Skills, 16*:369, 1963.

Overall, J. E., and C. J. Klett: *Applied Multivariate Analysis.* New York, McGraw-Hill, 1972.

Pandolf, K. B., and B. J. Noble: The effect of pedalling speed and resistance changes on perceived exertion for equivalent power outputs on the bicycle ergometer. *Med Sci Sports, 5*:132, 1973.

Pandolf, K. B., E. Cafarelli, B. J. Noble, and K. F. Metz: Perceptual responses during prolonged work. *Percept Mot Skills, 35*:975, 1972.

Pearson, R. G.: Scale analysis of a fatigue checklist. *J Appl Psychol, 41*:186, 1957.

Pearson, R. G., and G. E. Byars, Jr.: The development and validation of a checklist for measuring subjective fatigue. *USAF School Aviat Med Report No. 56-115*, 1956.

Pierson, W. R.: Fatigue, work decrement, and endurance in a simple repetitive task. *Br J Med Psychol, 36*:279, 1963a.

Pierson, W. R.: Isometric strength and occurrence of fatigue and work decrement. *Percept Mot Skills, 17*:470, 1963b.

Pierson, W. R., and A. Lockhart: Fatigue, work decrement and endurance of women in a simple repetitive task. *Aerospace Med, 35*:724, 1964.

Pierson, W. R., and P. J. Rasch: The determination of a representative score for reaction time and movement time. *Percept Mot Skills, 9*:107, 1959.

Pierson, W. R., and G. Q. Rich: Energy expenditure and fatigue during simple repetitive tasks. *Hum Factors, 9*:563, 1967.

Plateau, M. H.: Sur la mesure des sensations physique, et sur la loi qui lie l'intensité de ces sensations à l'intensité de la cause excitante. *Bull de l'Acad Roy Belg, 33*:376, 1872.

Poffenberger, A. T.: The effects of continuous work upon output and feelings. *J Appl Psychol, 12*:459, 1928.

Rowell, L. B.: Circulation. *Med Sci Sports, 1*:15, 1969.

Ruch, T. C., and H. D. Patton (Eds.): *Physiology and Biophysics.* Philadelphia, Saunders, 1967.

Saito, Y., K. Kogi, and S. Kashiwagi: Factors underlying subjective feelings of fatigue. *Journal of Science of Labour, 46*:205, 1970.

Schmale, H., H. Schmidtke, and A. Vukovich: Untersuchungen über den Grad der subjektiv gegebenen Beanspouchung bei Korperlicher arbeit. *Forschungs bericht des Landes Nordrhein-Westfalen, Nr 1261*, 1963.

Simonson, E., and N. Enzer: Physiology of muscular exercise and fatigue in disease. *Medicine, 21*:345, 1942.

Skinner, J. S., G. Borg, and E. R. Buskirk: Physiological and perceptual reactions to exertion of young men differing in activity and body size. In Franks, D. (Ed.): *Exercise and Fitness.* Chicago, The Athletic Institute, 1969.

Skinner, J. S., R. Mutsler, V. Bergsteinova, and E. R. Buskirk: The validity and reliability of a rating scale of perceived exertion. *Med Sci Sports, 5*:94, 1973a.

Skinner, J. S., R. Mutsler, V. Bergsteinová, and E. R. Buskirk: Perception of effort during different types of exercise and under different environmental conditions. *Med Sci Sports, 5*:110, 1973b.

Smith, G. M., L. D. Egbert, R. A. Markowitz, F. Môsteller, and H. K. Beecher: An experimental pain method sensitive to morphine in man: The submaximum effort tourniquet technique. *J Pharmacol Exp Ther, 154*:324, 1966.

Snyder, M., R. Schulz, and E. E. Jones: Expectancy and apparent duration as determinants of fatigue. *J Person Soc Psychol, 29:*426, 1974.

Stamper, D. A., R. A. Kinsman, and W. O. Evans: Subjective symptomatology and cognitive performance at high altitude. *Percept Mot Skills, 31:*247, 1970.

Stamper, D. A., R. T. Sterner, and R. A. Kinsman: Symptomatology subscales for the measurement of acute mountain sickness. *Percept Mot Skills, 33:*735, 1971.

Stevens, J. C., and W. S. Cain: Effort in isometric muscular contractions related to force level and duration. *Percept Psycholphys, 8:*240, 1970.

Stevens, J. C., and J. D. Mack: Scales of apparent force. *J Exp Psychol, 58:*405, 1959.

Stevens, S. S.: On the psychophysical law. *Psychol Rev, 64:*153, 1957.

Stevens, S. S.: The psychophysics of sensory function. *Am Sci, 2:*226, 1960.

Stevens, S. S., and E. H. Galanter: Ratio scales and category scales for a dozen perceptual continua. *J Exp Psychol, 54:*377, 1957.

Stevens, S. S., and H. B. Greenbaum: Regression effect in psychophysical judgement. *Percept Psycholphys, 1:*439, 1966.

Strauss, P. S., and J. Carlock: Effects of load-carrying on psychomotor performance. *Percept Mot Skills, 23:*315, 1966.

Thurstone, L. L., and E. J. Chave: *The Measurement of Attitudes.* Chicago, University of Chicago, 1929.

Tryon, R. C., and Bailey, D. E.: *Cluster Analysis.* New York, McGraw-Hill, 1970.

Wahlung, H.: Determination of the physical working capacity. *Acta Med Scand Suppl, 215,* 1948.

Walster, B., and E. Aronson: Effect of expectancy of task duration on the experience of fatigue. *J Exp Soc Psychol, 3:*41, 1967.

Weber, E. H.: De pulse, resorptione, auditu et tactu. Leip, Koehler, 1834.

Weiser, P. C., R. A. Kinsman, and D. A. Stamper: Task-specific symptomatology changes resulting from prolonged submaximal bicycle riding. *Med Sci Sports, 5:*79, 1973.

Weiser, P. C., D. A. Stamper, R. A. Kinsman, and J. P. Hannon: Relationship of heart rate increment during exercise to the time of exhaustion. *Fed Proc, 30:*372 (abstract), 1971.

Welford, A. T.: Fatigue and monotony. In Edholm, O. G. (Ed.): *The Physiology of Human Survival.* New York, Acad Pr, 1965.

Wijting, J. P., S. Wollack, and P. C. Smith: A factor analytic study of the subjective components of activation. *Percept Mot Skills, 31:*635, 1970.

Wolf, G.: Construct validation of measures of three kinds of experimental fatigue. *Percept Mot Skills, 24:*1067, 1967.

Wotzka, F., and E. Grandjean: Physiologische und psycholische Ermüdungsmessungen bei Flugverkehrsleitern. *Z Präventivmed, 13:*204, 1968.

Yoshitake, H.: Rating feelings of fatigue. *Journal of Science of Labour, 45:*422, 1969.

Yoshitake, H.: Relations between the symptoms and the feeling of fatigue. *Ergonomics, 14:*175, 1971.

SECTION SEVEN
CLOSING COMMENTS

Chapter 15

What Do We Call Fatigue?

S. HOWARD BARTLEY

INTRODUCTION

NOT EVERYONE MEANS the same thing when he uses the word *fatigue*. While this may be permissible in conversational language where words have several meanings, and where the immediate context determines the meaning, it is not permissible in a technical or scientific language. In a truly technical or scientific language, words get their meaning by definition, not by context. In such a vocabulary, words have only one meaning. No word is used to label two different classes of things, and no thing is given more than one label. With such a language, confusion is held to a minimum.

These principles are not strictly adhered to in much of the usage we give certain words. Fatigue is one very good example. No doubt one of the bases for this laxity in would-be technical language stems from the fact that it acquires its vocabulary from everyday conversational speech where strict meanings are not formally assigned to words. Words that started out to label the layman's observations became even more varied in their technical meanings after they were brought into the experimental laboratory. Or, not only more varied in meaning, they became markedly different in meaning, while the layman's meanings linger on. Thus, when the laboratory is given to studying problems, the diversity and vagueness increases whereas it ought to decrease.

It is characteristic of humans to be doing one thing while supposing they are doing another. The phrase "you know what I mean," is the substitute for individuals making clear to themselves and then to others what they mean. They seldom do anything to recognize and point out the lack of common meaning in the words they use. They simply take for granted that everyone means the same thing by using a given word, especially when it is prevalently used.

Fatigue is a term employed in the ways just described, and the present discourse is meant to rehearse this matter and implications and consequences involved.

The present discourse is a delineation of the diverse ways that the word fatigue has been used by various workers. Taken as a total this variety would appear not to be a very helpful thing in the promotion of human understanding, and thus the mere depiction of it may appear to be an indictment. The purpose, however, has been rather to present the idea of the desirability of coming to a mutual consent on the use of concepts and terms in the area at issue.

Accordingly, it has been thought best to omit specific examples of the practice outlined. To do so would greatly and unnecessarily extend the chapter, and furthermore the readers who are versed in the area will immediately recall examples of their own.

THE ORIGIN OF THE FATIGUE CONCEPT

We could begin by dealing with the matter ahistorically, which seems to be the way most authors think about it. But I will start with the way the concept of fatigue appears to have arisen in the first place. Like many other words, fatigue labelled a self-experienced condition in people. In fact, there were other words that labelled the same condition, so fatigue had synonyms or partial synonyms like *tiredness* and *weariness*. So the individual in everyday life would say either, "I'm tired," "I'm fatigued," or "I'm weary." But he went further than that. He wanted to account for his feelings, and so descriptive adjectives turned to nouns which were made to label causal conditions. Somehow or other, *fatigue* got to be the formal noun used for the *condition* in which he felt as just described. Fatigue has gotten to be the name for the condition as well as the experience that results. So, now, we do not find research called "tiredness" studies, but instead they are "fatigue" studies.

As the technical person and scientist pick up a problem, the details of condition begin to loom up and become the central or the only concern, and, in turn, even the "conditions for the condition" become attended to. Later, newcomers in research each arrive at the general problem area from very restricted and specific entrance points, so new centers of interest and understanding are brought in. From the purely analytical standpoint, this may be appropriate but as matters typically develop, origins and the interrelations between elements in the matter become lost sight of. Language manifests and promotes this.

THE CONCEPT EXTENDED

From the foregoing, one would suppose that fatigue is a concept that applies to humans and problems about it would lie in biology, not in areas beyond clarification of human condition and performance. Nevertheless, this has not been the case. Metals are said to fatigue. Often we profess to eschew anthropomorphisms, but here is one at work. We will pass up this usage by simply saying that if a word is needed for labelling performance failure in all systems, biological and nonbiological, could not some such term as *incapacitation* be used, since as far as we know it is not a term with a specific biological origin. Fatigue then would be a species of incapacitation, a kind of biological incapacitation, namely, the kind experienced in humans.

FATIGUE: PERCEPTUAL EXPERIENCE OR INCAPACITATION?

Of course, there is the problem of whether fatigue is to be used for the *experience,* or for the *incapacitation* itself. However, Simonson (1971) has used the term *fatigue* for "all processes resulting in a decrement of capacities." However, in actual practice, some authors have studied *change* in a selected body process during the individual's task performance as fatigue, assuming that it is a form of decrement of capacity, while in fact it may be an adaptive process instead. This problem was not resolved in man's original everyday vocabulary. I think it more appropriate, at this point, to use the term fatigue to label the experience syndrome, and find other terms to label conditions and processes.

FATIGUE AND IMPAIRMENT

Bartley and Chute (1947) made a distinction which is both logical and workable. The condition of incapacitation that arises in individuals by something happening to *intra-cellular* activity, such as in cases of anoxia and the like, they called *impairment.* They then used a term for conditions of incapacitation at *inter-cellular* levels. They called this *disorganization,* forms of which are substrates for fatigue, for anxiety, etc. It is apparent that cells need not be impaired in order for disorganization to occur in the brain, where an endless variety of patterns of activity can occur, and an emergent phenomena in some of these cases, we have the experiential syndromes of fatigue, etc. Who denies that one can feel fatigued quite immediately upon being confronted with certain kinds of obligations (tasks)? Mere confrontment as well as extended activity serve to evoke fatigue, so we cannot lean on the idea that prolonged activity is necessary for producing fatigue.

KINDS OF FATIGUE

One of the results of the prevalent outlook on fatigue is the notion that we can speak of *kinds* of fatigue. This is exemplified in classifying fatigue into *subjective, objective,* and *physiological.* Bills (1943) did this. Subjective fatigue was said to be a kind of experience, awareness, or feeling. Objective fatigue was exemplified in studies of work output. And, physiological fatigue was the kind involved where selected body processes were found to change during performance of a task. Simonson (1935) classified them into five categories: (1) accumulation of metabolites, (2) depletion of energy yielding substances, (3) changes in the state of substrate, (4) changes of regulations, and (5) transmission fatigue. Various other workers, particularly in Germany, have accepted these categories. These body processes have been of many kinds.

It is obvious that the subjective, objective and physiological categories are quite unlike each other, and that actually there is no suitable way of transposing from one to the other. The first category is ordinarily called *psychological*. I call it personalistic, a means whereby one bypasses the many naive notions of what is meant by psychological, and whereby the category is positioned in a taxonomy classifying matters pertaining to levels of organization in the body. Phenomena in this level are dealt with differently than are the subpersonalistic. The second (objective fatigue) pertains to work output and should simply be called that, else one is introducing a foreign category—a category pertaining not to a description of the organism (performer) but to products outside of him. The third category pertains simply to the nature of processes within the body, not the performer as a person or a unit.

This abuse brings us to pointing out that there are two references possible in dealing with organisms as units or persons. One is the *organism-centered* reference and the other is the *environmental centered* reference. It would seem obligatory to remain within the organism if it is the organism that is to be studied. Unfortunately some authors slip into the environment for their center of concern. Logically this rules them out as directly studying fatigue. Here we can say that the study of work decrement turns out not to be a study of fatigue as such.

Physiological fatigue involves subsystems within the organism. These may be taken as correlates of fatigue, just as work decrement may be, or they may be studies centered on the processes themselves. Here the definition and criterion of fatigue may be any one of a variety of things. Although such studies are called fatigue studies, the approaches used imply that sometimes a strict definition of fatigue is a secondary matter. With the lack of a single definition for fatigue such studies cannot always be well compared either with each other or used as references of comparison in fatigue studies of any kind.

As far back as 1921, the question of tests to measure fatigue was prominent. Muscio found that tests then in use did not all agree. Some would show an increase and others a decrease in the hypothetical thing called fatigue in the same situation. He concluded they were not all measuring the same thing and suggested abandoning the concept of fatigue altogether. Apparently, no one wanted to do this. However, taking Muscio's results seriously might lead to one or the other of four alternatives.

ALTERNATIVE ONE: to abandon fatigue or any other single label for the tests usually made for it.

ALTERNATIVE TWO: to choose whatever it is that one of the tests measures and call it fatigue and find other labels for whatever the other tests measure.

ALTERNATIVE THREE: to adopt a very general notion of what to call fatigue, such as changes in body processes that reduce their effectiveness. This would imply that fatigue is a generic concept applying to many processes and thus being manifested in many forms. The opposite of this alternative is to use the word incapacity for the *general* condition, and free fatigue to be used otherwise. This takes us back to Alternative One where the word, fatigue, is abandoned as a technical term, or to Alternatives Two and Four where one form of incapacitation is called fatigue.

ALTERNATIVE FOUR: to accept the idea that fatigue is a condition that only the individual can identify in himself, since it is a kind of experience. This alternative lies in the category already labelled as personalistic.

These categories are not purely theoretical and hypothetical. They are implied in various studies found in the literature. The trouble is that one writer uses one category and others use the others. This leaves the field in confusion. Few, if any, of the data dictate which category to use. And this is just the point, clarification will only come from arrival at some voluntary agreement about labelling and taxonomy.

Some years ago, I was called upon to review the work done in the name of fatigue. After gathering the material together, it seemed that about the best way to deal with the actual studies given the fatigue label was to classify them into four groups, as follows:

Class One Studies: (a) those studying cells under prolonged activity; (b) those investigating hormones and vitamins; (c) those dealing with drugs; (d) those varying diet; (e) those varying conditions such as oxygen availability, X-ray irradiation, etc.

Class Two Studies: focusing on changes in the function of various parts of the body, such as the visual or auditory systems, and the visceral systems.

Class Three Studies: studies of exertion of the individual as in various work situations.

Class Four Studies: studies of the kinds of performance decrement or deterioration in intellectual rather than exertional tasks.

An inspection of these groups indicates that they are quite different from each other. Whatever fatigue is, it must be something that is common to all the groups. The most obvious commonality is *change,* and this change is toward deterioration in activity. What the changes are in the first group is not made explicit, but obviously they represent quite a diversity. In the groups as a total, then it would seem that fatigue is simply another name for *incapacitation* and the question of human experience or awareness is entirely omitted.

It is not claimed that the groupings are complete, for some studies could have been found in which human sensation, perception and feelings were the objects of study or were at least considered as more than merely incidental. The groups as listed pretty well covered the kinds of studies that would be considered relevant by a physiologist.

One might ask the question of why can't such a list be taken as representing an appropriate view of fatigue, a view in which fatigue is simply a synonym for several other broad generic terms such as incapacitation, deterioration in function, and the like? In other words, what is wrong with the way *fatigue* as a word or concept is now used? This can be answered by what was said in the first part of this chapter. It violates the historic use of the term which should have priority over the indiscriminate variety of meanings that have gotten attached to the word by accretion and it involves several logical incompatibilities.

The very accretive process itself (i.e. the social process in the development of knowledge and understanding) is one in which the old and the new become illogically jumbled together and this breeds confusion and frustrates communication. Once the connotation of fatigue becomes as general as the words, change and incapacitation, it loses much of its original force and uniqueness. It means that those who used fatigue to indicate something about human experience (a kind of self-recognized condition) are pushed out of "house and home" and left to hunt a new term for the phenomena they are dealing with.

We continue to be brought back to the fact that fatigue began as a label for a human condition, and that it still has this as one connotation. The existence of plural connotations is not as sophisticated a practice as we should exhibit.

Physicists and others have recognized the need for standardization of terms and have brought a great deal of this about by mutual consent. The most obvious cases are those in which units of measurement are standardized. Biologists, where phenomena of various levels of organization are unavoidably being dealt with, might well concern themselves with concepts and a language that would possess as much internal consistency as possible.

BIBLIOGRAPHY

Bartley, S. H.: Fatigue and inadequacy. *Physiol Revs, 37*:301-324, 1957.

Bartley, S. H., and E. Chute: *Fatigue and Impairment in Man.* New York, McGraw-Hill, 1947; Reprinted, New York: Johnson Reprint Corp., 1969.

Bills, A. G.: *The Psychology of Efficiency.* New York, Harper, 1943.

Muscio, B.: Is a fatigue test possible? *Br J Psychol, 12*:31-46, 1921.

Simonson, E.: Der Heutige Stand der Theorie der Ermüdung. *Ergebn Physiol, 37*:299, 1935.

Simonson, E.: *Physiology of Work Capacity and Fatigue.* Springfield, Thomas, 1971.

Epilogue

HANS SCHAEFER

FATIGUE IS ONE of the most exciting and most mysterious phenomena profoundly affecting our very existence, as any reader can tell when he attempts to integrate the multifaceted aspects of fatigue presented in this book. Fatigue decides the outcome of our endeavors: success or failure, achievement or resignation, alertness or submergence in sleep or forgetfulness. At the same time, fatigue is the key for understanding the genius whose distinction often consists largely in an extraordinary memory and nearly absent fatiguability.

Whoever considers the possibilities of a physiological interpretation for psychological phenomena, will be more reserved in explaining the mechanisms of mental and psychological processes as he knows more of their fundamental basis. Probably every physiologist, unless he is mystically oriented, will admit that there cannot be anything in the consciousness of man which is not somehow related to biochemical-physical processes in the brain. However, as investigators in the natural sciences, we have to admit that this assumption itself has some mystical characteristics, as soon as one proceeds further than the crude relationship and mere recognition of the existence of a somatic basis for psychological processes. We know that certain psychological functions are closely related to neurophysiological processes; for instance, attention and vigilance which are determined by impulses conducted to the thalamus. However, the true detailed basis of these mental states which Bollnow described from phenomenal aspects and Gellhorn from neurophysiological aspects remains "in the dark."

The history of fatigue which I have lived through as physiologist, from Mosso's experiments to the metabolic theories, particularly lactic acid accumulation, was a chain of errors. The erroneous conclusions were drawn mainly on two levels: on the one hand the theories of metabolic causes for fatigue phenomena had to be revised, and then there was the controversy about the fatigue phenomenon itself (i.e. its definition) and its dependence on such metabolic processes that occur in prolonged activity. Such processes alone do not determine the fatigue phenomena. Rather, something else is involved, whose physiological correlate is still unknown and its clarification is complicated by two characteristic difficulties. The first is the fundamental impossibility in distinctly correlating identifiable somatic processes to all psychological processes. The machinery of the organic process is so complicated that a correlation matrix between seemingly simple psychological functions and the incredibly complex structure of cerebral processes cannot as yet be constructed. The second difficulty is due to the fact that the central nervous processes are more than enormously complex. They are also connected by feedback loops whose mechanisms cannot at present even be simulated by models.

A relatively simple principle of such feedback is illustrated by the connection between state of arousal and blood pressure (Heinemann, et al.). It functions in such a way that anything which increases the blood pressure, also increases drive, and a depressed level of drive in turn decreases the blood pressure, as is well known through a decreasing tonic sympathetic activity. Such processes, however, are only the very simplest illustration of feedback coupling among drive, emotional activity and psychological and somatic efficiency.

The somatic sensation, i.e. a feeling of having a body with qualities of fitness, of increased or reduced capabilities, and with a sensation of being embedded in a surrounding, mysterious, unexplainable world, is a universe full of subjective intrigue. It has been analysed by ingenious phenomenologists like Merleau-Ponty, Plügge, Herman Schmitz, and Erwin Strauss. The "Psychology of the Human World" (Strauss) deeply affects the performance capability of man. Such phenomena are accessible only to introspective self-recognition and cannot be translated into neurophysiology. Yet, they are, nevertheless, very real and no less useful than nerve action potentials.

This world especially has not yet been analysed with respect to the normal worker. To understand the phenomena of the working world an anthropology of working man is still missing. The anthropologists can depict the phenomena of a highly sophisticated, highly introspective person (with high level of reflections), however valuable their conclusions may be for giving reports. The world of mental states is little reflective and very elemental, almost subconscious by definition, and largely inaccessible to rational analysis.

The epilogue of a physiologist, therefore, viewing the complexity of the phenomena, ends with a contemplation of the rational limits. It would be a gross mistake to believe that this world of "not quite rational" is not physiology any more. On the contrary, it is here that the physiology, if at all, begins to be understandable again: in the world of simple neurohormonal causes of largely subconscious emotional processes. The science of fatigue has to do with both spheres: the rational world and the world of subconscious processes, which are probably more decisive for the general course of things than rationality. Both spheres, of course, can be explored only in a scientific way, and this is the very appeal of such a science of fatigue. The approach in these two volumes clearly illustrates these two worlds. Fatigue is perhaps the best example of a psychosomatic process that one can imagine. Its analysis expands our perspective, ultimately leading to the recognition that "There are more things in heaven and earth than are dreamt of in our philosophy" of fatigue.

BIBLIOGRAPHY

Bollnow, O. F.: *Der Wesen der Hemmungen.* Frankfurt A. M., Klostermann, 1968.

Gellhorn, E.: *Autonomic Imbalance and the Hypothalamus.* Minneapolis, U Minn Pr, 1957.

Gellhorn, E.: *Autonomic-Somatic Integrations.* Minneapolis, U Minn Pr, 1967.

Heinemann, H., H. Schaefer, and V. Sturm: Die Interferenz von Kardiovaskularen Antworten und Affektivem Verholten. *Schweiz Med Wochenschr, 100*:184, 1970.

Merleau-Pouty, M.: *Phenomenologie de la Perception.* Paris, 1945.

Plügge, H.: *Wohlbefinden und Missempfinden.* Tübingen, Niemeyer, 1962.

Schmitt, H.: *Der Gefuhlsraum System der Philosophie.* Bonn, Bouvier, 111/2, 1969.

Straus, E.: *Psychologie der Menschlichen Welt.* Heidelberg, Springer, 1960.

Author Index

A

Abele, G., 211, 216
Abrahams, J. P., 257, 263, 267
Acheson, G. H., 64, 102
Agarwal, G. C., 60, 99
Ahlborg, G., 38
Aizerman, M. A., 60, 79, 97
Akert, K., 67, 103
Albers, W. R., 211, 217
Allphin, W., 167, 171, 175
Allport, F. H., 328, 329
Alluisi, E. A., 217
Amassian, V. E., 73, 97
Amberg, E., 238, 250
American Recommended Practice of Industrial Lighting, 164, 171
American Standard Code of Lighting, 164, 171
American Standard Practice for School Lighting, 164, 171
Andersen, P., 77, 97
Anderson, D. A., 256, 258, 260, 271
Anderson, N. McL., 40
Andrejeva, E. A., 60, 79, 97
Andrew, W., 255, 257
Andrews, T. G., 173, 229, 236
Angeleri, F. A., 112, 132
Anonymous, 194, 216
Antoni, W., 324, 329
Aoyama, M., 67, 97
Appelberg, H., 78, 97
Appley, M. H., 307, 329
Arieff, A. J., 102
Armstrong, R. B., 38
Aronson, E., 309, 335, 359, 365, 405
Asami, T., 107, 122, 132
Asanuma, H., 80, 83, 97
Aschaffenburg, G., 238, 250
Aschoff, J., 301, 329
Ash, I. E., 308, 329
Ashworth, B., 131, 132
Askew, E. W., 16, 37
Astrand, P.-O., 8, 11, 15, 16, 18, 19, 20, 22, 24, 27, 37, 38, 266, 267, 390, 391, 400
Atkins, E., 104, 163, 171
Atkinson, J. W., 290, 291, 299, 300, 311, 315, 323, 329, 332

B

Babadjanian, M. G., 111, 132
Babadschanjan, M. G., 245, 250
Babin, W. L., 111, 132
Babloyantz, A., 333
Bailey, D. E., 382, 383, 405
Bain, G., 210, 217
Bakan, P., 210, 212, 215, 216
Baker, C. H., 213, 215, 216, 281
Baker, R. A., 202, 203, 216
Bakers, J. H., 344, 400
Balke, B., 16, 37
Ballard, G., 176, 189
Baltes, P. B., 259, 267, 270
Barber, T. X., 309, 329
Barborka, C. J., 98
Barcroft, J., 65, 97
Barcroft, M., 18, 37
Barker, D., 121, 132
Barnard, R. J., 37
Bar-Or, O., 391, 393, 399, 400
Barrera, S. E., 69, 102
Barron, D. H., 97
Bartemeir, L. H., 66, 103
Bartenwerfer, H., 285, 300, 313, 314, 322, 326, 329
Bartlett, C. S., 225, 234
Bartlett, F. C., 106-107, 112, 116, 132, 288, 289, 329
Bartley, S. H., 156, 165, 166, 170, 171, 173, 227, 234, 285, 287, 288, 298, 300, 313, 314, 329, 331, 358, 359, 374, 375, 398, 400, 402, 411, 414
Bartoshuk, A. K., 313, 329
Baschnagel, N. A., 109, 134
Basmajian, J. V., 391, 401
Basowitz, H., 262, 269
Bateson, G., 328, 329

Bauer, P. S., 38
Baumler, G., 242, 243, 244, 251
Baur, A., 222, 234
Beaver, W. L., 42
Beckett, S., 134
Beecher, H. K., 371, 401, 404
Behr, E., 248, 251
Beinert, R. L., 225, 234
Belbin, R. M., 264, 265
Belding, H. S., 392, 403
Belenkii, V. Ye., 78, 97
Bell, C. W., 403
Bellet, S., 275, 280
Bellia, G., 112, 132
Benton, R. W., 182, 185, 190
Benua, N. N., 257, 258
Berens, C., 159, 162, 171, 173, 222, 234
Berger, R. A., 84, 103, 107, 111, 135
Bergsteinova, V., 404
Bergstrom, J., 27, 28, 37, 40
Bergum, B. O., 314, 329
Berkowitz, B., 260, 267
Bernard, J., 85, 98
Bernhard, C. G., 77, 97
Bernyer, G., 340, 345, 347, 375, 401
Bertalanfafy, L., von, 328, 329
Bertrand, A. B., 280
Bevegard, B. G., 19, 31, 37
Bieber, I., 71, 76, 97
Bigland, B., 10, 37
Bigland-Ritchie, B., 20, 37
Bills, A. G., 211, 214, 216, 240, 241, 242, 243, 244, 251, 289, 329, 411, 414
Bintig, U., 264, 269
Bird, T. L., 332
Birney, R. C., 323, 329
Birren, J. E., 257, 260, 261, 262, 263, 265, 267, 271
Bishop, A., 76, 80, 97
Bitterman, M. E., 162, 167, 168, 170, 171, 174, 178, 188, 222, 225, 235

419

Black, J. E., 21, 37
Blankstein, S. S., 176, 181, 189, 190
Blatt, N., 159, 171
Blount, W. P., 161, 172
Bodansky, O., 188
Boden, Ch., 314, 330
Bohm, E., 77, 97
Bollnow, O. F., 415, 417
Bonde-Petersen, F., 20, 39, 402
Borchgrevink, C. F., 39
Borg, G., 31, 340, 341, 343, 344, 347, 366, 367, 391, 392, 395, 399, 400, 401, 404
Borges Dias, A., 225, 235
Bornemann, E., 285, 329
Boshes, B., 102
Bosma, J. F., 59, 79, 97
Bottiger, I., 29, 37
Botwinick, J., 114, 132, 260, 262, 263, 267, 268
Bouisset, S., 20, 37
Bourguignon, G., 176, 188, 216
Bowers, R., 37
Bracken, H., von, 232, 233, 235, 285, 316, 327, 329, 330
Branam, G., 37
Branks, J., 248, 251, 313, 330
Bransford, T., 276, 280
Braun, J. C., 279, 281
Braunwald, E., 38
Bredenkamp, J., 179, 181, 185, 188
Breen, L. Z., 264, 268
Bremer, F., 185, 188
Brengelmann, G. L., 41
Brewer, R. L., 332
Brinley, J. F., 268
Britten, R. H., 221, 237
Broadbent, D. E., 208, 213, 214, 215, 243, 244, 251, 279, 280, 314, 330
Brody, H., 255, 257
Brouha, L., 190
Brown, F. A., Jr., 301, 330
Brown, M., 102
Browne, R. C., 289, 330
Brozek, J., 158, 162, 163, 164, 167, 168, 169, 170, 172, 174, 177, 181, 182, 184, 188, 190, 221, 224, 225, 226, 235, 237, 319, 330

Bryan, J. F., 313, 332
Buchthal, F., 125, 132
Buckley, C. J., 362, 398, 399, 401
Bujas, Z., 183, 184, 188, 340, 347, 348, 363, 374, 377, 386, 390, 401
Bunning, E., 301, 330
Burdick, H., 329
Burge, E. L., 97
Burge, W. E., 88, 97, 136
Burgess, M., 248, 251
Burnham, W. H., 285, 330
Burns, N., 281
Burnstein, E., 312, 330
Busch, H., 158, 172, 178, 180, 181, 184, 185, 188
Busila, V., 103
Buskirk, E., 21, 37, 400, 404
Byars, G. E., Jr., 339, 360, 363, 374, 382, 398, 399, 404
Byrne-Quinn, E., 42

C

Cafarelli, E., 403, 404
Cain, W. S., 346, 347, 401, 405
Calapay, G. G., 112, 132
Caldwell, L. S., 368, 370, 371, 373, 375, 396, 400, 401, 403
Carlock, J., 363, 405
Carmichael, L., 161, 163, 170, 172, 221, 225, 235
Carns, M. L., 95, 99
Carpenter, G. C., 172
Carstocea, L., 112, 132, 133
Carterette, E. C., 227, 235
Casey, S., 217
Cattell, R. B., 261, 269, 307, 330
Chaffin, D. B., 126, 132
Chambers, W. W., 102
Chatel, J. C., 298, 330
Chave, E. J., 338, 405
Cheah, J. S., 119, 120, 127, 132
Cherepakhim, M. A., 88, 98
Chernilovskaya, F. M., 163, 172
Chin, N. K., 121, 132
Chown, S., 265, 269
Christensen, E. H., 27, 29, 37
Chute, E., 156 170, 171, 274, 275, 285, 329, 400, 411, 414

Cisler, L. E., 355, 387, 402
Cizek, P., 173
Clark, F. L., 264, 268
Clark, G. F., 189
Clark, R. A., 332
Clark, S. L., 103
Clausen, J. P., 21, 37
Clawson, B. J., 255, 257, 274, 280
Clay, M. H., 264, 266, 268
Cleghorn, R. A., 349, 403
Cliff, N., 337, 401
Clinton, M., 174
Close, R. I., 37
Clough, J. F. M., 79, 98
Cobb, L. A., 31, 37
Cobb, P. W., 276, 277, 278, 280
Cogan, D. G., 157, 172
Cogan, F. C., 157, 172
Coghill, G. E., 65, 98
Cohen, L. A., 75, 98
Coleman, T. G., 39
Collier, R. M., 91, 98
Collins, J. B., 166, 172, 224, 235
Collins, V. P., 274, 280
Cloquhoun, W. P., 197, 199, 200, 216, 280, 307, 330
Conrad, H. S., 259, 269
Cooper, C. J., 112, 132
Cope, M., 132
Costa, L. D., 112, 135
Costill, D. L., 28, 38
Cottrell, C. L., 171, 174
Courts, F. A., 248, 251, 313, 330
Craig, F. N., 16, 38
Craik, F. J. M., 262, 268
Creed, R. S., 63, 98
Cronbach, L. J., 367, 401
Crooker, T. G., 332, 353, 402
Crossman, E. R. F. W., 214, 216
Crovitz, E., 262, 268

D

Dadzio, W., 264, 269
Dahlstrom, H., 341, 375, 401
Dahm, J., 102
Danforth, W. H., 39
Dardano, J. F., 215, 216
Daric, J., 264, 268
Davey, C. P., 112, 132

Author Index

Davidson, W. Z., 315, 330
Davis, D. R., 249, 251, 300, 315, 330
Davis, R. C., 226, 235
Davis, S. W., 179, 189
Dearborn, W. F., 161, 163, 170, 172, 221, 225, 235
DeCharms, R., 293, 330
Decker, J. D., 65, 98
Deering, I. D., 102
Deese, J., 196, 213, 216
Dejours, P., 16, 17, 30, 38
De Lattre, J., 39
Della Corte, M., 333
Dellow, P. G., 101
Del Pozo, E. C., 70, 99
Dember, W. N., 317, 330
Demilia, L. A., 170, 172
Demmel, W., 225, 235
Denny-Brown, D. E., 65, 72, 94, 98
Deroanne, R., 40
De Robertis, E., 86, 98
Dill, D. B., 29, 31, 38
Diringshofen, H., von, 208, 216
Dirken, J. M., 401
Dix, M. R., 227, 235
Dobin, N. B., 102
Docktor, R., 394, 401
Doctor, H. J., 364, 403
Dodge, R., 165, 172
Doerr, H. O., 248, 251
Dohm, G. L., 37
Doll, E., 40
Donders, F. C., 112, 132
Doney, R. G., 280
Dornhorst, A. C., 18, 27
Doudlah, A. M., 92, 104
Dow, R. S., 102
Dowduff, M. D., 279, 281
Dowdy, R. P., 37
Downs, S., 262, 268
Dreher, G., 259, 269
Drew, G. C., 211, 216, 272, 280
Drinkwater, B. L., 333
Duffield, D. W., 98
Dujardin, J., 40
Duker, E., 210, 216
Duker, H., 179, 189, 210, 211, 216, 217, 238, 244, 251, 260, 268, 293, 319, 330
Dunne, A. C., 264, 268

Dureman, E. I., 314, 330
Durig, A., 221, 235

E

Eagan, C. J., 119, 120, 122, 127, 135
Eagles, J. B., 233, 235, 249, 251
Eason, R. G., 248, 251, 313, 330, 347, 401
Eastman, A. A., 280
Easton, T. A., 11, 58, 62, 75, 93, 95, 98, 106, 118, 121, 125
Ebashi, S., 9, 38
Eccles, J. C., 11, 38, 86, 87, 98
Eccles, R. M., 78, 98
Edgerton, V. R., 37
Edstrom, L., 121, 125, 134
Edwards, A. L., 360, 401
Edwards, H. T., 38
Edwards, R. H. T., 391, 393, 402
Egan, J. P., 227, 235
Egbert, L. D., 371, 404
Ehlers, Th., 320, 330
Ehrenstein, W., 228, 229, 235
Eisdorfer, C., 262, 268
Eisler, H., 344, 375, 402
Eitner, S., 266, 268
Ekblom, B., 22, 38, 391, 392, 393, 394, 399, 400, 402
Ekelund, L.-G., 30, 31, 38, 402
Ekman, G., 340, 341, 402
Elbel, E. R., 108, 111, 132
Elbel, H., 211, 217
Elias, R., 132
Elliot, E., 214, 217
Ellis, R. S., 255, 258
El'ner, A. M., 77, 78, 102
Emonet-Denand, F., 78, 97
Endo, K., 189
Endo, M., 38
Engel, W. K., 11, 41
Engels, J. B., 299, 330
Eno Foundation for Highway Traffic Control, 276, 277, 280
Enzer, N., 7, 41, 158, 174, 176, 177, 181, 182, 185, 189, 210, 218, 256, 258, 358, 404
Enzer, V., 319, 334
Epstein, S. E., 38

Erb, W. H., 117, 133
Erlemeier, N., 260, 270
Essen, B., 25, 41
Ettema, J. H., 251
Evans, O. W., 217
Evans, W. O., 382, 402, 405
Everts, E. V., 11, 38
Eysenck, H. J., 210, 217

F

Faber, I. E., 334
Fabrycky, J., 296, 330
Faloona, G. R., 37
Farr, S. D., 109, 134
Fatigue of Workers, 165, 172
Faulkner, J. A., 28, 38, 40
Feather, N. T., 308, 330
Fechner, G. T., 340, 402
Felig, P., 29, 38
Felpel, L. P., 67, 102
Ferree, C. E., 162, 172, 224, 235
Ferroni, A., 132
Festinger, L., 292, 330
Fidone, S. J., 77, 98
Filippov, B. G., 135
Filley, G. F., 42
Finkelman, I., 102
Finkle, J. R., 102
Fisch, H., 331
Fisch, R., 291, 331
Fischbein, E., 314, 331
Fischgold, H., 85, 98
Flandrois, R., 133
Fleishman, E. A., 300, 310, 331
Florek, H., 159, 168, 170, 172
Folkow, B., 18, 38
Foltz, E. E., 91, 98, 355, 358, 359, 374, 387, 402
Fomin, S. V., 98
Forbes, A., 87, 98
Forsaith, B., 264, 270
Fox, R. H., 219
Frankenhaeuser, M., 391, 402
Franklin, J. C., 162, 172
Frankstein, S. I., 101
Freedy, A., 332
French, E. G., 300, 331
French, J. D., 210, 217
Freud, S., 298, 331
Friedman, A. S., 260, 268
Friedman, S., 168, 172
Frohlich, F. W., 221, 235

Frolkis, V. V., 257, 258
Fruktov, J. M., 111, 133
Fry, G. A., 157, 171, 173
Fuhrer, 309
Fujihara, Y., 38
Fukuda, J., 173
Fukuda, T., 73, 75, 98
Fulton, J. F., 71, 75, 76, 97, 98, 100
Furakawa, T., 37

G

Gagge, A. P., 373, 375, 385, 397, 400, 402
Galanter, E. H., 344, 405
Gamberale, F., 367, 368, 375, 391, 393, 394, 399, 402
Gangleberger, J. A., 112, 133
Gardner, M. B., 227, 235
Garron, D. C., 307, 331
Garvey, W. D., 200, 217
Gawrila, L., 271
Gawrilescu, N., 112, 133
Gazzaniga, 75
Geldard, F. A., 157, 173
Gelfand, I. M., 56, 98
Gellhorn, E., 59, 79, 97, 99, 100, 101, 415, 417
Gerathewohl, S. J., 208, 217, 221, 235
Gerben, J. J., 391, 394, 400, 402
Gerbrandy, J., 119, 122, 127, 136
Gernandt, B. E., 66, 67, 99
Gibbons, D., 274, 281
Gilden, L., 112, 135
Gilman, S., 72, 78, 99, 104
Gilson, W. E., 133
Givener, I., 166, 173
Glanzer, M., 260, 268
Glaser, R., 260, 268
Glennon, J. A., 135
Goldbarg, A. N., 38, 391, 392, 393, 394, 399, 400, 402
Goldman, M. R., 133
Goldsmith, R., 219
Goldstein, L. G., 276, 279, 280
Gollnick, P. D., 12, 16, 28, 29, 38
Goralewski, G., 208, 217
Gottlieb, G. L., 60, 82, 99
Goubel, F., 20, 37

Gowing, J., 219
Graf, O., 211, 217, 226, 235, 238, 251
Graham, J. R., 225, 234
Graham-Brown, T., 62, 99
Granati, A., 132
Grandjean, E. P., 35, 39, 181, 185, 186, 189, 190, 286, 297, 304, 306, 314, 317, 320, 331, 335, 375, 377, 405
Granger, H. J., 39
Granick, S., 260, 268
Granit, R., 59, 99, 106, 221, 235
Grechow, J., 211, 217
Green, R. E., 260, 267
Green, R. F., 260, 268
Greenbaum, H. B., 346, 405
Greenberg, L. A., 170, 173
Gregor, R., 38
Gregory, M., 208, 216
Greisen, L., 227, 235
Griew, S., 264, 270
Griffith, J. W., 353, 374, 402
Grigg, P., 77, 99
Grillner, S., 82, 99
Grimby, G., 10, 21, 39
Grimby, L., 11, 39, 131, 132, 133
Grindley, W., 221, 235
Groll-Knapp, E., 112, 133
Gross, I. H., 298, 331, 358, 359, 398, 402
Grossman, J. L., 262, 269
Grossman, S. P., 11, 39
Grun, D., 39
Gualtierotti, T., 134
Guilford, J. P., 337, 338, 361, 402
Gunther, N., 228, 235
Gurfinkel, V. S., 97, 98
Guth, S. K., 276, 280
Gutin, B., 112, 133
Guttich, H., 259, 268
Guyton, A. C., 18, 39
Guzman, F. C., 70, 99

H

Haddy, F. J., 19, 39
Hafemann, G., 225, 235
Hagbarth, K.-E., 62, 99
Haggard, H. W., 170, 173
Haggendal, E., 39
Haggendal, J., 112, 133

Haider, M., 112, 133, 232, 235, 326, 331
Halberg, F., 301, 302, 304, 307, 331, 332, 334
Halberstam, J. L., 262, 271
Hale, H. B., 362, 402
Hall, K. R. L., 332, 353, 402
Haller, J. S., 299, 331
Halliday, A. M., 233, 235, 249, 251, 330
Halstead, W. C., 166, 173
Halverson, H. M., 76, 80, 99
Hamburger, V., 65, 98, 99
Hampton, I. F. G., 219
Hannerz, J., 10, 11, 39, 131, 133
Hannon, J. P., 41, 42, 385, 405
Hansen, O., 27, 29, 37
Harper, C. R., 211, 217
Harris, D. A., 362, 402
Harris, J. D., 227, 236
Hart, B. L., 64, 99
Hartley, L. H., 22, 29, 31, 39
Hartman, B. O., 362, 398, 399, 401, 402
Hartmann, E., 201, 217, 229, 230, 236
Hartridge, H., 158, 173, 222, 236
Hartson, L. D., 116, 133
Hashimoto, K. K., 181, 185, 186, 189, 320, 331
Hassler, R., 11, 40
Hastings, J. W., 331
Hathaway, S., 114, 133
Hauty, G. T., 361, 402
Havel, R. J., 15, 39
Hawkes, G. R., 217
Hayes, K. C., 90, 91, 93, 94, 95, 99, 107, 111, 112, 114, 116, 119, 120, 123, 124, 125, 127, 133, 134
Haywood, H. C., 312, 331
Head, H., 193, 217
Hecht, E., 208, 217
Heckhausen, H., 290, 291, 300, 323, 331
Heinemann, H., 416, 417
Hellebrandt, F. A., 90, 91, 92, 93, 95, 99-100, 104
Helmholtz, H., von, 108, 133, 221, 236
Helmreich, E., 13, 39

Hemphill, R. E., 298, 332, 353, 402
Henane, R., 89, 90, 94, 100, 101-102, 107, 118, 121, 123, 128, 129, 133, 134
Henatsch, E.-M., 102
Henatsch, H. D., 102
Hendler, R., 38
Hendley, C. D., 188
Henneman, E., 8, 9, 10, 27, 28, 33, 39, 128, 133
Henriksson, J., 20, 39, 391, 392, 393, 394, 395, 399, 402
Henschel, A., 266, 269
Hermansen, L., 37
Hernandez-Peon, R., 243, 251
Heron, A., 265, 269, 279, 280
Herwig, B., 226, 236
Hesser, C. M., 402
Heumann, G., 238, 251
Heuting, J. E., 364, 365, 399, 402
Heymans, C., 38
Hick, E. E., 244, 251
Hick, W. E., 214, 217
Hildebrandt, G., 301, 307, 332
Hildebrandt, J., 38
Hines, M., 75, 103
Hirsch, J. A., 222, 236
Hirsche, H., 23, 39
Hirsh, I. J., 227, 236
Hofbauer, H., 264, 269
Hoffmann, G., 211, 218, 274, 275, 280
Hofstetter, H. W., 159, 160, 173, 222, 236
Hogan, R. P., 39
Hokanson, J. E., 246, 248, 249, 251, 252
Holfeld, L., 225, 235
Halland, J. G., 214, 217
Holmgren, A., 20, 31, 38, 39
Holmqvist, B., 63, 78, 82, 93, 100
Holst, E., von, 228, 236
Holway, A. H., 157, 162, 173, 236
Hongo, T., 67, 78, 81, 97, 99, 100, 103
Horn, G., 86, 100
Horn, J. L., 261, 269
Hornstra, L., 315, 332
Horvath, S. M., 333

Hosman, J., 346, 402
Houk, J. C., 8, 39, 128, 133
House, J. L., 402
Houtz, S. J., 99
Howe, L., 159, 173
Huemme, U., 102
Huizing, H. C., 227, 236
Hulicka, I. M., 262, 269
Hull, C. L., 309, 362, 402, 403
Hultman, E., 12, 13, 14, 24, 37, 40
Hunt, C. C., 128, 133
Hurvich, L. M., 157, 162, 173, 236
Huston, R. L., 37
Huxley, H. E., 9, 40
Hyde, J., 79, 100
Hylan, J. P., 238, 251
Human, R., 214, 217, 244, 251

I

Ianuzzo, C. D., 38
Ingemann Jensen, J. H., 17, 40
Ishizuka, T., 182, 189
Iskander, A., 148, 149, 150, 151
Issekutz, A. C., 40
Issekutz, B., Jr., 15, 16, 28, 29, 40
Ito, T., 71, 100
Ives, J. E., 165, 173
Ives, J. H., 175, 221, 237
Ivy, A. C., 98, 210, 218
Iwama, K., 182, 183, 189

J

Jackson, D., 337, 403
Jacobs, M. J., 65, 100
Jacobsen, C. F., 98
Jankowska, E., 78, 82, 100
Jansen, G., 227, 236
Janssen, C. G. C., 364, 403
Jansson, E. D., 38
Jarrard, L. E., 308, 332
Jenik, P., 138, 142, 150
Jenkins, H. M., 196, 217
Jerison, H. J., 210, 217
Johnson, B. L., 120, 122, 128, 134
Johnson, D. A., 79, 99
Johnson, E. A., 331
Johnson, R. E., 190

Johnson, W. A., 362, 402
Johnson, W. P., 31, 37
Jokl, E., 122, 128, 134
Jokl, P., 122, 128, 134
Joly, R., 103
Jones, E. E., 334, 365, 366, 403, 405
Jones, H. E., 259, 269
Jones, L. G., 39
Jones, W. B., 19, 40
Jorfeldt, L., 37, 40
Joteyko, J., 91, 100
Jouvet, M., 251
Jung, F. T., 355, 387, 402
Jung, R., 11, 40

K

Kahler, R. L., 38
Kalsbeek, J. W. H., 245, 251
Kalveram, K. T., 320, 332
Kaminsky, G., 143, 150
Kamon, E., 392, 403
Kanabrocki, E. L., 301, 332
Kanouse, D., 366, 403
Kapri, M., 103
Karkovic, A., 183, 188
Karlsson, J., 13, 14, 25, 40
Karpatkin, S., 39
Karpovich, P. V., 89, 90, 93, 94, 104, 107, 118, 119, 120, 123, 135
Kashiwagi, S., 379, 404
Katinas, G. S., 302, 331
Kato, M., 67, 100
Kaufman, R. P., 135
Kawamura, T., 120, 123, 134
Kay, C., 391, 403
Kay, H., 262, 263, 269
Keevil-Rogers, P., 262, 269
Keiper, Ch., 258, 271, 281
Kelley, H. H., 366, 403
Kelso, A., 177, 184, 190
Kennard, M. A., 75, 76, 98, 100
Kennedy, J. L., 175
Kennedy, W. P., 161, 174
Keppler, D., 40
Kernell, D., 98
Kerr, W. A., 353, 402, 403
Kesert, B. H., 102
Kety, S. S., 256, 258
Keul, J., 14, 15, 16, 22, 40
Keys, A., 167, 169, 172, 174, 177, 179, 182, 188, 190, 224,

226, 235, 258, 319, 330
Khitum, S. A., 135
Kilborn, A., 38
Kilpatrick, F. P., 360, 401
Kimura, N., 123, 134
King, D. W., 12, 29, 38
Kinsman, R. A., 42, 286, 288, 292, 295, 300, 301, 306, 307, 332, 359, 375, 380, 382, 383, 384, 385, 387, 390, 399, 403, 405
Kirchner, W., 279, 280
Kirihara, S., 378, 403
Kirk, R. E., 208, 217
Kleitman, N., 233, 236, 304, 307, 332
Klemm, W. R., 71, 100
Klett, C. J., 339, 404
Kline, J. S., 42
Klinger, E., 290, 308, 312, 323, 332
Klix, F., 328, 332
Knehr, C. A., 162, 173
Knochel, J. P., 37
Knuttgen, H. G., 25, 40, 402
Kodat, V., 173
Kogi, K., 186, 189, 331, 379, 391, 398, 399, 403, 404
Kolb, S., 105
Korbsch, 233
Korchin, S. J., 262, 269
Kornetsky, G., 210, 217
Kostina, J. I., 132, 250
Kostyuk, P. G., 77, 101
Kotchen, T. A., 39
Kots, Ya. M., 59, 80, 82, 101
Koyal, S. N., 42
Koyl, L., 259, 269
Kraepelin, E., 238, 244, 251, 252, 285, 334
Krakov, 185
Kramer, K., 18, 40
Kraning, K. K., 41
Kreps, J. M., 265, 269
Krikorian, A. M., 99
Krivohlavy, J., 160, 173
Krkovic, A., 377, 401
Kroebel, W., 221, 236
Kroll, W., 89, 90, 91, 93, 101, 107, 111, 112, 114, 116, 117, 118, 122, 123, 134
Krouse, R., 97, 136
Kryshanowskaja, W. W., 271
Kryter, K. D., 227, 236

Kubota, K., 103
Kudina, L. P., 121, 135
Kudo, N., 97, 100
Kugelberg, E., 121, 125, 131, 132, 134
Kunigk, H., 264, 269
Kuno, M., 78, 101
Kupfmuller, K., 138, 150
Kurtz, J. I., 161, 173
Kuypers, H. G. J. M., 77, 101
Kyreileis, 221

L

Lacour, J., 39
Lagasse, P. P., 114, 134
Laird, D., 227, 236
Lambert, E. H., 123, 134
Lambertsen, C. J., 182, 189
Lampert, U., 267, 269
Lamy, M., 40
Lancaster, W. B., 159, 173
Landis, C., 189, 319, 332
Lapierre, J., 104, 136
Lapique, L., 176, 189
Larner, J., 12, 40
Lashley, K. S., 242, 252
Lassen, N. A., 21, 37
Lauer, A. R., 272, 277, 278, 279, 280
Laughlin, H. P., 298, 299, 315, 332
Laurig, W., 147, 150
Laursen, A. M., 77, 101
Lawrence, D. G., 77, 101
Lee, J., 334
Lee, R. H., 177, 189
Lefebvre, R., 104, 136
Lehr, D. J., 314, 329
Lehr, U., 259, 261, 269, 271, 308, 334
Lenzi, R., 132
Levinson, E. J., 38
Lewis, H. E., 219
Liddell, E. G. T., 98
Lighting for School Buildings, 164, 171
Linderholm, H., 391, 401
Lindsley, D. B., 286, 332
Ling, T. H., 102
Linquette, Y., 103
Lion, K. S., 167, 173
Lipak, J., 89, 101
Lippold, O. C. J., 10, 20, 37, 40, 115, 126, 134

Lisin, V. V., 82, 101
Liske, E., 211, 217
Liu, C. N., 102
Livingston, R. B., 67, 103
Lloyd, A. J., 366, 368, 369, 370, 371, 373, 375, 390, 395, 396, 397, 400, 403
Lloyd, D. P. C., 77, 101
Lober, P. H., 255, 258, 274, 280
Lochner, W., 189
Locke, E. A., 310, 311, 313, 332
Lockhart, A., 297, 333, 352, 404
Loeb, M., 210, 217
Loewenfeld, I. E., 185, 186, 187, 189, 224
Lombard, W. P., 118, 119, 120, 134
London, P., 309, 332
Long, H. A., 216, 280
Loofbourrow, G. N., 59, 101
Lottig, H., 208, 217
Lowe, H., 262, 269
Lowell, E. L., 332
Lowenstein, O., 166, 173, 185, 186, 187, 189, 224
Lucaccini, L. F., 314, 332
Luce, G. G., 301, 304, 332
Luce, R. D., 340, 403
Luchian, O., 133
Luckiesh, M., 161, 162, 163, 166, 168, 170, 173, 221, 225, 236
Ludwig, D., 300, 333
Lund, J. P., 66, 101
Lund, S., 99
Lundberg, A., 62, 78, 98, 100, 101
Luparello, T. J., 384, 387, 403
Lurie, A. A., 189
Lybrand, W. A., 167, 173, 229, 236
Lyman, J., 332

M

Macarez, J. A., 89, 94, 100, 101, 121, 123, 128, 129, 133, 134
Maciaszek, A., 108, 112, 114, 115, 226, 136
Mack, J. D., 343, 346, 405

Mackworth, J. F., 196, 210, 217
Mackworth, N. H., 193, 194, 196, 205, 210, 213, 217, 218
MacNeill, M., 219
Maddi, S. R., 307, 332
Magni, F., 82, 102
Magoun, H. W., 112, 135, 185, 189, 212, 218
Maling, H. M., 64, 102
Malomsoki, J., 109, 110, 111, 134, 135
Mamzashuili, M. I., 132, 250
Manni, E., 69, 102
Marcus, A., 315, 333
Marechal, R., 41
Maresca, M., 333
Margaria, R., 119, 120, 134
Markowitz, R. A., 371, 404
Marsden, C. D., 126, 129, 134
Mart'yanov, V. A., 82, 101
Masius, E., 267, 268
Mason, J. W., 39
Masters, A. M., 120, 134
Mateescu, R., 132
Mateev, D., 114, 134
Matsumoto, A., 67, 102
Maxwell, A. R., 280
Maxwell, L. C., 40
Mayne, R., 138, 150
Mayo, T. B., Jr., 353, 402
Mazzi, 221
McBaim, W. N., 208, 218
McCandless, B., 233, 234, 236
McClaskey, E. B., 366, 368, 369, 370, 371, 396, 400, 403
McClelland, D. C., 286, 288, 290, 291, 296, 318, 324, 330, 332, 333
McCormick, E. J., 307, 333
McCouch, G. P., 62, 67, 102
McCullough, R. E., 42
McDonald, W. I., 78, 99
McFann, H. H., 334
McFarland, R. A., 157, 160, 162, 173, 208, 218, 225, 232, 236, 267, 269, 270, 272, 275, 278, 279, 280
McGavach, Th., 255, 258
McGrath, S. D., 349, 363, 403
McLachlan, R. S., 101
McNelis, J. F., 280
McNelly, G., 339, 362, 363, 374, 398, 403

McNelly, F. W., Jr., 290, 308, 312, 332
McTaggart, W. G., 280
Mead, L. C., 175
Mederos, L. O., 134
Megirian, D., 66, 99
Meier-Ewert, K., 67, 102
Melcher, A., 402
Meltzer, H., 300, 333
Menzer, J., 371, 373, 375, 396, 403
Merkel, J., 214, 218, 244, 252
Merleau-Ponty, M., 416, 417
Merton, P. A., 106, 114, 115, 117, 126, 134
Messick, S., 337, 403
Metz, K. F., 403, 404
Meyer, D. L., 70, 102, 103
Meyer, M. F., 227, 236
Meyers, C. R., 109, 111, 134
Micko, H. Ch., 195, 196, 198, 200, 218
Mihaila, I., 133
Miles, C. C., 259, 270
Miles, W. R., 259, 270
Miles, W., 155
Miller, G. A., 226, 236
Miller, H. I., 40
Miller, J. G., 243, 252
Minzat, I., 331
Mitsuihashi, T., 379, 403
Moen, P., 301, 333
Monnier, M., 112, 113, 134
Monsson, C. D., 136
Mora, G., 299, 333
Morgan, W. P., 309, 323, 333, 391, 395, 400, 403
Mori, S., 67, 102
Morrison, D. F., 260, 268
Morrison, H. W., 330
Morton, H. B., 126, 134
Moruzzi, G., 112, 135, 185, 189, 212, 218
Mosel, J. N., 280
Moseley, A. L., 234, 236
Moss, F. K., 161, 162, 166, 168, 170, 173
Moss, F. M., 221, 225, 236
Mosso, A., 285, 333
Mosteller, F., 371, 404
Motokawa, K., 182, 183, 189
Mougey, E. H., 39
Mouillac-Baudevin, J., 78, 104

Mountcastle, V. B., 121, 135
Mucher, H., 180, 189, 313, 318, 333
Muller-Lyer, 229
Munson, N., 92, 104
Munsterberg, H., 285, 289, 333
Muravov, I. V., 257, 258
Murphy, D. B., 218
Murray, H. A., 290, 323, 333
Murray, J. A., 9, 41
Murrell, K. F. H., 264, 270
Muscio, B., 321, 333, 412, 414
Mutsler, R., 404
Myers, T. I., 218

N

Nack, G., 229, 236
Nagy, A. N., 172
Naimark, A., 39
Narasaki, S., 160, 173
Nash, D., 40
National Research Council: Conference on Visual Fatigue, 155, 174
Naumenko, A. I., 257, 258
Neal, G. L., 210, 218
Nehrke, M. F., 260, 270
Neil, E., 38
Nelson, W., 331
Nemessuri, M., 111, 135
Nesselroade, J. R., 259, 270
Newlin, E. P., 217
Nicholis, G., 333
Nicholson, W. M., 315, 333
Nisbett, R. E., 366, 403
Niven, J. R., 338, 403
Noble, B. J., 391, 392, 393, 399, 403, 404
Nobuko, T., 173
Nordesjo, L.-O., 40
Nordheden, B., 402
Norrsell, U., 101
Nowlis, H., 382, 403
Nowlis, V., 382, 403
Nunney, D. N., 359, 360, 374, 390, 399, 404
Nyberg-Hansen, R., 77, 102
Nystrom, C. L., 119, 120, 135

O

Obal, F., 40
O'Banion, K., 387, 403
Oden, M. H., 260, 271

O'Doherty, B., 267, 269
Ohtsuki, I., 38
Okhrimenko, A. P., 112, 136
Olechowsky, R., 262, 270
Olson, C. B., 10, 28, 33, 39
Oppel, 229
Oppenheim, R., 99
Orlovski, G. N., 69, 82, 102, 103
Orme, J. E., 301, 333
Ormond, E., 196, 216
Orne, M. T., 309, 333
Oscarsson, O., 81, 100, 102
Oshima, M., 179, 189
Oster, G., 275
Otis, A. B., 22, 41
Overall, J. E., 339, 404
Owen, S. G., 189
Owens, W. A., 260, 270

P

Pacella, B. L., 67, 102
Padykula, H. A., 41
Pafnote, M., 133
Pal'tsev, Ye. I., 59, 77, 78, 97, 102
Pampu, I., 331
Pandolf, K. B., 391, 392, 393, 395, 399, 400, 403, 404
Pang, M., 132
Parrish, A. M., 99
Partridge, M. J., 99
Paterson, D. G., 163, 174
Patton, H. D., 390, 391, 404
Paul, P., 15, 16, 27, 28, 29, 40
Pauli, R., 238, 243, 252
Pavlina, Z., 340, 347, 401
Pavlova, G. A., 82, 102
Payne, R. B., 361, 402
Pearson, R. G., 210, 218, 339, 360, 362, 363, 374, 382, 398, 399, 404
Peele, R., 298, 330
Pennington, L. L., 39
Perl, E. R., 78, 101
Pernow, B., 37, 39
Person, R. S., 121, 135
Petajan, J. A., 119, 120, 122, 127, 135
Peter, J. B., 37
Peterson, B. W., 67, 102
Petit, J. M., 40
Petruschkat, R., 329
Petz, B., 183, 188, 377, 401
Phillippson, M., 64, 80, 102

Phillips, C. G., 98
Phillips, W. H., 109, 111, 135
Pickett, R. M., 217
Pierson, W. R., 297, 333, 337, 351, 352, 353, 374, 404
Pirnay, F., 21, 22, 40, 41
Plateau, M. H., 340, 404
Platt, F. N., 272, 280
Plugge, H., 416, 417
Poffenberger, A. T., 360, 374, 398, 404
Poggendorf, 229
Poklekowsky, G., 138, 150
Pollock, L. J., 71, 102
Ponder, E., 161, 174
Popesco, P., 133
Post, B., 402
Poulton, E. C., 225, 236
Powesland, P., 264, 270
Preobrazhenskaya, I., 262, 270
Preston, J. B., 59, 77, 98, 104
Prichard, J. S., 83, 93, 103, 119, 135
Prigogine, I., 328, 333
Procacci, P., 307, 333
Prokop, L., 224, 236
Prokop, O., 224, 236
Provost, R., 279
Pruen, B., 166, 172, 224, 235
Pushkar, D., 219
Pyzik, S. W., 102

Q

Quarter, J., 315, 333
Quensel, W., 40
Quimby, J. T., 174
Quo, Sung-Ken, 88, 89, 103, 118, 135

R

Radermecker, R., 41
Rand, G., 162, 172, 224, 235
Ranson, S. W., 103
Rascano, V., 84, 103
Rasch, P. J., 351, 404
Raven, P. B., 333
Rechtmann, M. B., 101
Redfearn, J. W. T., 126, 134, 233, 235, 249, 251, 330
Reeves, T. J., 19, 40
Reid, C., 114, 135
Reinberg, A., 301, 303, 333
Reinfrank, R. F., 120, 127, 135

Reitman, W., 330
Reitnauer, P. G., 222-224, 237
Report No. 178: Summary of Fort Knox driver study, 277, 281
Report No. 318: Camp Lee driver study, 277, 278, 281
Resnikoff, P., 403
Rey, J. P., 181, 184, 189
Rey, P., 180, 181, 184, 186, 189
Rich, G. Q., 352, 404
Richardson, I. M., 264, 270
Richter, C. P., 66, 75, 103, 305, 333, 334
Ricketts, P. T., 39
Ricks, D. F., 307, 335
Riemann, H., 228, 237
Riss, W., 65, 81, 103
Rivers, W. H. R., 238, 252, 285, 334
Robbin, J. S., 268
Roberts, E. M., 104
Roberts, M. B. V., 84, 103
Roberts, T. D. M., 71, 103
Robinson, B. F., 38
Robinson, S., 16, 24, 41
Rodahl, K., 8, 11, 15, 16, 18, 19, 20, 22, 27, 37, 40, 390, 391, 400
Rohmert, W., 137, 138, 144, 147, 148, 149, 150, 151
Rohrer, H., 225, 237
Rosenblum, M., 73, 97
Rosenbrock, 147
Ross, S., 173, 200, 218, 229, 236
Roth, E., 262, 270
Rougier, G. Y., 90, 103
Rowan, M. P., 30, 41
Rowell, L. B., 18, 19, 21, 22, 24, 31, 41, 367, 404
Rozeske, J., 273
Ruch, F. L., 262, 270
Ruch, T. C., 390, 391, 404
Rudinger, G., 260, 270
Rudolph, G., 167, 174
Runge, W., 331
Russel, A., 286, 294, 307, 322, 326, 334
Rutenfranz, J., 137, 147, 148, 149, 151
Ryan, A. T., 178, 188
Ryan, T. A., 167, 168, 170, 171, 174

S

Saito, Y., 379, 403, 404
Saldanha, E. L., 221, 237
Saltin, B., 22, 24, 25, 31, 37, 38, 39, 40, 41, 373, 402
Sanada, Y., 71, 100
Sandow, A., 9, 41
Sansom, W., 219
Sansoucy, H., 104, 136
Santa Maria, D. L., 114, 135
Sarason, I. G., 316, 334
Sarphati, H. R., 364, 365, 399, 402
Schade, M., 95, 99
Schaefer, H., 33, 35, 41, 286, 306, 314, 317, 327, 334, 417
Schaefer, K.-P., 70, 102, 103
Schaffer, H. R., 94, 103
Schaie, K. W., 259, 270
Scherrer, H., 251
Scheving, L. E., 332
Schimmel, H., 112, 135
Schlaich, K., 148, 150
Schlein, E. M., 37
Schmalbruch, H., 125, 132
Schmale, H., 340, 344, 347, 348, 375, 400, 404
Schmalt, H. D., 331
Schmidt, C. F., 258
Schmidt, H. H., 265, 266, 270
Schmidt, R. A., 114, 135
Schmidtke, H., 33, 41, 107, 150, 158, 170, 174, 177, 178, 179, 181, 184, 190, 195, 196, 198, 200, 201, 204, 211, 214, 218, 225, 231, 237, 238, 243, 244, 247, 249, 252, 278, 286, 295, 314, 322, 334, 340, 344, 375, 404
Schmitt, O. H., 281, 302, 334
Schmitz, H., 416, 417
Schmitz-Scherzer, R., 259, 269
Schneider, H., 263, 270
Schneider, P., 114, 136
Schnore, M. M., 262, 269
Schober, H., 221, 237
Schonpflug, W., 307, 334
Schott, D., 103
Schulz, R., 334, 365, 405
Schwab, R. S., 83, 93, 103, 119, 135, 311, 334
Scott, J. B., 19, 39
Sears, T. A., 77, 97
Seashore, R. H., 210, 218

Sechenov, I. M., 91, 103
Sells, S. B., 159, 171
Semrowich, W. L., 38
Severin, F. V., 69, 103
Shambes, G. M., 60, 92, 103, 104
Sharkey, B. J., 394, 401
Shatolov, A. M., 135
Shaw, W. A., 313, 334
Sheerer, N., 84, 103, 107, 111, 135
Shek, M. P., 166, 174
Shekelle, R. B., 307, 331
Shepherd, J. T., 19, 31, 37
Shepherd, R. E., 38
Shepherd, R. J., 391, 403
Sherrington, C. S., 62, 73, 84, 85, 87, 88, 98, 99, 103, 243, 252
Shibuya, T., 189
Shik, M. L., 69, 103
Shimamura, M., 67, 99, 103
Shimazu, H., 78, 103
Shirley, M. M., 76, 80, 104
Shore, M. F., 248, 252
Siegert, 221
Siemens, M., 225, 237
Sime, W. E., 403
Simmerman, H., 170, 174, 221, 237
Simonson, E., 7, 9, 14, 15, 16, 17, 19, 20, 21, 23, 24, 28, 30, 33, 41, 83, 84, 87, 91, 104, 107, 114, 119, 121, 135, 142, 151, 158, 162, 163, 164, 167, 168, 169, 170, 172, 174, 176, 177, 179, 181, 182, 183, 184, 185, 187, 188, 189, 190, 205, 210, 218, 221, 224, 225, 226, 235, 237, 255, 256, 258, 260, 263, 264, 266, 271, 274, 275, 281, 286, 306, 310, 319, 334, 358, 404, 411, 414
Simonson, S., 151
Sinden, R. H., 173
Singer, J. J., 133
Singer, R., 196, 213, 218
Sipowicz, R. R., 202, 216
Sjoeberg, H., 402
Skinner, J. S., 391, 392, 393, 399, 400, 404
Skyarchik, E. L., 135
Smirnov, K. M., 135
Smith, G. M., 371, 404
Smith, J. L., 60, 104

Smith, K. R., 205, 218
Smith, P. C., 300, 334, 371, 373, 378, 396, 403, 405
Smith, R. P., 370, 375, 400, 401
Smith, S., 208, 218
Sneed, T. W., 37
Snyder, M., 309, 334, 365, 405
Sobel, I., 264, 271
Sodal, I. E., 42
Sokolov, K. T., 257, 258
Sokolova, V. N., 132
Sokolow, A., 151
Sokolowa, W. N., 250
Solowjewa, W. P., 221, 237
Solway, E., 162, 171
Sorge, R. W., 109, 111, 135
Sorokin, B., 377, 401
Sothern, R. 331
Soule, R. G., 38
Spaeth, J. L., 264, 268
Sparks, K., 37, 38
Speakman, D., 267, 271
Spector, S., 403
Spence, K. W., 315, 334
Spieth, S., 257, 258
Spieth, W., 260, 268
Spinelli, D., 134
Sremec, B., 340, 347, 363, 401
Stackhause, S., 281
Staffeld, C., 275
Stainsby, W. N., 22, 41
Stamper, D. A., 42, 332, 359, 375, 380, 382, 383, 384, 385, 387, 390, 399, 403, 405
Stanford, J. F., III, 362, 402
Stark, E. K., 159, 171
Stark, L., 60, 99
Stehenskaja, E., 271
Stein, E. M., 38
Stein, J. M., 41
Stein, R. B., 11, 41, 60, 104, 106, 135
Steinhaus, A. H., 177, 184, 190
Stenberg, J., 22, 31, 41
Stenson, H. H., 217
Sternberg, M., 117, 118, 119, 135
Sterner, R. T., 382, 405
Stevens, J. C., 343, 346, 347, 401, 405
Stevens, S. S., 337, 338, 340, 341, 343, 344, 346, 405
Stier, F., 141, 151

Stolwijk, J. A. J., 373, 402
Stoney, S. D., Jr., 97
Strange Petersen, E., 40
Strauss, E., 416, 417
Strauss, P. S., 363, 405
Stroud, M. W., 189
Strughold, H., 224, 237
Stull, G. A., 114, 135
Sturm, V., 417
Suci, G. J., 279, 281
Suzuki, K., 182, 184, 190
Szmodis, I., 109, 110, 111, 134

T

Taggart, P., 274, 281
Talbott, J. H., 38
Talland, G. A., 263, 271
Tan, B. Y., 119, 120, 127, 132
Tanaka, R., 82, 97, 100, 104
Tanji, J., 67, 100
Tarnecki, R., 102
Tausch, R., 228, 237
Taylor, A. H., 173
Taylor, A. W., 38
Taylor, E. W., 9, 41
Taylor, F. V., 217
Taylor, H. L., 21, 41
Taylor, M. A., 334
Taylor, W. G., 226, 236
Tchirkov, V. J., 132
Teevan, R. C., 329
Teichner, W. H., 108, 135
Tenney, S. M., 344, 400
Terman, L. M., 260, 271
Terry, H. L., 97, 136
Terzuolo, C., 185, 188
Thieman, T. J., 371, 395, 396, 403
Thomae, H., 259, 271, 308, 334
Thompson, L. R., 114, 175, 221, 237
Thompson, L. W., 132
Thompson, N., 263, 267, 268
Thompson, W. D., 97
Thorn, G. S., 170, 174
Thorndike, E., 285, 286, 292, 314, 334
Thurstone, L. L., 338, 405
Tiffin, J., 307, 333
Tigay, E. L., 102
Tinker, M. A., 162, 163, 165, 170, 174, 225, 237
Tipton, C. M., 89, 90, 93, 94, 104, 107, 118, 119, 120, 123, 135
Tong, Y. L., 305, 331, 334
Tonnesen, K. H., 21, 41
Topal, J. R., 353, 402
Tower, S. S., 77, 104
Travis, R. C., 167, 175
Trense, E., 179, 184, 190
Troger, A., 266, 268
Troland, L. T., 164, 175
Trouton, D. S., 217
Tryon, R. C., 382, 383, 405
Tschirkow, W. J., 250
Tsetlin, M. L., 98
Tune, G. S., 267, 270, 280
Turner, C., 38
Tussing, L., 229, 237
Tuttle, W. W., 118, 199, 120, 135
Tyler, D. B., 249, 252

U

Uemura, K., 59, 104
Ukhtomsky, A. A., 176, 190
Ulich, E., 137, 147, 148, 151
Underdahl, L. O., 134
Unger, R. H., 37

V

Vaida, I., 133
Valins, S., 366, 403
Van der Meulen, J. P., 72, 104
Vasilenko, D., 77, 101
Vassilev, I. G., 112, 135
Vaughan, H. G., 112, 135
Vedel, J. P., 78, 104
Vejby-Christensen, H., 40
Vendsalu, A., 112, 136
Verdy, M., 89, 104, 119, 120, 127, 136
Vernon, P. E., 260, 271
Vidacek, S., 340, 347, 363, 401
Viets, H. R., 100
Villoz, 114
Visser, P., 364, 402
Viteles, M. S., 205, 218
Vodanovic, M., 340, 347, 401
Voigt, J., 234, 237
Volkov, S. M., 257, 258
Voor, J. H., 371, 395, 396, 403
Voorhoeve, P. E., 77, 78, 101, 105
Voss, G., von, 238, 252
Vroom, V. H., 300, 308, 335
Vuco, J., 126, 134
Vukovich, A., 340, 344, 375, 404

W

Wachholder, K., 158, 172, 178, 180, 181, 184, 185, 188
Wagner, Ch., 144, 151
Wahlung, H., 367, 405
Wahren, I., 37
Wahren, J., 38
Wald, G., 155, 188, 190
Wallace, J. G., 277, 281
Waller, J. A., 274, 281
Waller, W. H., 39, 69, 104
Walster, B., 309, 335, 359, 365, 405
Wang, Shu-Mao, 177, 190
Ward, D. C., 280
Ward, J. E., 83, 97
Ward, W. D., 227, 236
Ware, J. R., 202, 216
Warmolts, J. R., 11, 41
Wasserman, K., 30, 42
Waterland, J. C., 90, 91, 92, 99-100, 104
Weaver, S. J., 312, 331
Weber, A., 9, 42
Weber, E. H., 340, 405
Weber, M., 291, 335
Weber, R. A., 170, 175, 221, 222, 237
Wedensky, N. E., 176, 190
Weil, H., 232, 237
Weil, J. V., 17, 18, 42
Weiner, B., 366, 403
Weiner, H., 73, 97, 200, 218
Weisendanger, M., 114, 136
Weiser, P. C., 13, 14, 15, 16, 26, 29, 30, 31, 41, 42, 286, 288, 292, 295, 301, 306, 307, 332, 359, 375, 380, 382, 383, 387, 390, 391, 395, 396, 399, 400, 403, 405
Weiss, A. D., 112, 113, 114, 122, 136, 268
Welford, A. T., 112, 136, 214, 218, 260, 263, 267, 270, 271, 278, 279, 280, 281, 289, 310, 313, 314, 316, 331, 335, 336, 405
Wendel, H., 189
Wendland, J. P., 188, 190

Wendt, H. W., 292, 295, 296, 307, 318, 322, 326, 328, 329, 330, 333, 335
Wenger, E., 99
Wenzel, H. G., 205, 218
Werdinius, B., 112, 133
Wessman, A. E., 307, 335
West, W. D., 280
Westerman, R. F., 119, 122, 127, 136
Weston, H. C., 168, 175, 221, 237
Westphal, C. F. O., 117, 137
Wetstone, H. J., 135
Wever, R., 302, 306, 335
Wherry, F. E., 39
Whipp, S. N., 42
White, C. T., 248, 251
White, L. R., 165, 175, 221, 237
White House Conference on Aging, 259, 271
Wicker, G., 307, 334
Wickwire, G. C., 120, 136
Wieding, H., 210, 217
Wiesendanger, M., 77, 101

Wieland, H., 225, 237
Wiener, E. L., 196, 218
Wigertz, O., 402
Wijting, J. P., 378, 383, 405
Wilkinson, R. T., 203, 205, 218, 219
Williams, C., 38
Williams, E. R., 159, 173
Wilson, V. J., 67, 104-105
Wilson, W. H., 227, 237
Winchell, P., 182, 183, 188, 190
Windle, W. F., 62, 65, 97, 105
Winkelmann, A., 102
Winsman, F. R., 402
Witte, N. D., 266, 271
Witte, N. K., 112, 136
Wittkower, E. D., 349, 403
Wojtczak-Jarosz, J., 108, 112, 114, 115, 116, 136
Wolf, G., 301, 335, 377, 378, 379, 382, 383, 399, 405
Wolfbein, S. L., 264, 271
Wollack, S., 378, 405
Wood, C. G., 249, 252
Wood, G. A., 112, 113, 136

Woods, J. J., 20, 37
Woods, J. N., 72, 105
Woodworth, R. S., 108, 136
Wotzka, F., 181, 190, 375, 377, 405
Wotzka, G., 304, 335
Wright, S., 321, 335

Y

Yamanaka, H., 189
Yokota, T., 77, 105
York, D. H., 78, 105
Yoshida, M., 67, 104
Yoshitake, H., 380, 405
Yurchenko, A. S., 112, 136

Z

Zajonc, R. B., 312, 330
Zaretsky, H. H., 262, 271
Zelazo, N. A., 105
Zelazo, P. R., 73, 105
Zimmerli, W., 109, 134
Zimnitzkaya, L. P., 135
Zivin, I., 102
Zoppi, M., 333
Zubek, J. P., 208, 219

Subject Index

A

Achievement motivation, 286-287
  see also Motivation and fatigue
Acquisition of information, disturbance of, *see* Information acquisition, disturbance of
Aerobic work, *see* Motor and metabolic support systems
Aging, 255
  cerebral atherosclerosis, 255, 256, 257
  cerebral flow and fusion frequency of flicker, 256
  driving performance, 272-280
    accident statistics, 272-275
      age of licensed drivers and time of day, 273
      arterial hypertension and diabetes, 274, 275
      cause of accidents, 273-274
      coronary heart disease, 274-275
      driving experience and exposure, 272-273
      driving habits and dropout, 272, 274
    reaction times and information utilization, 278-280
      age restriction in driver licensing, 279
      fatigue, 278
      Harvard Vigilance Test, 278
      handicaps of the older driver, compensation for, 279
      motor coordination, 278, 279
      need for research, 280
      short-term memory, 278, 279
    vision, 275-278
      auditory acuity and accident rate, 277-278
      dark adaptation thresholds, 275-276
      daylight driving, 276
      visual acuity and accident rate, 276-277
  functional changes during work, 256
  industrial countries, 259
  learning, 261-262
    experimental research, 261
    findings of experimental studies, 262
  light physical, sedentary and mental work, 255
    streneous mental work, 256
  mental abilities, 259-261
    age and cohort effects, 260
    "crystallized" intelligence, 261
    decrease in, 259, 260
    "disuse hypothesis," 260
    ecological conditions, 261
    education, 260
    "fluid" intelligence, 261
    health, 260
      coronary disease and performance, 260-261
    longitudinal studies, 260
    "occupational transfer effect," 260
    "primary process of aging," 261
    socioeconomic status, 260
  moderate and heavy physical work, 255
  muscle strength, decrease in, 255-256
  neural cell mass, decrease in, 255, 257
  physical exercise, 255
    beneficial effect of, 257
    ischemic responses to, 255
  psychomotor skills, 257, 263-264
    complexity of task, 263
    definition of, 263
    deterioration of performance, 257
    health, 263
    pre-motor and motor time, differentiation of, 263-264
    speed of information processing and response, 263
  White House Conference on Aging, 259
  work productivity and, 264-267
    accident rate and absenteeism, 267
    attention and concentration, demand for, 266
    attitudes of society, 265
    job requirements, 265
    measurement, problems of, 264
    physical stress, 266
      impairments and physical handicaps, 266-267
    promotion, 265
    qualification, 265
      age distribution of workers with different, 265-266
    type of work, 265
    working conditions, 264-265

Arm, mechanical functioning system of, *see* Motor coordination
ATP regeneration, *see* Metabolic support system regulation
Audition, *see* Information acquisition, disturbance of
Automobile driving, *see* Aging, driving performance

B

Babinski reflex, 64
Babinski-Weil Test, 90
Biophysical models for studying work and fatigue, *see* Work and fatigue, biophysical models for studying
Blink rate, 161-162
  see also Visual fatigue, ease of seeing studies
Blocking, *see* Information acquisition, disturbance of
Blood supply, *see* Metabolic support system regulation

C

CFF (or FFF), *see* Critical or fusion frequency of flicker
Chain reflexes, *see* Reflexes
Coitus reflex, *see* Reflexes, spinal
Color fatigue, 157-158
  see also Visual fatigue, sensory studies
Conflict studies, *see* Visual fatigue
Coordination, *see* Motor coordination
Critical (CFF) or fusion (FFF) frequency of flicker, 158, 176-186
  amphetamine and Pervitin, 176, 184
  categories of work, 177
  changes in, 176, 177
  controversial results of studies, 176-177, 177-178, 184-186
    central sympathetic stimulation, 184-185
      central sympathomimetic drugs, 184
      pupil reflex, 185
      tasks requiring concentration, 185
    diurnal variations of the CFF, 184
    in occupational work, 184, 185-186
    lack of standardization of CFF determination technique, 184
    possible reasons for, 184-186
  drop of, 176
  electrical stimulation of the eye, 182-184
    intermittent electrical stimulation, 183-184
      advantages of, 183
    rectangular electric pulses, 182
      indicator voltage values, 183
      types of work investigated, 182-183

  general state of excitability of the CNS, 176, 177, 181
  increase of CFF, 179, 184-185
  index of general fatigue, 176-177
  mental work, 178, 179-181
    arithmetic problems, 179
    decrease of CFF, 179, 181
      reduction of, 179-180
    tapping test, 181
    task severity, 179-180
      Duker test, 179-180
      Orbeli phenomenon, 180, 185
    visual-mental task (Bourdon test), 180-181
  physical work, 182
    cerebral ischemia, 182
    depression of CFF, 182
  sedentary or light physical work, 177-179
    day shift and night shift, 177, 179
    decrease of CFF, 177-178, 179
    noise, 179
    reading, 178-179
    sympathomimetic drugs, 179, 184
    work interruptions, 177
  subjective fatigue, 176
  see also Visual fatigue, sensory studies

D

Dark adaptation, 188
Driving an automobile, *see* Aging, driving performance
Dyspnea, 18, 24

E

Ease of seeing studies, *see* Visual fatigue
Ergographic studies, *see* Visual fatigue
Expectancy, 308-309
  see also Motivation and fatigue
Extension reflex, crossed, *see* Reflexes, spinal
Extensor thrust reflex, *see* Reflexes, spinal

F

Fatigue
  achievement motivation, 286-287, 290-291
    imagery method, 290-291
    methodology of, 186-187
    questionnaires and rating scales, 291
    socialization practices, 291
  age and, *see* Aging
  as a potentially motivational problem, 285-287
    see also Motivation and fatigue
  cardiovascular system and its feedback control, 19
  categories of, 411-412

circadian and other chronobehavioral factors, 301-308
 circannual phenomena, 307
 circatrigintan phenomena, 307
 "dynamic source traits," 307
 exhaustion feelings and motivation, 301-302
  exhaustion type descriptions, 302-303, 305, 306
  motivation states pattern, 303, 305, 306
  phase lag, 305
  psychomotor tasks, 303-304
  spectral analysis of time series and cosine fitting procedure, 302, 305-306
  studies in rodents, 304-305
 free-running cycles, 306-307
 industrial environments and controlled studies, 307
 interindividual variability, 306
 long range "phase" studies of human behavior, 307-308
 long-term changes, studies of, 307
 menstrual cycle in females, 307
 P-technique, 307
concept of, 43-44
 extended, 410-411
 origin of, 410
cultural-religious influences and values, 291-297
 achievement orientation score, 293-294
 emphasis in subjective experience and research, 291-292
 fatigue experience studies, 292-294, 295, 296-297
  avoidance motivation and exhaustion, 293-294, 295, 296-297
  female subjects, 295, 296-297
  male subjects, 292-294, 296
  Protestants, Roman Catholics and Anglican subjects, 296-297
 motivational factors, 292
 orthogonal factor analyses, 297
 projection mechanism, 294
 Protestant or Socialist work ethics, 292
  achievement motivation, 292, 295-296
 value questionnaire, 292-293
 work related attitudes of the individual, 294
definition of, 7, 83, 88, 221, 287-290, 409-414
 alternatives for abandoning the concept of fatigue, 412-413
 behavioristic approach, 288
 classification of categories, 411-412
 classification of fatigue studies, 413

conversational language, 409
coordination of subunits and temporal aspects, 289
determinable changes in the expression of an activity, 288-289
extended origin of fatigue, 410-411
impairment and fatigue, 411
incapacitation, 410-411, 413
interaction with motivation, 289-290
intrusion of stimuli during performance of a task, 289
label for a human condition, 414
need for standardization of terms, 414
objective fatigue, 411
 work output, 412
origin of the fatigue concept, 410
perceptual experience or incapacitation, 411
performance decrement and fatigue, 288
physiological fatigue, 411
 nature of processes within the body, 412
 organism-centered and environmental-centered reference, 412
plural connotations of fatigue, 414
self-experienced condition, 410
"subjective" fatigue, 287-288
 psychological fatigue, 412
systems approach, 289
vagueness of, 287
disorganization of psychological and physiological processes, 377
dyspnea, 18
emotional, 298-299
 see also Motivation and fatigue
emotional and personal history factors, 297-301
 chronic subjective fatigue, 298
 emotional fatigue, 298-299
 incentive-fatigue ratio, 299
 individual variation, 300
 monotony, 300
 motivation, 299-300
 neurasthenia, 298, 300
  definition of, 298-299
  treatment of, 299
 personality dispositions, 300
 sleep deprivation, 298, 299
entropic processes in, 328
history of fatigue research, 285-287
 chain of errors, 415-416
 see also Motivation and fatigue
maximal work fatigue, 36
motivation and, see Motivation and fatigue
negentropic processes in, 328

occurrence of, 7
    sites of, 83
  origin of term, 156
  predicting effects of performance upon, *see* Motivation and fatigue
  production of, 156
  prolonged work, 18
    submaximal aerobic work, 27
  psychological criteria of, 106-107
  psychosomatic process in, 416-417
  reaction times, reflex times and, *see* Reaction times, reflex times and fatigue
  reflexes upon, effect of, *see* Reflexes
  reflex loop gain compensation for, *see* Reaction times, reflex times and fatigue
  sedentary work, 33
  "Stimmungsermüdung," concept of, 33-35
  subjective, 298
    chronic, 298
    definition of, 287-288, 411
    measurement of, *see* Symptomatology, subjective
    neurasthenia, 298-299
    symptoms of, 336
    see also Symptomatology, subjective
  submaximal work fatigue, 36
  visual methods for measurement of, *see* Critical or fusion frequency of flicker, *see* Dark adaptation, *see* Pupillography
  see also Symptomatology, subjective
  see also Visual fatigue
  see also Work and fatigue
Feedback, arousal and blood pressure, 416
  characteristics of behavior of, 50-51
  classical closed loop negative, 50
  dimensional and scaling closure, 47-48
  duality of feed-forward and, 45, 46
    classical concepts of life systems, 46-47
  illustration of, 416
  loop response time, problem of, 50
  negative, 45
    asymptomatic conformity, 51
    definition of, 45-46
    objectives, 51
  origin of, 45
  positive, 46
    combination with negative feedback, 51
    confusion with feed-forward control, 51
    objectives, 51
  servo system, 46
Feed-forward, 45
  advantage of, 50
  characteristics of behavior, 50, 51
  confusion with positive feedback control, 51
  definition of, 46
  target of, 51
Flexion reflex, *see* Reflexes, spinal
Frequency of flicker, *see* Critical or fusion frequency of flicker

G

General fatigue, *see* Symptomatology, subjective

H

Harvard step test, 89
Harvard Vigilance Test, 278

I

"Ideenflucht," 238
  see also Information processing, disturbance of
Illusion, optical, *see* Information acquisition, disturbance of
Illusions and hallucinations, *see* Information acquisition, disturbance of
Incentive, 311-314
  see also Motivation and fatigue
Information acquisition, disturbance of, 220-234
  audition, 226-228
    auditory fusion frequency, measurement of, 226-227
    noise and work capacity, 227
    upper frequency threshold, 226
    variations of auditory reception, 226, 227
  blocking, 232-233
    extreme mental work, 232-233
  correct reception of environmental stimuli, conditions for, 220
  illusions, optical, 228-229
    analytical perception of objects, 228
      alcohol intoxication, 228
    experiments with industrial workers, 228-229
    geometric-optical deceptions, 228
    "Gestaltpsychologie," 228
  illusions and hallucinations, 233-234
    examples, 233-234
    primitivisation of perception processes, 234
    prolonged sleep deprivation, 233-234
    psychophysical stress, 233
    visual hallucinations, 234

ocular muscle function, 222-226, 227
  accommodation, range of, 222
  accommodation, time course of, 222-224
  blinking rate, 225-226
  fusion, range of, 225
  performance in strenuous visual work at different stimulation levels, 226
  pupillary reflex fatigue, 224
  strabismus divergens, 224
    development of, 224-225
  voluntary horizontal eye movements, rate of, 225
perceptual disturbance, 227, 228-234
  blocking, 232-233
  cerebral location of, 232
  degree of wakefulness, 229-232
  illusions, optical, 228-229
  illusions and hallucinations, 233-234
  negative after-images, time course of, 232
  see also Information acquisition, disturbance of, *individual disturbances*
vision, 220-222, 227
  adaptation, process of, 221
  fatigue, 220, 227
    adaptation and, differentiation between, 221
    cause of, 221
    definition of, 221
  visual receptors, 221, 227
    color recognition, 222
    fusion frequency of flicker, 222
    visual acuity, 221, 222
    visual field, 221-222
wakefulness, degree of, 229-232
  automobile accidents and fatigue, 229
  recognition threshold, 229-231
  signal detection theory, 231
  experiments, 231-232
Information processing, disturbance of, 238-250
  choice reaction situations, 244-249
    choice reaction time experiments, 244-246
      results of, 246-247
    physical exertion and mental performance, 248-249
      cerebral ischemia, 249
    reaction time in, 244
      choice alternatives, 244
      training and fatigue, effect of, 244-245
    work duration on mental performance, effect of, 245-246
    decision-making tasks, 247-248
  classical investigations, 238

faulty association of stimuli-memory and behavioral patterns, 238
"Ideenflucht," 238
internal, 238
mental work, 238
quantitative analysis of, 238-240
  limit of prolonged performance, 239
  recovery time for compensation of fatigue, 239-240
regulation of social behavior, 249-250
  examples, 249
  external stress, 249
  inadequate, 249
  intensive mental load, 249
  planned fatigue prophylaxis, 249-250
task-unrelated associations, 238
transient reactivity failure, 240-244
  blocking of central nervous processes, 240
  cause of, 240
  experiments, 240-241
    frequency of blocks and duration of, 241
  forced autonomic pauses, 241
  information theory explanation, 242-244
    one-channel perception, 243-244
    orientation reactions, 243
    overload-inhibition, 243
    "Partial Moment Criterion," 242-243
    psychological analysis, 242
  mental block, 240, 241
  periodic failures of central integration mechanisms, 242
  see also Information acquisition, disturbance of

K

Key cluster analysis, 375, 377
  see also Symptomatology, subjective, multidimensional analysis of

M

Metabolic support system regulation, 12-19
  prolonged (supra) maximal aerobic endurance capacity, 24-25
    ATP regeneration, 24-25
    ATP regeneration-contraction coupling, 25
    dyspnea, 24
    fundamental problem during, 24
    oxygen delivery, 24
  submaximal aerobic work, 27-32
    ATP regeneration, 27-29
      fat oxidation, 27, 28
      fat oxidation and carbohydrate, 27

motor unit recruitment, 28
muscle glycogen, role of, 28
"weak legs," 28-29
blood supply, 30-32
cardiovascular functions, alteration of, 31-32
cardiovascular system, control of, 30-31
sympathetic nervous system, 30
substrate supply, 29-30
ventilation, 30
transition to higher work levels, 12-19
ATP regeneration, 12-15
ADP, 12
anaerobic glycolysis, 14, 15
immediate, 12-13
intermediary metabolic pathways, 12
metabolic sources of, 12-14
muscular contractions, 12
myokinase and creatine phosphokinase, 13-14, 15
oxygen supply, 16
pyruvate and fatty acid oxidation in mitochondria, 14-15
substrate supply, 15-16
blood supply, 18-19
central circulatory responses to walking, 19
components of muscle blood supply system, 18
inadequate, 19
muscle blood flow, 18-19
visceral blood flow, 19
substrate supply, 15-16
FFA entry into muscle, 15
FFA mobilization, 15-16
muscle glycogen, 16
storage sites, 15
ventilation, 16-18
fast and slow component of ventilatory increase, 17-18
increase in, 16, 17
oxygen supply, 16
respiratory changes, 16-17
see also Motor and metabolic support systems
Motivation and fatigue, 285-328
achievement motivation, 286-287, 290-291
see also Fatigue, achievement motivation
cognitive aspects, 316-317
effects on performance and fatigue, 316-317
information processing, 317
inhibitory-activating neurophysiological system, 317
stimulation and arousal, 316-317
definitional issues, 287-290
see also Fatigue, definition of
determinants of fatigue from outside the task setting, 290-308
achievement motivation, 290-291
circadian and other chronobehavioral factors, 301-308
cultural-religious influences and values, 291-297
emotional and personal history factors, 297-301
see also Fatigue, *individual determinants*
entropic and negentropic processes, 328
expectancy, 308-309
duration of tasks, 309
effect on performance and fatigue, 308-309
intention, 311
motivational theories, 308
perceptions of necessary exertion, 308
fatigue as a potentially motivational problem, 285-287
achievement motivation, 286-287
First Law of Thermodynamics, 287
function of motivation, 286
historical note on, 285-287
improvements in psychological methodology, 286
lack of motivation measures, 286
societal values, 287
First Law of Thermodynamics, 287, 328
incentive, 311-314
arousal and performance, 313-314
definition of, 311
effects on performance and fatigue, 311-314
example of, 311-312
goals for performance, 312-313
individual motivational orientation, 312
intention, 311
tension level and performance, 313-314
type of performance and its context, 312
vigilance studies, 314
logic of potential fatigue indicators, 321-323
fatigue test, 321
impossibility of, 321
prediction of performance, 322
validation, 321-322
improvements in fatigue research, 322
performance prediction, 323-328
block diagram of variables, 327-328
crude projection hypothesis, 326
physiological indicators, 326
rating scales, 323-324

Subject Index

approach and avoidance, 323, 324, 325, 326
  contrast phenomenon, 326
  examples of, 324-326
  problems of, 324
  "self" and "other" assessment, 324-325, 326
  time trends of ratings, 326-327
Thematic Apperception Test, 323
predicting effects of performance upon fatigue, 317-321
  arousal parameters, 318
  factor analysis, 320
  motivation and arousal study, 318
    network of results, 319-320
    relevant variables, 318-319
  path analysis, 321
stress and anxiety, 315-316
  arousal level and performance, 315
  effects on performance and fatigue, 315-316
  ego-involvement and motivating instructions, 316
  stimulus situation, 315-316
suggestion, 308, 309-311
  ability, interaction with level of, 310
  effects on performance and fatigue, 308, 309-311
  hypnosis, 309-310
  hypnotic and waking performances, differences between, 310
  intention, 310-311
  motivational suggestions, 309, 310
  static work, measuring, 310
Motor and metabolic support systems, 5-36
  adaptations of, 7, 8, 36
  fatigue, definition and occurrence of, 7
  fatigue, manifestation of, 35-36
  maladjustments of feedback regulation of, 7, 35-36
  maximal (and supramaximal) aerobic work, 19-25, 36
    definition of, 36
    maximal aerobic power, 20-22
      blood circulation and capillary tissue-mitochondria oxygen exchange, 21
      determination of, 20
      limiting factors of, 20, 21, 22
      maximal aerobic endurance capacity and, 20
      motor unit activity, 20
      muscle blood flow, 21-22
      muscle mass, 20
      muscle oxygen extraction, 22
      muscle oxygen utilization, 21
      pulmonary ventilation and alveolar-blood oxygen exchange, 21
      stroke volume, 21, 22
      variation in, 20
    prolonged (supra) maximal aerobic endurance capacity, 22-25
      metabolic support system, 22-23
      metabolic support system regulation, 24-25
      motor system regulation, 23-24
      training on work, effect of, 22
    tasks, type of, 20
    work performance, determination of, 19
  organization and control of, 5-7
    components and subsystems of performance, 5-6
    functional control, 6
  sedentary work, 32-35, 36
    ATP regeneration, 33
    definition of, 32, 36
    factors limiting, 32, 33
    motor unit activity, 33
    motor unit recruitment, 33
    "Stimmungsermüdung," concept of, 33-35
    substrate and oxygen supply, 33
    ventilation, 33
  submaximal aerobic work, 25-32, 36
    definition of, 25
    factors limiting, 25, 32
    metabolic support system regulation, 27-32
    motor system regulation, 25-27
  transition to higher work levels, 8-19
  see also Metabolic support system regulation
  see also Motor system regulation
Motor coordination, 137-150
  aspects of, 137
  classification of components of, 142-143
  control loops, internal and external, 138
  coordination of body limbs and muscle groups, 143
  disciplines studying, 137
  evaluation of, 144-145
    measures used for, 144
    scale of degrees of motor coordination, 145-147
  in space and time, 142-147
    classification of coordination components, 142-143
    cyclographic analysis of working movements, 143-144
    hand-eye-movement coordination, 147

output capacity criteria, 144
performance and strain measures, 144-145
piano playing task, 144
scale of degrees of motor coordination, 145-147
example, 147
mechanical functioning system of the arm, 138-142
biochemical computer analysis, 139-142
example, 141-142
energy consumption and movement frequency, 139-142
individual types of movements, 138-139
energy consumption and movement frequency, 139-141
example, 141-142
individual movement type, determination of, 138-139
load (stress) and strain, relation between, 138
mechanical load factors, classification of, 138
model of research in, 144
psychomotor skills, 137
definition of, 137-138
sensory and motor aspects, 138
spatial coordination, 142-143
spatial and time coordination, 143
time coordination, 143
trainability of, 137, 147-150
active, mental and observative training, 147
heart rate, 149
physical and nonphysical fraction, 149-150
intentional basic tension, 150
interrupted training, 147
heart rate, 149-150
positive effects of, 148
massed training, 147-148
heart rate, 149-150
performance, 148-149
tracking experiments, 149
Motor performance, components and subsystems of, 5-6
factors limiting, 8
maintenance of, 12
motor feedback controlling system, 11
see also Performance
Motor system regulation, 8-12
prolonged (supra) maximal aerobic endurance capacity, 23-24
impairment of the working fiber's contractile state, 23-24
motor unit activity, 23
submaximal aerobic work, 25-27
Golgi tendon organs, 26, 27
mechanoreceptors, 26, 27
muscle spindles, 26-27
steady-state work, 25-26
"weak muscles," 26, 27
transition to higher work levels, 8-12
components of the motor system, 8, 12
degradations of muscle contraction, 10
"follow-up-length-servo" control, 11
higher motor center activity, 11, 12
immediate adaptation, 9, 11
interneurons, 11
intersegmental reflexes, 11, 12
locomotion, commencement of, 12
mechanoreceptors, 11, 12
motoneurons, 11
motorfeedback control, 11, 12
motor unit activity, 8-9
motor unit recruitment, 9-10, 11-12
muscle excitation and contraction coupling mechanism for, 9
muscle fibers, characteristics of, 9
velocity of muscle contraction, 10-11
see also Motor and metabolic support systems
Muscle blood supply system, 18
Muscle excitation and contraction, 9
Muscle fibers, characteristics of, 9
Muscle servo, 60
see also Reflexes, stretch reflex

N

Neurasthenia, 298
definition of, 298-299
treatment of, 299

O

Ocular muscle function, see Information acquisition, disturbance of

P

Perceptual disturbance, see Information acquisition, disturbance of
Performance, components and subsystems of, 5-6
maximal aerobic work, 19
origin and control of, 5
supporting system, 6
see also Motor and metabolic support systems, organization and control of
Performance prediction, 323-328
see also Motivation and fatigue

Phillippson's reflex, *see* Reflexes, spinal
Plantar reflex, *see* Reflexes, spinal
Psychomotor skills, 137-138
   see also Motor coordination
Psychophysical studies, *see* Symptomatology, subjective
Pupillography, 186-187
   intermittent photic stimulation, 186
   mental work and pupil reflex, 186-187
      restitution phenomenon, 187
   Orbeli phenomenon, 186
   phases of pupil reflex, 186
   restoration of pupillary reflex, 186

R

Reaction times, reflex times and fatigue, 106-131
   acute fatiguing exercise, 107
   fractioned reaction time, 112-117
      breakdown of skilled performance, 116-117
      central and peripheral components, differentiation between, 113-114
         locus of fatigue, determination of, 114
      changes in muscle's contractile properties, 114
      experimental methods, 112-114
      local muscular fatigue effects, 116
      locus of fatigue, determination of, 114
      prolonged work, 114-115
         abortive reactions, 115
         muscular fatigue, 115-116
   fractioned reflex times, 122-125
      achilles tendon reflex, 123
         conventional assessment of, 123-124
         voluntary and involuntary response, 124-125
      fractioned voluntary response times and, 122
      achilles tendon reflex, 124-125
      compensatory adjustment of the central nervous system, 123
      patellar reflex, 122-123
      motoneuron recruitment, 125
      patellar reflexes, 122-123
      phasic and tonic motor units, 125
      reflex latency and reflex motor time, 122
      temperature effects, 125
   psychological criteria of fatigue, 106-107
   reaction time (RT) lags, 107
   reflex fatigue, 106
   reflex loop gain compensation, 125-131
      achilles tendon reflex, augmenting effect of exercise on, 126-127, 128-129
      electromyographic records, 126
      flexor pollicis longus, tension records of, 126
      follow-up servomechanism mode of control, 126
      fusimotor system, 125
      future research, 130-131
      Golgi tendon organ influence on muscle contraction, 128
      intramuscular temperature effects, 128
      length or tension servo-loops, alterations in the gain of, 128
      motoneuron recruitment, 126-127
      muscle spindle sensitivity to stretch, 125, 126
         motoneuron recruitment, 126, 127
         sympathetic stimulation, 128
      muscular work, 126
      sympathetic nervous system, 128
   simple reaction times and fatigue, 108-112
      changes in RT, 108-109, 110, 111-112
      isotonic and isometric exercises, 111
      local muscular exercise, 111
      local neuromuscular impairment, 110-111
      muscular exertion, 108
         competitive exercises, 108-109
         changes in nervous activity, 109-110
      prolonged physical and mental work, 112
   tendon reflexes, 106, 107, 117-122
      achilles tendon reflex, 120
         local neuromuscular fatigue, 120
      characteristics of different tendon reflexes, 120-121
         fiber type composition of muscle groups, 121
         muscle groups, 120-121
      local muscular fatigue, 119-120
      local muscular impairment, 121
      local neuromuscular fatigue, 120
      measurement of reflex parameters, 118
      muscular activity, 118
         fitness of subject, 119, 120, 121
         potentiation of reflex contraction, 118-119
         reflex depression, 118, 119-120
      patellar reflex, 117
         muscular exercise, effect of, 118, 119
      reflex depression, 118, 119
         fitness of subject, 119
         local muscular fatigue, 119-120
         mechanisms underlying, 121
         patellar reflex, 118, 120, 121
      reflex fatigue, 118

reflex potentiation, 118-119
  achilles tendon reflex, 120, 121, 122
  fitness of subject, 119
  increased intramuscular temperature, 122
  local muscular fatigue, 119-120
  mechanisms underlying, 121-122
  patellar reflex, 119
"reflex time," indiscriminate use of, 118
stimulation technique and measurement employed, 121
temperature effects, 122
use as diagnostic and research tools, 117-118
voluntary response to stimulus, ability of, 106
Reflexes, 55-97
  basic alphabet of movement, 66
  central nervous system control, 57
  chain reflexes, 57
  coordination, 55
  decerebrate preparation, 66-72
    capacity to right, stand and walk, 69, 70
    decerebrate rigidity, 66
    hierarchical conceptualization of CNS, 72
    jump reflex in the hypothalamic cat, 70
    labyrinthine acceleratory reflexes, 70
    labyrinthine positional reflexes, 70
    locomotion, 69
      midbrain and pons pyramid stimulation, 69-70
    long spinal reflexes, 66-67
    progression of neuraxial transections, 71
      phylogenetic progression, 72
      progression of motor capability, 71-72
    righting reflexes, 70-71
      body-on-body, 71
      body-on-head, 71
      grasp reflex, 71
      labyrinthine, 70-71
      neck, 71
      optical, 71
    spinal reflexes, 66
    tonic neck and tonic labyrinthine reflexes, 67
      elicitation and mediation, pattern of, 67-69
  definition of term, 57
  facilitation and inhibition of, 95
  fatigue and, 83-95
    active pauses, effect of, 91
    Babinski-Weil test, 90
    bimanual exercise, 93
    central nervous system, 83-84
    cyclo-ergometer, 89

definition of fatigue, 83, 88
fatigue of voluntary movement, 84
fatigue-compensatory mechanism of gamma loop gain, 91
functional decortication, 90
Harvard step test, 89
hierarchy tree, 95-97
indirect learning or cross education, 91
isometric exercise, 90
isotonic exercise, 90, 91
Jendrassik maneuver, 89, 93
mental fatigue, 88, 89-90
  balancing and tendon reflexes, 90
  synaptic fatigue, 89
normal movement, 90
patellar and achilles tendon reflex thresholds, 88-89, 90
physical fatigue, 88-89, 90
reflex fatigue, 84-88
  see also Reflex fatigue
reflex recruitment, 93-94, 97
reflex thresholds, 88-89
  control experiments, 89, 90
  synaptic fatigue, 89-90
suggestions for research, 94-95
synergistic cocontraction, 91
tonic neck reflex pattern, 92
  shoulder girdle and arms, movements of, 92-93
unimanual fatigue, 93
immobility reflex, 71
intact animal, 72-76
  forced grasping, 75
    body position in space, 75-76
    grasp reflex and, 76
  grasp reflex, 76
  hopping reactions, 72-73
    cerebral cortex, 73
    positive supporting reaction, 72
  phylogeny and ontogeny, 76
    movement in initial stages of, 76
  placing reactions, 72
    cerebral cortex, 73
    proprioceptive placing reflex, 73
  postural reflex, 75
  power grip, 76
  reflex walking, 73
  tonic neck, tonic labyrinthine and righting reflexes, 73
    chain reflexes, 74
    coordination of movement, 75
    movement patterns, 73-74
    naturalness of, 75
    volitional control, 74-75

learned, 57
movements, composition of, 55-56
  synergies, 56-57
origin of term, 57
prerequisites for voluntary movement, 65-66
reduction of motor activities to small components, 57-58
spinal reflexes, 62-66
  clasp knife reaction, 63-64
    muscle servo, 64
  coitus reflex, 64
  crossed extension reflex, 63
  extensor thrust reflex, 63
  fetal movements, 65
  flexion reflex, 62
    control centers, 63
    crossed extension reflex, 63
    local sign, 62-63
    patterns of, 62, 63
  neuraxial transections, 64-65
  Phillippson's reflex, 64
  plantar reflex, 64
  recovery of function after CNS damage, 65-66
  reflex stepping, 64
  reflex walking, 64
  rhythm generators, 64
  righting reflexes, 64
  scratch (scalptor) reflex, 64
  shake reflex, 64
  spinal preparation, 62
  stretch reflex, 62
stretch reflex, 58-62
  clasp knife reaction, 60
  double reciprocal inhibition, 59
  gamma fusimotor system, 59-60
    alpha-gamma linkage, 59, 60
  importance of, 62
  length control, 59
  "match point," 59
  mediation of, 58
  monosynaptic relations, 58-59
  motoneuron threshold, 62
  motoneural recruitment, 59
  muscle servo, 60
  polysynaptic relations, 59
  reciprocal inhibition, 59
  uses of, 60
supraspinal control of, 76-83
  alpha-gamma coactivation, 77
  cerebellar frontal lobe damage, 78
  composition of movements, 83
  grips and grasps, phylogenetic and ontogenetic progression of, 80
    pyramidal projections to motoneurons, 80-81
  interneurons of reflex arcs, facilitation and inhibition of, 78-79, 81
    organized movements, 79-80
    pyramidal projections to motoneurons, 80-81
  pyramidal tract, 78
  myotatic loop gain, regulation of, 82
  parallel reflex paths, 82-83
  presynaptic terminals of afferent fibers, interneuron, vestibular nuclei, 81-82
  pyramidal system damage, 77-78
  volitional movement, 77
synergies, 56, 57-58
  composition of movements, 56-57
  definition, 56
  value of concept of reflexes as, 57-58
  "type" movements, 58
  unlearned, 57
  volitional movement, 72
  see also Reaction times, reflex times and fatigue
Reflex fatigue, 84-88, 106
  cascade hypothesis, 87-88
  conduction in the reflex arc, 85
  definition of, 84
  development of, 85
    flexion reflex, 85, 87
    scratch reflex, 85-86, 87-88
  earthworm fatigue, 84-85
  effect of, 106
  flexion reflex, 85, 87
  localization of fatigue of volitional movement, 84
  mammalian, 85
  mechanism of, 86
  neuromuscular fatigue, 86

S

Symptomatology, subjective, 336-400
  differentiation, degree of, 389
  feeling tone, 355-358, 387
  General Fatigue, 383-384, 385, 387, 399
    pyramidal schema, 387-389
  measurement of subjective qualities, 336, 377-386
    multidimensional analysis, 374-386
    nondimensional, single point measures, 349-355
    psychophysical studies, 339-349
    scaling techniques, 337-339
    self-report techniques, 336
    unidimensional rating scales, 355-374

see also Symptomatology, subjective, individual measurements
multidimensional analysis of, 374-386, 387
  air traffic controllers, study of, 375-377
  difference between identifiable types of individuals, 385-386
  factor analysis, 375, 379
    varimax factor analysis, 377-378
  fatigue categories, identification of, 377-378
    subjective effort, 377-378
    tapping and tracking tasks, 377
  individual mental tests, 377
  industrial fatigue in Japan, 378-380
    fatigue scale, 379
    frequency of symptoms, 379, 380
    work situations, 379-380
  key cluster analysis, 375, 377, 382
  Physical Activity Questionnaire (PAQ), 380
    fatigue category, composition of, 383-385, 399
    General Fatigue, 383, 384, 399
    Leg Fatigue, 383, 384-385, 399
    motivation category, 383, 385
    identification and labelling of symptom categories, 382-383
    Initial Adjective Checklist, 380-382
    instructions to subjects of study, 382
    key cluster analysis, 382
    Modified Adjective Checklist, 382
    ordinal scale, 382
    Sperical Analysis diagram, 383
    task aversion category, 383, 385
  rating scales, critical flicker fusion and tapping tests, 375-377
  rationale for the application of, 375
  subjective and behavioral measures, change of, 377
  varimax factor analysis, 377-378
nondimensional, single point measures, 349-355
  aircraft crews, study of, 349-351
  characteristic of, 349
  criticism of, 354-355
  reaction time task, 351
    female P.E. students, 352-353
    male medical students, 351-352
    motivation and cooperation, 352-353
  "tear ballot," 353
  verbal report, 349
  weight-holding task, 353-354
performance and, 336, 337
psychophysical studies, 339-349
  classical psychophysics, history of, 340

force and duration on perceived force, effects of, 346-347, 347-348
  constant effort task, 347
  physiological processes, 347
limitation of, 348-349
magnitude estimation technique, 341, 344, 346
magnitude production technique, 341, 344
perception of effort and levels of stimulus, 340
power function, 340-341
power function for force exerted, 340
  application of, 340
  constant effort task, 347
  dynamic work, 344-345
  fatigue and EMG activity, 348
  force and duration, effects of, 346-347, 347-348
  hysteresis, 343
  magnitude production and estimation technique, 344
  negative task, 348
  perceived heaviness of lifted weights, 345-346
  positive task, 348
  ratio estimation method, 341-343, 343-344
  ratio production method, 341, 343, 343-344, 345-346
  static work, 344, 345, 346
ratio scaling, 339, 341
ratio estimation methods, 341
  application of, 341
  perception of force exerted during work, 341-343, 343-344
ratio production methods, 341
  application of, 341
  dynamic work, 344-345
  perceived heaviness of lifted weights, 345-346
  perception of force exerted during work, 341, 343-344
surface electromyography, 347
task requirements, 346
time-course for fatigue, 346
psychophysiological aspects of, 389-397
  fatigue, 390-391
    heart rate and EMG, 390
    isometric work, 390
    Leg Fatigue, 391
  pain, 395-397
    biofeedback, 396-397
    EMG changes, 395, 396
    isometric hand dynamometer task, 395-396

self-paced technique, 395, 396
perceived effort, 391-395
    autonomic blocking drugs, 392-393
    hypoxia, 394-395
    motor systems feedback, 393, 394, 395
    prolonged work, 395
    RPE and work task, 393-394
    RPE-heart rate relationship, 391-392
    RPE scale, 366-367, 391-395
    training, 394
    see also Symptomatology, subjective, unidimensional rating scales
thermal discomfort, 397
pyramidal schema of levels of subjective reports, 387-389, 397-398
    functions of, 389
    work task, 397-398
research inadequacies in, 336
scaling techniques, 337-339
    characteristics of scales, 338-339
    interval scales, 338-339
    nominal scales, 338
    ordinal scales, 337, 339
    psychophysics, psychological assessment and psychometric scales, 337
    ratio scales, 339
self-report techniques, 336
summary and conclusions, 397-400
symptoms of subjective fatigue, 336, 387
task requirements, 398-400
    mental work and light submaximal work, 398
    moderate or heavy work, 398
        categories of subjective symptomatology, 398
        fatigue category, composition of, 399
        pain and perceived effort expended, 400
        perceived effort expended, 400
        rating of perceived effort, 399-400
        thermal sensations, 400
undifferentiated fatigue, 358-360, 386, 387
    subordinate report of, 389
    see also Symptomatology, subjective, unidimensional rating scales
unidimensional rating scales, 355-374, 399-400
    example of an early study, 355-358
    exertion, 366-370
        effort perceived, 366-368
        effort expended, 368-370
        effort expended and mean task time, 369-370
        heart rates and rating scale of perceived effort, 367-368
        rating scale of perceived effort, 366-367, 399-400

        self-paced technique, 368-369
    feeling tone, 355, 387
        work performance and prework, 355-358
    pain, 370-373, 400
        interval timing, 371, 373
        isometric hand dynamometer task, 371-373, 395-396
        self-paced and irregular ratings, 371, 373
        task time, effort expended and intensity of, 370-371, 371-373
    thermal discomfort, 373-374, 400
        physiological measurements, 374
        seven-point scale, 374
        work performance and, 373-374
    tiredness, 360-366
        aeromedical studies, 362
        block turning task, 362-363
        eleven-point rating scale, 363-364
        external and internal physiological cues, 365-366
        external information about work load level, 364, 365
        external information on subjective reports, effects of, 365
        five-point scale, 363
        identification of factors contributing to subjective feelings of, 363
        interval scale construction, 360-361, 362-363
        interval scale application, 361-362, 362-363
        McNelly's scale, 362-363
        nine-point rating scale, 362
        Pearson's checklist, 361-362
        portages with various loads, 363-364
        prolonged mental work, 360
        static work, 364-365
        Tichener's "stimulus error," 364
        work load and individual postwork ratings of, 364
    undifferentiated fatigue, 358-360
        rating scale for evaluation of housework, 358-359
        rating scale for evaluation of fatigue in male students, 359-360
work categories, 398

T

Tendon reflexes, see Reflexes
    see also Reaction times, reflex times and fatigue

V

Ventilation, see Metabolic support system regulation

Vigilance, 193-216
  activation theory of, 212, 215
  block theory of, 211-212, 214
  definition of, 193
  degree of preceding work load, 202-205
    heavy muscular work, 204-205
    sleep deprivation on signal detection, effect of, 202
      environment with low level stimulation, 203-204
      experiments, 202-203
  drugs, effect of, 209-211
    alcohol, 210-211
    amphetamine, 210
    tranquilizers and depressants, 210
  expectation theory of, 213-214, 215
  external stress factors, 205-209
    climatic stress and performance level, 205
      experiments, 205-208
    hypoxia and performance level, 208
    individual variation, 208
    noise and performance level, 208
  filter theory of, 213, 215
  inhibition theory of, 213, 215
  motivation theory of, 314
  observer performance in stimuli depressed environment, 193
    laboratory experiments, 194-195
    performance motivation, 195
    radar observers during war, 193-194
  psychophysiological variable of level of, 214
  reinforcement theory of, 213, 215
  self-stimulation theory of, 212-213
  signal classification, 196
  signal intensity, 200-201
    Bunse-Roscoe equation for threshold, 200
    demand for high, 200-201
    preceding load work and necessary, 201
    reaction time to acoustic stimuli, 201
    suprathreshold stimuli, 200
  signal interactions, 199-200
  signal type and frequency, 196-199
    critical signals and observer performance, 196-197
    neutral and noncritical signals and observer performance, 196
    noncritical additional signals and observer performance, 196-197
    occupational therapy, 197
    variables affecting quality of observation, 198-199
  theories of, 211-216
    see also Vigilance theories
Vigilance theories, 211-216
  vigilance decline as result of adaptation, 212-216
    activation theory, 212, 215
    activity and performance, discrimination of types of, 214
    detection and identification of a signal, 214
    expectation theory, 213-214, 215
    filter theory, 213, 215
    inhibition theory, 213, 215
    learning of time discriminations, 215
    prediction of experimental results, 215 216
    reinforcement theory, 213, 215
    self-stimulation theory, 212-213
    unlearning, theories of, 215
  vigilance decline as result of fatigue, 211
    blocking theory, 211-212, 214
Vision, see Aging, driving performance
  see Information acquisition, disturbance of
  see Visual fatigue
Visual fatigue, 155-171
  body mechanisms, 155-156
  concepts of fatigue, 156
  conflict studies, 165-166
    contraction and relaxation of muscles, 165
    fixation, 165, 166
    pupillary reflexes, 165
      dark and light reflex, 166
      intermittent photic stimulation, 165-166
      ocular discomfort, 165, 166
  ease of seeing studies, 161-165
    basal metabolism and illumination level, 162
    blink rate, 161-162
      conditions of illumination, 161, 162, 163
      fatigue and, 162
      stress, 162
    convergence reserve, 161
    criteria, 161
    critical flicker frequency and illumination levels, 163
    pupil area, 162
    qualitative features of illumination, 164
    reading and illumination levels, 161
      efficiency and fatigue in reading, 162-163, 165
      general reading level, 164
      preadaptation levels, 165
      recommended illumination, 164-165
    visual task performance, fatigue and illumination levels, 163-164, 165
      sources of illumination, 164
    working efficiency and illumination level, 163

ergographic studies, 159-160
  accommodative ergograph investigations, 159-160
  ergograph, 159
  fatigue curves, 160
  motor processes within the eye, 159
fatigue studies, 155
  categories of, 156-157
human activity, categories of, 170
literature on, 170
National Research Council Conference on, 155
nonvisual functions, 168-170
  changes in, 168
    eye position, 168-169
  meals on visual performance and fatigue, effects of, 169-170
  muscle tension, 168
  muscular and mental exertion, 169
sensory studies, 157-159
  changes in sensed intensity, 157
  color fatigue, 157
    disappearance times, 157-158
    forms of, 157-158
    recovery times, 158
  critical (CFF) or fusion (FFF) frequency of flicker test, 158-159
    chronic visual fatigue, 159
    strenuous visual work, 158
  fixed posture, 157
  reduction in visual performance, 157
symptomatic studies, 160-161
  exercising the eyes, 160
  phorias, 160
  reading, 161
visual task performance studies, 166-168
  binocular visual field, microchanges in, 168
  cost of performance and efficiency, concepts of, 167
  infants, 168
  jump fixation task, 167
  Landolt ring test, 166
  perceptual organization, 167-168
  photic stimulation, 167
  scanning test, 166

test for experimental investigation of visual performance and fatigue, 167
transfer of one performance to another, 167

W

Work, concept of, 43
  maximal (supramaximal) aerobic, see Motor and metabolic support systems
  sedentary, see Motor and metabolic support systems
  submaximal aerobic, see Motor and metabolic support systems
Work and fatigue, aging, psychological aspects of, see Aging
  biophysical models for studying, 43-52
    algorithmic system, 43, 49
    communication, 44-45
    concept of time, 44
    concept of, 43-44
    control and supervisory systems, 45
    dimensional and scaling closure, principle of, 47-48
    feedback and feed-forward systems, 45-46
      characteristics of behavior of, 50-51
      see also Feedback
      see also Feed-forward
    feed-forward and feedback duality, 45, 46
      classical concepts of life systems, 46-47
    feed-up feed-down control of internal linguistics, 50, 51
    hierarchical feed-up, feed-down class of adaptive modifications, 48-49
      information and control structure of biological systems, 49
      repertoire of internal linguistic paths within the organism, 50
    nondestructive assessment of a system, 52
    problems of definition, 43
    systems status measures of control loop parameters, 52
    transduction, dimensions and scales, 51-52
  motor and metabolic support systems during, see Motor and metabolic support systems
  subjective symptomatology during, see Symptomatology, subjective

DATE DUE			
DEC 1 '80			
MAR 15 '82			
OCT 3			
GAYLORD			PRINTED IN U S A

JULIA TUTWILER LIBRARY
LIVINGSTON UNIVERSITY
DATE BOOK IS DUE BACK

This book is due back on or before the last date stamped in back. If it is returned after that date, the borrower will be charged a daily fine. In checking the book out the borrower assumes responsibility for returning it.

NO "OVER-DUE" NOTICE WILL BE SENT OUT FROM THE LIBRARY.